# Advanced Research in Sclerosis

# Advanced Research in Sclerosis

Editor: Billy Patterson

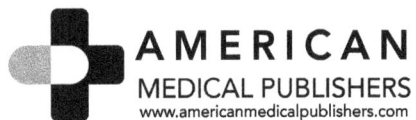

**AMERICAN**
MEDICAL PUBLISHERS
www.americanmedicalpublishers.com

**AMERICAN**
MEDICAL PUBLISHERS
www.americanmedicalpublishers.com

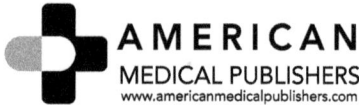

**Cataloging-in-Publication Data**

Advanced research in sclerosis / edited by Billy Patterson.
p. cm.
Includes bibliographical references and index.
ISBN 978-1-63927-207-5
1. Multiple sclerosis. 2. Multiple sclerosis--Research. 3. Multiple sclerosis--Immunological aspects. I. Patterson, Billy.
RC377 .A28 2022
616.834--dc23

American Medical Publishers,
41 Flatbush Avenue,
1st Floor, New York,
NY 11217, USA

ISBN 978-1-63927-207-5 (Hardback)

# Contents

Preface.................................................................................................................................IX

Chapter 1    **Sex disparities in systemic sclerosis-associated pulmonary
arterial hypertension**..................................................................................... 1
Christopher R. Pasarikovski, John T. Granton, Adrienne M. Roos, Saghar Sadeghi,
Amie T. Kron, John Thenganatt, Jakov Moric, Cathy Chau and Sindhu R. Johnson

Chapter 2    **Subclinical dermal involvement is detectable by high frequency ultrasound
even in patients with limited cutaneous systemic sclerosis**................................ 8
A. Sulli, B. Ruaro, V. Smith, S. Paolino, C. Pizzorni, G. Pesce and M. Cutolo

Chapter 3    **Tie2 as a novel key factor of microangiopathy in systemic sclerosis**................15
Falk Moritz, Janine Schniering, Jörg H. W. Distler, Renate E. Gay, Steffen Gay,
Oliver Distler and Britta Maurer

Chapter 4    **Mir-155 is overexpressed in systemic sclerosis fibroblasts and is required for
NLRP3 inflammasome-mediated collagen synthesis during fibrosis**................26
Carol M. Artlett, Sihem Sassi-Gaha, Jennifer L. Hope,
Carol A. Feghali-Bostwick and Peter D. Katsikis

Chapter 5    **Survival and quality of life in incident systemic sclerosis-related pulmonary
arterial hypertension**....................................................................................34
Kathleen Morrisroe, Wendy Stevens, Molla Huq, David Prior, Jo Sahhar,
Gene-Siew Ngian, David Celermajer, Jane Zochling, Susanna Proudman
and Mandana Nikpour

Chapter 6    **Limited cutaneous systemic sclerosis skin demonstrates distinct molecular
subsets separated by a cardiovascular development gene expression signature**.........44
Emma C. Derrett-Smith, Viktor Martyanov, Cecilia B. Chighizola, Pia Moinzadeh,
Corrado Campochiaro, Korsa Khan, Tammara A. Wood, Pier Luigi Meroni,
David J. Abraham, Voon H. Ong, Robert Lafyatis, Michael L. Whitfield and
Christopher P. Denton

Chapter 7    **Sustained benefit from combined plasmapheresis and allogeneic mesenchymal
stem cells transplantation therapy in systemic sclerosis**................................54
Huayong Zhang, Jun Liang, Xiaojun Tang, Dandan Wang, Xuebing Feng,
Fan Wang, Bingzhu Hua, Hong Wang and Lingyun Sun

Chapter 8    **Systemic sclerosis associated interstitial lung disease – individualized
immunosuppressive therapy and course of lung function: results of
the EUSTAR group**......................................................................................61
Sabine Adler, Dörte Huscher, Elise Siegert, Yannick Allanore, László Czirják,
Francesco DelGaldo, Christopher P. Denton, Oliver Distler, Marc Frerix,
Marco Matucci-Cerinic, Ulf Mueller-Ladner, Ingo-Helmut Tarner,
Gabriele Valentini, Ulrich A. Walker, Peter M. Villiger and Gabriela Riemekasten

Chapter 9    Characterization of inflammatory cell infiltrate of scleroderma skin: B cells
             and skin score progression ............................................................................................... 73
             Silvia Bosello, Cristiana Angelucci, Gina Lama, Stefano Alivernini,
             Gabriella Proietti, Barbara Tolusso, Gigliola Sica, Elisa Gremese and
             Gianfranco Ferraccioli

Chapter 10   The effects of upper and lower limb exercise on the microvascular reactivity
             in limited cutaneous systemic sclerosis patients........................................................... 84
             A. Mitropoulos, A. Gumber, H. Crank, M. Akil and M. Klonizakis

Chapter 11   Prospective evaluation of the capillaroscopic skin ulcer risk index in systemic
             sclerosis patients in clinical practice................................................................................. 95
             Ulrich A. Walker, Veronika K. Jaeger, Katharina M. Bruppacher,
             Rucsandra Dobrota, Lionel Arlettaz, Martin Banyai, Jörg Beron,
             Carlo Chizzolini, Ernst Groechenig, Rüdiger B. Mueller, François Spertini,
             Peter M. Villiger and Oliver Distler

Chapter 12   Quantitative videocapillaroscopy correlates with functional respiratory
             parameters: a clue for vasculopathy as a pathogenic mechanism for lung
             injury in systemic sclerosis.............................................................................................. 102
             Alfredo Guillén-Del-Castillo, Carmen Pilar Simeón-Aznar,
             Eduardo L. Callejas-Moraga, Carles Tolosa-Vilella, Serafín Alonso-Vila,
             Vicente Fonollosa-Pla and Albert Selva-O'Callaghan

Chapter 13   Characterization of the HLA-DRβ1 third hypervariable region amino acid
             sequence according to charge and parental inheritance in systemic sclerosis ............ 111
             Coline A. Gentil, Hilary S. Gammill, Christine T. Luu, Maureen D. Mayes,
             Dan E. Furst and J. Lee Nelson

Chapter 14   The association of low complement with disease activity in
             systemic sclerosis.............................................................................................................. 117
             James Esposito, Zoe Brown, Wendy Stevens, Joanne Sahhar, Candice Rabusa,
             Jane Zochling, Janet Roddy, Jennifer Walker, Susanna M. Proudman and
             Mandana Nikpour

Chapter 15   Epstein-Barr virus lytic infection promotes activation of Toll-like receptor 8
             innate immune response in systemic sclerosis monocytes............................................. 129
             Antonella Farina, Giovanna Peruzzi, Valentina Lacconi, Stefania Lenna,
             Silvia Quarta, Edoardo Rosato, Anna Rita Vestri, Michael York,
             David H. Dreyfus, Alberto Faggioni, Stefania Morrone, Maria Trojanowska and
             G. Alessandra Farina

Chapter 16   Intestinal dysbiosis is common in systemic sclerosis and associated with
             gastrointestinal and extraintestinal features of disease ............................................... 143
             Kristofer Andréasson, Zaid Alrawi, Anita Persson, Göran Jönsson and Jan Marsal

Chapter 17   Multiplex serum protein analysis reveals potential mechanisms and markers
             of response to hyperimmune caprine serum in systemic sclerosis................................ 151
             Niamh Quillinan, Kristina E. N. Clark, Bryan Youl, Jeffrey Vernes,
             Deirdre McIntosh, Syed Haq and Christopher P. Denton

Chapter 18    **The 5-HT1A receptor agonist buspirone improves esophageal motor function and symptoms in systemic sclerosis: a 4-week, open-label trial** ...................................................... 161
George P. Karamanolis, Stylianos Panopoulos, Konstantinos Denaxas, Anastasios Karlaftis, Alexandra Zorbala, Dimitrios Kamberoglou, Spiros D. Ladas and Petros P. Sfikakis

Chapter 19    **miR-155 in the progression of lung fibrosis in systemic sclerosis** ...................................................... 167
Romy B. Christmann, Alicia Wooten, Percival Sampaio-Barros, Claudia L. Borges, Carlos R. R. Carvalho, Ronaldo A. Kairalla, Carol Feghali-Bostwick, Jessica Ziemek, Yu Mei, Salma Goummih, Jiangning Tan, Diana Alvarez, Daniel J. Kass, Mauricio Rojas, Thiago Lemos de Mattos, Edwin Parra, Giuseppina Stifano, Vera L. Capelozzi, Robert W. Simms and Robert Lafyatis

Chapter 20    **Exercise echocardiography for the assessment of pulmonary hypertension in systemic sclerosis** ...................................................... 180
Rui Baptista, Sara Serra, Rui Martins, Rogério Teixeira, Graça Castro, Maria João Salvador, José António Pereira da Silva, Lèlita Santos, Pedro Monteiro and Mariano Pêgo

Chapter 21    **B cell depletion therapy upregulates Dkk-1 skin expression in patients with systemic sclerosis: association with enhanced resolution of skin fibrosis** ...................................................... 191
Dimitrios Daoussis, Athanassios Tsamandas, Ioannis Antonopoulos, Alexandra Filippopoulou, Dionysios J. Papachristou, Nicholaos I. Papachristou, Andrew P. Andonopoulos and Stamatis-Nick Liossis

**Permissions**

**List of Contributors**

**Index**

# Preface

An autoimmune disorder in which the connective tissue of the body gets affected is known as systemic sclerosis or systemic scleroderma. It is classified into two forms - non-systemic and systemic. The systemic condition can be limited or diffuse. Limited scleroderma is characterized by Raynaud's phenomenon, sclerodactyly, telangiectasia, esophageal dysfunction and calcinosis. Diffuse scleroderma, in contrast, can cause pulmonary, musculoskeletal, renal and gastrointestinal complications. The prognosis of systemic sclerosis is different for the diffuse and limited forms of the disease. So far, the underlying cause of sclerosis is not understood. There is no cure for scleroderma but its symptoms are managed with therapy. This book provides significant information of the modern research dimensions in systemic sclerosis to help develop a good understanding of its assessment and clinical management. It explores all the important aspects of systemic sclerosis in the present day scenario. For someone with an interest and eye for detail, this book covers the most significant topics in immunology.

This book is a comprehensive compilation of works of different researchers from varied parts of the world. It includes valuable experiences of the researchers with the sole objective of providing the readers (learners) with a proper knowledge of the concerned field. This book will be beneficial in evoking inspiration and enhancing the knowledge of the interested readers.

In the end, I would like to extend my heartiest thanks to the authors who worked with great determination on their chapters. I also appreciate the publisher's support in the course of the book. I would also like to deeply acknowledge my family who stood by me as a source of inspiration during the project.

**Editor**

# Sex disparities in systemic sclerosis-associated pulmonary arterial hypertension

Christopher R. Pasarikovski[1], John T. Granton[2], Adrienne M. Roos[1], Saghar Sadeghi[1], Amie T. Kron[1], John Thenganatt[3], Jakov Moric[4], Cathy Chau[1] and Sindhu R. Johnson[1,3,5*]

## Abstract

**Background:** The impact of male sex as a determinant of health outcomes in systemic sclerosis-associated pulmonary arterial hypertension (SSc-PAH) is controversial. The primary objective of this study was to evaluate the effect of sex on survival in patients with SSc-PAH. The secondary objectives were to evaluate the effect of sex on age of PAH diagnosis, time from SSc diagnosis to PAH diagnosis, and SSc disease manifestations.

**Methods:** Sex-based disparities were evaluated in a cohort of SSc-PAH patients with a primary outcome of time from PAH diagnosis to all-cause mortality. Secondary outcomes were differences in age of diagnosis, disease duration, and SSc manifestations. Survival differences were evaluated using Kaplan-Meier and Cox proportional hazard models.

**Results:** We identified 378 SSc-PAH (58 males, 320 females) patients, with a female:male ratio of 5.5:1. Males had a shorter mean ± standard deviation time from SSc diagnosis to PAH diagnosis (1.7 ± 14 versus 5.5 ± 14.2 years); shorter PAH duration (3.5 ± 3.1 versus 4.7 ± 4.2 years), increased frequency of renal crisis (19 % versus 8 %, relative risk (RR) 2.33, 95 %CI 1.22, 4.46), interstitial lung disease (67 % versus 48 %, RR 1.41, 95 %CI 1.14, 1.74), and diffuse subtype (40 % versus 22 %, RR 1.84, 95 %CI 1.26, 2.69). Males appeared to have decreased 1-, 2-, 3-, and 5-year survival (83.2 %, 68.7 %, 53.2 %, 45.6 %) compared to females (85.7 %, 75.7 %, 66.4 %, 57.4 %). However, there was no difference in mortality between sexes (HR 1.43 (95 %CI 0.97, 2.13).

**Conclusions:** Sex disparities appear to exist in the frequency of PAH, time to PAH diagnosis, PAH disease duration and SSc disease burden. However, male sex does not independently impact SSc-PAH survival.

**Keywords:** Systemic sclerosis, Scleroderma, Pulmonary arterial hypertension, Sex, Survival, Scleroderma renal crisis

## Background

Systemic sclerosis (SSc) is a systemic autoimmune rheumatic disease characterized by vasculopathy and fibrosis that primarily affects females with a female:male ratio 3–4:1 [1]. Sex hormones likely play an important role in the observed female preponderance in SSc [2]. Although female prevalence is high, several authors have reported that male sex is associated with decreased survival [3–7]. Male sex has been associated with an increased risk of mortality in SSc patients above that observed for males in the general population [7].

SSc-associated pulmonary arterial hypertension (SSc-PAH) is a leading cause of SSc-related mortality, with a prevalence of approximately 7 % [8]. Little is known about the effect of sex on disease onset, time to PAH diagnosis, and survival in patients with SSc-PAH [9, 10]. In a cohort study of 259 SSc-PAH patients, male sex was associated with increased risk of mortality (hazard ratio (HR) 2.2, 95 % confidence interval (CI) 1.35, 3.55) [11]. However, in another cohort study of 152 SSc-PAH patients, male sex was not an independent risk factor for mortality (HR 2.02, 95 %CI 0.65, 6.2) [12]. Furthermore, sex was not

* Correspondence: sindhu.Johnson@uhn.ca
[1]Toronto Scleroderma Program, Mount Sinai Hospital, Toronto Western Hospital, Division of Rheumatology, Department of Medicine, Faculty of Medicine, University of Toronto, Ground Floor, East Wing, Toronto Western Hospital, 399 Bathurst Street, Toronto, ON M5T 2S8, Canada
[3]University Health Network Pulmonary Hypertension Programme, Toronto General Hospital, Division of Respirology, Department of Medicine, Faculty of Medicine, University of Toronto, Toronto, ON, Canada
Full list of author information is available at the end of the article

an independent risk factor in a cohort of patients with connective tissue disease-associated PAH (22 % of whom had SSc-PAH) and idiopathic PAH (IPAH) (HR 0.78, 95 %CI 0.40, 1.51) [13]. Using data from the REVEAL registry, Benza et al. found that men >60 years of age had poorer 1-year survival compared to females (HR 2.2, 95 %CI 1.6, 3.0) [14]. This finding was confirmed by Shapiro et al., who reported sex differences in 2-year survival from enrolment in the REVEAL registry among men diagnosed with group I PAH aged >60 years (HR 1.67, 95 %CI 1.28, 2.17) [15]. They also noted that male sex was associated with poorer survival for the IPAH subgroup of group I PAH patients across all age groups [15]. Humbert et al. reported that among patients with IPAH, familial, and anorexigen-associated PAH, females had better survival (HR 0.52, 95 %CI 0.30, 0.88 [16]. However, Fisher et al. reported that there was no significant difference between males and females in 3-year survival for patients diagnosed with IPAH and SSc-PAH combined [17].

Thus, the current literature on the effect of sex on SSc-PAH is limited and conflicted. The effect of sex on age of onset, time to diagnosis, disease duration, disease manifestations and survival in SSc-PAH is not well understood. The aim of this study is to improve our understanding of the sex-based disparities in SSc-PAH. The primary objective of this study was to evaluate the effect of sex on survival in patients with SSc-PAH. The secondary objectives were to evaluate the effect of sex on age of PAH diagnosis, time from SSc diagnosis to PAH diagnosis, and SSc disease manifestations.

## Methods

### Patients

The University Health Network Pulmonary Hypertension Programme has the largest published single-center longitudinal cohort in Canada [18]. Patients are prospectively followed every 6 to 12 months using a standardized protocol. Adult SSc-PAH patients seen between 1998 and January 1, 2014 were included if they fulfilled the American College of Rheumatology (ACR) – European League Against Rheumatism (EULAR) classification criteria for SSc [19], and had PAH confirmed by catheterization with a mean pulmonary artery pressure (mPAP) >25 mm Hg, pulmonary capillary wedge pressure (PCWP) <15 mm Hg and pulmonary vascular resistance (PVR) >3 Wood units on catheterization [20]. Patients with another etiology for PAH (e.g. human immunodeficiency virus, anorexigen use, portal hypertension, congenital cardiac abnormalities) were excluded.

### Exposure

Sex was defined as self-reported biological and physiological characteristics at birth, and characterized as male or female. Gender (roles, behaviours, activities, and attributes that a given society considers appropriate) was not assessed. Patients were excluded from analysis if they had a known history of sex chromosome abnormalities or had undergone sex reassignment surgery.

### Outcome

The primary outcome of the study was the time from PAH diagnosis to death from all causes. Patients who were alive as of June 1, 2014 were censored. PAH diagnosis was defined as the date of right heart catheterization. SSc diagnosis was defined as the date a diagnosis of SSc was made by a physician. Dates of death were obtained from the clinic chart, hospital electronic record or obituary. Secondary outcomes included sex differences in age at PAH diagnosis, time from SSc diagnosis to PAH diagnosis, PAH disease duration, subtype of SSc (limited, diffuse), and SSc manifestations (Raynaud's phenomenon, digital ulceration, esophageal dysmotility, telangiectasia, interstitial lung disease (bibasilar reticular abnormalities with minimal ground-glass on high-resolution computerized tomography (CT) of the thorax) and serology (centromere, topoisomerase I (ScL-70); RNA polymerase III was not available). Comorbidities (coronary artery disease, hypertension, diabetes, hyperlipidemia, atrial fibrillation, and stroke), medications (warfarin, calcium channel blocker, endothelin receptor antagonist, prostaglandin analogue, and phosphodiesterase inhibitors), pulmonary function and hemodynamic measurements were compared.

### Analysis

All statistical analysis was done using RStudio (version 0.98.932, R Foundation for Statistical Computing, 2012). The Shapiro-Wilk statistic was used to test for normality. Continuous data were not normally distributed. Baseline characteristics for males and females were analyzed using standardized differences, and a difference of 25 % was considered significant. Use of standardized differences is a method of comparing two groups, independent of sample size. For dichotomous variables we also reported the relative risk (RR). Survival data were plotted using Kaplan-Meier curves and significance was tested using the log-rank test. Independent predictors of survival were evaluated using Cox regression analysis. Hazard ratios (HR) are reported with 95 % confidence intervals (95 % CI). University Health Network (12-5253-AE) and Mount Sinai Hospital (12-0233-C) research ethics board approvals were obtained for the conduct of this study. The ethics boards waived the need for consent, as this was a retrospective study with a high mortality rate.

## Results

### SSc-PAH patient characteristics

A total of 1142 charts were reviewed and 378 SSc-PAH patients were identified of whom 58 (15.3 %) were male

**Table 1** SSc-PAH baseline characteristics by sex

| SSc patient characteristics | Males n = 58 | Females n = 320 | Standardized difference |
|---|---|---|---|
| Age at PAH diagnosis, y, mean (SD) | 54.5 (11.0) | 57.3 (13.0) | 0.05 |
| Time from SSc to PAH diagnosis, y, mean (SD) | 1.7 (14.0) | 5.5 (14.2) | 0.93[a] |
| PAH disease duration, y, mean (SD) | 3.5 (3.1) | 4.7 (4.2) | 0.29[a] |
| SSc manifestations | | | |
| Diffuse subtype, n (%) | 23 (40 %) | 69 (22 %) | 0.40[a] |
| Raynaud's phenomenon, n (%) | 56 (97 %) | 302 (94 %) | 0.10 |
| Telangiectasia, n (%) | 46 (79 %) | 224 (70 %) | 0.22 |
| Renal crisis, n (%) | 11 (19 %) | 26 (8 %) | 0.32[a] |
| Esophageal dysmotility, n (%) | 51 (88 %) | 276 (86 %) | 0.05 |
| Digital ulcers, n (%) | 16 (28 %) | 120 (38 %) | 0.21 |
| Interstitial lung disease, n (%) | 39 (67 %) | 153 (48 %) | 0.40[a] |
| ScL-70 antibody, n (%) | 10 (17 %) | 36 (11 %) | 0.17 |
| Anticentromere antibody, n (%) | 9 (15 %) | 49 (17 %) | 0.06 |
| Cardiopulmonary measures | | | |
| 6MWD, m, mean (SD) | 344.3 (140.9) | 324.5 (154.6) | 0.06 |
| WHO functional class III-IV, n (%) | 24 (41 %) | 124 (39 %) | 0.05 |
| mPAP, mmHg, mean (SD) | 44.9 (20.5) | 40.7 (21.7) | 0.10 |
| mPVR, dyn · s/cm$^5$, mean (SD) | 705.0 (710.5) | 584.7 (552.9) | 0.19 |
| Cardiac output L/min, mean (SD) | 4.2 (2.4) | 3.3 (1.6) | 0.26[a] |
| PCWP, mmHg, /mean (SD) | 13.3 (6.2) | 9.5 (6.2) | 0.33[a] |
| BNP pg/mL, mean (SD) | 203.0 (266.9) | 245.9 (481.3) | 0.19 |
| FVC, % predicted | 79.3 (17.4) | 76.1 (24.6) | 0.04 |
| FEV1, % predicted | 80.3 (18.2) | 78.2 (26.1) | 0.03 |
| DLCO, ml/min/mmHg | 52.1 (19.7) | 55.3 (19.5) | 0.06 |
| Right ventricular enlargement | | | |
| Normal | 40 (69 %) | 250 (78 %) | 0.21 |
| Mild | 5 (9 %) | 24 (8 %) | 0.04 |
| Moderate | 10 (17 %) | 35 (11 %) | 0.18 |
| Severe | 3 (5 %) | 11 (3 %) | 0.09 |
| Right ventricular dysfunction | | | |
| Normal | 39 (67 %) | 249 (78 %) | 0.23 |
| Mild | 5 (9 %) | 26 (8 %) | 0.02 |
| Moderate | 12 (21 %) | 38 (12 %) | 0.24 |
| Severe | 2 (3 %) | 7 (2 %) | 0.07 |

**Table 1** SSc-PAH baseline characteristics by sex *(Continued)*

| Comorbidities | | | |
|---|---|---|---|
| Coronary artery disease, n (%) | 12 (21 %) | 40 (13 %) | 0.22 |
| Hypertension, n (%) | 13 (22 %) | 88 (28 %) | 0.12 |
| Diabetes mellitus, n (%) | 5 (9 %) | 21 (7 %) | 0.08 |
| Hyperlipidemia, n (%) | 8 (14 %) | 26 (8 %) | 0.18 |
| Atrial fibrillation, n (%) | 6 (10 %) | 28 (9 %) | 0.05 |
| Peripheral vascular disease, n (%) | 3 (5 %) | 19 (6 %) | 0.03 |
| Stroke, n (%) | 2 (3 %) | 15 (5 %) | 0.06 |

*SSc-PAH* systemic sclerosis-associated pulmonary arterial hypertension, *ScL-70* topoisomerase I, *6MWD* 6-minute walk test, *WHO* World Health Organization, *mPAP* mean pulmonary artery pressure, *mPVR* mean pulmonary vascular resistance, *PCWP* pulmonary capillary wedge pressure, *BNP* brain natriuretic peptide, *FVC* forced vital capacity, *FEV1* forced expiratory volume 1, *DLCO* diffusing capacity of the lungs for carbon monoxide
[a]Denotes standardized difference greater than 25 %

and 320 (84.7 %) were female. All patients fulfilled the ACR-EULAR classification criteria for SSc. The female:-male ratio was 5.5:1. The mean age at diagnosis was 54.5 ± 11.0 years for males and 57.3 ± 13.0 years for females. Males had a shorter mean time from SSc diagnosis to PAH diagnosis (1.7 ± 14 versus 5.5 ± 14.2 years; standardized difference 93 %) and shorter PAH disease duration (3.5 ± 3.1 versus 4.7 ± 4.2 years, standardized difference 29 %). Males had an increased frequency of renal crisis (19 % versus 8 %, relative risk (RR) 2.33, 95 %CI 1.22, 4.46), interstitial lung disease (67 % versus 48 %, RR 1.41, 95 %CI 1.14, 1.74) and diffuse cutaneous disease (40 % versus 22 %, RR 1.84, 95 %CI 1.26, 2.69). Adjusting for the presence of interstitial lung disease had marginal to no effect on the effect of male sex on pulmonary hypertension age of diagnosis, time from SSc diagnosis to PAH diagnosis and pulmonary hypertension disease duration. There were no significant differences between males and females in the presence of Raynaud's phenomenon, telangiectasia, digital ulcers, esophageal dysmotility, serology, 6-minute walk distance, World Health Organization (WHO) functional class, brain natriuretic peptide levels, comorbidities and medications (Table 1).

### SSc-PAH survival
There were 32 deaths (55 %) among males and 155 deaths (48 %) among females. The 1-, 2-, 3-, and 5-year survival estimates were 83.2 %, 68.7 %, 53.2 %, 45.6 % for males, and 85.7 %, 75.7 %, 66.4 %, 57.4 % for females (Table 2). The unadjusted median survival time for males was 3.8 years compared to a median survival of 6.5 years for females. There was no significant difference in Kaplan-Meier survival curves, log-rank test *p* = 0.07 (Fig. 1). The unadjusted HR for the effect of male sex on survival was 1.43 (95 %CI 0.97, 2.13). After adjusting for baseline differences

**Table 2** SSc-PAH survival estimates by sex

| Sex | Survival | | | | |
|---|---|---|---|---|---|
| | 1-year (95 %CI) | 2-year (95 %CI) | 3-year (95 %CI) | 5-year (95 %CI) | Median years |
| Male | 83.2 % (73.8 %, 93.9 %) | 68.7 % (57.1 %, 82.8 %) | 53.2 % (40.7 %, 69.4 %) | 45.6 % (33.1 %, 62.8 %) | 3.8 |
| Female | 85.7 % (81.8 %, 89.7 %) | 75.7 % (71.0 %, 80.8 %) | 66.4 % (61.7 %, 72.7 %) | 57.4 % (51.7 %, 63.7 %) | 6.5 |

*SSc-PAH* systemic sclerosis-associated pulmonary arterial hypertension

disease subtype and interstitial lung disease, the HR for male sex was attenuated to 1.27 (95 %CI 0.85, 1.90).

A sensitivity analysis was performed to explore the effect of PAH age of diagnosis >60 years that had been reported by others. There was no significant difference in survival curves between this subset of males and females, log-rank test 0.86 (Fig. 2). The unadjusted HR for the effect of male sex on survival in those aged 60 years or older was 1.06 (95 %CI 0.55, 2.07). There was a statistically significant difference in survival curves for those with an age of PAH diagnosis less than 60 years of age (log-rank test $p = 0.03$, Fig. 3) with a male sex unadjusted HR of 1.70 (1.04, 2.80). After adjusting for baseline differences in disease subtype in this subset, the HR for male sex was attenuated to 1.44 (95 %CI 0.85, 2.46).

## Discussion

We have found that sex disparities appear to exist in SSc-PAH. PAH is more common in females with SSc, yet males have a shorter time from SSc to PAH diagnosis, shorter PAH disease duration and increased burden of SSc disease. Despite these differences, male sex does not independently impact SSc-PAH mortality. To our

knowledge, this is the largest study to examine the impact of sex in SSc-PAH.

The female to male ratio for SSc-PAH of 5.5:1, is higher than the reported sex ratios for SSc in general, ranging between 3–4:1 [7]. This suggests that PAH is an SSc disease manifestation that occurs more frequently in females. However, males with SSc-PAH have an increased frequency of other serious SSc disease manifestations, notably, scleroderma renal crisis, diffuse cutaneous disease and interstitial lung disease. Furthermore, we found males had a shorter time from SSc diagnosis to PAH diagnosis, with the average male time to SSc-PAH diagnosis more than 3 years earlier than females. In a Japanese cohort study by Kasukawa et al. it was reported that a shortened average time between SSc and SSc-PAH diagnosis was associated with an increase in mortality [21]. Together with our findings, this may suggest that although PAH is less frequent in males, they may have more aggressive disease. The differential time to PAH diagnosis may also be reflective of sex-based differences is health-seeking behaviours and/or access to care [7].

We found that females tended to have better short- and long-term survival rates compared to males. However, sex

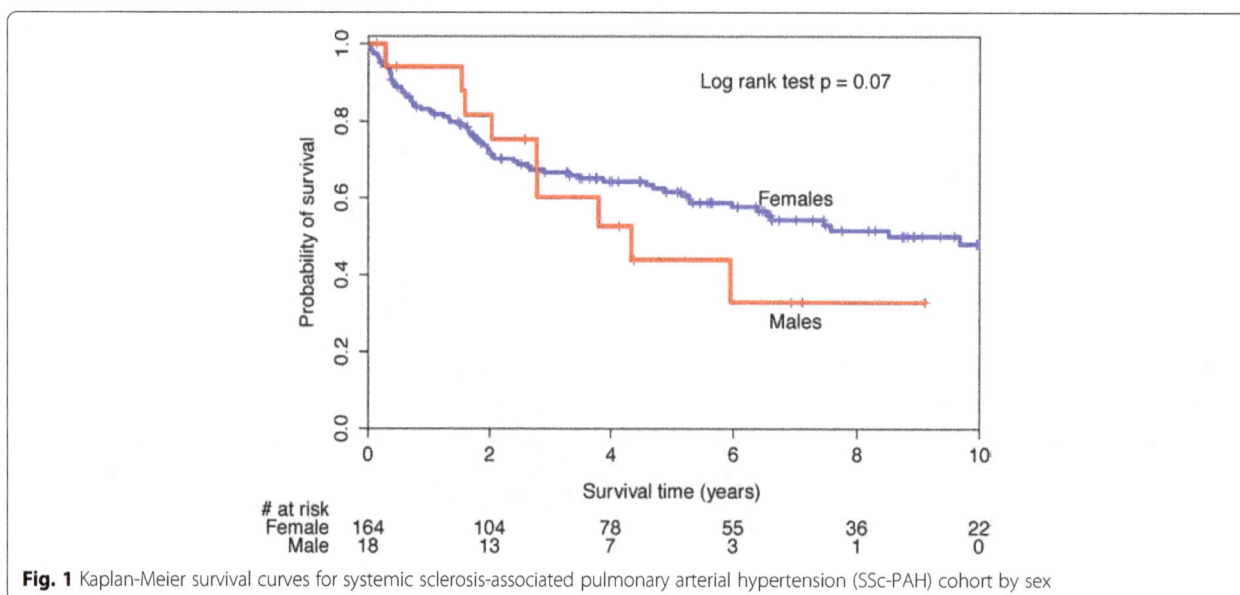

**Fig. 1** Kaplan-Meier survival curves for systemic sclerosis-associated pulmonary arterial hypertension (SSc-PAH) cohort by sex

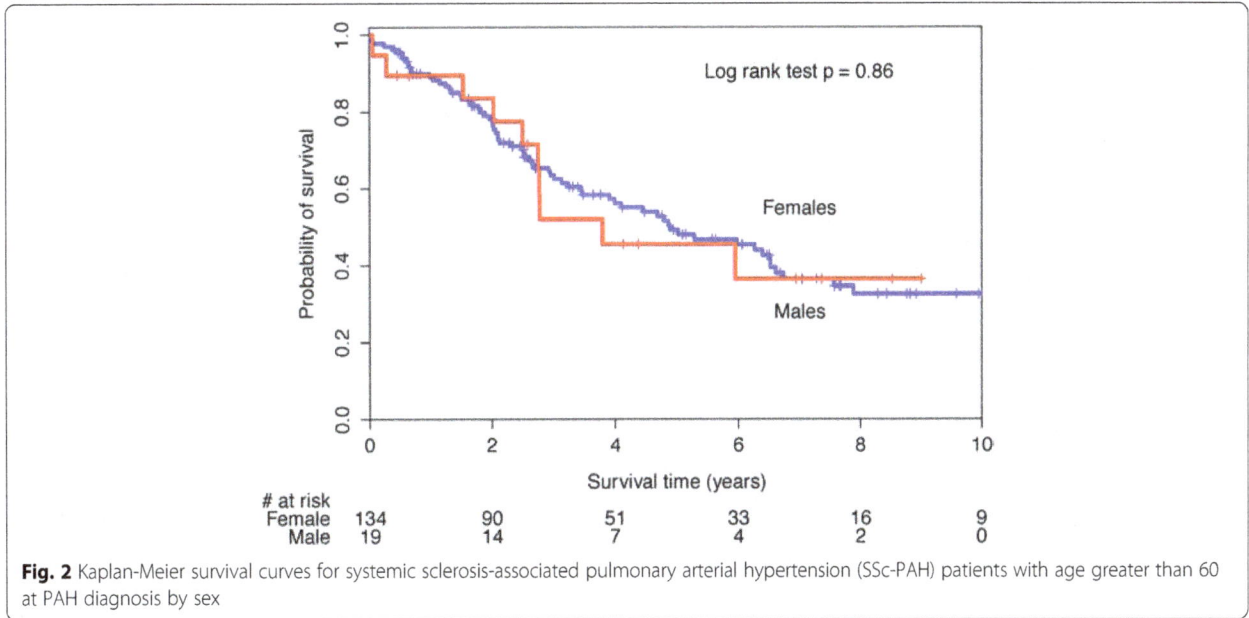

**Fig. 2** Kaplan-Meier survival curves for systemic sclerosis-associated pulmonary arterial hypertension (SSc-PAH) patients with age greater than 60 at PAH diagnosis by sex

was not found to be an independent factor for survival in SSc-PAH patients. Condliffe et al. reported that male sex was associated with decreased survival in a cohort of 259 patients with SSc-PAH [11]. MacGregor et al. reported that although male sex was not an independent risk factor, there was a trend toward increased death in male patients with SSc-PAH [12]. In both studies, survival curves for males and females were not provided so graphical comparisons to our findings could not be made. Visual inspection of our Kaplan-Meier curves suggests differential survival between sexes, particularly in the long term. The lack of statistical significance may be related to insufficient

power. However, accounting for baseline difference between sexes attenuated the HR toward a null effect. This suggests that perceived differences in survival between sexes in the full cohort are likely attributable to the baseline differences in measured and unmeasured confounders.

When examining SSc-PAH patients with an age of PAH diagnosis greater than 60 years, we found no significant difference in survival between the sexes. Examination of the Kaplan-Meier curves in this subset of patients, illustrates considerable overlap of the survival curves. It has been hypothesized that because post-menopausal female patients have lost the cardio-protective effect of estrogen,

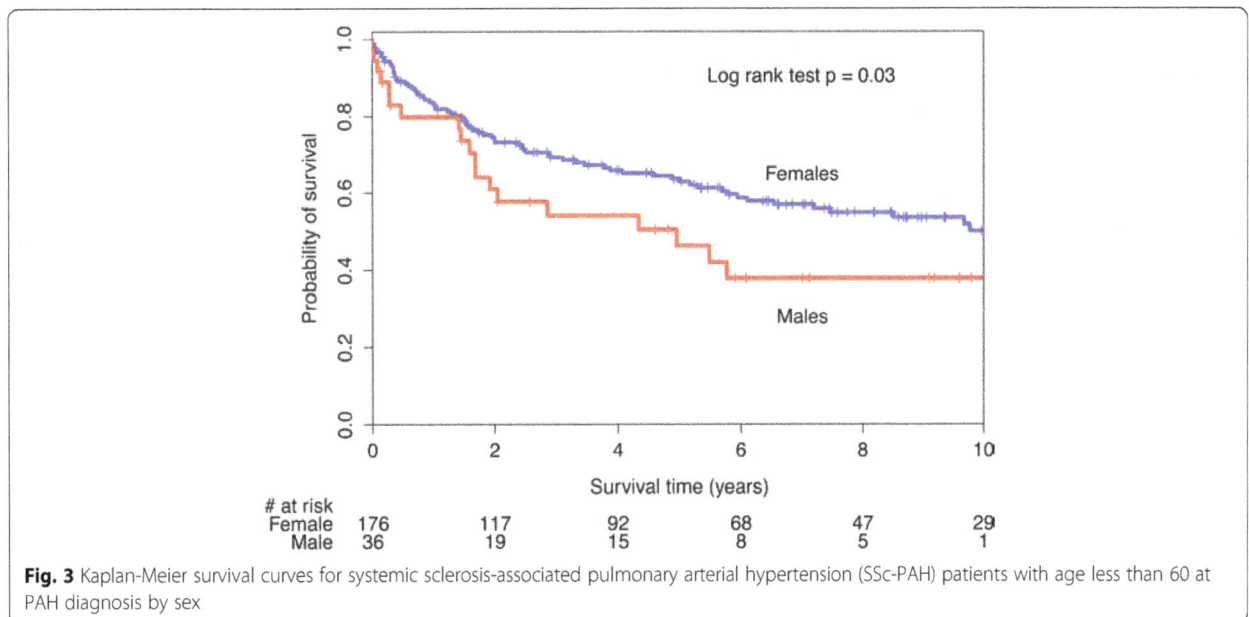

**Fig. 3** Kaplan-Meier survival curves for systemic sclerosis-associated pulmonary arterial hypertension (SSc-PAH) patients with age less than 60 at PAH diagnosis by sex

right ventricular adaptation is no longer possible. When we evaluated survival in those with an age of PAH diagnosis less than age 60 years, there appeared to be sex-based differences in survival. However the adjusted analysis suggested that these perceived differences were attributable to difference in other baseline characteristics. It may be that the observed differences in SSc-PAH survival between sexes reported in other studies may be attributable to unmeasured confounders.

A potential limitation of this study is the limited power to detect small differences in survival. A larger sample size would allow us to detect if male sex has a small, independent effect on survival. To our knowledge, this is the largest study to evaluate the effect of sex on survival in SSc-PAH, and we had sufficient power to detect moderate to large effects. A second potential limitation is our ability to evaluate all aspects of SSc disease burden. Although we were able to evaluate centromere and ScL-70 antibodies, we did not have the ability to evaluate other scleroderma-specific antibodies including RNA polymerase III. In addition, interstitial lung disease was present in a subset of patients. It should be noted that these patients had mild disease, evidenced by bibasilar reticulations on CT thorax. This may reflect a referral bias at our center as SSc patients with moderate to severe interstitial lung disease, or pulmonary hypertension attributable to interstitial lung disease are not seen on our Pulmonary Hypertension Clinic, but rather in the Interstitial Lung Disease Clinic. As such, patients with moderate to severe interstitial lung disease or pulmonary hypertension attributable to interstitial lung disease were not included in this analysis. Findings from this study should not be generalized to those patients. In addition, we did not collect smoking data. A third potential limitation of our study was the inability to account for sex-based differences in the psycho-social determinants of health outcomes. Our cohort study occurs within the context of a universal health care system, however it is possible that inequitable outcomes may occur. These may be related to sex-based differences in health-seeking behaviors and access to care, which were beyond the scope of this study. Future investigators may consider accounting for these factors. Finally, our survival analysis was limited to all-cause mortality. Since we did not have access to death certificates, we were not able to report cause-specific mortality. However there is controversy regarding the validity of cause-specific mortality obtained from death certificates [22]. As such, our use of all-cause mortality reflects a more conservative approach.

## Conclusions
Sex-based disparities appear to exist in the frequency of PAH, time to PAH diagnosis, PAH disease duration, and SSc disease burden. However, male sex does not independently impact SSc-PAH survival. Similarly, male sex does not independently affect survival in those diagnosed with SSc-PAH after the age of 60. Further research is needed to understand the basis for the differential frequency of PAH and time to diagnosis.

### Abbreviations
95%CI: 95 % Confidence interval; ACR: American College of Rheumatology; CT: Computerized tomography; EULAR: European League Against Rheumatism; HR: Hazard ratio; IPAH: Idiopathic pulmonary arterial hypertension; mPAP: Mean pulmonary artery pressure; PAH: Pulmonary arterial hypertension; PCWP: Pulmonary capillary wedge pressure; PVR: Pulmonary vascular resistance; RR: Relative risk; ScL-70: Topoisomerase I; SSc: Systemic sclerosis; WHO: World Health Organization.

### Competing interests
Dr. Sindhu Johnson has been awarded a Canadian Institutes of Health Research Clinician Scientist Award and is supported by the Freda Fejer Fund and the Oscar and Eleanor Markovitz Scleroderma Research Fund. Dr. Granton has received funding from Pfizer for research support for an investigator-led research study, from Actelion as a site investigator for clinical trials, as member of a Data Safety Monitoring Committee and for support of education programs through the hospital foundation, and from Ikaria as a site investigator for a clinical trial and as member of a steering committee. Saghar Sadeghi is supported by a Canadian Rheumatology Association-Roche Summer Studentship. Dr. Thenganatt has participated in advisory boards for Pfizer and Actelion. Dr. Moric has participated in advisory boards for Actelion and Intermune, and been a speaker for Actelion and Eli Lily. None of the authors have non-financial conflicts of interest to disclose.

### Authors' contributions
CRP participated in study design, developed the protocol, collected data, conducted statistical analysis and drafted the manuscript. JTG participated in study design, collected data, participated in interpretation of the results and drafted the manuscript. AMR participated in study design, assisted with protocol development, assisted with statistical interpretation and assisted with manuscript preparation. SS participated in study design, assisted with protocol development, assisted with statistical interpretation and assisted with manuscript preparation. ATK assisted with protocol development, data collection and cleaning, survival status verification, and assisted with manuscript preparation. JT contributed to study design, data verification, participated in interpretation of the results and assisted with manuscript preparation. JM contributed to study design, data verification, participated in interpretation of the results and assisted with manuscript preparation. CC assisted with protocol development and research ethics board submission, data collection, data cleaning, survival status verification, and assisted with manuscript preparation. SRJ conceived of the study, developed the protocol, collected the data, conducted statistical analysis and drafted the manuscript. All authors read and approve the final manuscript.

### Author details
[1]Toronto Scleroderma Program, Mount Sinai Hospital, Toronto Western Hospital, Division of Rheumatology, Department of Medicine, Faculty of Medicine, University of Toronto, Ground Floor, East Wing, Toronto Western Hospital, 399 Bathurst Street, Toronto, ON M5T 2S8, Canada. [2]University Health Network Pulmonary Hypertension Programme, Toronto General Hospital, Divisions of Respirology and Critical Care Medicine, Department of Medicine, Faculty of Medicine, University of Toronto, Toronto, ON, Canada. [3]University Health Network Pulmonary Hypertension Programme, Toronto General Hospital, Division of Respirology, Department of Medicine, Faculty of Medicine, University of Toronto, Toronto, ON, Canada. [4]University Health Network Pulmonary Hypertension Programme, Toronto General Hospital, Division of Respirology, Women's College Hospital, Department of Medicine, Faculty of Medicine, University of Toronto, Toronto, ON, Canada. [5]Institute of Health Policy, Management and Evaluation, University of Toronto, Toronto, ON, Canada.

## References

1. Chifflot H, Fautrel B, Sordet C, Chatelus E, Sibilia J. Incidence and prevalence of systemic sclerosis: a systematic literature review. Semin Arthritis Rheum. 2008;37:223–35. doi:10.1016/j.semarthrit.2007.05.003.
2. Pennell LM, Galligan CL, Fish EN. Sex affects immunity. J Autoimmun. 2012;38:J282–91. doi:10.1016/j.jaut.2011.11.013.
3. Mayes MD, Lacey Jr JV, Beebe-Dimmer J, Gillespie BW, Cooper B, Laing TJ, et al. Prevalence, incidence, survival, and disease characteristics of systemic sclerosis in a large US population. Arthritis Rheum. 2003;48:2246–55. doi:10.1002/art.11073.
4. Hachulla E, Carpentier P, Gressin V, Diot E, Allanore Y, Sibilia J, et al. Risk factors for death and the 3-year survival of patients with systemic sclerosis: the French ItinerAIR-Sclerodermie study. Rheumatology. 2009;48:304–8. doi:10.1093/rheumatology/ken488.
5. Hissaria P, Lester S, Hakendorf P, Woodman R, Patterson K, Hill C, et al. Survival in scleroderma: results from the population-based South Australian Register. Intern Med J. 2011;41:381–90. doi:10.1111/j.1445-5994.2010.02281.x.
6. Kuo CF, Luo SF, Yu KH, Chou IJ, Tseng WY, Chang HC, et al. Cancer risk among patients with systemic sclerosis: a nationwide population study in Taiwan. Scand J Rheumatol. 2012;41:44–9. doi:10.3109/03009742.2011.618145.
7. Hussein H, Lee P, Chau C, Johnson SR. The effect of male sex on survival in systemic sclerosis. J Rheumatol. 2014;41:2193–200. doi:10.3899/jrheum.140006.
8. Mukerjee D, St George D, Coleiro B, Knight C, Denton CP, Davar J, et al. Prevalence and outcome in systemic sclerosis associated pulmonary arterial hypertension: application of a registry approach. Ann Rheum Dis. 2003;62:1088–93.
9. Johnson SR, Swiston JR, Granton JT. Prognostic factors for survival in scleroderma associated pulmonary arterial hypertension. J Rheumatol. 2008;35:1584–90.
10. Johnson SR, Granton JT. Pulmonary hypertension in systemic sclerosis and systemic lupus erythematosus. Eur Respir Rev. 2011;20:277–86. doi:10.1183/09059180.00003811.
11. Condliffe R, Kiely DG, Peacock AJ, Corris PA, Gibbs JS, Vrapi F, et al. Connective tissue disease-associated pulmonary arterial hypertension in the modern treatment era. Am J Respir Crit Care Med. 2009;179:151–7. doi:10.1164/rccm.200806-953OC.
12. MacGregor AJ, Canavan R, Knight C, Denton CP, Davar J, Coghlan J, et al. Pulmonary hypertension in systemic sclerosis: risk factors for progression and consequences for survival. Rheumatology. 2001;40:453–9.
13. Zhang R, Dai LZ, Xie WP, Yu ZX, Wu BX, Pan L, et al. Survival of Chinese patients with pulmonary arterial hypertension in the modern treatment era. Chest. 2011;140:301–9. doi:10.1378/chest.10-2327.
14. Benza RL, Miller DP, Gomberg-Maitland M, Frantz RP, Foreman AJ, Coffey CS, et al. Predicting survival in pulmonary arterial hypertension: insights from the Registry to Evaluate Early and Long-Term Pulmonary Arterial Hypertension Disease Management (REVEAL). Circulation. 2010;122:164–72. doi:10.1161/CIRCULATIONAHA.109.898122.
15. Shapiro S, Traiger GL, Turner M, McGoon MD, Wason P, Barst RJ. Sex differences in the diagnosis, treatment, and outcome of patients with pulmonary arterial hypertension enrolled in the registry to evaluate early and long-term pulmonary arterial hypertension disease management. Chest. 2012;141:363–73. doi:10.1378/chest.10-3114.
16. Humbert M, Sitbon O, Chaouat A, Bertocchi M, Habib G, Gressin V, et al. Survival in patients with idiopathic, familial, and anorexigen-associated pulmonary arterial hypertension in the modern management era. Circulation. 2010;122:156–63. doi:10.1161/CIRCULATIONAHA.109.911818.
17. Fisher MR, Mathai SC, Champion HC, Girgis RE, Housten-Harris T, Hummers L, et al. Clinical differences between idiopathic and scleroderma-related pulmonary hypertension. Arthritis Rheum. 2006;54:3043–50. doi:10.1002/art.22069.
18. Johnson SR, Granton JT, Tomlinson GA, Grosbein HA, Le T, Lee P, et al. Warfarin in systemic sclerosis-associated and idiopathic pulmonary arterial hypertension. A Bayesian approach to evaluating treatment for uncommon disease. J Rheumatol. 2012;39:276–85. doi:10.3899/jrheum.110765.
19. van den Hoogen F, Khanna D, Fransen J, Johnson SR, Baron M, Tyndall A, et al. 2013 classification criteria for systemic sclerosis: an American College of Rheumatology/European League against Rheumatism collaborative initiative. Ann Rheum Dis. 2013;72:1747–55. doi:10.1136/annrheumdis-2013-204424.
20. Hoeper MM, Bogaard HJ, Condliffe R, Frantz R, Khanna D, Kurzyna M, et al. Definitions and diagnosis of pulmonary hypertension. J Am Coll Cardiol. 2013;62(25 Suppl):D42–50. doi:10.1016/j.jacc.2013.10.032.
21. Kasukawa R, Nishimaki T, Takagi T, Miyawaki S, Yokohari R, Tsunematsu T. Pulmonary hypertension in connective tissue disease. Clinical analysis of sixty patients in multi-institutional study. Clin Rheumatol. 1990;9:56–62.
22. Johansson LA, Westerling R. Comparing hospital discharge records with death certificates: can the differences be explained? J Epidemiol Community Health. 2002;56:301–8.

# Subclinical dermal involvement is detectable by high frequency ultrasound even in patients with limited cutaneous systemic sclerosis

A. Sulli[1], B. Ruaro[1], V. Smith[2], S. Paolino[1], C. Pizzorni[1], G. Pesce[3] and M. Cutolo[1*]

## Abstract

**Background:** The aim of the study was to detect by skin high-frequency ultrasound (US) possible subclinical skin involvement in patients affected by limited cutaneous systemic sclerosis (lcSSc), in those skin areas apparently not affected by the disease on the basis of a normal modified Rodnan skin score (mRSS). Differences in dermal thickness (DT) in comparison with healthy subjects were investigated.

**Methods:** Fifty patients with lcSSc (age $62 \pm 13$ years (mean $\pm$ SD), disease duration $5 \pm 5$ years) and 50 sex-matched and age-matched healthy subjects (age $62 \pm 11$ years) were enrolled. DT was evaluated by both mRSS and US at the usual 17 skin areas (zygoma, fingers, dorsum of the hands, forearms, upper arms, chest, abdomen, thighs, lower legs and feet). Non-parametric tests were used for the statistical analysis.

**Results:** Subclinical dermal involvement was detected by US even in the skin areas in patients with lcSSc, who had a normal local mRSS. In addition, statistically significantly higher mean DT was found in almost all skin areas, when compared to healthy subjects ($p < 0.0001$ for all areas). In particular, DT was significantly greater in patients with lcSSc than in healthy subjects in four out of six skin areas with a normal mRSS (score $= 0$) (upper arm, chest and abdomen), despite the clinical classification of lcSSc.

**Conclusions:** This study strongly suggests that subclinical dermal involvement may be detectable by US even in skin areas with a normal mRSS in patients classified as having lcSSc. This should be taken into account during SSc subset classification in clinical studies/trials.

**Keywords:** Systemic sclerosis, Dermal thickness, High-frequency ultrasound, Rodnan skin score, Nailfold videocapillaroscopy

## Background

Systemic sclerosis (SSc) is a connective tissue disorder characterized in the early stages by microvascular damage, with progressive fibrosis and skin impairment, the latter being a marker for disease classification and activity [1–6]. Skin involvement may be recognized and studied using the modified Rodnan skin score (mRSS), the validated method used to evaluate the severity of skin thickening in SSc, and to distinguish between patients with either limited (lcSSc) or diffuse (dcSSc) cutaneous involvement [2–4, 7]. As per definition, the affected skin is confined to the extremities (hands, forearms, feet, lower legs and face) in lcSSc, whilst it is also present on upper arms, chest, abdomen and thighs in dcSSc [4].

The mRSS has some drawbacks, as it is unable to identify slight alterations in skin thickness and has high intra-observer and inter-observer variability [3, 8–10]. Conversely, several studies report the utility of high-frequency ultrasound (US) for early identification of skin involvement in patients with SSc [11–15]. US may

* Correspondence: mcutolo@unige.it
[1]Research Laboratory and Academic Division of Clinical Rheumatology, Department of Internal Medicine, University of Genova, Viale Benedetto XV, n° 6, AOU IRCCS San Martino, 16132 Genova, Italy
Full list of author information is available at the end of the article

identify the different skin layers and offers a wide range of values for measurement of dermal thickness (DT), compared with the semi-quantitative mRSS scale comprising only 4 integer values. However, mRSS and US do not measure exactly the same properties of the skin. The mRSS measures skin thickness, texture and fixation, while US accurately measures the DT, even if it is difficult to differentiate between oedema and fibrosis [11, 16, 17].

The aim of this study was to use US to detect possible subclinical skin involvement in patients with lcSSc, in those skin areas apparently not affected on the basis of a normal local mRSS, looking for differences in DT in comparison with healthy subjects.

## Methods
### Study population
Fifty patients with lcSSc (age 62 ± 13 (mean ± SD) years, mean disease duration 5 ± 5 years), classified on the basis of a normal mRSS (score = 0) at the upper arms, chest, abdomen and thighs, were enrolled during routine clinical follow up [7]. Patients with SSc met either the American College of Rheumatology (ACR)/European League Against Rheumatism (EULAR) 2013 criteria for SSc, or the LeRoy's criteria for the classification of early SSc, and gave written informed consent to enter the study [1, 4]. Ethics approval was obtained from the local ethical board. Complete medical history was recorded, and clinical examination was carried out in all patients (the most important clinical findings are reported in Table 1).

Treatments received by patients included mainly aspirin, vasodilators, immunomodulatory drugs and endothelin-1 receptor inhibitors; there were no restriction criteria

related to therapy for inclusion of patients in the study, due to the cross-sectional nature of the investigation and the limited presence of possible bias in the primary endpoint.

Fifty sex-matched and age-matched healthy control subjects (CNT) (mean age ± SD 62 ± 13 years) were also evaluated after giving informed consent. US was performed in both patients with SSc and in healthy subjects, as described subsequently. Patients and healthy subjects with presence of lower extremity oedema, which could confound both mRSS and US assessment, were excluded.

### Skin high-frequency ultrasound
Skin US was performed in both patients with lcSSc and in healthy subjects to measure DT at the level of all 17 skin areas that are evaluated by the mRSS (at exactly the same spots), and the values were recorded in millimetres [12, 13] (see Fig. 1).

An ultrasound system equipped with an 18-MHz probe was used (MyLab 25, Esaote, Genoa, Italy). A high-frequency probe offers considerably good resolution, allowing the distinction between the epidermis, dermis and subcutaneous layers of skin, and measurement of DT [18]. In particular, DT was measured on the B-mode image by an electronic caliper included with the software, identifying the upper surface epidermis-dermis and the lower layer dermis-subcutis [12]. The same operator (BR) performed the US evaluations in all individuals, blinded to the mRSS.

### Modified Rodnan skin score
The severity of skin involvement was quantified by the mRSS in each individual. It was performed in the

**Table 1** Clinical findings in patients with systemic sclerosis (SSc) and healthy control subjects (CNT)

| | Age (years) | BMI (kg/m$^2$) | ANA pattern (cen/spe + nuc/spe) | ENA (Scl70/RNAP/neg) | RP duration (years) | SSc duration (years) | MES (score) | US-DT total (mm) | mRSS total (score) |
|---|---|---|---|---|---|---|---|---|---|
| CNT (n = 50) mean ± SD | 64.9 ± 15.1 | 22.3 ± 1.9 | - | - | - | - | 0 | 14.7 ± 0.5 | 0 |
| lcSSc (n = 50) mean ± SD | 62.5 ± 12.7 | 22.4 ± 1.8 | 33/11/6 | 11/1/5 | 12.1 ± 11.6 | 5.3 ± 4.9 | 3.2 ± 2.5 | 17.2 ± 1.7 | 4.8 ± 2.6 |
| SSc vs CNT p value* | n.s. | n.s. | - | - | - | - | - | <0.0001 | <0.0001 |
| Early (n = 21) mean ± SD | 61.3 ± 12.8 | 22.3 ± 2.0 | 14/5/2 | 5/0/2 | 6.6 ± 4.5 | 3.1 ± 3.5 | 0.7 ± 0.5 | 16.2 ± 1.0 | 3.2 ± 1.8 |
| Active (n = 16) mean ± SD | 58.6 ± 9.6 | 22.1 ± 1.5 | 12/2/2 | 3/1/0 | 13.0 ± 13.4 | 4.3 ± 3.7 | 4.4 ± 1.3 | 17.7 ± 1.2 | 5.0 ± 2.2 |
| Late (n = 13) mean ± SD | 69.2 ± 14.0 | 23.0 ± 2.3 | 7/4/2 | 3/0/3 | 20.0 ± 13.0 | 10.0 ± 5.0 | 6.0 ± 1.1 | 18.2 ± 2.0 | 7.3 ± 2.4 |
| E vs A vs L p value** | n.s. | n.s. | n.s. | n.s. | 0.002 | 0.0002 | <0.0001 | 0.0005 | <0.0001 |

*RP* Raynaud's phenomenon, *MES* microangiopathy evolution score, *DT* dermal thickness (ultrasound evaluation), *mRSS* modified Rodnan skin score, *SD* standard deviation, *E* Early, *A* Active, *L* Late (patterns of microangiopathy on nailfold videocapillaroscopy), *lcSSc* limited cutaneous systemic sclerosis, *BMI* body mass index, *ANA* antinuclear antibodies, *cen* centromeric, *spe + nuc* speckled and nucleolar, *spe* speckled, *ENA* extractable nuclear antigen antibodies, *Scl70* anti-topoisomerase antibodies, *RNAP* anti-RNA polymerase III autoantibodies, *neg* ENA-negative. *Mann-Withney U test. **Kruskal-Wallis test

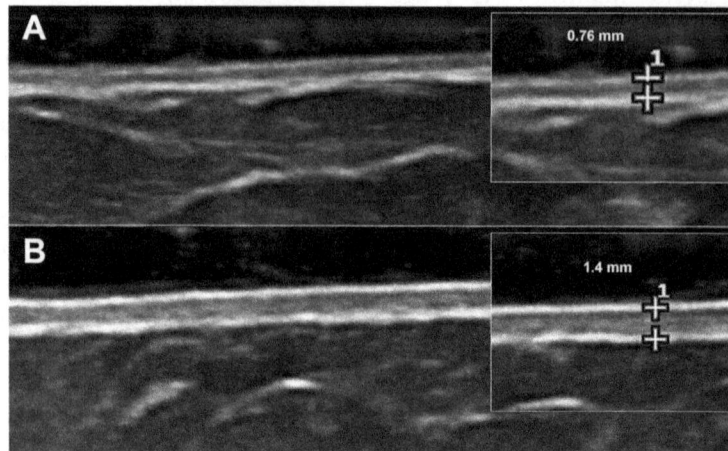

**Fig. 1** Example of measurement of dermal thickness by skin high-frequency ultrasound (18 MHz probe) in a healthy subject (**a**) and in a patient with systemic sclerosis (**b**) at the level of the abdomen

codified seventeen skin areas (zygoma, fingers, dorsum of the hands, forearms, upper arms, chest, abdomen, thighs, lower legs and feet) [7]. Skin thickness was assessed by palpation, and marked on a scale as 0 (normal), 1 (weak), 2 (intermediate) or 3 (severe skin thickening). In this study only patients classified as affected by lcSSc were enrolled (mRSS = 0 at the arms, chest, abdomen and thighs). The same operator (SP) assessed the mRSS in all subjects, blinded to the US assessment. Both mRSS and US were performed the same day in all patients with SSc.

### Nailfold videocapillaroscopy
Nailfold videocapillaroscopy (NVC) was performed using an optical probe, equipped with a × 200 contact lens, connected to image analysis software (Videocap, DS Medica, Milan, Italy) to classify patients with SSc into the proper pattern of microangiopathy (as early, active or late), and to calculate the microangiopathy evolution score (MES), as previously reported [19–22]. The same operator (CP) performed all NVC evaluations.

### Statistical analysis
Non-parametric tests were used for the statistical analysis. In particular, the Mann-Whitney $U$ test was performed to compare unpaired groups of variables, and the Kruskal-Wallis test was used to compare continuous variables with nominal variables with more than two levels. The Spearman rank correlation test was employed to identify relationships between variables, along with linear regression tests. $P$ values lower than 0.05 were considered statistically significant. The results are reported as mean with standard deviation (SD) and confidence intervals (CI).

### Results
The clinical features of patients with SSc and healthy subjects are reported in Table 1. Subclinical dermal involvement was detected by US even in areas of skin areas in patients with lcSSc who had local normal mRSS in those areas. When compared with healthy subjects, patients with lcSSc had a statistically significant higher mean DT in all skin areas ($p < 0.0001$ for all) except the thighs, where DT was greater in patients with lcSSc than in healthy subjects but the difference was not statistically significant ($p = 0.16$ and $p = 0.14$, respectively for the right and left thigh) (see Table 2 and Fig. 2 for further statistical data).

Of interest, DT was also significantly higher in four out of six skin areas where the mRSS was normal (score = 0) (upper arms, chest and abdomen). Moreover, at the level of the upper arms, chest and abdomen the mean DT in patients with lcSSc was higher than mean DT plus three standard deviations in the healthy subjects, and thus was above the normal range (99.73% probability) (see Table 2 for CI).

In particular, almost 75% of patients with SSc had DT beyond the normal range in the aforementioned skin areas (instead of the expected 5% of patients allowing for possible variation from the normal range), despite their classification as having lcSSc; furthermore, 46–74% of patients had DT above the 99.73% CI upper limit in the aforementioned skin areas) (see also Table 2).

As was predictable, the sum of the DT values for the 17 areas of skin assessed by either US or the mRSS was significantly higher in patients with SSc than in the control group (Table 1). There was statistically significant positive correlation between total US-DT and mRSS-DT values ($r = 0.37$, $p = 0.04$).

There was no statistically significant correlation between DT and the duration of either SSc ($p = 0.7$) or

**Table 2** Dermal thickness in healthy subjects and patients classified as affected by limited cutaneous systemic sclerosis (lcSSc) on the basis of a normal Rodnan skin score at the upper arms, chest, abdomen and thighs

| Dermal thickness | Healthy subjects | | | | | Patients with lcSSc | Patients with lcSSc with DT >2SD | Patients with lcSSc with DT >3SD |
|---|---|---|---|---|---|---|---|---|
| | Mean ± SD (mm) | Mean + 2SD (mm) | Mean + 3SD (mm) | 95% CI lower, upper | 99.73% CI lower, upper | Mean ± SD (mm) | Number (%) (out of 50) | Number (%) (out of 50) |
| Right finger | 0.70 ± 0.05 | 0.80 | 0.85 | 0.69, 0.72 | 0.68, 0.72 | 0.88 ± 0.14 | 32 (64) | 25 (50) |
| Left finger | 0.70 ± 0.06 | 0.82 | 0.88 | 0.69, 0.72 | 0.68, 0.72 | 0.88 ± 0.14 | 32 (64) | 28 (56) |
| Right hand | 0.71 ± 0.06 | 0.83 | 0.89 | 0.69, 0.72 | 0.68, 0.73 | 0.84 ± 0.12 | 23 (46) | 13 (26) |
| Left hand | 0.71 ± 0.06 | 0.83 | 0.89 | 0.69, 0.73 | 0.69, 0.74 | 0.86 ± 0.16 | 24 (48) | 18 (36) |
| Right forearm | 0.77 ± 0.05 | 0.87 | 0.92 | 0.75, 0.78 | 0.75, 0.79 | 0.98 ± 0.19 | 32 (64) | 28 (56) |
| Left forearm | 0.77 ± 0.05 | 0.87 | 0.92 | 0.75, 0.78 | 0.75, 0.79 | 0.99 ± 0.19 | 34 (68) | 30 (60) |
| Right upper arm | 0.82 ± 0.07 | 0.96 | 1.03 | 0.80, 0.83 | 0.79, 0.84 | 1.06 ± 0.16 | 37 (74) | 23 (46) |
| Left upper arm | 0.82 ± 0.06 | 0.94 | 1.00 | 0.80, 0.83 | 0.79, 0.84 | 1.07 ± 0.16 | 39 (78) | 25 (50) |
| Chest | 1.11 ± 0.03 | 1.17 | 1.20 | 1.11, 1.12 | 1.10, 1.13 | 1.23 ± 0.17 | 35 (70) | 24 (48) |
| Abdomen | 1.11 ± 0.02 | 1.15 | 1.17 | 1.11, 1.12 | 1.11, 1.12 | 1.28 ± 0.18 | 37 (74) | 37 (74) |
| Right thigh | 1.13 ± 0.21 | 1.55 | 1.76 | 1.08, 1.18 | 1.05, 1.21 | 1.18 ± 0.23 | 0 | 0 |
| Left thigh | 1.14 ± 0.20 | 1.54 | 1.74 | 1.08, 1.19 | 1.05, 1.22 | 1.18 ± 0.23 | 1 (2) | 0 |
| Right lower leg | 0.92 ± 0.04 | 1.00 | 1.04 | 0.91, 0.93 | 0.90, 0.93 | 1.03 ± 0.13 | 25 (50) | 16 (32) |
| Left lower leg | 0.92 ± 0.05 | 1.02 | 1.07 | 0.90, 0.93 | 0.90, 0.93 | 1.03 ± 0.10 | 21 (42) | 16 (32) |
| Right foot | 0.87 ± 0.04 | 0.95 | 0.99 | 0.86, 0.88 | 0.86, 0.89 | 0.96 ± 0.13 | 24 (48) | 17 (34) |
| Left foot | 0.88 ± 0.04 | 0.96 | 1.00 | 0.87, 0.89 | 0.86, 0.89 | 0.97 ± 0.11 | 25 (50) | 15 (30) |
| Zygoma | 0.66 ± 0.05 | 0.76 | 0.81 | 0.65, 0.67 | 0.64, 0.68 | 0.85 ± 0.10 | 38 (76) | 32 (64) |

Mean values, standard deviations (SD) and both 95% and 99.73% confidence intervals (CI) are reported. Of interest, patients with lcSSc had dermal thickness (DT) values greater than the normal range in healthy subjects (see mean +2SD and +3SD, and upper 95% and 99.73% CI reporting, respectively, the 5% and 0.27% chance that healthy subjects might have a dermal thickness above the range), also in those areas where the mRSS was zero

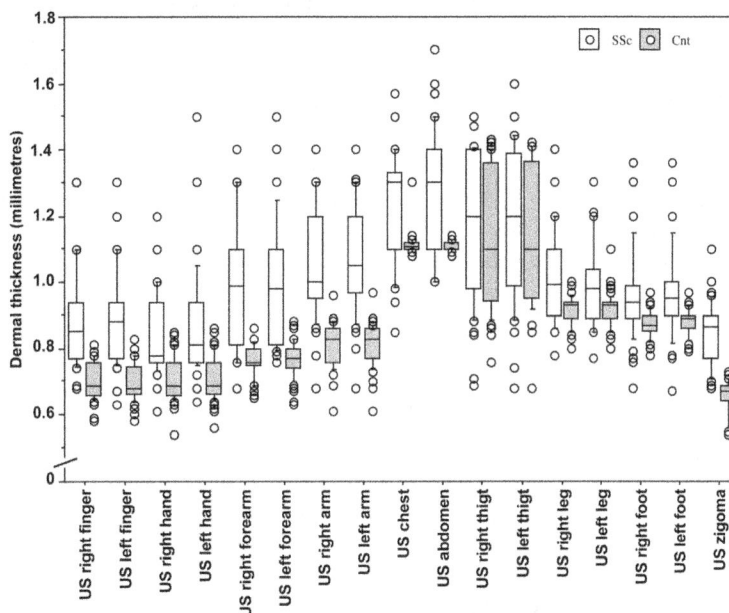

**Fig. 2** Dermal thickness evaluated by skin high-frequency ultrasound (*US*) in patients with systemic sclerosis (*SSc*) and healthy control subjects (*CNT*) (SSc vs CNT: *p* < 0.0001 for all, with the exclusion of thigh). Data are presented as box plots for different skin areas, with the 5th, 10th, 50th (median), 90th, 95th percentiles

Raynaud's phenomenon (RP) ($p = 0.6$). Neither was there any statistically significant correlation between DT and organ involvement (gastrointestinal tract, lung, heart, kidney or occurrence of digital ulcers) in our cohort of patients with lcSSc.

Patients with lcSSc who were positive for anti-centromere antibodies had lower DT ($17.07 \pm 1.65$ mm) than patients with anti-Scl-70 ($17.78 \pm 1.89$ mm) or anti-RNA polymerase III ($19.30 \pm 0.0$ mm), but the difference was not statistically significant ($p = 0.40$) (however the population was small and unbalanced in terms of the autoantibody profile). Dermal thickness, as evaluated by both US and the mRSS, was significantly higher in those patients with lcSSc who had the "late" pattern of micro-angiopathy on NVC and an elevated microangiography evolution score (MES) (see Table 1). The intra-operator reproducibility was 92% (95%CI 0.87–0.96) for mRSS and 96% (95% CI 0.94–0.97) for US.

## Discussion

The present investigation demonstrates, for the first time, that skin high frequency US is able to identify sub-clinical dermal involvement even in the skin areas where the mRSS is normal, in patients classified as affected by lcSSc. Skin involvement in SSc is critical for the initial diagnosis and it also has prognostic relevance [2, 3].

Cutaneous manifestations are clinically recognized and studied by the mRSS, the validated method to assess the severity of skin involvement in SSc [5, 7, 9]. The extension of skin involvement, evaluated by mRSS, is the parameter for classification of the disease into different subsets, characterized by either limited or diffuse skin involvement [2, 4]. This classification is largely used in clinical trials/studies.

Patients with lcSSc may have increased DT at the extremities, forearms, lower legs and face, but not at the upper arms, chest, abdomen and thighs, which characterizes the patients affected by dcSSc, as assessed by mRSS [2, 3, 7]. Therefore, the present US study of the skin brings important information to be considered when the patients are classified as being affected by lcSSc.

The subclinical skin involvement in patients with lcSSc is further supported in the present study by showing that mean DT values were beyond the normal DT value of the sex-matched and age-matched healthy control subjects (calculated as mean DT value plus three standard deviations, 99.73% CI upper limit): about 50% of individual patients had DT values above the 99.73% CI upper limit, and about 75% above the 95% CI upper limit (standard normal range) at the arms, chest and abdomen.

These observations seem to have a genetic and patho-physiological background, as recent studies carried out by gene microarray analysis suggested that in patients with SSc the clinically unaffected skin shares peculiar gene signatures and pathological aspects, similar to the overt clinically affected skin [23, 24]. More recently, clustering analysis revealed two prominent transcriptomes in skin biopsies from patients with SSc: the keratin and fibro-inflammatory signatures [25]. Interestingly, in both patients with dcSSc and patients with lcSSc, hyalinised collagen and myofibroblasts were identified even in skin that was not clinically involved, without significant differences between lcSSc and controls [26, 27].

Further possible applications of integrating skin US analysis with the mRSS in patients with SSc could originate from the recent observation that the baseline mRSS was the strongest predictor of skin improvement, independent of disease duration [28]. These findings also seem to link to the report that patients with either lcSSc or dcSSc may display similar organ/laboratory involvement in clinical studies [29–32]. Altogether these reports seem to suggest that US may identify skin involvement earlier than the mRSS in apparently unaffected skin areas in patients with lcSSc. This is also supported by other studies, which demonstrated that US is able to identify the oedematous phase preceding palpable skin involvement in the early stage of SSc [11, 12, 18].

One limitation to the present study might be the small cohort of enrolled patients, due to having recruitment at a single centre, and the larger standard deviation in DT observed in both patients and healthy subjects at the thighs might justify the absence of statistically significant differences between the two groups at this level. Furthermore, the US evaluation was made by only one operator, and so inter-rater reliability was not assessed.

Another limitation might be the 18-MHz probe employed to assess DT, due to its good but sub-optimal performance in analysing the skin; modern higher frequency probes (20–24 MHz) may allow easier identification of the dermal boundaries, reducing measurement error. Once again, the greater variation in DT observed at the thighs might be related to a slightly blurred image obtained with our 18-MHz probe at this level.

A further limitation may be linked to the fact that the patients with SSc were analysed without considering therapeutic management; however, the aim of the present study was to assess possible subclinical skin involvement in individual patients with lcSSc and ongoing treatments should not influence the results. Finally, DT may vary at different ages and according to premenopausal or postmenopausal status [33]; however, this bias was avoided by enrolling sex-matched and age-matched subjects.

By considering the capability of US to detect skin involvement in the early and subclinical stages of SSc, skin

US might be proposed as a further important tool for the clinical assessment of the disease. Of note, skin US may be considered a notable and acceptable technique for clinical research into the pathogenesis of the disease and treatment effects, as it represents a non-invasive and safe approach [34].

As this was a cross-sectional study, data on future worsening of DT (evaluated by both the mRSS and US) or progression from lcSSc to dcSSc are not provided. Further studies should investigate this matter. In terms of the feasibility of skin US, it is more time-consuming than mRSS assessment as it takes about 20–25 minutes including skin image capture and manipulation to measure DT. However, the examination is well-accepted by patients, and it do not imply further expense if the device is the same already employed to assess musculoskeletal apparatus during routine clinical practice.

## Conclusions

In conclusion, this study strongly suggests that subclinical dermal involvement may be detectable by skin high-frequency ultrasound even in patients classified as having lcSSc on the basis of the mRSS clinical evaluation. This should be taken into consideration during subset classification in clinical studies/trials.

### Abbreviations
CI: Confidence intervals; CNT: Controls, healthy subjects; dcSSc: Diffuse cutaneous systemic sclerosis; DT: Dermal thickness; IQR: Interquartile range; lcSSc: Limited cutaneous systemic sclerosis; MES: Microangiopathy evolution score; mRSS: Modified Rodnan skin score; NVC: Nailfold videocapillaroscopy; SD: Standard deviation; SSc: Systemic sclerosis; US: High-frequency ultrasound

### Acknowledgements
B. Ruaro is supported by grants from the Italian Society of Rheumatology (SIR) 2015. V. Smith is Senior Clinical Investigator of the Research Foundation - Flanders (Belgium) (FWO) (1802915 N).

### Funding
This study was financially supported by funding of the Research Laboratory and Academic Division of Clinical Rheumatology of the University of Genova, Italy.

### Authors' contributions
AS participated in study conception and design, analysis and interpretation of data and writing the manuscript, and performed the statistical analysis. BR participated in study conception and design, analysis and interpretation of data, writing the manuscript, patient selection and acquisition of data. SP and CP participated in patient selection and assessment and acquisition of data, and helped to revise the manuscript. VS participated in study analysis and interpretation of data and writing the manuscript. GP carried out autoantibody detection and revised the manuscript. MC participated in study conception and design and analysis and interpretation of data, and writing he manuscript. All authors read and approved the final manuscript.

### Competing interest
The authors declare that they have no competing interests.

### Author details
[1]Research Laboratory and Academic Division of Clinical Rheumatology, Department of Internal Medicine, University of Genova, Viale Benedetto XV, n° 6, AOU IRCCS San Martino, 16132 Genova, Italy. [2]Department of Rheumatology, Ghent University Hospital, Department of Internal Medicine, Ghent University, Ghent, Belgium. [3]Laboratory of Autoimmunity, Department of Internal Medicine, University of Genova, IRCCS A.O.U, San Martino, Genoa, Italy.

### References
1. Krieg T, Takehara K. Skin disease: a cardinal feature of systemic sclerosis. Rheumatology. 2009;48:iii14–8.
2. Cutolo M, Sulli A, Smith V. Assessing microvascular changes in systemic sclerosis diagnosis and management. Nat Rev Rheumatol. 2010;6:578–87.
3. van den Hoogen F, Khanna D, Fransen J, Johnson SR, Baron M, Tyndall A, et al. 2013 classification criteria for systemic sclerosis: an American college of rheumatology/European league against rheumatism collaborative initiative. Ann Rheum Dis. 2013;72:1747–55.
4. LeRoy EC, Meedsger Jr TA. Criteria for the classification of early systemic sclerosis. J Rheumatol. 2001;28:1573–6.
5. Medsger Jr TA, Silman AJ, Steen VD, Black CM, Akesson A, Bacon PA, et al. A disease severity scale for systemic sclerosis: development and testing. J Rheumatol. 1999;26:2159–67.
6. Valentini G, Della Rossa A, Bombardieri S, Bencivelli W, Silman AJ, D'Angelo S, et al. European multicentre study to define disease activity criteria for systemic sclerosis. II. Identification of disease activity variables and development of preliminary activity indexes. Ann Rheum Dis. 2001;60:592–8.
7. Clements P, Lachenbruch P, Siebold J, White B, Weiner S, Martin R, et al. Inter and intraobserver variability of total skin thickness score (modified Rodnan TSS) in systemic sclerosis. J Rheumatol. 1995;22:1281–5.
8. Hachulla E, Launay D. Diagnosis and classification of systemic sclerosis. Clinic Rev Allerg Immunol. 2011;40:78–83.
9. Kaldas M, Khanna PP, Furst DE, Clements PJ, Kee Wong W, Seibold JR, et al. Sensitivity to change of the modified Rodnan skin score in diffuse systemic sclerosis—assessment of individual body sites in two large randomized controlled trials. Rheumatology. 2009;48:1143–6.
10. Czirják L, Nagy Z, Aringer M, Riemekasten G, Matucci-Cerinic M, Furst DE. The EUSTAR model for teaching and implementing the modified Rodnan skin score in systemic sclerosis. Ann Rheum Dis. 2007;66:966–9.
11. Kaloudi O, Bandinelli F, Filippucci E, Conforti ML, Miniati I, Guiducci S, et al. High frequency ultrasound measurement of digital dermal thickness in systemic sclerosis. Ann Rheum Dis. 2010;69:1140–3.
12. Moore TL, Lunt M, McManus B, Anderson ME, Herrick AL. Seventeen-point dermal ultrasound scoring system-a reliable measure of skin thickness in patients with systemic sclerosis. Rheumatology. 2003;42:1559–63.
13. Sulli A, Ruaro B, Alessandri A, Pizzorni C, Cimmino MA, Zampogna G, et al. Correlation between nailfold microangiopathy severity, finger dermal thickness and fingertip blood perfusion in systemic sclerosis patients. Ann Rheum Dis. 2014;73:247–51.
14. Hesselstrand R, Carlestam J, Wildt M, Sandqvist G, Andréasson K. High frequency ultrasound of skin involvement in systemic sclerosis - a follow-up study. Arthritis Res Ther. 2015;17:329.
15. Akesson A, Hesselstrand R, Scheja A, Wildt M. Longitudinal development of skin involvement and reliability of high frequency ultrasound in systemic sclerosis. Ann Rheum Dis. 2004;63:791–6.
16. Czirják L, Foeldvari I, Muller-Ladner U. Skin involvement in systemic sclerosis. Rheumatology. 2008;47:v44–5.
17. Kissin EY, Merkel PA, Lafyatis R. Myofibroblasts and hyalinized collagen as markers of skin disease in systemic sclerosis. Arthritis Rheum. 2006;54:3655–60.
18. Hesselstrand R, Scheja A, Wildt M, Akesson A. High-frequency ultrasound of skin involvement in systemic sclerosis reflects oedema, extension and severity in early disease. Rheumatology. 2008;47:84–7.
19. Cutolo M, Sulli A, Pizzorni C, Accardo S. Nailfold videocapillaroscopy assessment of microvascular damage in systemic sclerosis. J Rheumatol. 2000;27:155–60.
20. Sulli A, Pizzorni C, Smith V, Zampogna G, Ravera F, Cutolo M. Timing of transition between capillaroscopic patterns in systemic sclerosis. Arthritis Rheum. 2012;64:821–5.
21. Sulli A, Secchi ME, Pizzorni C, Cutolo M. Scoring the nailfold microvascular changes during the capillaroscopic analysis in systemic sclerosis patients. Ann Rheum Dis. 2008;67:885–7.

22. Ruaro B, Sulli A, Pizzorni C, Paolino S, Smith V, Cutolo M. Correlations between skin blood perfusion values and nailfold capillaroscopy scores in systemic sclerosis patients. Microvasc Res. 2016;105:119–24.
23. Pendergrass SA, Lemaire R, Francis IP, Mahoney JM, Lafyatis R, Whitfield ML. Intrinsic gene expression subsets of diffuse cutaneous systemic sclerosis are stable in serial skin biopsies. J Invest Dermatol. 2012;132:1363–73.
24. Frost J, Ramsay M, Mia R, Moosa L, Musenge E, Tikly M. Differential gene expression of MMP-1, TIMP-1 and HGF in clinically involved and uninvolved skin in South Africans with SSc. Rheumatology. 2012;51:1049–52.
25. Assassi S, Swindell WR, Wu M, Tan FD, Khanna D, Furst DE, et al. Dissecting the heterogeneity of skin gene expression patterns in systemic sclerosis. Arthritis Rheumatol. 2015;67:3016–26.
26. Van Praet JT, Smith V, Haspeslagh M, Degryse N, Elewaut D, De Keyser F. Histopathological cutaneous alterations in systemic sclerosis: a clinicopathological study. Arthritis Res Ther. 2011;13(1):R35.
27. Smith V, Van Praet JT, Vandooren B, Van der Cruyssen B, Naeyaert JM, Decuman S, et al. Rituximab in diffuse cutaneous systemic sclerosis: an open-label clinical and histopathological study. Ann Rheum Dis. 2010;69: 193–7.
28. Dobrota R, Maurer B, Graf N, Jordan S, Mihai C, Kowal-Bielecka O, et al. Prediction of improvement in skin fibrosis in diffuse cutaneous systemic sclerosis: a EUSTAR analysis. Ann Rheum Dis. 2016;75:1743–8.
29. Sulli A, Soldano S, Pizzorni C, Montagna P, Secchi ME, Villaggio B, et al. Raynaud's phenomenon and plasma endothelin: correlations with capillaroscopic patterns in systemic sclerosis. J Rheumatol. 2009;36:1235–9.
30. Scheja A, Wildt M, Wuttge DM, Hesselstrand R. Progressive capillary loss over a decade in patients with systemic sclerosis, in particular in patients with early digital ischaemic manifestations. Scand J Rheumatol. 2011;40: 457–61.
31. Pakozdi A, Nihtyanova S, Moinzadeh P, Ong VH, Black CM, Denton CP. Clinical and serological hallmarks of systemic sclerosis overlap syndromes. J Rheumatol. 2011;38:2406–9.
32. Hanitsch LG, Burmester GR, Witt C, Hunzelmann N, Genth E, Krieg T, et al. Skin sclerosis is only of limited value to identify Patients with SSc with severe manifestations-an analysis of a distinct patient subgroup of the German Systemic Sclerosis Network (DNSS) Register. Rheumatology. 2009; 48:70–3.
33. Vinet E, Bernatsky S, Hudson M, Pineau CA, Baron M, Canadian Scleroderma Research Group. Effect of menopause on the modified Rodnan skin score in systemic sclerosis. Arthritis Res Ther. 2014;16(3):R130.
34. Cutolo M, Sulli A. Therapy. Optimized treatment algorithms for digital vasculopathy in SSc. Nat Rev Rheumatol. 2015;11:569–71.

# Tie2 as a novel key factor of microangiopathy in systemic sclerosis

Falk Moritz[1,2], Janine Schniering[1], Jörg H. W. Distler[3], Renate E. Gay[1], Steffen Gay[1], Oliver Distler[1] and Britta Maurer[1*]

## Abstract

**Background:** The angiopoietin(Ang)/Tie2 system is a key regulator of vascular biology. The expression of membrane bound (mb) Tie2 and Ang-1 ensures vessel stability, whereas Ang-2, inducible by vascular endothelial growth factor (VEGF), hypoxia, and inflammation, acts as an antagonist. Tie2 signalling is also attenuated by soluble Tie2 (sTie2), the extracellular domain of the receptor, which is shed upon stimulation with VEGF. Herein, we investigate the role of Ang/Tie2 in the peripheral vasculopathy in systemic sclerosis (SSc) including animal models.

**Methods:** The expression of Ang-1/-2 and Tie2 in skin/serum of SSc patients was compared with healthy controls by immunohistochemistry (IHC)/ELISA. Expression of Ang/Tie2 was analysed in different animal models: VEGF transgenic (tg) mice, hypoxia model, bleomycin-induced skin fibrosis, and tight skin 1 (TSK1) mice.

**Results:** In SSc, dermal microvessels abundantly expressed Ang-2, but not Ang-1 compared with healthy controls. The percentage of mbTie2+ microvessels was profoundly decreased whereas the levels of sTie2 were increased already in early disease. Both in skin and sera of SSc patients, the Ang1/2 ratio was reduced, being lowest in patients with digital ulcers indicating vessel destabilizing conditions. We next studied potential influencing factors in animal models. The VEGF tg mouse model, the hypoxia, and the inflammation-dependent bleomycin model all showed a similar dysregulation of Ang/Tie2 as in SSc, which did not apply for the non-inflammatory TSK1 model.

**Conclusion:** Peripheral microvasculopathy in SSc results from a complex dysregulation of angiogenic signalling networks including the VEGF and the Ang/Tie2 system. The profoundly disturbed Ang-/Tie-2 balance might represent an important target for vascular therapeutic approaches in SSc.

**Keywords:** Microvasculopathy, Systemic sclerosis, Angiopoietins, Tie2

## Background

Microvascular injury due to dysregulation of angiogenic factors such as vascular endothelial growth factor (VEGF) and hypoxia [1–4] is a very early pathogenic event in systemic sclerosis (SSc) [5]. The Angiopoietin(Ang)/Tie2 system is a key regulator of angiogenesis. The binding of Ang-1, produced by vascular smooth muscle cells and other perivascular cells, to the membrane-bound (mb) Tie2 receptor on endothelial cells (EC) is crucial for vessel stability. Tie2 activation promotes vessel assembly and maturation by mediating survival signals for EC and regulating the recruitment of pericytes [6]. Ang-2, inducible

in EC by VEGF, hypoxia, and inflammation [6–8], antagonizes the Ang-1/Tie2 pathway by competing with Ang-1. Both ligands bind to Tie2 with similar affinity. Under physiologic conditions, the levels of Ang-1 exceed those of Ang-2, thereby ensuring the quiescent state of the vasculature. Increased levels of Ang-2 are associated with vascular remodelling [9]. Furthermore, the effects of Ang-2 are VEGF-dependent. In the absence of VEGF, Ang-2 has vessel destabilizing effects and induces regression of microvessels [10, 11]. In the presence of VEGF, Ang-2 induces angiogenesis with endothelial cell proliferation, migration and disruption of the vascular basement membrane due to the increased expression of matrix metalloproteinases [12]. Thus, the Ang-1/-2 ratio determines the functional status of the local vasculature. In contrast to mbTie2, little

* Correspondence: britta.maurer@usz.ch
[1]Department of Rheumatology, University Hospital Zurich, Gloriastrasse 25, 8091 Zurich, Switzerland
Full list of author information is available at the end of the article

is known about soluble Tie2 (sTie2), the extracellular domain of the Tie2 receptor, which is released by proteolytic cleavage by matrix metalloproteases upon stimulation with VEGF in a process also referred to as shedding [13, 14]. sTie2 is detectable in healthy individuals, and increased serum concentrations were measured in cardiovascular diseases, diabetic retinopathy [15], and SSc [16, 17].

Previous studies supported an equal affinity of Ang-1 and Ang-2 for the Tie2 receptor [10, 11, 13]. Interestingly, a recent study reported a higher affinity of Ang-1 to sTie2, which indicates that sTie2 might shift the Ang-1/Ang-2 ratio in favour of Ang-2 thereby inducing destabilization and regression of microvessels [18]. Other studies suggest competitive binding to mbTie2 thereby blocking access for Ang-1/-2 with inhibition of downstream signalling [6]. The scheme in Fig. 1 summarizes the current concept of the role of Ang/Tie2 in vascular remodelling.

In the present study, we assessed alterations of the Ang/Tie2 system in SSc-associated dermal microvasculopathy and in different animal models of SSc.

## Methods

### Patients

Serum samples were obtained from patients with limited cutaneous (lc) SSc (n = 21) and diffuse cutaneous (dc) SSc patients (n = 13) fulfilling the LeRoy criteria [19], patients with early SSc not yet fulfilling the LeRoy criteria (= pre-SSc) (n = 12), and from age- and sex-matched healthy donors (n = 40). The patients were 56.2 ± 11.6 years old, the majority was female (75%). The average disease duration was 6.3 ± 4.64 years. All patients had Raynaud's phenomenon, 68% had a history of digital ulcers, 37% had current digital ulcers, and 93% had teleangiectasias. The majority of patients were ANA positive (88.3%). A total of 39% were positive for anti-Scl-70, 44% for anti-centromere, and 2% for anti-

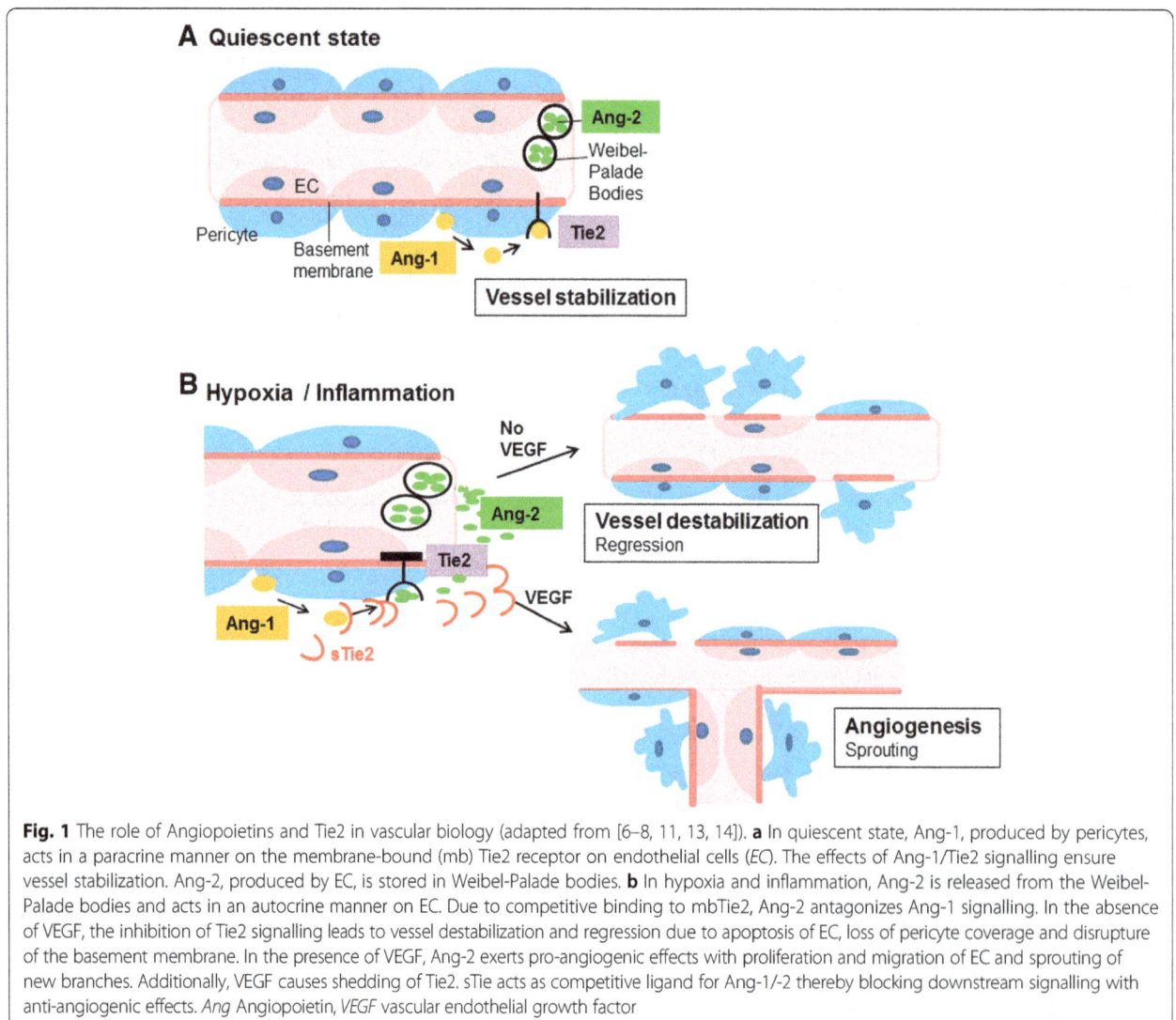

**Fig. 1** The role of Angiopoietins and Tie2 in vascular biology (adapted from [6–8, 11, 13, 14]). **a** In quiescent state, Ang-1, produced by pericytes, acts in a paracrine manner on the membrane-bound (mb) Tie2 receptor on endothelial cells (*EC*). The effects of Ang-1/Tie2 signalling ensure vessel stabilization. Ang-2, produced by EC, is stored in Weibel-Palade bodies. **b** In hypoxia and inflammation, Ang-2 is released from the Weibel-Palade bodies and acts in an autocrine manner on EC. Due to competitive binding to mbTie2, Ang-2 antagonizes Ang-1 signalling. In the absence of VEGF, the inhibition of Tie2 signalling leads to vessel destabilization and regression due to apoptosis of EC, loss of pericyte coverage and disrupture of the basement membrane. In the presence of VEGF, Ang-2 exerts pro-angiogenic effects with proliferation and migration of EC and sprouting of new branches. Additionally, VEGF causes shedding of Tie2. sTie acts as competitive ligand for Ang-1/-2 thereby blocking downstream signalling with anti-angiogenic effects. *Ang* Angiopoietin, *VEGF* vascular endothelial growth factor

RNA-polymerase III. The majority of patients had an active pattern in the nailfold capillaroscopy, whereas 33% showed a late, and 17% an early, pattern [20]. Skin biopsies were obtained by punch biopsies from involved skin at the forearms from 24 of the above mentioned SSc patients (13 lcSSc, 11 dcSSc) and from 19 of the above mentioned healthy controls. All participants had signed a consent form approved by the local institutional review boards. The study had been approved by the cantonal ethics committee Zurich.

## Animals

### VEGF tg mice

To investigate the effect of VEGF on Ang/Tie2, VEGF homo- (+/+) ($n = 8$) and heterozygous (+/−) ($n = 9$) transgenic (tg) mice and wildtype (wt) littermates ($n = 6/9$) were analysed. VEGF tg mice have been described previously [21]. Briefly, in VEGF tg mice, the murine VEGF164 gene which is the murine equivalent to VEGF-A165, was cloned into a human keratin 14 promoter expression cassette which had previously been shown to selectively target transgene expression to basal keratinocytes of the skin [21]. VEGF tg mice were on the FVB background.

### Hypoxia model

Four- to six-week-old female C57BL/6 mice (n = 3) were exposed to systemic normobaric hypoxia by substitution of oxygen with nitrogen in a closed Perspex chamber using a Digamix 2 M 302/a-F pump (H. Woesthoff GmbH, Bochum, Germany) at a flow rate of 37 l/min. When mice were placed into the chamber, $O_2$ fractions were decreased gradually from 21 to 6% within 1 h and mice were kept in the hypoxic chamber for additional 24 to 48 h. In parallel, nine littermates were kept under normoxic conditions. The experimental set-up was described previously [4].

### Bleomycin-induced skin fibrosis in mice

The bleomycin model is a frequently used model of chemically induced dermal fibrosis. The bleomycin-induced skin fibrosis in mice is considered as an animal model that mimics early, pro-inflammatory stages of skin fibrosis in SSc. Skin fibrosis was induced in 6- to 8-week-old C57/BL6 mice (n = 4) by local injections of bleomycin for 21 days as previously described [22]. Briefly, 100 μl of bleomycin dissolved in 0.9% sodium chloride (NaCl) at a concentration of 0.5 mg/ml was administered every other day by subcutaneous injections in defined areas of the upper back. Subcutaneous injections of 100 μl 0.9% NaCl were used in a second group (n = 4) as controls.

### TSK1 mice

Compared to the bleomycin model, tight skin 1 (TSK1) mice [23] are considered as a late-stage, non-inflammatory model of skin fibrosis in SSc. Due to a dominant mutation of the fibrillin 1 gene, TSK1 mice develop an increased dermal and especially hypodermal thickness. TSK1 mice were interbred with pa/pa mice in which a recessive mutation (pa) induces a light grey colour of the fur and pink eyes. Because the fibrillin 1 gene is genetically linked to the pa gene, mice can be screened for the tsk1 mutation based on the colour of eyes and fur. All mice with black fur and eyes carry the dominant tsk1 mutation and are heterozygous for the pa mutation. In contrast, mice with grey fur and pink eyes do not carry the tsk1 mutation, but are homozygous for the mutated pa gene. Apart from changing the skin colour, the pa mutation does not alter skin physiology and has no impact on skin fibrosis [23]. In the current experiments, four TSK1 and four pa/pa mice were analysed.

The animal protocols were approved by the cantonal veterinary office Zurich.

## Immunohistochemistry

Murine and human skin samples were fixed in 4% formalin and embedded into paraffin as described previously [24]. For immunohistochemistry, 5 μm thick sections of human and murine skin were used. Immunohistochemical double stainings were performed in sequential order. On the first day, after pre-treatment with citrate buffer, the slides were incubated with primary rabbit polyclonal von Willebrand Factor (vWF) antibody (Abcam, Cambridge, UK) at room temperature for 1 h, followed by incubation with biotin-labelled secondary goat anti-rabbit antibody (Jackson ImmunoResearch, Soham, UK). Staining was visualized with ABC phosphatase kit (Vector Laboratories, Burlingame, CA, USA) and developed using Vector blue. After additional heat-mediated treatment with citrate buffer, sections were incubated with primary rabbit polyclonal Ang-1 or Ang-2 antibodies (Abcam) overnight at 4 °C, followed by incubation with biotin-labelled secondary goat anti-rabbit antibodies (Jackson ImmunoResearch). Stainings were visualized using an ABC peroxidase kit and developed using DAB (Vector Laboratories). The sequential staining with Tie2 was performed similarly with the exception that no additional heat-mediated removal was required on the second day since the primary Tie2 antibody was mouse monoclonal (Abcam). Isotype-matched IgGs were used as negative controls.

## Analysis of skin sections

The analyses of all immunohistochemical stainings were performed by two independent examiners who were blinded with regard to the different groups. All slides were analysed twice by each examiner. In case of a variation of the results >10%, the respective slides were re-assessed to reach consensus. Pictures were taken with a slide scanner (Zeiss Axio Scan.Z1), using Zen lite software (blue edition 2.3) (Carl Zeiss Microscopy GmbH, Jena, Germany).

For the semi-quantitative analysis of microvessel density, pictures of five randomly chosen high power fields (HPF)/slide were taken. Then, vWF+ blood vessels (dermal microvessels) were counted. Either the ratio or the percentage of Ang-1+, Ang-2+, or Tie2+ blood vessels was determined by assessing their numbers referred to the total number of vWF+ microvessels/HPF using the respective double stainings. Blood vessel density was assessed in the dermis without the epidermal and the subdermal layers, except for the TSK1 mice in which the hypodermis was analysed. The number/percentage of microvessels was then calculated for each group using GraphPad Prism software (GraphPad Software Inc., San Diego, CA, USA).

### ELISA
Serum concentrations of Ang-1/-2 and sTie2 were measured using the colorimetric sandwich ELISA technique (Quantikine; R&D Systems, Abingdon, UK).

### Real-time PCR
Biopsy specimens (0.5 cm2) were homogenized with TissueLyser (Qiagen, Basel, Switzerland). Total RNA was isolated using the RNeasy Mini Kit (Qiagen, Hombrechtikon, Switzerland) and reverse transcribed into complementary DNA (cDNA) with random hexamers [25]. Expression of murine Ang-1, Ang-2, TEK (= Tie), and 18S rNA was measured using TaqMan Gene Expression Assays (Applied Biosystems, Basel, Switzerland). qPCR was performed using a 7500 Real-Time PCR System (Applied Biosystems). All qPCR experiments were performed in duplicate.

### Cell culture, reagents, stimulation assay, and analysis
Human dermal microvascular endothelial cells (HMVEC-d adult, Cambrex, Rockland, ME, USA) were cultured in six-well plates in endothelial cell medium (EGM-2 MV, Lonza, Basel, Switzerland), and passages 3–8 were used for analysis. After 24 h of serum reduction, HMVECs were stimulated for 12, 24, and 48 h with recombinant VEGF-A165 (R&D Systems) at concentrations of 2.5, 5, and 10 ng/ml. Controls were exposed to equivalent dosages of the carrier protein BSA [26]. sTie was measured by ELISA as described above in cell culture supernatants. The percentage of Tie2+ cells was evaluated using flow cytometry analysis (FACS) according to the instructions of the manufacturer. Briefly, HMVECs were washed with PBS, detached with trypsin/0.5% EDTA and centrifuged at $200 \times g$ for 5 min. Afterwards cell pellets were

resuspended and incubated for 15 min at room temperature with the primary Tie2 antibody. Isotype-matched IgGs were used as negative controls. The analysis was performed using the FACScan flow cytometer (Becton Dickinson, Mansfield, MA, USA). Data were analysed with CellQuest software (Becton Dickinson Immunocytometry Systems, San Jose, CA, USA).

### Statistical analysis
For statistical analysis, GraphPad Prism software (version 5.01) was employed (GraphPad Software Inc.). Normal distribution of data was examined using the Kolmogorov-Smirnov test. For parametric non-related data, expressed as mean ± standard error of the mean (SEM), the unpaired two-tailed $t$ test was used. Nonparametric non-related data, expressed as median$_{(Q1, Q3)}$ were analysed employing the Mann-Whitney $U$ test. $P$ values less than 0.05 were considered statistically significant.

Information on the histology and assessment of skin fibrosis in the bleomycin model and the measurement of collagen contents by hydroxyproline assay is provided in Additional file 1 supplemental methods.

## Results
### Dysregulation of the Ang/Tie2 system in the dermal microvasculopathy in SSc
In skin biopsies of SSc patients, the microvascular density was generally reduced compared with healthy controls (ratio of vWF+ vessels/HPF 27.3$_{(24,38)}$ vs. 45.5$_{(31,60)}$; $p = 0.001$; Fig. 2a, b). Dermal capillaries of SSc patients expressed Ang-2 more abundantly than healthy controls (Fig. 2a, b) (ratio of Ang-2+/vWF+ microvessels/HPF 1.7$_{(1.3,2.5)}$ vs. 1.1$_{(0.8,1.3)}$; $p = 0.01$). Most impressively, the percentage of mbTie2-positive microvessels was strongly and consistently decreased in the skin of SSc patients compared with healthy controls (median$_{(quartile range)}$ 3.8$_{(1,6)}$% vs. 87$_{(78,99)}$%; $p < 0.001$) (Fig. 2a, b). The expression of Ang-1 did not differ in dermal capillaries of SSc patients compared with healthy controls (Fig. 2a). In the analysed sections, no difference in the expression of Ang-1/-2 or Tie2 could be observed between lcSSc or dcSSc. Furthermore, to evaluate whether the changes on tissue level were reflected on systemic level, we additionally measured the serum levels of Ang-1, Ang-2, and sTie2. To evaluate whether the loss of mbTie2 in dermal microvessels might be due to shedding [13], we assessed the serum levels of sTie2, which is the soluble, cleaved, extracellular domain of the Tie2 receptor. Indeed, sTie2 levels of SSc patients were higher than those of healthy controls (mean ± SEM 9.6 ± 1.7 ng/ml) without differences between the lcSSc or dcSSc subsets (16.7 ± 7.5, 13.6 ± 1.7 ng/ml; $p < 0.01$) (Fig. 3a). In accordance with the shedding hypothesis, treatment of human dermal microvascular endothelial cells (HMVECs)

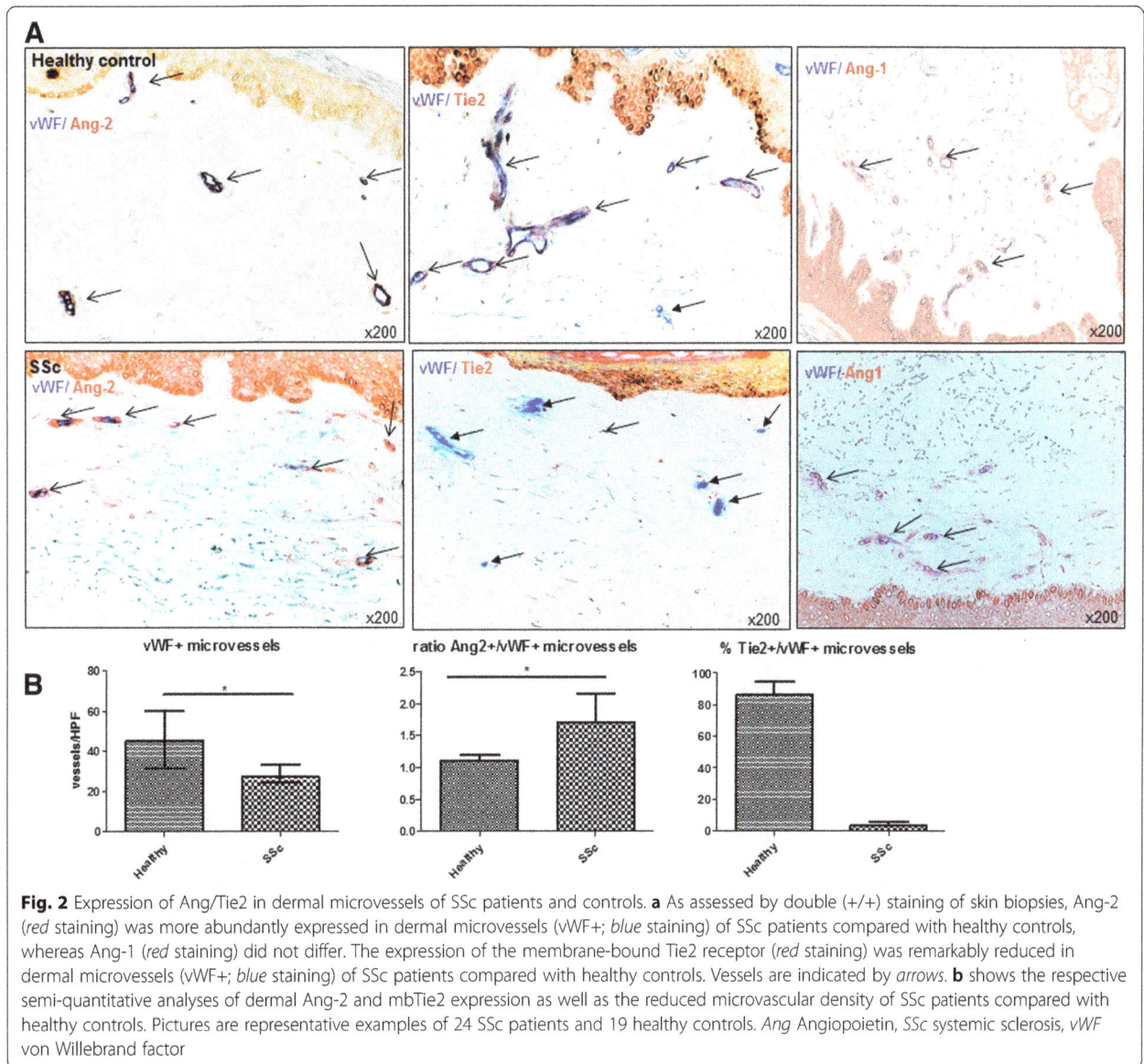

**Fig. 2** Expression of Ang/Tie2 in dermal microvessels of SSc patients and controls. **a** As assessed by double (+/+) staining of skin biopsies, Ang-2 (*red* staining) was more abundantly expressed in dermal microvessels (vWF+; *blue* staining) of SSc patients compared with healthy controls, whereas Ang-1 (*red* staining) did not differ. The expression of the membrane-bound Tie2 receptor (*red* staining) was remarkably reduced in dermal microvessels (vWF+; *blue* staining) of SSc patients compared with healthy controls. Vessels are indicated by *arrows*. **b** shows the respective semi-quantitative analyses of dermal Ang-2 and mbTie2 expression as well as the reduced microvascular density of SSc patients compared with healthy controls. Pictures are representative examples of 24 SSc patients and 19 healthy controls. *Ang* Angiopoietin, *SSc* systemic sclerosis, *vWF* von Willebrand factor

with increasing dosages of VEGF for 12 h reduced the numbers of Tie2-positive cells by 9.6, 20.2, and 25.1% whereas in parallel there was an increase of the sTie2 concentration in the supernatants by 47 to 57% (Fig. 3b). Serum Ang-2 levels were increased in both lcSS and dcSSc patients as compared with healthy controls ($1.4 \pm 0.2$ and $1.5 \pm 0.3$ vs. $0.3 \pm 0.02$ ng/ml; $p < 0.01$) whereas the Ang-1 levels where remarkably lower ($18.4 \pm 5.7$ and $32.9 \pm 10.3$ vs. $68.4 \pm 5.4$ ng/ml; $p < 0.01$) (Fig. 3a). Irrespective of the cutaneous subtype, in the whole group of SSc patients with established disease, the serum levels of Ang-1 ($23.9 \pm 5.3$), Ang-2 ($1.5 \pm 0.2$), and sTie2 ($17.9 \pm 1.1$) differed significantly from healthy controls ($p < 0.001$, respectively). The imbalance towards Ang-2 in patients with lcSSc and dcSSc resulted in a strongly reduced Ang-1/-2 ratio as compared with healthy controls (13:1 and 23:1 vs. 221:1,

respectively; $p < 0.05$. Interestingly, SSc patients with digital ulcers had a significantly lower Ang-1/Ang-2 ratio as compared with those without ($2.4_{(2,3)}$ vs. $7.2_{(7,9)}$; $p < 0.02$). In contrast, patients with teleangiectasias had a significantly higher Ang-1/Ang-2 ratio ($1.9 \pm 0.4$ vs. $1.3 \pm 0.08$; $p < 0.05$) than those without. Most importantly, in patients with pre-SSc, serum levels of Ang-1/-2 already differed significantly from healthy controls ($35.5 \pm 8.8$ vs. $68.4 \pm 5.4$ ng/ml and $0.9 \pm 0.2$ vs. $0.3 \pm 0.02$ ng/ml; $p < 0.02$) (Fig. 3a). Serum levels of sTie2 were as high as in patients with established disease and thus remarkably elevated compared with healthy controls ($14.4 \pm 1.9$ vs. $9.6 \pm 1.8$ ng/ml; $p = 0.01$) (Fig. 3a). Of note, in line with previous results [2, 3], pre-SSc patients also had significantly elevated serum VEGF levels compared with healthy controls ($481_{(120,559)}$ vs. $101_{(10,169)}$; $p = 0.01$), which were as high as

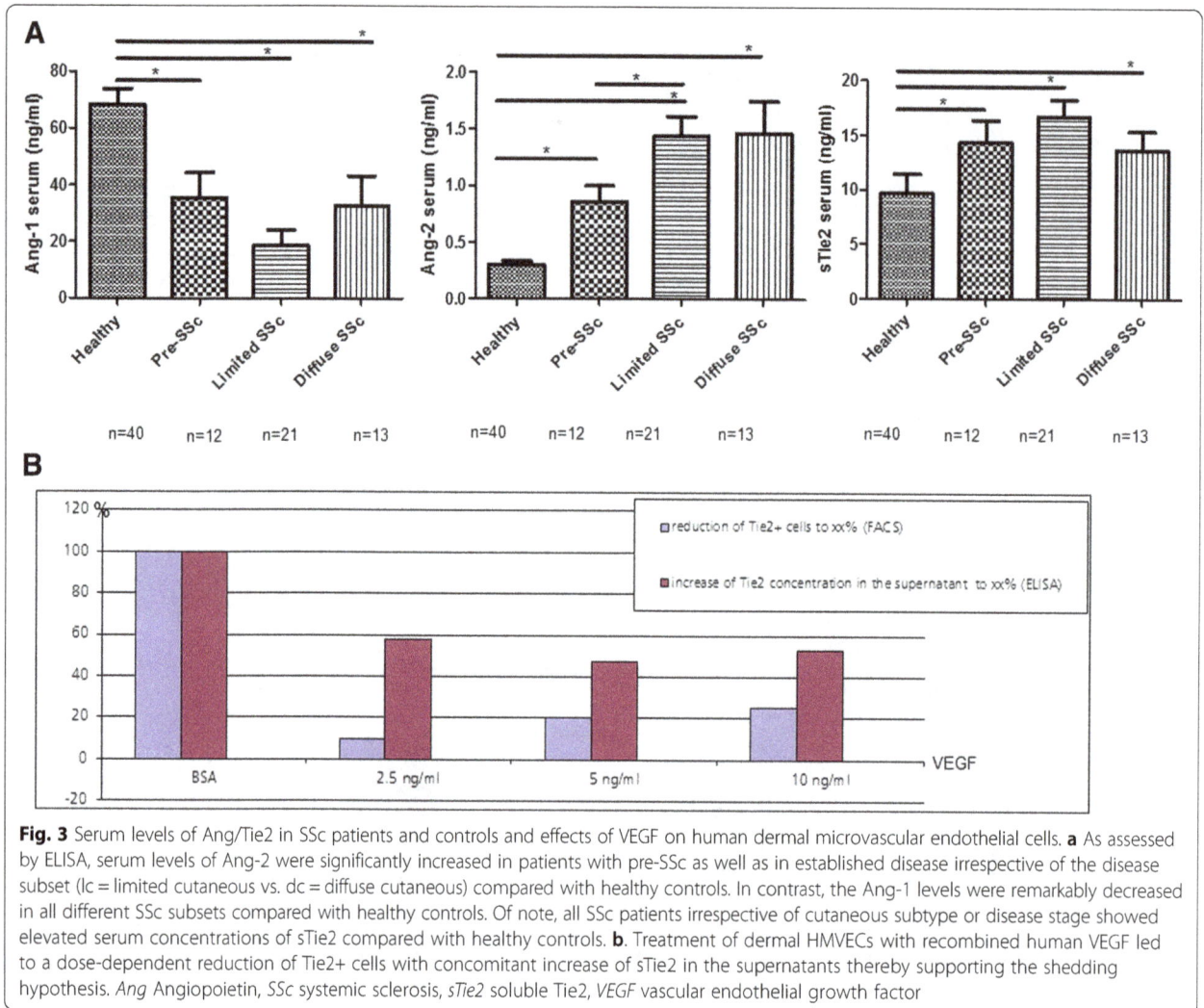

**Fig. 3** Serum levels of Ang/Tie2 in SSc patients and controls and effects of VEGF on human dermal microvascular endothelial cells. **a** As assessed by ELISA, serum levels of Ang-2 were significantly increased in patients with pre-SSc as well as in established disease irrespective of the disease subset (lc = limited cutaneous vs. dc = diffuse cutaneous) compared with healthy controls. In contrast, the Ang-1 levels were remarkably decreased in all different SSc subsets compared with healthy controls. Of note, all SSc patients irrespective of cutaneous subtype or disease stage showed elevated serum concentrations of sTie2 compared with healthy controls. **b**. Treatment of dermal HMVECs with recombined human VEGF led to a dose-dependent reduction of Tie2+ cells with concomitant increase of sTie2 in the supernatants thereby supporting the shedding hypothesis. *Ang* Angiopoietin, *SSc* systemic sclerosis, *sTie2* soluble Tie2, *VEGF* vascular endothelial growth factor

in patients with established disease (lcSSc $412_{(250,609)}$ and dcSSc $634_{(404,941)}$ pg/ml).

In summary, we observed a severe disturbance in the expression of Ang-1 and Ang-2 as well as of Tie2 in the skin and sera of patients SSc.

### Potential influences on the Ang/Tie2 expression in vivo

To assess which pathogenic factors in SSc might affect the expression of Ang/Tie2, we evaluated pathophysiologically different animal models of SSc. First, we studied the Ang/Tie2 system in a vascular model of SSc, using the VEGF tg mice since VEGF plays a key role in SSc-associated microvasculopathy and has been suggested to strongly influence the effects of Ang/Tie2 on vascular remodelling [6, 13] (Fig. 1). As previously shown, VEGF tg mice develop a proliferative vasculopathy with tortuous and dilated capillaries with increased vessel wall thickness reminiscent of both the capillary changes observed in SSc [1] and in Ang-2-overexpressing mice [11]. In VEGF+/+ tg mice as compared with VEGF+/- tg

mice, chronically high levels of VEGF dampen the proangiogenic effects of VEGF [1], which is similarly observed in SSc patients with a chronically elevated VEGF levels and insufficient angiogenesis [2, 3].

In VEGF-+/- and VEGF+/+ tg mice, a higher proportion of dermal microvessels (vWF+) expressed Ang-2 compared with wt mice (% of Ang-2+/vWF+ microvessels/HPF $100_{(78,100)}$ and $100_{(100,100)}$ vs. $36.7_{(0,57)}$; $p = 0.004$, $p = 0.0003$) (Fig. 4a), whereas Ang-1 was reduced (% of Ang-1+/vWF+ microvessels/HPF $0_{(0,50)}$ and $20_{(0,50)}$ vs. $75_{(66.7,75)}$; $p = 0.04$, $p = 0.05$) (Fig. 4b). Of note, expression of mbTie2 was remarkably reduced in the dermal capillaries (vWF+) of both VEGF+/- and VEGF+/+ tg mice as compared with controls (% of Tie2+/vWF+ microvessels/HPF $50_{(25,100)}$ and $16.7_{(0,50)}$ vs. $100_{(88.3,100)}$; $p = 0.03$, $p = 0.0006$) (Fig. 4c). These observations are in line with previous data showing that VEGF tips the balance towards Ang-2 and decreases the local expression of mbTie2 [27]. Furthermore, the decreased Ang-1/-2 ratio with a strong concomitant loss of

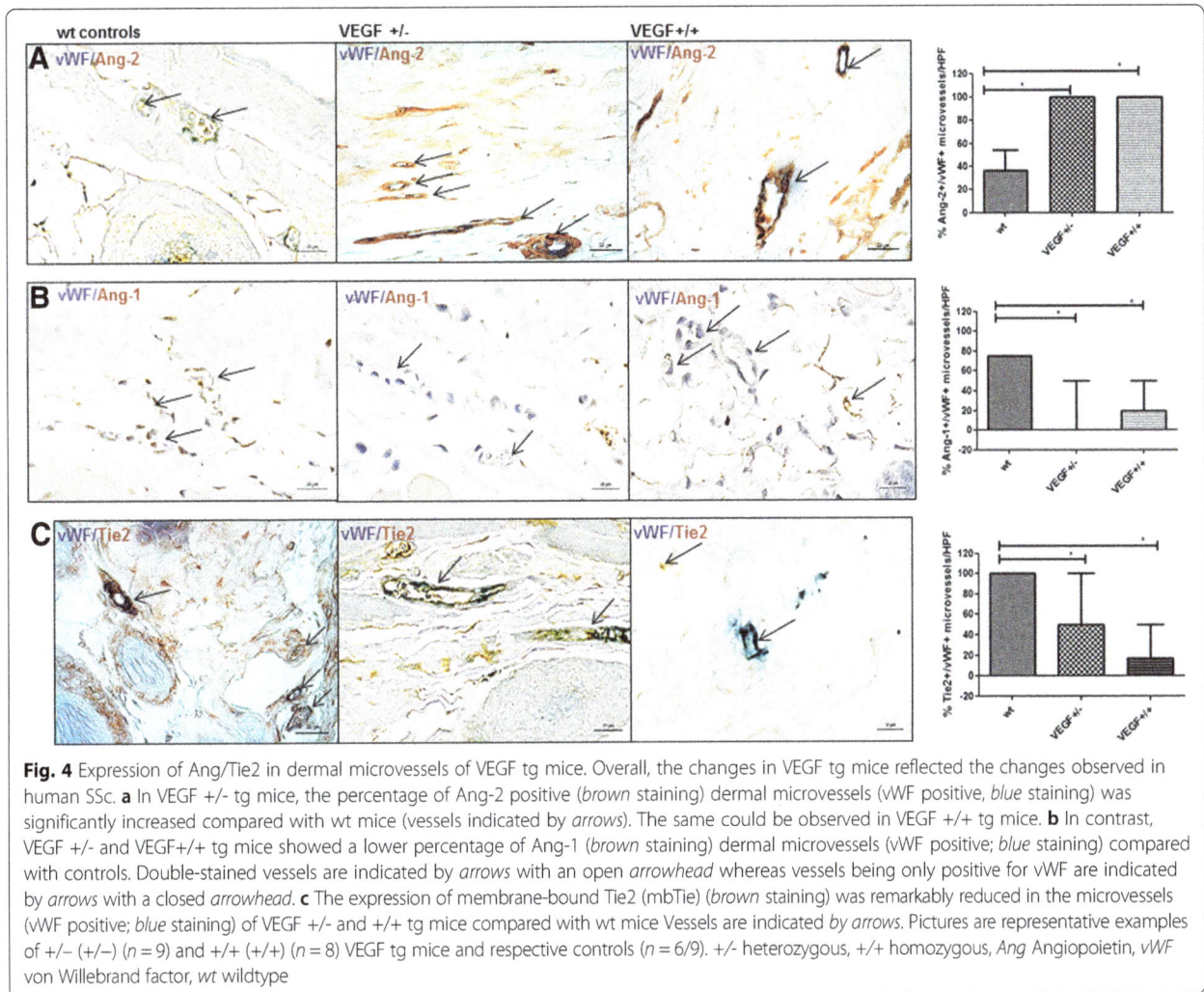

**Fig. 4** Expression of Ang/Tie2 in dermal microvessels of VEGF tg mice. Overall, the changes in VEGF tg mice reflected the changes observed in human SSc. **a** In VEGF +/- tg mice, the percentage of Ang-2 positive (*brown* staining) dermal microvessels (vWF positive, *blue* staining) was significantly increased compared with wt mice (vessels indicated by *arrows*). The same could be observed in VEGF +/+ tg mice. **b** In contrast, VEGF +/- and VEGF+/+ tg mice showed a lower percentage of Ang-1 (*brown* staining) dermal microvessels (vWF positive; *blue* staining) compared with controls. Double-stained vessels are indicated by *arrows* with an open *arrowhead* whereas vessels being only positive for vWF are indicated by *arrows* with a closed *arrowhead*. **c** The expression of membrane-bound Tie2 (mbTie) (*brown* staining) was remarkably reduced in the microvessels (vWF positive; *blue* staining) of VEGF +/- and +/+ tg mice compared with wt mice Vessels are indicated *by arrows*. Pictures are representative examples of +/- (+/−) (*n* = 9) and +/+ (+/+) (*n* = 8) VEGF tg mice and respective controls (*n* = 6/9). +/- heterozygous, +/+ homozygous, *Ang* Angiopoietin, *vWF* von Willebrand factor, *wt* wildtype

mbTie2 in chronic VEGF exposure in vivo mirrored the observed changes in SSc (Fig. 2).

Tissue hypoxia is a known phenomenon in SSc [2, 4]. To evaluate whether hypoxia might contribute to the dysbalance of the Ang/Tie2 system in SSc, we analysed the tissue expression in hypoxic compared to normoxic mice. Whereas the expression of Ang-1 mRNA did not change, Ang-2 and Tie2 mRNA transcripts increased on the tissue level in hypoxia ($2.4 \pm 0.4$-fold; $p = 0.027$ and $2.6 \pm 0.8$-fold; $p = 0.042$) compared to normoxia (Additional file 2). Our data are in accordance with previous studies showing that hypoxia increases the expression of Ang-2 [6]. Since Ang-2 blocks Tie2 signalling, this ultimately leads to vessel destabilization and regression [6].

Since inflammation is another characteristic pathogenic feature in early stages of SSc, we next assessed the expression levels of Ang/Tie2 in the model of bleomycin-induced skin fibrosis [28] since it mimics early, inflammatory stages of SSc [29]. Treatment with bleomycin resulted in significant skin fibrosis as measured by increase in dermal thickness (mean $\pm$ SEM $1.5 \pm 0.05$-fold) and hydroxyproline contents ($1.6 \pm 0.1$-fold; $p < 0.05$ each) (Additional file 3). Interestingly, there was a trend towards a higher percentage of Ang-2+ dermal microvessels (vWF+) in bleomycin-challenged mice vs. saline-treated controls (% of Ang-2+/vWF+ microvessels/HPF $95.8 \pm 2.7$ vs. $65 \pm 15$; $p = 0.08$) (Fig. 5a). No differences were observed for the expression of Ang-1 in controls and bleomycin-treated mice (% of Ang-1+/vWF+ microvessels/HPF $66.7_{(66.7,75)}$ vs. $100_{(66.7,100)}$; $p = 0.3$) (Fig. 5b). The expression of mbTie2 in dermal capillaries (vWF+) was lower in bleomycin-treated mice vs. saline-treated controls (% of Tie2+/vWF+ microvessels/HPF $50_{(33,75)}$ vs. $100_{(94,100)}$; $p = 0.002$) (Fig. 5c). These observations are in line with recent data giving evidence of that in inflammatory conditions, the expression of Ang-2 is increased whereas the expression of mbTie2 is decreased [7].

Finally, we investigated the dermal expression of Ang/Tie2 in an inflammation-independent, late-stage model

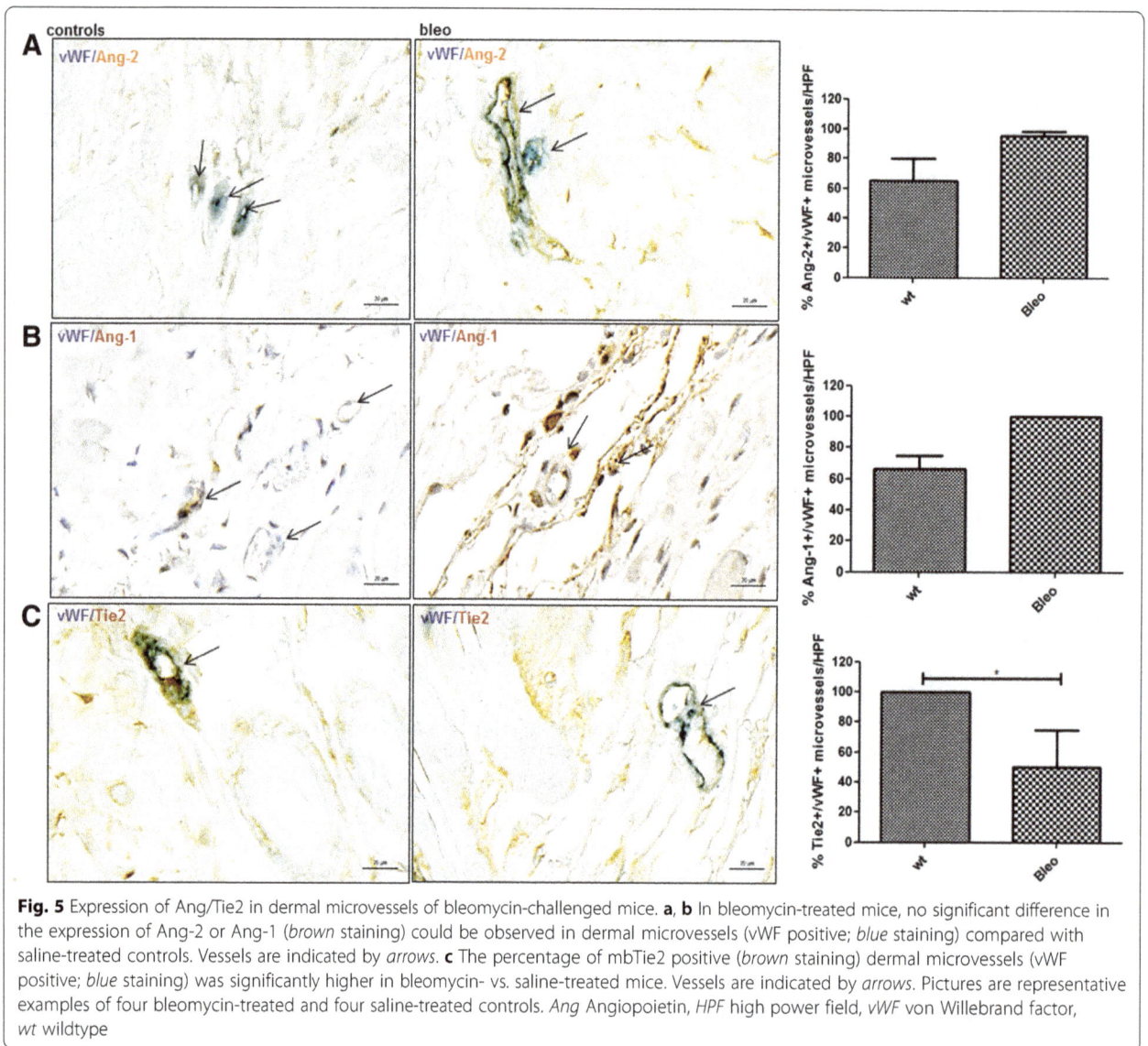

**Fig. 5** Expression of Ang/Tie2 in dermal microvessels of bleomycin-challenged mice. **a, b** In bleomycin-treated mice, no significant difference in the expression of Ang-2 or Ang-1 (*brown* staining) could be observed in dermal microvessels (vWF positive; *blue* staining) compared with saline-treated controls. Vessels are indicated by *arrows*. **c** The percentage of mbTie2 positive (*brown* staining) dermal microvessels (vWF positive; *blue* staining) was significantly higher in bleomycin- vs. saline-treated mice. Vessels are indicated by *arrows*. Pictures are representative examples of four bleomycin-treated and four saline-treated controls. *Ang* Angiopoietin, *HPF* high power field, *vWF* von Willebrand factor, *wt* wildtype

of SSc, the TSK1 model [30]. In TSK1 mice, the expression of Ang-2 in capillaries (vWF+) was not changed compared with pa/pa controls ($100_{(50,100)}$ vs. $100_{(88,100)}$; $p = 0.9$) (Fig. 6a). No statistically significant difference was observed in TSK1 mice vs. pa/pa controls neither for Ang-1 (% of Ang-1+/vWF+ microvessels/HPF $0_{(0,25)}$ vs.$25_{(0,75)}$; $p = 0.2$) nor for mbTie2 (% of Tie2+/vWF+ microvessels/HPF $58.4_{(13,67)}$ vs. $100_{(0,100)}$, $p = 0.2$) (Fig. 6b, c) although there was a tendency to a reduction of Tie2 + microvessels in TSK1 mice.

## Discussion

In SSc, peripheral microvasculopathy is a key pathogenic event. Our results suggest that a dysbalance of Ang/Tie2 might contribute to the vascular changes. An excess of Ang-1 – as herein observed on tissue and serum level – is known to induce vascular remodelling

by blocking Tie2 signalling on EC [6, 10, 11] (Fig. 1). Interestingly, SSc patients with digital ulcers showed a significantly lower Ang-1/-2 ratio as compared with those without, which further underlines the potential clinical relevance of the observed alterations although the low number of patients and the heterogeneity of the disease warrant some caution in the interpretation of these results. Depending on the absence/presence of VEGF [6, 13], the destabilization of vessels might then lead to regression or (disorganized) sprouting (Fig. 1), both well-described events in SSc microvasculopathy. Moreover, the substantial loss of mbTie2 on dermal microvessels in SSc with concomitant increase in sTie2, which also competes with Ang-1, further impairs Tie2 signalling (Fig. 1). Notably, treatment of dermal HMVECs with VEGF led to a dose-dependent reduction of Tie2+ cells with concomitant increase of sTie2 in

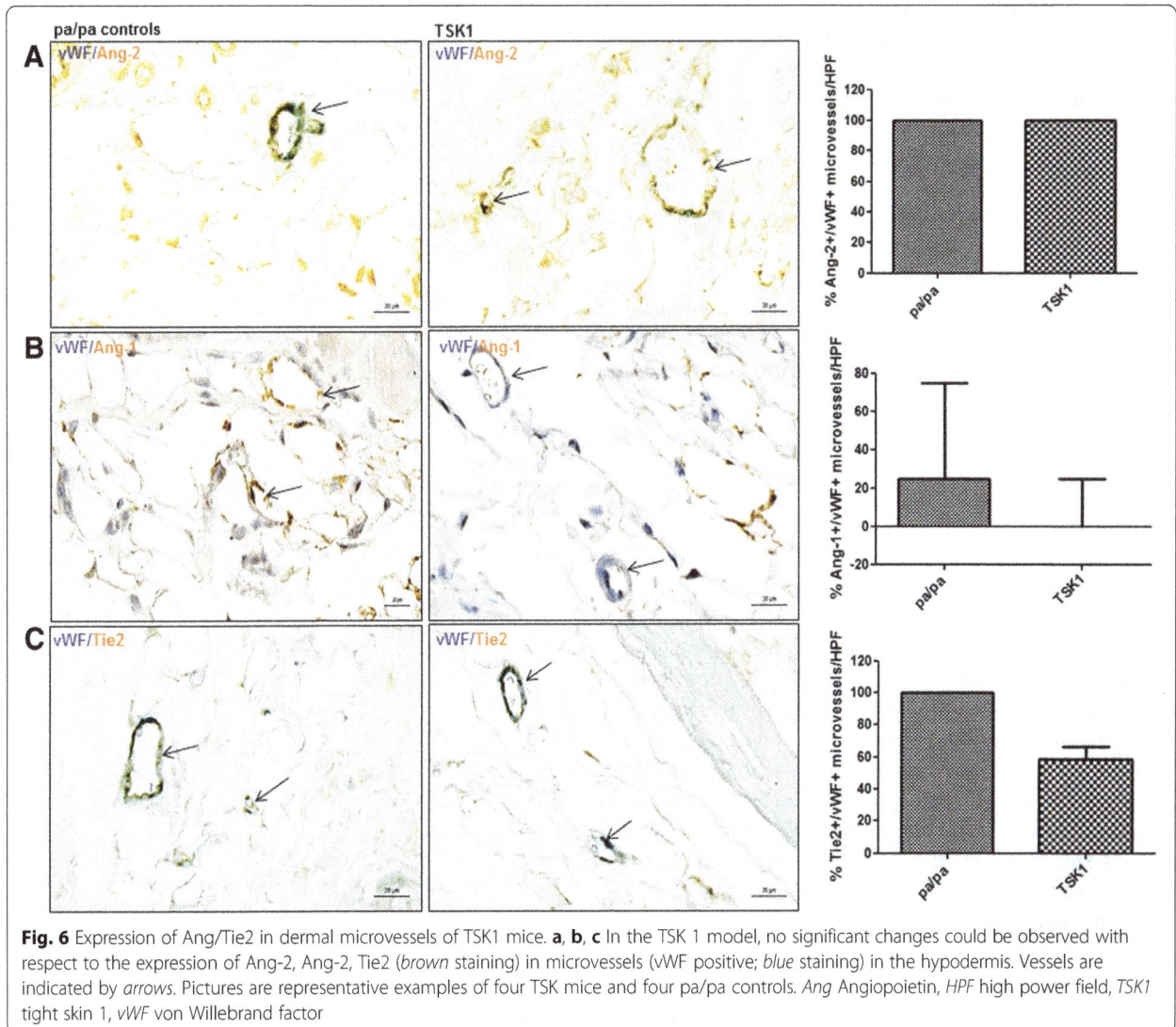

**Fig. 6** Expression of Ang/Tie2 in dermal microvessels of TSK1 mice. **a**, **b**, **c** In the TSK 1 model, no significant changes could be observed with respect to the expression of Ang-2, Ang-2, Tie2 (*brown* staining) in microvessels (vWF positive; *blue* staining) in the hypodermis. Vessels are indicated by *arrows*. Pictures are representative examples of four TSK mice and four pa/pa controls. *Ang* Angiopoietin, *HPF* high power field, *TSK1* tight skin 1, *vWF* von Willebrand factor

the supernatants thereby supporting the shedding hypothesis. Interestingly, a similar dysbalance of Ang-1/-2, sTie2, and VEGF levels was already observed in pre-SSc patients as in patients with established disease indicating that the disturbance of angiogenic signalling networks is an early pathogenic event.

Our data on the expression of angiopoietins and Tie2 in dermal microvessels of SSc patients extend previous, partially conflicting results on the systemic levels of Ang-1/-2 and sTie2 in SSc. Interestingly, all available studies [16, 31–33] as well as our own data found increased systemic levels of Ang-2 without differences regarding lcSSc or dcSSc subtypes [32, 33]. Data on Ang-1 are more ambiguous. Whereas Michalska et al. reported a similar reduction of Ang-1 levels and the Ang-1/Ang-2 ratio in SSc [16], the study by Dunne et al. showed an increase of Ang-1 in the dcSSc subset, but not the combined SSc group as compared with healthy

controls [32]. However, apart from discrepancies that might arise from studying such a heterogeneous disease, these differences might also be attributed to the use of plasma [32] instead of serum. Similar to our observations, the serum levels of sTie2 were found to be elevated by Noda et al [17] and Dunne et al. [32], however, the latter study only demonstrating significant differences in the lcSSc subgroup. The study by Gerlicz et al. showed a trend towards higher levels of sTie2 in both SSc subsets compared with healthy controls, yet the data were not statistically significant [33]. But again, all these studies including our own have only analysed very limited numbers of patients. Therefore, the observed changes of serum/plasma angiopoietin and sTie2 levels in SSc and particularly their correlation with clinical (vascular) features warrant a standardized and systematic evaluation in a large, multicentre cohort. Apart from the fact that in most published studies not all three parameters (Ang-1, Ang-2, sTie2) have been simultaneously analysed, some of the current discrepancies of the association with clinical vascular features might arise from differences such as treatment (vasodilating agents, immunosuppressive drugs), the definitions of ulcers and nailfold capillaroscopy patterns used, but also biobank-related issues such as different processing and/or storage of blood samples and use of different ELISA assays. Thus, although the current available data support a dysbalance of the Ang/Tie2 system in SSc, the clinical implications have yet to be elucidated including the performance of more detailed functional in vitro experiments.

Our in vivo data derived from the different animal models, which closely mirrored the changes observed in SSc patients, suggested that VEGF, hypoxia, and inflammation might play a role in the dysbalance of the Ang/Tie2 system in SSc.

## Conclusions

Thus, our data extend the previous concept of peripheral microangiopathy in SSc [1–4, 34] giving novel evidence on tissue level of an even more complex dysregulation of angiogenic key players. The dysregulation of the Ang/Tie-2 system appears to be specific for vascular and inflammatory conditions, as the non-vascular and inflammation-independent TSK1 model did not reflect the changes observed in the human disease. This further underlines that for proof of concept studies the appropriate choice of an animal model that closely reflects the situation of the human disease, is of outmost importance [35]. However, for the development of targeted treatment strategies those interactions and their biologic relevance will first have to be carefully and thoroughly studied in suitable preclinical settings including detailed functional experiments and specific animal models.

## Additional files

**Additional file 1:** Supplemental methods (DOC 43 kb)

**Additional file 2: Figure S1.** Induction of skin fibrosis in the murine bleomycin skin model. (A) shows the increase in dermal thickness upon bleomycin treatment (HE staining) whereas (B) depicts the increased deposition of extracellular matrix proteins (Sirius Red staining). (C) and (D) show the semi-quantitative analysis of dermal thickness measurements and of hydroxyproline contents. Pictures are representative examples of four bleomycin-treated and four saline-treated controls. (TIF 71 kb)

**Additional file 3: Figure S2.** Changes of the expression of angiopoietins and Tie2 in chronic hypoxia in vivo. (A) shows no effect of hypoxia on the levels of Ang-1 mRNA, whereas Ang-2 (B) and Tie2 mRNA transcripts (C) increased compared to normoxia. RNA from three mice kept in hypoxia and nine mice kept in normoxia were analysed by qRT-PCR. (TIF 371 kb)

## Abbreviations
+/-: Heterozygous; +/+: Homozygous; Ang: Angiopoietin; dc: Diffuse cutaneous; EC: Endothelial cells; HMVEC: Human microvascular endothelial cell; HPF: High power field; IHC: Immunohistochemistry; lc: Limited cutaneous; mb: Membrane bound; SEM: Standard error of the mean; SSc: Systemic sclerosis; sTie2: Soluble Tie2; tg: Transgenic; TSK1: Tight skin 1; VEGF: Vascular endothelial growth factor; vWF: von Willebrand factor; wt: Wildtype

## Acknowledgements
The authors thank Maria Comazzi for the excellent technical support. Imaging was performed with a slide scanner (Zeiss Axio Scan.Z1, software: Zen lite, blue edition 2.3) provided and maintained by the Center for Microscopy and Image Analysis, University of Zurich.

## Authors' contributions
FM has made substantial contributions to the conception of the study and the acquisition, analysis and the interpretation of data and was involved in drafting the manuscript. JS was centrally involved in the acquisition and analysis of data and in revising the manuscript. JHWD, RG, and SG made contributions to the conception and design of the study, in the interpretation of the data and the revision of the manuscript. OD was involved in the conception and design of the study, the interpretation of data and in drafting and revising the manuscript. BM made substantial contributions to conception and design of the study, was centrally involved in the acquisition, analysis and interpretation of data, and in drafting and revising the manuscript. All authors have given final approval of the version to be published.

## Competing interests
FM had Articulum Fellowship program (Pfizer), congress funding from Roche, Lilly, Medac
JHWD has consultancy relationships and/or has received research funding from Actelion, Anamar, BMS, Celgene, Bayer Pharma, Boehringer Ingelheim, JB Therapeutics, Sanofi-Aventis, Novartis, UCB, GSK, Array Biopharma and Active Biotech in the area of potential treatments of SSc and is stock owner of 4D Science. OD had a consultancy relationship and/or has received research funding from 4 D Science, Actelion, Active Biotec, Chemom AG, Bayer, Biogenldec, BMS, Boehringer Ingelheim, ChemomAb, EpiPharm, espeRare foundation, Genentech/Roche, GSK, Inventiva, Lilly, medac, MedImmune, Pharmacyclics, Pfizer, Sanofi, Serodapharm, and Sinoxa in the area of potential treatments of scleroderma and its complications. In addition, Patent licensed: mir-29 for the treatment of systemic sclerosis. Speaker's fees from AbbVie, iQone Healthcare, and Mepha.
BM had grant/research support from AbbVie, Protagen, EMDO, Novartis, congress support from Pfizer, Roche, and Actelion. Patent licensed: mir-29 for the treatment of systemic sclerosis.
All others were supported by their respective institutions.

## Author details
[1]Department of Rheumatology, University Hospital Zurich, Gloriastrasse 25, 8091 Zurich, Switzerland. [2]Department of Oncology, St. Georg Hospital, Leipzig, Germany. [3]Department of Internal Medicine 3, University Hospital, Erlangen, Germany.

## References
1. Maurer B, Distler A, Suliman YA, Gay RE, Michel BA, Gay S, Distler JH, Distler O. Vascular endothelial growth factor aggravates fibrosis and vasculopathy in experimental models of systemic sclerosis. Ann Rheum Dis. 2014;73(10):1880–7.
2. Distler O, Distler JH, Scheid A, Acker T, Hirth A, Rethage J, Michel BA, Gay RE, Muller-Ladner U, Matucci-Cerinic M, et al. Uncontrolled expression of vascular endothelial growth factor and its receptors leads to insufficient skin angiogenesis in patients with systemic sclerosis. Circ Res. 2004;95(1):109–16.
3. Distler O, Del Rosso A, Giacomelli R, Cipriani P, Conforti ML, Guiducci S, Gay RE, Michel BA, Bruhlmann P, Muller-Ladner U, et al. Angiogenic and angiostatic factors in systemic sclerosis: increased levels of vascular endothelial growth factor are a feature of the earliest disease stages and are associated with the absence of fingertip ulcers. Arthritis Res. 2002;4(6):R11.

4. Distler JH, Jungel A, Pileckyte M, Zwerina J, Michel BA, Gay RE, Kowal-Bielecka O, Matucci-Cerinic M, Schett G, Marti HH, et al. Hypoxia-induced increase in the production of extracellular matrix proteins in systemic sclerosis. Arthritis Rheum. 2007;56(12):4203–15.

5. Distler JH, Gay S, Distler O. Angiogenesis and vasculogenesis in systemic sclerosis. Rheumatology. 2006;45 Suppl 3:iii26–27.

6. Thomas M, Augustin HG. The role of the Angiopoietins in vascular morphogenesis. Angiogenesis. 2009;12(2):125–37.

7. Milam KE, Parikh SM. The angiopoietin-Tie2 signaling axis in the vascular leakage of systemic inflammation. Tissue Barriers. 2015;3(1-2):e957508.

8. Scholz A, Plate KH, Reiss Y. Angiopoietin-2: a multifaceted cytokine that functions in both angiogenesis and inflammation. Ann N Y Acad Sci. 2015;1347:45–51.

9. Vajkoczy P, Farhadi M, Gaumann A, Heidenreich R, Erber R, Wunder A, Tonn JC, Menger MD, Breier G. Microtumor growth initiates angiogenic sprouting with simultaneous expression of VEGF, VEGF receptor-2, and angiopoietin-2. J Clin Invest. 2002;109(6):777–85.

10. Scharpfenecker M, Fiedler U, Reiss Y, Augustin HG. The Tie-2 ligand angiopoietin-2 destabilizes quiescent endothelium through an internal autocrine loop mechanism. J Cell Sci. 2005;118(Pt 4):771–80.

11. Maisonpierre PC, Suri C, Jones PF, Bartunkova S, Wiegand SJ, Radziejewski C, Compton D, McClain J, Aldrich TH, Papadopoulos N, et al. Angiopoietin-2, a natural antagonist for Tie2 that disrupts in vivo angiogenesis. Science. 1997;277(5322):55–60.

12. Etoh T, Inoue H, Tanaka S, Barnard GF, Kitano S, Mori M. Angiopoietin-2 is related to tumor angiogenesis in gastric carcinoma: possible in vivo regulation via induction of proteases. Cancer Res. 2001;61(5):2145–53.

13. Findley CM, Cudmore MJ, Ahmed A, Kontos CD. VEGF induces Tie2 shedding via a phosphoinositide 3-kinase/Akt dependent pathway to modulate Tie2 signaling. Arterioscler Thromb Vasc Biol. 2007;27(12):2619–26.

14. Reusch P, Barleon B, Weindel K, Martiny-Baron G, Godde A, Siemeister G, Marme D. Identification of a soluble form of the angiopoietin receptor TIE-2 released from endothelial cells and present in human blood. Angiogenesis. 2001;4(2):123–31.

15. Makinde T, Agrawal DK. Intra and extravascular transmembrane signalling of angiopoietin-1-Tie2 receptor in health and disease. J Cell Mol Med. 2008;12(3):810–28.

16. Michalska-Jakubus M, Kowal-Bielecka O, Chodorowska G, Bielecki M, Krasowska D. Angiopoietins-1 and -2 are differentially expressed in the sera of patients with systemic sclerosis: high angiopoietin-2 levels are associated with greater severity and higher activity of the disease. Rheumatology (Oxford). 2011;50(4):746–55.

17. Noda S, Asano Y, Aozasa N, Akamata K, Yamada D, Masui Y, Tamaki Z, Kadono T, Sato S. Serum Tie2 levels: clinical association with microangiopathies in patients with systemic sclerosis. J Eur Acad Dermatol Venereol. 2011; 25(12):1476–9.

18. Yuan HT, Khankin EV, Karumanchi SA, Parikh SM. Angiopoietin 2 is a partial agonist/antagonist of Tie2 signaling in the endothelium. Mol Cell Biol. 2009;29(8):2011–22.

19. LeRoy EC, Black C, Fleischmajer R, Jablonska S, Krieg T, Medsger Jr TA, Rowell N, Wollheim F. Scleroderma (systemic sclerosis): classification, subsets and pathogenesis. J Rheumatol. 1988;15(2):202–5.

20. Cutolo M, Sulli A, Pizzorni C, Accardo S. Nailfold videocapillaroscopy assessment of microvascular damage in systemic sclerosis. J Rheumatol. 2000;27(1):155–60.

21. Detmar M, Brown LF, Schon MP, Elicker BM, Velasco P, Richard L, Fukumura D, Monsky W, Claffey KP, Jain RK. Increased microvascular density and enhanced leukocyte rolling and adhesion in the skin of VEGF transgenic mice. J Invest Dermatol. 1998;111(1):1–6.

22. Akhmetshina ADC, Pileckyte M, Maurer B, Axmann R, Jüngel A, Zwerina J, Gay S, Schett G, Distler O, Distler JH. Dual inhibition of c-abl and PDGF receptor signaling by dasatinib and nilotinib for the treatment of dermal fibrosis. FASEB J. 2008;22:2214–22.

23. Siracusa LD, McGrath R, Ma Q, Moskow JJ, Manne J, Christner PJ, Buchberg AM, Jimenez SA. A tandem duplication within the fibrillin 1 gene is associated with the mouse tight skin mutation. Genome Res. 1996;6(4):300–13.

24. Distler JHJA, Huber LC, Schulze-Horsel U, Zwerina J, Gay RE, Michel BA, Hauser T, Schett G, Gay S, Distler O. Imatinib mesylate reduces production of extracellular matrix and prevents development of experimental dermal fibrosis. Arthritis Rheum. 2007;56:311–22.

25. Distler JH, Jungel A, Huber LC, Schulze-Horsel U, Zwerina J, Gay RE, Michel BA, Hauser T, Schett G, Gay S, et al. Imatinib mesylate reduces production of extracellular matrix and prevents development of experimental dermal fibrosis. Arthritis Rheum. 2007;56(1):311–22.

26. Ball SG, Shuttleworth CA, Kielty CM. Vascular endothelial growth factor can signal through platelet-derived growth factor receptors. J Cell Biol. 2007; 177(3):489–500.

27. Findley CM, Cudmore MJ, Ahmed A, Kontos CD. VEGF induces Tie2 shedding via a phosphoinositide 3-kinase/Akt-dependent pathway to modulate Tie2 signaling. Arterioscler Thromb Vasc Biol. 2007;27(12):2619–26.

28. Akhmetshina A, Venalis P, Dees C, Busch N, Zwerina J, Schett G, Distler O, Distler JH. Treatment with imatinib prevents fibrosis in different preclinical models of systemic sclerosis and induces regression of established fibrosis. Arthritis Rheum. 2009;60(1):219–24.

29. Beyer C, Schett G, Distler O, Distler JH. Animal models of systemic sclerosis: prospects and limitations. Arthritis Rheum. 2010;62(10):2831–44.

30. Green MC, Sweet HO, Bunker LE. Tight-skin, a new mutation of the mouse causing excessive growth of connective tissue and skeleton. Am J Pathol. 1976;82(3):493–512.

31. Riccieri V, Stefanantoni K, Vasile M, Macri V, Sciarra I, Iannace N, Alessandri C, Valesini G. Abnormal plasma levels of different angiogenic molecules are associated with different clinical manifestations in patients with systemic sclerosis. Clin Exp Rheumatol. 2011;29(2 Suppl 65):S46–52.

32. Dunne JV, Keen KJ, Van Eeden SF. Circulating angiopoietin and Tie-2 levels in systemic sclerosis. Rheumatol Int. 2013;33(2):475–84.

33. Gerlicz Z, Dziankowska-Bartkowiak B, Dziankowska-Zaborszczyk E, Sysa-Jedrzejowska A. Disturbed balance between serum levels of receptor tyrosine kinases Tie-1, Tie-2 and angiopoietins in systemic sclerosis. Dermatology. 2014;228(3):233–9.

34. Manetti M, Guiducci S, Romano E, Ceccarelli C, Bellando-Randone S, Conforti ML, Ibba-Manneschi L, Matucci-Cerinic M. Overexpression of VEGF165b, an inhibitory splice variant of vascular endothelial growth factor, leads to insufficient angiogenesis in patients with systemic sclerosis. Circ Res. 2011;109(3):e14–26.

35. Maurer B, Distler A, Dees C, Khan K, Denton CP, Abraham D, Gay RE, Michel BA, Gay S, Hw Distler J, et al. Levels of target activation predict antifibrotic responses to tyrosine kinase inhibitors. Ann Rheum Dis. 2013;72(12):2039–46.

# Mir-155 is overexpressed in systemic sclerosis fibroblasts and is required for NLRP3 inflammasome-mediated collagen synthesis during fibrosis

Carol M. Artlett[1*], Sihem Sassi-Gaha[1], Jennifer L. Hope[1,2], Carol A. Feghali-Bostwick[3] and Peter D. Katsikis[1,2]

## Abstract

**Background:** Despite the important role that microRNAs (miRNAs) play in immunity and inflammation, their involvement in systemic sclerosis (SSc) remains poorly characterized. miRNA-155 (miR-155) plays a role in pulmonary fibrosis and its expression can be induced with interleukin (IL)-1β. SSc fibroblasts have activated inflammasomes that are integrally involved in mediating the myofibroblast phenotype. In light of this, we investigated whether miR-155 played a role in SSc and if its expression was dependent on inflammasome activation.

**Methods:** miR-155 expression was confirmed in SSc dermal and lung fibroblasts by quantitative polymerase chain reaction (PCR). Wild-type and NLRP3-deficient murine fibroblasts were utilized to explore the regulation of miR-155 during inflammasome activation. miR-155-deficient fibroblasts and retroviral transductions with a miR-155 expression or control vectors were used to understand the contribution of miR-155 in fibrosis.

**Results:** miR-155 was significantly increased and the highest expressing miRNA in SSc lung fibroblasts. Its expression was dependent on inflammasome activation as miR-155 expression could be blocked when inflammasome signaling was inhibited. In the absence of miR-155, inflammasome-mediated collagen synthesis could not be induced but was restored when miR-155 was expressed in miR-155-deficient fibroblasts.

**Conclusions:** miR-155 is upregulated in SSc. These results suggest that the inflammasome promotes the expression of miR-155 and that miR-155 is a critical miRNA that drives fibrosis.

**Keywords:** Fibrosis, NLRP3 inflammasome, miR-155, Systemic sclerosis, IL-1

## Background

Systemic sclerosis (SSc) is a chronic autoimmune disease. It is characterized by uncontrolled fibrosis that is directly related to the morbidity and mortality of the disease [1]. Fibrotic lesions in SSc have persistently activated myofibroblasts and these cells mediate the excessive deposition of collagen in the dermis and visceral organs and display vascular abnormalities [2–4]. Patients typically present with an autoantibody profile that often defines disease progression and organ involvement [5, 6]. We recently found that activation of the inflammasome orchestrates

the increased collagen synthesis in SSc fibroblasts [7]. We also found that inhibition of inflammasome signaling significantly abrogated the myofibroblast phenotype [7]. Based on these findings, we concluded that inflammasome activation plays a significant role in the pathogenesis of SSc fibrosis.

MicroRNAs (miRNAs) have been shown to regulate gene expression and specific miRNAs have been reported to be involved in SSc fibrosis [8–10]; however, little is known about the regulation of specific miRNAs during fibrosis. miRNA-155 (miR-155) has been identified as having immune regulatory functions and plays a critical role in innate and adaptive immune responses [11–14]. Increased miR-155 has been associated with liver [15] and lung fibrosis [16] and an additional study

* Correspondence: Carol.artlett@drexelmed.edu
[1]Department of Microbiology and Immunology, Drexel University College of Medicine, 2900 Queen Lane, Philadelphia, PA 19129, USA
Full list of author information is available at the end of the article

has shown that the downregulation of miR-155 at wound sites abrogates fibrosis [17]. miR-155 can be induced by interleukin (IL)-1β [18] and transforming growth factor (TGF)-β1 [19]. In light of the observation that IL-1β induces miR-155 and because we found that IL-1β processing by the inflammasome is elevated in SSc fibroblasts [7], we investigated whether miR-155 was overexpressed in SSc cells and whether its expression requires activation of the inflammasome. In some of these studies, bleomycin was used to activate the inflammasome and induce IL-1 processing and secretion and we used this molecule to further explore the contribution of the inflammasome activation to miR-155 expression in fibrosis. The results of these studies demonstrate that SSc fibroblasts have increased synthesis of miR-155, and that miR-155 expression is dependent on inflammasome activation. Importantly, miR-155 is required for collagen production following inflammasome activation as cells devoid of miR-155 cannot produce collagen in a fibrotic setting. This suggests that miRNAs are involved in the pathogenesis of SSc and, in particular, miR-155 may be an essential regulator of SSc fibrosis downstream of inflammasome activation.

## Methods

### Human subjects

Primary fibroblast strains were derived from SSc lung ($n = 9$) and normal lung ($n = 5$) explants. The lung fibroblasts lines were derived from Caucasian SSc patients aged 46–52 years (eight female, one male) with nonspecific interstitial pneumonia, that is usual interstitial pneumonia with or without pulmonary arterial hypertension. Control lung fibroblast lines were established from Caucasian normal individuals (three female, two male) aged 25–76 years who had all died due to head trauma. SSc skin-derived fibroblasts ($n = 5$) were established from Caucasian SSc patients with diffuse disease aged 40–50 years (four female, one male), with Scl-70 or RNA polymerase autoantibodies. Normal dermal fibroblasts ($n = 6$) were obtained from Coriell Repositories, Camden, NJ, USA ($n = 4$) or obtained from Pittsburgh ($n = 2$) and were derived from Caucasian and one Black individual aged 16–80 years of age. All of the SSc patients fulfilled the preliminary criteria for the classification of SSc [20, 21]. All human-derived fibroblasts were tested between passages 3 and 6.

### Cell culture

Normal human primary dermal fibroblasts ($n = 4$) and SSc primary dermal fibroblasts ($n = 5$) or normal human primary lung fibroblasts ($n = 3$) and SSc primary lung fibroblasts ($n = 3$) (750,000 cells/dish) were cultured in Dulbecco's modified Eagle's medium (DMEM; Mediatech Inc., Manassas, VA, USA) supplemented with 10% fetal bovine serum (FBS; Mediatech) and 1% penicillin/

streptomycin (Mediatech). In the additional experiments, SSc fibroblasts were exposed to 20 μM caspase-1 inhibitor (Z-YVAD(OMe)-FMK (YVAD); Enzo Life Sciences, Plymouth Meeting, PA, USA) for 48 h. RNA was isolated using the Qiagen miRNeasy kit and the culture media was reserved for hydroxyproline assays according to Artlett et al. [7].

Fibroblasts cell lines from murine skin explants were established from NLRP3-deficient mice, miR-155-deficient mice, and wild-type C57BL/6 mice as previously described [7]. All fibroblasts derived from the knockout mice were on a C57BL/6 background. miR-155-deficient mice were a kind gift from Dr. Martin Turner (Babraham Institute, UK).

### miR-155 expression

miR-155 expression was measured by quantitative real-time polymerase chain reaction (RT-PCR) normalized to SNORD44 for human fibroblasts or SNORD47 for mouse fibroblasts using primers purchased from Quanta Biosciences, Gaithersburg, MD, USA. Total miRNA was reverse transcribed with qScript miRNA cDNA reaction kit (Quanta Biosciences) and quantified with PerfectCT SYBR Green Supermix (Quanta Biosciences) according to the manufacturer's instructions.

### Fibroblast transduction

Retroviruses were produced in the Platinum-E cell line (Cell Biolabs). The miR-155-expressing MigR1-miR-155-gfp retrovirus was provided by E. Vigorito (Babraham Institute, UK). A MigR1-control-gfp retrovirus that expressed scrambled miR-155 sequence was used as the control. miR-155-deficient cells were transduced as previously described [14] but modified for fibroblasts. Briefly, fibroblasts at 50% confluency were treated with 8 μg/ml polybrene and retrovirus, centrifuged at 2000 g for 90 min, incubated at 37°C for 4 h, and then fresh media was added. Some of the dishes received 10 μM bleomycin or 50 ng/ml IL-1 receptor antagonist (IL-1RA) at 0 and 24 h post-transduction, and were then recovered for hydroxyproline analyses. Transduction efficiency of both retroviral constructs was determined by green fluorescent protein (GFP) expression to be approximately 10% using flow cytometry.

### Western blotting

Fibroblasts (C57BL/6 and miR-155KO) were cultured as described with or without 10 μM bleomycin; 200 μg of whole cell lysate was size fractionated on an 8% SDS polyacrylamide gel and the proteins transferred to a PVDF membrane (ThermoFisher Scientific, Waltham, MA, USA). Nonspecific binding sites were blocked with 5% skim milk and then probed with rabbit-anti-mouse TGF-β1 or β-actin (Santa Cruz Biotechnologies, Santa

Cruz, CA, USA) overnight at 4°C. The membrane was washed and incubated with goat-anti-rabbit-HRP (Jackson Immunoresearch, West Grove, PA, USA). The horseradish peroxidase (HRP) signal was developed with SuperSignal Chemiluminescent Substrate (ThermoFisher Scientific). Band densities were quantified using ImageQuant LAS4000. TGF-β1 bands were normalized to the β-actin levels.

### Statistical analyses

The Mann Whitney $t$ test or Wilcoxon matched-pairs signed-rank test were used to analyze the data by GraphPad Prism 7. A $p$ value <0.05 was considered significant.

## Results

### miRNA-155 is overexpressed in SSc dermal and lung fibroblasts

miR-155 has been reported to be elevated in fibrosis and we wanted to determine whether this was a relevant miRNA for SSc. We found the relative expression of miR-155 in SSc lung fibroblasts ($n = 9$) to be 3.65-times more than that of normal lung fibroblasts ($n = 5$) ($p < 0.01$; Fig. 1a). We also found that SSc dermal fibroblasts ($n = 5$) had twice the relative expression of miR-155 than normal dermal fibroblasts ($n = 6$) ($p = 0.04$; Fig. 1b). These findings suggest that the increased miR-155 expression in fibroblasts may be contributing to fibrosis.

### miRNA-155 is induced by inflammasome activation

We have previously shown that SSc fibroblasts have an activated inflammasome [7] and it has been reported that miR-155 expression can be induced by IL-1β [18]. We therefore wanted to determine whether inflammasome activation could be inducing miR-155. SSc fibroblasts ($n = 7$) were cultured with the inflammasome inhibitor YVAD for 48 h. We found that in the presence of the caspase-1 inhibitor miR-155 was significantly reduced ($p = 0.03$; Fig. 2a). Further confirming our previous findings, total collagen synthesis was also significantly reduced when caspase-1 was inhibited with YVAD ($p < 0.01$; Fig. 2b). These data suggest that miR-155 expression is dependent on caspase-1 activation and that miR-155 upregulation could correlate with collagen production in SSc.

In addition, because we found the NLRP3 inflammasome to be integral in SSc fibrosis [7], we explored whether NLRP3-deficient fibroblasts (NLRP3KO) could express miR-155. B6 and NLRP3KO fibroblasts were cultured with bleomycin ± YVAD, and miR-155 expression was measured. In the wild-type B6 fibroblasts, the relative expression of miR-155 was induced with bleomycin ($p = 0.01$; Fig. 2c) and the induced expression of miR-155 could be abolished with YVAD ($p = 0.02$;

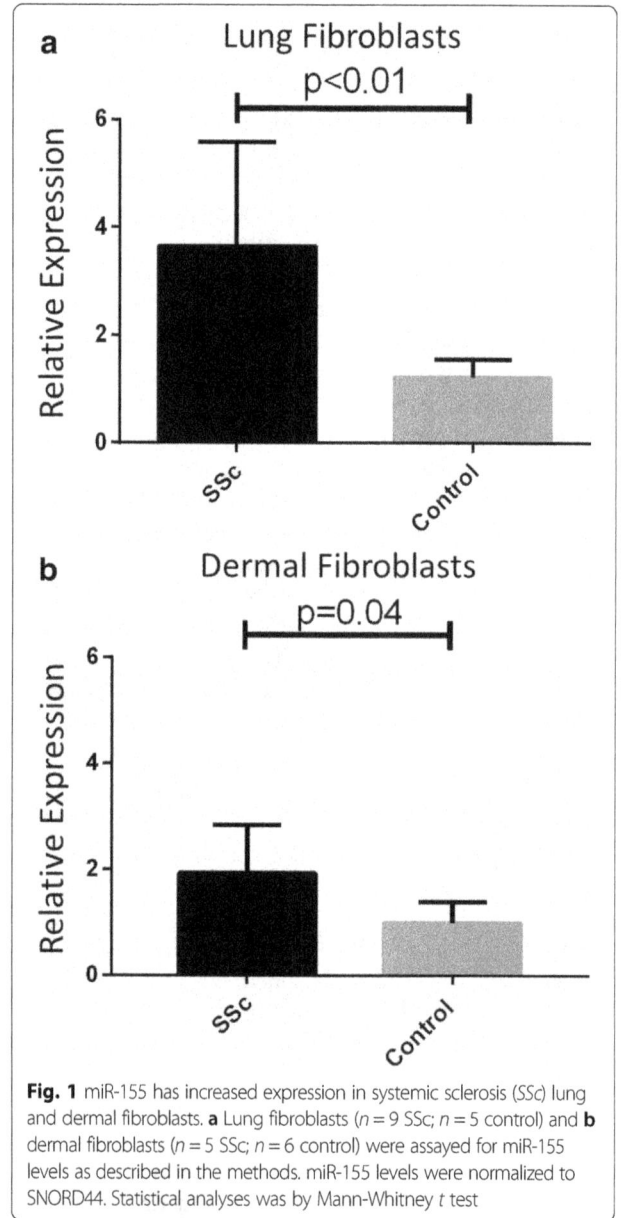

**Fig. 1** miR-155 has increased expression in systemic sclerosis (*SSc*) lung and dermal fibroblasts. **a** Lung fibroblasts ($n = 9$ SSc; $n = 5$ control) and **b** dermal fibroblasts ($n = 5$ SSc; $n = 6$ control) were assayed for miR-155 levels as described in the methods. miR-155 levels were normalized to SNORD44. Statistical analyses was by Mann-Whitney $t$ test

Fig. 2c). Furthermore, miR-155 was not expressed in NLRP3KO fibroblasts ($p = 0.01$; Fig. 2c) and could not be induced at all with bleomycin ($p = 0.01$; Fig. 2c). Correspondingly, we then examined hydroxyproline levels and found that bleomycin induced collagen ($p < 0.01$; Fig. 2d) and YVAD blocked this process ($p < 0.01$; Fig. 2d). These data suggest that the NLRP3 inflammasome and caspase-1 may play a role in miR-155 expression in fibroblasts.

### miRNA-155 is required for inflammasome-driven collagen synthesis

Having established that both miR-155 expression and collagen production by fibroblasts were upregulated by inflammasome activation, it was important to determine

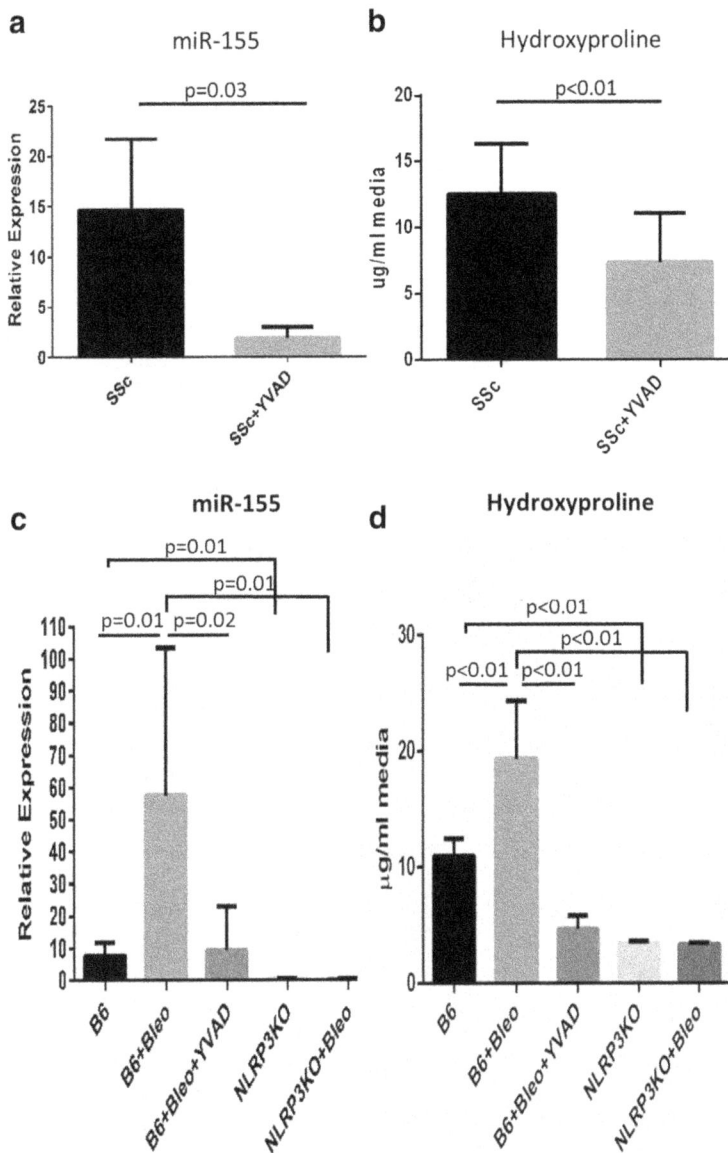

**Fig. 2** miR-155 expression requires the NLRP3 inflammasome. **a** Systemic sclerosis (*SSc*) lung fibroblasts (*n* = 7) were treated with 20 μM YVAD for 48 h. miRNA was extracted and the resulting cDNA was assayed for miR-155 levels normalized to SNORD44. **b** Hydroxyproline was measured in the culture supernatants from **a**. Statistical analyses for **a** and **b** used the Wilcoxon ranked paired *t* test. **c** In mouse cells, miR-155 expression was induced with 20 μM bleomycin (*Bleo*) + 20 μM YVAD for 48 h and analyzed for miR-155 expression normalized to SNORD47. Data are presented as the average from two independent experiments with three replicates (*n* = 6 for each condition) + SEM. **d** Hydroxyproline was measured from the culture supernatants from **c**. Statistical analyses for **c** and **d** used the Mann-Whitney *t* test

whether miR-155 expression was required for collagen production during fibrosis. To address this, we first tested whether miR-155KO fibroblasts responded to bleomycin. We found that, unlike the B6 fibroblasts responding to bleomycin ($p < 0.01$; Fig. 3a), bleomycin did not induce collagen synthesis in the miR-155KO fibroblasts ($p < 0.001$; Fig. 3a).

To directly confirm this observation and to prove that miR-155 facilitates fibrosis, we transduced miR-155KO fibroblasts with a miR-155 retroviral expression vector or the retroviral control vector and then stimulated the fibroblasts with bleomycin. When cells were transduced with the control vector, collagen synthesis could not be induced with bleomycin (Fig. 3b). However, after restoration of miR-155 in the miR-155KO fibroblasts, there was a significant induction of total collagen, even without bleomycin stimulation ($p = 0.03$; Fig. 3b) and this effect was further enhanced with bleomycin ($p < 0.001$; Fig. 3b). These data indicate that miR-155 is required for fibrosis.

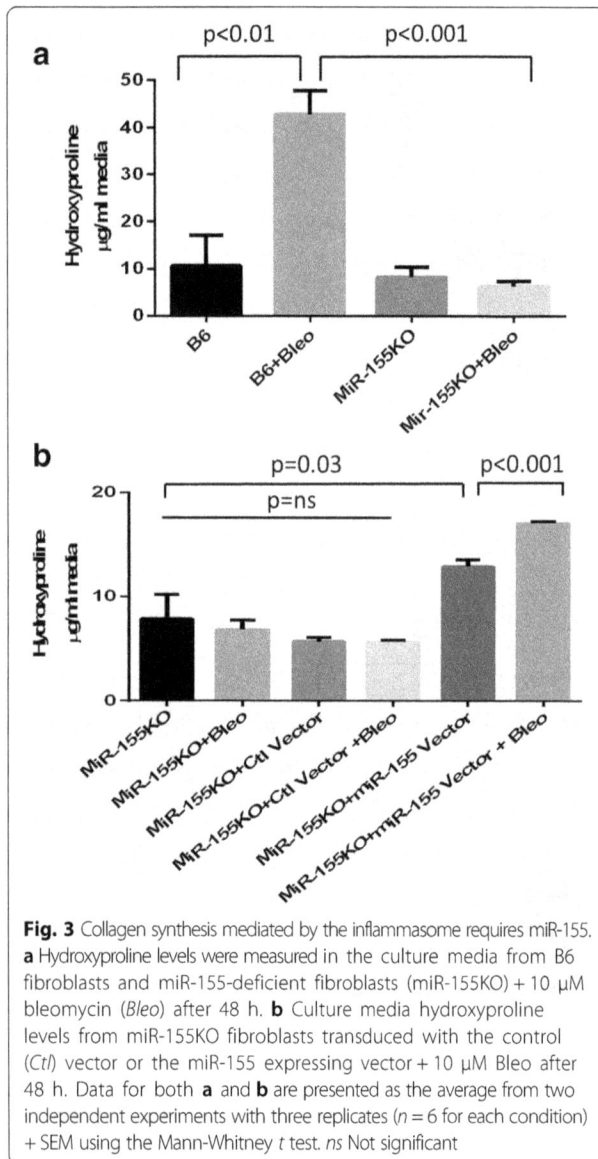

**Fig. 3** Collagen synthesis mediated by the inflammasome requires miR-155. **a** Hydroxyproline levels were measured in the culture media from B6 fibroblasts and miR-155-deficient fibroblasts (miR-155KO) + 10 μM bleomycin (*Bleo*) after 48 h. **b** Culture media hydroxyproline levels from miR-155KO fibroblasts transduced with the control (*Ctl*) vector or the miR-155 expressing vector + 10 μM Bleo after 48 h. Data for both **a** and **b** are presented as the average from two independent experiments with three replicates (*n* = 6 for each condition) + SEM using the Mann-Whitney *t* test. *ns* Not significant

### miRNA-155 modulates fibrosis via IL-1 signaling

We found increased hydroxyproline when miR-155 was overexpressed in fibroblasts; however, only 10% of the fibroblasts were transduced by the miR-155 retrovirus (data not shown). This suggested that there might be an indirect mechanism driving the miR-155-mediated fibrotic response. IL-1 has been reported to promote miR-155 expression, and so we questioned whether miR-155 could promote IL-1 transcription that synergizes with the activation of the inflammasome; we therefore blocked the IL-1 receptor with its antagonist (IL-1RA). In repeat experiments, in the absence of miR-155, IL-1RA had no effect on hydroxyproline levels (Fig. 4a); however, in the presence of miR-155, IL-1RA completely abrogated bleomycin-induced hydroxyproline ($p < 0.01$; Fig. 4a). In addition, the spike in the level of hydroxyproline that was

observed when miR-155KO fibroblasts were transduced with the miR-155 vector (without bleomycin stimulation) was also via a mechanism that entailed IL-1, as this spike was abolished with IL-1RA ($p < 0.01$; Fig. 4a).

Confirming the data by Pottier et al. [18], we found that the addition of IL-1 to fibroblasts induced miR-155 in a dose-dependent manner (Fig. 4b). However, we found this expression was not transient in fibroblasts and that miR-155 expression was still elevated at 48 h at the time point when total miRNA was isolated for the other experiments. Taken together, these data suggest that in fibroblasts activation of the inflammasome is involved in IL-1-mediated expression of miR-155 and that miR-155 synergizes with the inflammasome to drive collagen synthesis during fibrosis. Furthermore, these data also imply that miR-155 provides a feed-forward mechanism promoting IL-1 transcription that can lead to upregulated collagen synthesis via IL-1 receptor signaling and further miR-155 expression.

We also found that miR-155 was necessary for increased TGF-β1 protein levels. We stimulated C57BL/6 and the miR-155KO fibroblasts with bleomycin and measured TGF-β 1 protein levels in fibroblasts. We found that there was a significant induction of TGF-β1 in the B6 fibroblasts; however in the miR-155KO TGF-β1 could not be induced. This suggests that miR-155 is driving TGF-β1 expression and contributing to the fibrotic pathology in these cells.

### Discussion

miR-155 has been studied previously in other fibrotic conditions; however, little is known about its regulation in SSc fibrosis. Pottier et al. [18] reported that miR-155-overexpressing fibroblasts had increased motility on collagen gels suggesting that this miRNA could help to mediate wound closure, whereas the knockdown of miR-155 during wound healing abrogated fibrosis. A recently published study reports on the role of miR-155 in SSc fibrosis [22]; however, this study did not explore what caused the increase in miR-155 in SSc fibroblasts but investigated the downstream responses mediated by miR-155. Yan et al. [22] found that miR-155 regulated the Akt and Wnt/β-catenin pathways. Our study further confirms and helps to define the crucial role of miR-155 in SSc fibrosis.

miR-155 expression is upregulated by IL-1 and we explored this observation in light of our recent finding that IL-1 and the inflammasome plays a significant role in SSc fibrosis [7]. We found that miR-155 expression in SSc fibroblasts is driven by inflammasome activation since inhibition of the inflammasome signaling cascade with a caspase antagonist abolished miR-155 expression and, in turn, significantly lowered collagen (Fig. 2). Our previous study used bleomycin to activate the inflammasome and upregulate collagen via IL-1 expression [7]; therefore, in these studies, we used bleomycin to activate the inflammasome and to determine the role of the

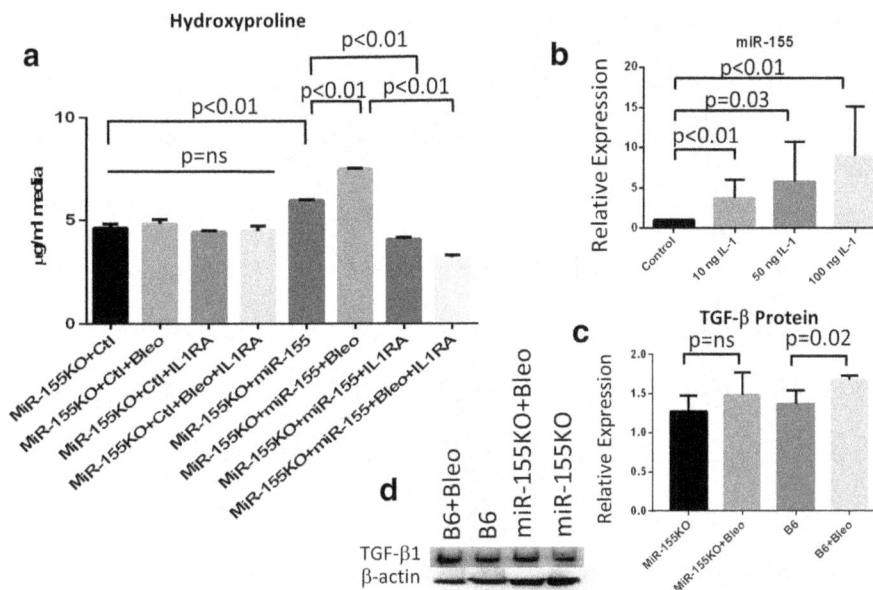

**Fig. 4** miR-155 regulates fibrosis via interleukin-1 (*IL-1*) and IL-1 induces miR-155. **a** miR-155KO fibroblasts were transduced with the miR-155 expression vector or the control (*Ctl*) vector. Some of the dishes received 10 μM bleomycin (*Bleo*) at 0 h and some of the cells also received 50 ng/ml IL-1 receptor antagonist (*IL-1RA*) at 0 and 24 h. Media was recovered after 48 h and hydroxyproline was measured (*n* = 9 replicates). **b** Dose-dependent induction of miR-155 in fibroblasts (*n* = 7 replicates). **c** Graphical representation of transforming growth factor beta (*TGF-β*) levels in miR-155KO and B6 cells ± bleo. **d** Representative Western blot (one of three samples independently tested). Data are presented as averages + SEM using the Mann-Whitney *t* test. *ns* Not significant

NLRP3 inflammasome in miR-155 expression. Thus, to further confirm the role of the inflammasome in miR-155 expression, we show for the first time that NLRP3KO fibroblasts cannot induce miR-155 expression when stimulated with bleomycin (Fig. 2c). Taken together, this suggests that the NLRP3 inflammasome is required for miR-155 expression. We next asked whether miR-155 participates in fibrosis and found that bleomycin cannot induce collagen synthesis in the miR-155KO fibroblasts (Fig. 3a), whereas the restoration of miR-155 using a viral vector resulted in increased collagen (Fig. 3b). IL-1 was found to induce miR-155 expression (Fig. 4b) and the synthesis of collagen in miR-155-sufficient fibroblasts, and that this was mediated via IL-1 since IL-1RA abolished these findings (Fig. 4a).

Previous research by Kong et al. [19] found that TGF-β1 upregulated the expression of miR-155, leading to altered SMAD signaling; however, another study found miR-155 to be decreased by TGF-β [18]. While the data from these findings are confounding, they suggest that the expression of miR-155 by TGF-β could be dependent on the pathological setting, e.g., fibrosis vs. wound healing, and the cells they are directly acting in. We found that, in the absence of miR-155, TGF-β was not induced, supporting the findings by Zhang et al. that miR-155 can induce TGF-β expression [23].

The data presented here imply that blockade of the IL-1 receptor or sequestration of IL-1 from the circulation could be of therapeutic benefit to SSc patients. Drugs such as kineret, rilonacept, or ilaris may prove efficacious for this, as yet, untreatable pathology. Currently, there is a placebo-controlled clinical trial underway to determine whether rilonacept could be used to treat SSc. Rilonacept sequesters IL-1 from the circulation using an antibody that binds and inactivates IL-1. Administration of IL-1RA, which blocks IL-1 from binding its receptor, has been used in various human and animal studies to prevent various organ fibroses [24–29] and it is further suggested that blockade of IL-1 signaling may also be beneficial. Furthermore, elevated IL-1 or decreased IL-1RA has been directly associated with fibrosis. Decreased expression of IL-1RA has been found in idiopathic pulmonary fibrosis and this has been specifically linked to the single nucleotide polymorphism at rs2637988 which controls expression of the gene [30, 31]. Children deficient in IL-1RA have chronic inflammation that can lead to fibrosis of the lungs or vertebra, if they survive long enough [32]. Further supporting this observation, the uncontrolled expression of IL-1 in Familial Mediterranean Fever or Muckle-Wells Syndrome has been associated with an increased risk for peritoneal fibrosis [33, 34].

## Conclusions

These data imply that miR-155 is a critical regulator in the fibrotic process and that miR-155 expression requires the NLRP3 inflammasome processing of IL-1 leading to fibrosis. Thus, we propose that the inflammasome is the initiator causing IL-1 transcription and autocrine signaling that drives the expression of miR-155 via an IL-1 signaling mechanism (Fig. 5). miR-155 synergizes with the inflammasome to induce a positive

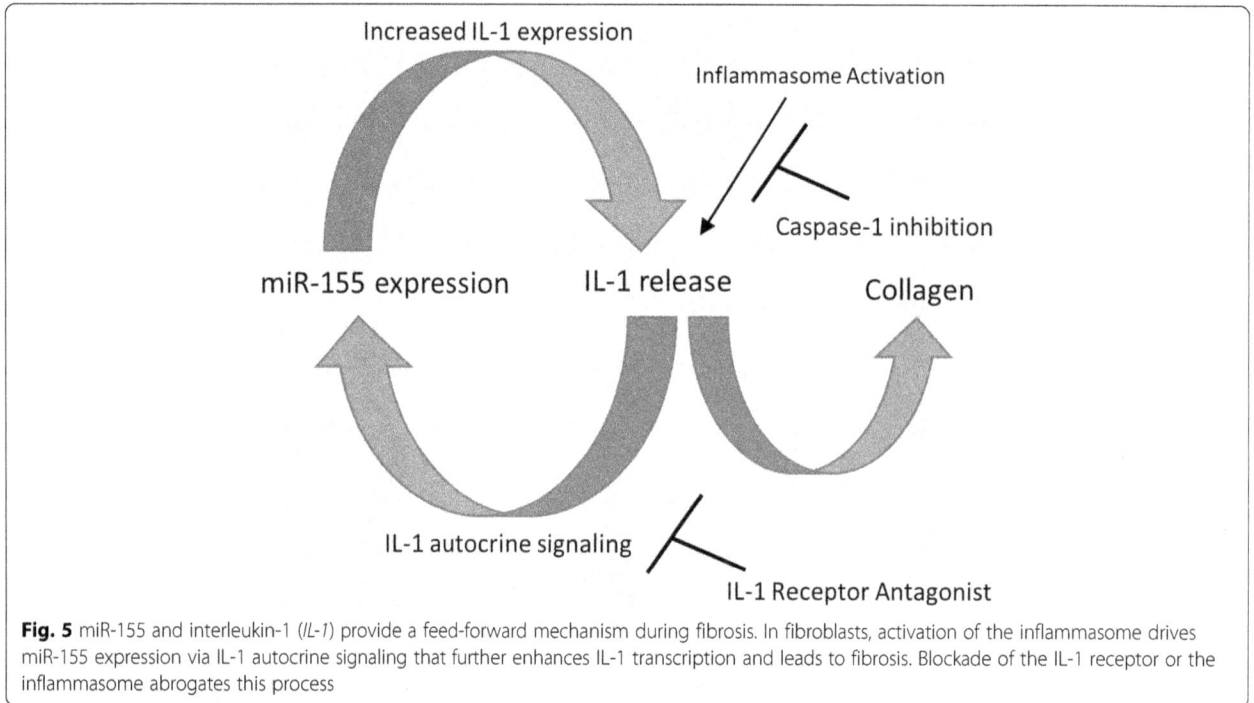

**Fig. 5** miR-155 and interleukin-1 (*IL-1*) provide a feed-forward mechanism during fibrosis. In fibroblasts, activation of the inflammasome drives miR-155 expression via IL-1 autocrine signaling that further enhances IL-1 transcription and leads to fibrosis. Blockade of the IL-1 receptor or the inflammasome abrogates this process

feed-forward signal that further promotes IL-1 release and autocrine signaling leading to continual collagen expression. Inhibiting either the IL-1 receptor with its antagonist or the inflammasome with YVAD breaks this cycle, and abrogates miR-155 expression and fibrosis.

### Abbreviations
B6: C57BL6; IL: Interleukin; IL-1RA: interleukin-1 receptor antagonist; miR-155: MicroRNA-155; miRNA: MicroRNA; NLRP3: NOD-like receptor family, pyrin domain containing 3; NLRP3KO: NLRP3-deficient; SSc: Systemic sclerosis; TGF: Transforming growth factor; YVAD: Z-YVAD(OMe)-FMK

### Acknowledgements
This work was funded by a research award from the Scleroderma Foundation to CMA and by NIH AR061271 to CAF-B.

### Authors' contributions
CMA conceived and designed the experiments, analyzed the data, and wrote the manuscript; SS-G performed the experiments and revised the manuscript; CAF-B established explants from SSc and normal fibroblasts and revised the manuscript; JLH generated retroviral vectors and performed flow cytometry and revised the manuscript; PDK conceived and designed the experiments and wrote the manuscript. All authors listed have read the manuscript for content and have approved the final version.

### Competing interests
The authors declare that they have no competing interests.

### Author details
[1]Department of Microbiology and Immunology, Drexel University College of Medicine, 2900 Queen Lane, Philadelphia, PA 19129, USA. [2]Department of Immunology, Erasmus University Medical Center, Rotterdam, The Netherlands. [3]Division of Rheumatology & Immunology, Medical University of South Carolina, Charleston, SC, USA.

### References
1. Varga J. Systemic sclerosis: an update. Bull NYU Hosp Jt Dis. 2008;66:198–202.
2. Kirk TZ, Mark ME, Chua CC, Chua BH, Mayes MD. Myofibroblasts from scleroderma skin synthesize elevated levels of collagen and tissue inhibitor of metalloproteinase (TIMP-1) with two forms of TIMP-1. J Biol Chem. 1995;270:3423–8.
3. Abraham DJ, Eckes B, Rajkumar V, Krieg T. New developments in fibroblast and myofibroblast biology: implications for fibrosis and scleroderma. Curr Rheum Rep. 2007;9:136–43.
4. Tomasek JJ, Gabbiani G, Hinz B, Chaponnier C, Brown RA. Myofibroblasts and mechano-regulation of connective tissue remodelling. Nat Rev. 2002;3:349–63.
5. Meyer OC, Fertig N, Lucas M, Somogyi N, Medsger Jr TA. Disease subsets, antinuclear antibody profile, and clinical features in 127 French and 247 US adult patients with systemic sclerosis. J Rheumatol. 2007;34:104–9.
6. Parodi A, Drosera M, Barbieri L, Rebora A. Scleroderma subsets are best detected by the simultaneous analysis of the autoantibody profile using commercial ELISA. Dermatology. 2002;204:29–32.
7. Artlett CM, Sassi-Gaha S, Rieger JL, Boesteanu AC, Feghali-Bostwick CA, Katsikis PD. The inflammasome activating caspase-1 mediates fibrosis and myofibroblast differentiation in systemic sclerosis. Arthritis Rheum. 2011;63:3563–74.
8. Kawashita Y, Jinnin M, Makino T, Kajihara I, Makino K, Honda N, Masuguchi S, Fukushima S, Inoue Y, Ihn H. Circulating miR-29a levels in patients with scleroderma spectrum disorder. J Dermatol Sci. 2011;61:67–9.
9. Maurer B, Stanczyk J, Jungel A, Akhmetshina A, Trenkmann M, Brock M, Kowal-Bielecka O, Gay RE, Michel BA, Distler JH, et al. MicroRNA-29, a key regulator of collagen expression in systemic sclerosis. Arthritis Rheum. 2010;62:1733–43.
10. Li C, He H, Zhu M, Zhao S, Li X. Molecular characterisation of porcine miR-155 and its regulatory roles in the TLR3/TLR4 pathways. Dev Comp Immunol. 2012;39:110–6.
11. Vigorito E, Perks KL, Abreu-Goodger C, Bunting S, Xiang Z, Kohlhaas S, Das PP, Miska EA, Rodriguez A, Bradley A, et al. microRNA-155 regulates the generation of immunoglobulin class-switched plasma cells. Immunity. 2007;27:847–59.
12. Thai TH, Calado DP, Casola S, Ansel KM, Xiao C, Xue Y, Murphy A, Frendewey D, Valenzuela D, Kutok JL, et al. Regulation of the germinal center response by microRNA-155. Science. 2007;316:604–8.
13. O'Connell RM, Kahn D, Gibson WS, Round JL, Scholz RL, Chaudhuri AA, Kahn ME, Rao DS, Baltimore D. MicroRNA-155 promotes autoimmune inflammation by enhancing inflammatory T cell development. Immunity. 2010;33:607–19.

14. Gracias DT, Stelekati E, Hope JL, Boesteanu AC, Doering TA, Norton J, Mueller YM, Fraietta JA, Wherry EJ, Turner M, et al. The microRNA miR-155 controls CD8(+) T cell responses by regulating interferon signaling. Nat Immunol. 2013;14:593–602.

15. Bala S, Csak T, Saha B, Zatsiorsky J, Kodys K, Catalano D, Szabo G. The pro-inflammatory effects of miR-155 promote liver fibrosis and alcohol-induced steatohepatitis. J Hepatol. 2016;64:1378–87.

16. Zheng L, Xu CC, Chen WD, Shen WL, Ruan CC, Zhu LM, Zhu DL, Gao PJ. MicroRNA-155 regulates angiotensin II type 1 receptor expression and phenotypic differentiation in vascular adventitial fibroblasts. Biochem Biophys Res Commun. 2010;400:483–8.

17. Yang LL, Liu JQ, Bai XZ, Fan L, Han F, Jia WB, Su LL, Shi JH, Tang CW, Hu DH. Acute downregulation of miR-155 at wound sites leads to a reduced fibrosis through attenuating inflammatory response. Biochem Biophys Res Commun. 2014;453:153–9.

18. Pottier N, Maurin T, Chevalier B, Puissegur MP, Lebrigand K, Robbe-Sermesant K, Bertero T, Lino Cardenas CL, Courcot E, Rios G, et al. Identification of keratinocyte growth factor as a target of microRNA-155 in lung fibroblasts: implication in epithelial-mesenchymal interactions. PLoSOne. 2009;4:e6718.

19. Kong W, Yang H, He L, Zhao JJ, Coppola D, Dalton WS, Cheng JQ. MicroRNA-155 is regulated by the transforming growth factor beta/Smad pathway and contributes to epithelial cell plasticity by targeting RhoA. Mol Cell Biol. 2008;28:6773–84.

20. Masi AT, Rodnan GP, Medsger TA, Altman RD, D'Angelo WA, Fries JF, LeRoy EC, Kirsner AB, Mackenzie AH, McShane DJ, et al. Preliminary criteria for the classification of systemic sclerosis (scleroderma) Subcommittee for Scleroderma Criteria of the American Rheumatism Association Diagnostic and Therapeutic Criteria Committee. Arthritis Rheum. 1980;23:581–90.

21. LeRoy EC, Black CM, Fleischmajer R, Jablonska S, Krieg T, Medsger TA, Rowell N, Wollheim F. Scleroderma (systemic sclerosis): classification, subsets and pathogenesis. J Rheumatol. 1988;15:202–5.

22. Yan Q, Chen J, Li W, Bao C, Fu Q. Targeting miR-155 to treat experimental scleroderma. Sci Rep. 2016;6:20314.

23. Zhang D, Cui Y, Li B, Luo X, Li B, Tang Y. miR-155 regulates high glucose-induced cardiac fibrosis via the TGF-beta signaling pathway. Molec BioSystems. 2016;13:215–24.

24. Brown CA, Toth AP, Magnussen B. Clinical benefits of intra-articular anakinra for arthrofibrosis. Orthopedics. 2010;33:877.

25. Magnussen RA, Brown CA, Lawrence TJ, Toth AP. Intra-articular anakinra for the treatment of persistent inflammation and arthrofibrosis following anterior cruciate ligament reconstruction. Duke Orthopedic J. 2011;1:51–6.

26. Lan HY, Nikolic-Paterson DJ, Mu W, Vannice JL, Atkins RC. Interleukin-1 receptor antagonist halts the progression of established crescentic glomerulonephritis in the rat. Kidney Int. 1995;47:1303–9.

27. Gasse P, Mary C, Guenon I, Noulin N, Charron S, Schnyder-Candrian S, Schnyder B, Akira S, Quesniaux VFJ, Lagente V, et al. IL-1R1/MyD88 signaling and the inflammasome are essential in pulmonary inflammation and fibrosis in mice. J Clin Invest. 2007;117:3786–99.

28. Aouba A, Georgin-Lavialle S, Pagnoux C, Martin Silva N, Renand A, Galateau-Salle F, Le Toquin S, Bensadoun H, Larousserie F, Silvera S, et al. Rationale and efficacy of interleukin-1 targeting in Erdheim-Chester disease. Blood. 2010;116:4070–6.

29. Adam Z, Szturz P, Buckova P, Cervinkova I, Koukalova R, Rehak Z, Krejci M, Pour L, Zahradova L, Hajek R, et al. Interleukin-1 receptor blockade with anakinra provided cessation of fatigue, reduction in inflammation markers and regression of retroperitoneal fibrosis in a patient with Erdheim-Chester disease—case study and a review of literature. Vnitr Lek. 2012;58:313–8.

30. Barlo NP, van Moorsel CH, Korthagen NM, Heron M, Rijkers GT, Ruven HJ, van den Bosch JM, Grutters JC. Genetic variability in the IL1RN gene and the balance between interleukin (IL)-1 receptor agonist and IL-1beta in idiopathic pulmonary fibrosis. Clin Exp Immunol. 2011;166:346–51.

31. Korthagen NM, van Moorsel CH, Kazemier KM, Ruven HJ, Grutters JC. IL1RN genetic variations and risk of IPF: a meta-analysis and mRNA expression study. Immunogenetics. 2012;64:371–7.

32. Aksentijevich I, Masters SL, Ferguson PJ, Dancey P, Frenkel J, van Royen-Kerkhoff A, Laxer R, Tedgard U, Cowen EW, Pham TH, et al. An autoinflammatory disease with deficiency of the interleukin-1-receptor antagonist. N Eng J Med. 2009;360:2426–37.

33. Berkun Y, Ben-Chetrit E, Klar A, Ben-Chetrit E. Peritoneal adhesions and intestinal obstructions in patients with familial Mediterranean fever—are they more frequent? Semin Arthritis Rheum. 2007;36:316–21.

34. Paydas S, Gokel Y. Different renal pathologies associated with hypothyroidism. Renal Fail. 2002;24:595–600.

# 5

# Survival and quality of life in incident systemic sclerosis-related pulmonary arterial hypertension

Kathleen Morrisroe[1,2], Wendy Stevens[2], Molla Huq[1,2], David Prior[1], Jo Sahhar[3], Gene-Siew Ngian[3], David Celermajer[4], Jane Zochling[5], Susanna Proudman[6,7], Mandana Nikpour[1,2*] and the Australian Scleroderma Interest Group (ASIG)

## Abstract

**Background:** Pulmonary arterial hypertension (PAH) is a leading cause of mortality in systemic sclerosis (SSc). We sought to determine survival, predictors of mortality, and health-related quality of life (HRQoL) related to PAH in a large SSc cohort with PAH.

**Methods:** We studied consecutive SSc patients with newly diagnosed (incident) World Health Organization (WHO) Group 1 PAH enrolled in a prospective cohort between 2009 and 2015. Survival methods were used to determine age and sex-adjusted standardised mortality ratio (SMR) and years of life lost (YLL), and to identify predictors of mortality. HRQoL was measured using the Short form 36 (SF-36) instrument.

**Results:** Among 132 SSc-PAH patients (112 female (85%); mean age 62 ± 11 years), 60 (45.5%) died, with a median (±IQR) survival time from PAH diagnosis of 4.0 (2.2–6.2) years. Median (±IQR) follow up from study enrolment was 3.8 (1.6–5.8) years. The SMR for patients with SSc-PAH was 5.8 (95% CI 4.3–7.8), with YLL of 15.2 years (95% CI 12.3–18.1). Combination PAH therapy had a survival advantage ($p < 0.001$) compared with monotherapy, as did anticoagulation compared with no anticoagulation ($p < 0.003$). Furthermore, combination PAH therapy together with anticoagulation had a survival benefit compared with monotherapy with or without anticoagulation and combination therapy without anticoagulation (hazard ratio 0.28, 95% CI 0.1–0.7). Older age at PAH diagnosis ($p = 0.03$), mild co-existent interstitial lung disease (ILD) ($p = 0.01$), worse WHO functional class ($p = 0.03$) and higher mean pulmonary arterial pressure at PAH diagnosis ($p = 0.001$), and digital ulcers ($p = 0.01$) were independent predictors of mortality.

**Conclusions:** Despite the significant benefits conferred by advanced PAH therapies suggested in this study, the median survival in SSc PAH remains short at only 4 years.

## Background

Systemic sclerosis (SSc) is a multisystem autoimmune disease, which occurs worldwide with a prevalence ranging from 7/million to 489/million and an incidence ranging from 0.6/million/year to 122/million/year [1]. SSc is characterized by vasculopathy and excessive collagen production, leading to skin and internal organ fibrosis. As there are no effective disease-modifying agents or cure, there is substantial morbidity and mortality in this disease.

Despite an improvement over the last three decades, morbidity and mortality in SSc remain high. This is highlighted in a recent large study showing an age and sex adjusted standardised mortality ratio (SMR) of 4.06 for newly diagnosed SSc patients, with 22.4 and 26.0 years of life lost (YLL) in women and men, respectively [2]. Cardiorespiratory manifestations, in particular pulmonary arterial hypertension (PAH), are the leading cause of SSc-related death [3].

PAH occurs with a prevalence of 8–15% in SSc patients [4, 5]. It is characterised by abnormal vascular

* Correspondence: m.nikpour@unimelb.edu.au
[1]Department of Medicine, The University of Melbourne at St Vincent's Hospital, 41 Victoria Parade, Fitzroy, 3065 Melbourne, Victoria, Australia
[2]Department of Rheumatology St Vincent's Hospital, 41 Victoria Parade, Fitzroy, 3065 Melbourne, Victoria, Australia
Full list of author information is available at the end of the article

proliferation and remodelling, vasoconstriction and thrombosis of the pulmonary vasculature, leading to elevated pulmonary vascular resistance (PVR), ultimately resulting in right heart failure and death [6]. PAH is often asymptomatic in the early phases. Once symptomatic, the average life expectancy without treatment has been 2–3 years [6]. Consequently, annual screening with algorithms incorporating transthoracic echocardiogram (TTE) and pulmonary function tests (PFTs) is recommenced [7].

Historically, treatment options for patients with SSc-PAH are limited [6]. However, in the past decade, with the introduction of new advanced pulmonary vasodilator therapies used as monotherapy or combination therapy, improvement in symptoms, function and survival has been demonstrated [8, 9]. Currently, there are seven PAH-specific therapeutic agents with regulatory approval available for use in Australia. These agents target the prostacyclin pathway (epoprostenol and iloprost), nitric oxide pathway (sildenafil and tadalafil) or the endothelin pathway (ambrisentan, macitentan and bosentan). Although not available for use in Australia, Riociguat is available in other countries. In Australia, the Pharmaceutical Benefit Scheme (PBS) subsidises monotherapy with one of these agents if prescribed by a physician in a government-designated PAH treatment centre. Once on therapy, patients must demonstrate stability or improvement relative to baseline parameters on two tests (6 minute walk distance (6MWD), TTE or repeat right heart catheterization (RHC)). The PAH-specific therapy can be changed if the patient fails to maintain stability on the aforementioned tests. Combined PAH-specific therapy, using two or more drugs with different modes of action can only occur by compassionate access through hospital pharmacies or the manufacturers, or at patients' own expense. Anticoagulation in the treatment of PAH is a contentious issue in SSc, with some studies showing a survival benefit in patients with idiopathic PAH (iPAH) and connective tissue disease (CTD)-associated PAH [10, 11] and others not showing a survival benefit [12]. Furthermore anticoagulation in SSc is not without risk.

Despite an improvement in survival with these therapies, survival in SSc-PAH remains well below that of iPAH and CTD-PAH [13] with one-year, two-year and three-year survival of 90%, 78% and 56%, respectively compared with one-year, three-year and five-year survival in idiopathic PAH of 92%, 75% and 66%, respectively [13, 14]. Survival in incident SSc-PAH may be below this as these figures are derived from incident and prevalent SSc-PAH cohort data, introducing a survival bias. Not only does SSc-PAH affect patient survival, it also has a significant impact on patients' functional capacity and health-related quality of life (HRQoL) [15, 16].

We sought to determine survival and HRQoL related to incident SSc-PAH in a large cohort of Australian SSc patients, and to identify predictors of mortality.

## Methods

### Patient cohort

All patients fulfilled either the American College of Rheumatology criteria for SSc or Leroy and Medsger criteria for SSc [17, 18]. Patients included in this analysis were from the Australian Scleroderma Cohort Study (ASCS). The ASCS is a prospective multi-centre study of risk and prognostic factors for cardiopulmonary outcomes in SSc. The ASCS compromises 13 Australian centres and has been approved by the human research ethics committee of each of the participating hospitals (St. Vincent's Hospital, Melbourne Royal Adelaide Hospital, Monash Medical Centre, Royal Perth Hospital, The Queen Elizabeth Hospital, Sunshine Coast Rheumatology, Prince Charles Hospital, John Hunter Hospital, Royal North Shore Hospital, Royal Prince Alfred Hospital, St George Hospital, Canberra Rheumatology and the University of Tasmania). All patients provide written informed consent at recruitment.

### Inclusion and exclusion criteria

All patients were screened annually for PAH with PFTs and TTE. Any patient identified as at high risk of developing PAH, defined as systolic pulmonary arterial pressure ($sPAP_{TTE}$) of at least 50 mmHg and/or diffusing lung capacity for carbon monoxide (DLCO) <50% predicted with forced vital capacity (FVC) >85% predicted, without adequate explanation on high-resolution computer tomography (HRCT) of the chest or ventilation-perfusion (V/Q) scan of lung or both, underwent RHC.

We included all consecutive adult (age >18 years) SSc patients from the ASCS between June 2009 and June 2015, who were diagnosed with World Health Organization (WHO) Group 1 PAH on RHC (mean pulmonary arterial pressure (mPAP) of at least 25 mmHg and pulmonary arterial wedge pressure (PAWP) <15 mmHg) [19].

Patients were excluded if they had WHO Group 2 or 3 pulmonary hypertension or Group 1 PAH but with co-existing ILD with FVC <60% and abnormal HRCT of the chest. V/Q scanning was used to exclude pulmonary hypertension due to chronic thromboembolism.

### Data collection

Patient demographics, clinical variables and cardiac and pulmonary assessments were obtained from the ASCS database. All physical examination and investigation data were collected within one month of the first RHC, before starting pulmonary vasodilator therapy. Clinical manifestations and autoantibody status were defined as present, if ever present from SSc diagnosis. Scleroderma disease onset and disease duration were defined from the date of onset of the first non-Raynaud manifestation. Autoantibodies measured included anti-nuclear antibodies (ANA), antibodies to extractable nuclear antigens (ENA), anti-RNA polymerase III antibodies, anti-Scl-70 antibody and antiphospholipid antibodies (APLA). TTE was performed according to standardised procedures only at tertiary centres with expertise. Pulmonary involvement was assessed by PFTs and HRCT.

Patient-reported outcome measures were collected annually, including the SSc-specific health assessment questionnaire (SHAQ) and the Medical Outcomes Study Short Form-36 (SF-36), a functional assessment tool and a health-related quality of life measurement tool, respectively, which are both well-validated for use in SSc [20]. These patient-reported outcomes (PROs) were chosen as they are collected annually for each patient in the ASCS.

Demographics and clinical manifestations were compared between SSc patients who developed and those that did not develop PAH. Furthermore, PRO scores were compared between these two groups.

### Outcome variables

The principal outcome variable was all-cause mortality. The date of death was recorded. Where data were available, the exact cause of death was recorded. Patient status (alive or dead) at the time of censoring (January 2016) was confirmed by checking with the treating physician and verified against hospital records. The secondary outcome variables that we evaluated were the most recent SHAQ score and the physical and mental component scores of the SF-36 (PCS and MCS) following PAH treatment.

### PAH therapy and other medications

All specific PAH therapies (endothelin receptor antagonists (ERA), phosphodiesterase-5-inhibitors (PDE5) and prostacyclin analogues) and their combinations (monotherapy or combination therapy) were prescribed at the discretion of the managing physician(s) and these medications were recorded at each visit. Use of other therapeutic agents such as anticoagulation (including indication, date of initiation and target international normalised ratio (INR) for warfarin, date and reason for cessation of anticoagulation), antiplatelet agents, hydroxychloroquine (HCQ), mycophenolate mofetil (MMF), hormone replacement therapy (HRT) and proton pump inhibitors (PPIs) were also at the discretion of the managing physician(s) and were recorded.

### Statistical analysis

Patient characteristics at baseline are presented as mean ± standard deviation for continuous variables and as number (percentage) for categorical variables. All-cause mortality was used for analyses because causes of death could not always be confidently ascribed. Kaplan-Meier (K-M) curves were used to estimate survival in patients with SSc-PAH. One-year, two-year and three-year survival were assessed; date of RHC diagnosis of PAH was considered the baseline from which survival was measured. The log-rank and Wilcoxon tests were used to compare survival curves. The SMR was calculated using the observed deaths in our SSc cohort and the expected deaths in the Australian population, which was sourced from the Australian Bureau of Statistics (ABS). YLL was also calculated based on Australian life expectancy using ABS data.

After testing to ensure proportionality of hazard, Cox proportional hazards regression analyses were used to determine univariable and multivariable predictors of mortality. All variables a with $p$ value $\leq 0.1$ in univariable analysis or variables with clinical face validity were selected for inclusion in multivariable analysis. The results were reported as hazard ratios (HR) with accompanying 95% confidence intervals (CI). Mixed effect linear regression was used to identify and quantify determinants of the SHAQ score and the PCS and MCS of the SF-36 following PAH treatment. A two-tailed $p$ value $\leq 0.05$ was considered statistically significant. All statistical analyses were performed using STATA 14.0 (StataCorp LP, College Station, TX, USA).

## Results

### Patient characteristics

Of the 1578 SSc patients enrolled in ASCS, 132 patients were diagnosed with incident Group 1 SSc-PAH and included in this study. Patient characteristics by PAH status are summarised in Additional file 1: Table S1. SSc-PAH patient characteristics and haemodynamic measurements are summarised in Table 1. Our SSc-PAH cohort compromised predominantly women (84.9%) with limited disease subtype (limited cutaneous systemic sclerosis (lcSSc) (68.9%) and a mean (IQR) follow-up duration of 3.8 (1.6–5.8) years since ASCS recruitment. At PAH diagnosis, the mean SSc disease duration was 14.1 ± 11.9 years, with no difference between disease subtypes ($p = 0.40$). Anti-centromere ANA was the most common autoantibody detected (51.6%), followed by APLA (30%). Anti-Scl-70 was infrequent (7.4%).

Despite annual screening, the majority of patients at PAH diagnosis were in WHO functional class II (17.4%) or class III (59.9%) with a mean baseline 6MWD of 326.1 (±105.5) m. Hemodynamics measured at the time of PAH diagnosis showed moderate PAH with an mPAP of 35.6 (± 10.4) mmHg, mean right atrial pressure (mRAP) of 8.3 (± 4.3) mmHg and mean cardiac index (mCI) of 3.2 (± 1.9) L/min/m². Mean DLCO at PAH

**Table 1** Characteristics of patients with SSc-PAH

| Characteristic | Mean (± SD), number (percent) or median (IQR) |
|---|---|
| Total number of patients | 132 |
| Female | 112 (85%) |
| Age at PAH diagnosis, years | 62.3 (± 10.9) |
| Disease duration[a] at PAH diagnosis, years | 14.1 (± 11.9) |
| Status at censoring | |
| Alive | 70 (53.0%) |
| Dead | 60 (45.5%) |
| Withdrawn | 1 (0.8%) |
| Unable to contact | 1 (0.8%) |
| Race | |
| Caucasian | 112 (84.9%) |
| Asian | 6 (4.6%) |
| Aboriginal-Islander | 1 (0.8%) |
| Hispanic | 1 (0.8%) |
| Follow-up duration[b], years (median (IQR)) | 3.8 (1.6–5.8) |
| Survival from PAH diagnosis, years (median (IQR)) | 4.0 (2.2–6.2) |
| Disease duration[a] at PAH diagnosis, years | 14.4 ± 12.1 |
| Disease subtype | |
| Limited | 91 (68.9%) |
| Diffuse | 30 (22.7%) |
| MCTD | 7 (5.3%) |
| Autoantibody status | |
| Anti-centromere pattern ANA | 63 (51.6%) |
| Antiphospholipid antibodies (>ULN) | 33 (30%) |
| RNA polymerase III positive | 8 (11.4%) |
| Scl 70 positive | 9 (7.4%) |
| WHO functional class at time of PAH diagnosis | |
| Class I | 3 (2.3%) |
| Class II | 23 (17.4%) |
| Class III | 79 (59.9%) |
| Class IV | 12 (9.1%) |
| Baseline 6MWD, m | 326.13 (±105.5) |
| Baseline mRAP, mmHg | 8.3 (± 4.3) |
| Baseline mPAP, mmHg | 35.6 (± 10.4) |
| Baseline PAWP, mmHg | 10.5 (± 3.4) |
| Baseline mCI, L/min/m2 | 3.2 (± 1.9) |
| Baseline PVR, Wood units | 8.7 (± 3.8) |
| Presence of a pericardial effusion at PAH diagnosis | 24 (18.2%) |
| Mean DLCO, % predicted mL/min/mmHg | 46.6 (± 13.5) |
| Mean DLCO/VA, % predicted mL/min/mmHg | 56.7 (± 20.2) |
| Medical therapy | |
| Pulmonary vasodilator therapy[c] | |
| Monotherapy | 91 (68.9%) |
| Combination therapy | 41 (31.1%) |
| Warfarin therapy[d] | 37 (28.5%) |

**Table 1** Characteristics of patients with SSc-PAH *(Continued)*

| | |
|---|---|
| Hydroxychloroquine therapy[d] | 12 (9.1%) |
| Antiplatelet agent[c] | 48 (36.9%) |
| Mycophenolate mofetil therapy[d] | 7 (5.4%) |
| Hormone replacement therapy[d] | 16 (12.3%) |
| Proton pump inhibitor[d] | 105 (80.8%) |
| Home oxygen[d] | 28 (21.5%) |

*Abbreviations*: *SSc* systemic sclerosis, *PAH* pulmonary arterial hypertension, *MCTD* mixed connective tissue disease, *ANA* antinuclear antibody, *ULN* upper limit of normal, *WHO* World Health Organization, *6MWD* six-minute walk distance, *mRAP* mean right atrial pressure, *mPAP* mean pulmonary arterial pressure, *PAWP* pulmonary artery wedge pressure, *PVR* peripheral vascular resistance, *mCI* mean cardiac index, *DLCO* diffusing capacity of the lung for carbon monoxide, *DLCO/VA* DLCO adjusted for alveolar volume
[a]Disease duration from first non-Raynaud manifestation
[b]Follow-up duration was defined as years from study enrollment
[c]Monotherapy is treatment with a single PAH-specific therapy. Combination therapy is treatment with more than one specific PAH agent from different classes at one time
[d]Treatment ever following the diagnosis of PAH

diagnosis was 46.6% (± 13.5) predicted, and DLCO corrected for alveolar volume (DLCO/VA) was 56.7% (± 20.2) predicted. A pericardial effusion was present at PAH diagnosis in 18.2% of patients.

### Specific PAH therapy

All patients were treated with at least one specific PAH medication. Considering the Australian PBS regulations, in our study, the majority of patients (68.9%) were treated with monotherapy (including sequential therapy) and 31.1% with combination therapy (two or more advanced PAH therapies at the same time). Six patients received upfront combination therapy at the time of PAH diagnosis. The remainder of patients (31 patients (26.5%)) on combination therapy received additional therapy as "add-on" therapy due to functional deterioration. Medications were altered at physician discretion based on failure of the specific PAH therapy or adverse effects.

As monotherapy, bosentan (68.1%) was the most commonly prescribed drug followed by sildenafil (15.9%). Other monotherapy prescribed and its frequency included ambrisentan (8.7%), macitentan (2.9%) and sitaxentan (before its withdrawal) (2%). The most common combination was bosentan and sildenafil (49.1%) followed by bosentan and tadalafil (12.3%). Supplemental home oxygen was used by 21.5% of patients.

Patients treated with combination therapy compared with monotherapy had more severe PAH reflected by a higher mPAP (39.4 (± 11.9) vs. 34.1 (± 10.4) mmHg, $p = 0.007$), mPVR (6.2 (± 3.2) vs. 4.3 (± 2.5) Wood Units, $p = 0.003$), lower DLCO percent than predicted (41.4 (± 11.8) vs. 49.7 (± 13.5), $p = 0.003$) and the presence of a pericardial effusion (36.6% vs. 11.3%, $p = 0.001$) at PAH diagnosis. There was also a trend towards more digital ulcers (68.3% vs. 49.4%, p = 0.06) at PAH diagnosis in those commenced on combination therapy compared with monotherapy. There was no difference in mRAP ($p = 0.37$), mCI (2.7 (± 0.9) vs. 3.5 (± 2.1) L/min/m2, $p = 0.21$), age at PAH diagnosis ($p = 0.38$) or disease subtype ($p = 0.47$) (Additional file 1: Table S2) in combination versus monotherapy.

### Anticoagulation and other medical therapies

In our cohort of SSc-PAH patients, 28.5% were anticoagulated with warfarin, 36.9% were on an antiplatelet agent, 80.8% on a PPI, 12.3% on HRT, 9.1% on HCQ and 5.4% on MMF (for treatment of their skin disease). Nine patients were on both warfarin and aspirin concurrently.

In those who were treated with warfarin, 54.1% were initiated on warfarin specifically for the treatment of PAH and 45.9% were placed on warfarin for another indication following the diagnosis of PAH. Eleven PAH patients had to cease their anticoagulation after their PAH diagnosis due to complications of warfarin therapy including gastrointestinal bleeding (which accounted for 58.3% of reasons for stopping warfarin) and difficulty monitoring the INR (INR target 1.5–2.5).

Patients on anticoagulation had more severe PAH reflected by higher mPVR (6.2 (± 3.6) vs. 4.5 (± 2.5) Wood units, $p = 0.02$), lower mCI (2.4 (± 0.7) vs. 3.7 (± 1.8) L/min/m2, $p = 0.007$), shorter 6MWD (291.3 (± 100.3) vs. 340.2 (± 104.9) m, $p = 0.01$), lower mDLCO (42.3 (± 12.5) vs. 48.6 (± 13.5) mL/min/mmHg, $p = 0.05$) and the presence of a pericardial effusion (36.1% vs. 12.9%, $p = 0.003$) at PAH diagnosis. There was no difference in mRAP ($p = 0.19$), mPAWP ($p = 0.99$), mDLCO/VA (50.0 (± 21.8) vs. 59.4 (±19.3) mL/min/mmHg, $p = 0.21$), mPAP (39.5 (± 14.1) vs. 34.5 (±9.3) mmHg, age at PAH diagnosis ($p = 0.88$), disease subtype ($p = 0.85$) or presence of digital ulcers ($p = 0.94$) (Additional file 1: Table S2) in those who were anticoagulated compared with those who were not.

Of note, 37.5% of patients (6 patients) with a known history of gastric antral vascular ectasia (GAVE), defined as characteristic vascular lesions seen on endoscopy, but without recent bleeding, were anticoagulated with warfarin, while only 27.2% of patients (31 patients) with PAH and no history of GAVE were anticoagulated. This further highlights that many factors, not only GAVE, influence an individual physician's decision to prescribe anticoagulation in this group of patients.

### Survival in SSc-PAH

SSc-PAH had a significant impact on survival ($p < 0.001$) (Fig. 1). Over a median (± IQR) follow-up of 3.8 (1.6–5.8) years from study enrolment, 60 (45.5%) patients died with a median (± IQR) survival time from PAH diagnosis of 4.0 (2.2–6.2) years. One-year, two-year,

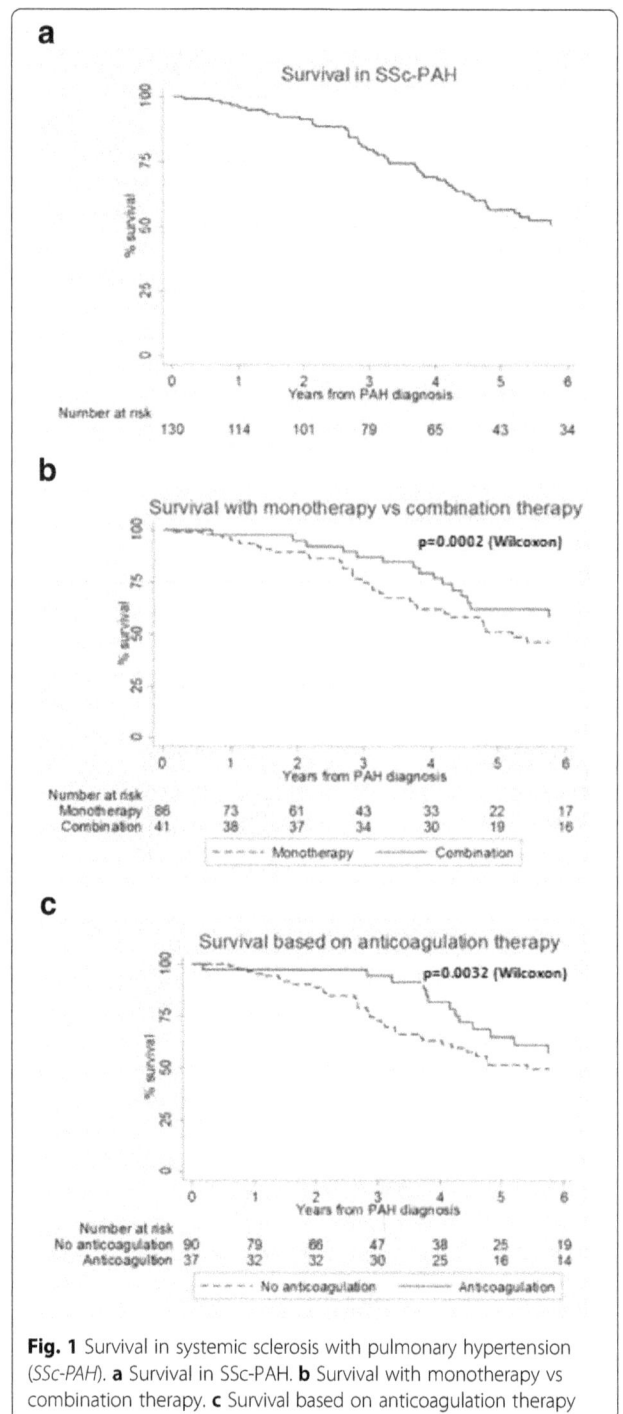

**Fig. 1** Survival in systemic sclerosis with pulmonary hypertension (*SSc-PAH*). **a** Survival in SSc-PAH. **b** Survival with monotherapy vs combination therapy. **c** Survival based on anticoagulation therapy

three-year and five-year survival was 87.8%, 78.3%, 61.7% and 32.2%, respectively. The age and sex adjusted SMR for patients with SSc-PAH compared with mortality in the general population was 5.8 (95% CI 4.3–7.3). The overall YLL for both male and female patients due to SSc-PAH was 15.2 years (95% CI 12.3–18.1). Men had higher YLLs than women (17.0 years (95% CI 7.7–23.0) compared with 15.4 years (13.8–20.3)). The majority of deaths were directly related to PAH (70%), with PAH being a significant contributor in the remaining causes of death (malignancy (13.3%), gastrointestinal complication (10%), renal (3.3%), and infection (3.3%)).

In univariable analysis (Additional file 1: Table S3), factors associated with mortality included the presence of calcinosis ever, worse WHO functional class, shorter 6MWD, higher mPAP and mPVR and lower DLCO at PAH diagnosis, home oxygen use and lack of PPI use.

Independent predictors of mortality in SSc-PAH in multivariable hazards regression analysis are summarised in Table 2. To ensure model stability, a desired ratio of independent-to-outcome variables was set at one to ten. Older age at PAH diagnosis (HR 1.1, 95% CI 1.0–1.1, $p = 0.03$), presence of mild ILD (HR 2.8, 95% CI 1.4–5.6, $p = 0.01$), worse WHO functional class (HR 2.0, 95% CI 1.1–3.9, $p = 0.03$), higher mPAP at PAH diagnosis (HR 1.1, 95% CI 1.0–1.1 mmHg, $p = 0.001$) and presence of digital ulcers ever (HR 3.1, 95% CI 1.4–7.2, $p = 0.01$) were predictive of mortality. The 6MWD was not predictive of mortality. Using PAH monotherapy as our reference group, the addition of anticoagulation to monotherapy was associated with a trend towards survival benefit ($p = 0.09$). Additionally, PAH combination therapy (all cases were a combination of a PDE5 inhibitor and an ERA) also showed a trend towards a survival benefit compared with monotherapy alone ($p = 0.10$). Furthermore, combination PAH therapy, together with anticoagulation, provided the most significant survival advantage with a 72% reduction in mortality compared with pulmonary vasodilator monotherapy alone (HR 0.28, 95% CI 0.1–0.7, $p = 0.01$).

Kaplan-Meier survival curves (Fig. 1) depict the survival advantage with combination PAH therapy

compared with monotherapy ($p < 0.001$) and anticoagulation compared with no anticoagulation ($p < 0.003$). Mean time ($\pm$ SD) to death was longer for patients who were anticoagulated than those who were not (5.4 ($\pm$ 2.5) vs. 3.5 ($\pm$ 2.1), $p = 0.001$) and for those on PAH combination therapy compared to those on monotherapy (5.2 ($\pm$ 2.8) vs. 3.5 ($\pm$ 1.9), $p = 0.02$). There was no difference in mean time to death in those with and without APLA on anticoagulation ($p = 0.68$) or those with limited versus diffuse disease subtypes ($p = 0.56$).

### Patient-reported outcome measures in SSc-PAH

In relation to physical function, patients with SSc-PAH had significantly lower SHAQ scores indicating significant functional limitation in their daily activities compared with SSc patients without PAH (Table 3). Determinants of a better SHAQ score using mixed

**Table 2** Independent predictors of mortality in SSc-PAH determined by multivariable Cox proportional hazard regression analysis

| Characteristic | Hazard ratio (95% CI) | P value |
|---|---|---|
| Age at diagnosis of PAH, years | 1.1 (1.0–1.1) | 0.03 |
| ILD on HRCT (FVC >60%) | 2.8 (1.4–5.6) | 0.01 |
| WHO functional class | 2.0 (1.1–3.9) | 0.03 |
| Pulmonary arterial pressure at PAH diagnosis, mmHg | 1.1 (1.0–1.1) | 0.001 |
| Digital ulcers present ever | 3.1 (1.4–7.2) | 0.01 |
| Specific PAH therapies and anticoagulation | | |
| Vasodilator monotherapy only | reference | reference |
| Vasodilator monotherapy and anticoagulation | 0.39 (0.1–1.2) | 0.09 |
| Vasodilator combination therapy only | 0.49 (0.2–1.2) | 0.10 |
| Vasodilator combination therapy and anticoagulation | 0.28 (0.1–0.7) | 0.01 |

*Abbreviations*: *SSc* systemic sclerosis, *PAH* pulmonary arterial hypertension, *WHO* world health organization, *ILD* interstitial lung disease, *HRCT* high-resolution computer tomography. *FVC* forced vital capacity, *6MWD* six-minute walk distance, *mRAP* mean right atrial pressure, *mPAP* mean pulmonary arterial pressure, *HCQ* hydroxychloroquine

**Table 3** Patient-reported outcomes in patients with SSc-PAH compared to patients with SSc without PAH

| Outcomes | PAH | No PAH | P value |
|---|---|---|---|
| SHAQ domain[a] | | | |
| Patient number | 132 | 1447 | |
| Total score | 3.2 ± 1.7 | 3.3 ± 2.1 | 0.74 |
| Breathing | 4.9 ± 2.5 | 2.3 ± 2.4 | <0.001 |
| Digital ulcers | 1.9 ± 2.5 | 1.4 ± 2.4 | 0.02 |
| Intestinal | 2.8 ± 2.5 | 2.2 ± 2.4 | 0.002 |
| Patient global assessment | 5.1 ± 2.2 | 3.6 ± 2.4 | <0.001 |
| Pain | 3.9 ± 2.6 | 3.4 ± 2.6 | 0.03 |
| Vascular (RP) | 3.3 ± 2.5 | 2.7 ± 2.5 | 0.01 |
| SF-36 domain[b] | | | |
| Physical functioning | 35.7 ± 23.8 | 57.5 ± 28.9 | <0.001 |
| Role limitation, physical | 27.2 ± 39.1 | 49.2 ± 43.4 | <0.001 |
| Role limitation, emotional | 55.9 ± 44.9 | 67.3 ± 40.4 | 0.05 |
| Social functioning | 64.2 ± 27.7 | 70.5 ± 26.9 | 0.07 |
| Mental health | 66.1 ± 21.1 | 68.9 ± 20.2 | 0.28 |
| Energy/vitality | 38.6 ± 22.2 | 47.1 ± 24.1 | 0.01 |
| Bodily pain | 55.3 ± 28.8 | 60.7 ± 27.9 | 0.10 |
| General health perception | 36.6 ± 20.5 | 46.2 ± 22.7 | 0.01 |
| Physical component score | 31.7 ± 8.7 | 38.9 ± 11.6 | <0.001 |
| Mental component score | 46.3 ± 10.7 | 46.3 ± 10.4 | 0.48 |

Systemic sclerosis (SSc)-specific health assessment questionnaire (SHAQ) and Medical Outcomes Study Short Form-36 (SF-36) values are based on the average of all instrument scores collected annually in the database. For those with pulmonary hypertension (PAH), this includes only those scores that have been collected since PAH diagnosis. For those without PAH this includes all scores within the database for these patients. Raynaud's phenomenon (RP)
[a]The SHAQ is a generic instrument measuring functional outcome validated for use in SSc. The score ranges from 0 to 10, with 0 being no functional limitation and 10 being severe functional limitation
[b]The SF-36 form is a 36-item scale that measures eight domains of health status. The final score is standardised to the general population normative score of 50. The final score for each domain lies between 0 and 100, with 0 being the worst possible health and 100 the best possible health

effects linear regression included older age at PAH diagnosis (coefficient −0.1, 95% CI 0.1 to 0.1, $p = 0.02$) while the presence of GIT manifestations (coefficient 0.7, 95% CI −2.7 to −0.1, $p = 0.04$) was associated with a worse SHAQ score over time. Neither PAH-specific therapy nor anticoagulation was associated with a significant change in the total SHAQ score after treatment (Table 4).

SSc-PAH patients had lower HRQoL scores across a number of domains of the SF-36 at PAH diagnosis, particularly in physical functioning, role-physical and general health and vitality, compared with the US normative mean of 50, indicating decreased HRQoL [21] and significantly lower SF-36 scores than SSc patients without PAH (Table 3). Determinants of worse SF-36 PCS using mixed effects linear regression included the presence of digital ulcers (coefficient −3.7, 95% CI −7.2 to

−0.1, $p = 0.04$) and warfarin therapy (coefficient −3.7, 95% CI −7.1 to −0.3; $p = 0.03$). The presence of GIT manifestations was associated with better SF-36 PCS score (coefficient 4.7, 95% CI 0.9 to 8.6, $p = 0.01$). Combination therapy was not associated with a significant change in PCS scores after treatment (Table 4). Determinants of improved SF-36 MCS using mixed effects linear regression included treatment with combination PAH therapy (coefficient 5.2, 95% CI 1.3–9.1, $p = 0.01$) (Table 4).

## Discussion

In our SSc-PAH cohort, the median overall survival was only 4 years with mortality of 45.5% over a follow-up period from study enrolment averaging 3.8 years. The one-year, two-year and three-year survival was 87.8%, 78.3% and 61.7%, respectively. Our results are similar to those in a recent French study (90%, 78% and 50% survival) and lower than in a recent American study (93%, 88% and 75%), both of which also prospectively studied survival in a cohort with incident SSc-PAH [13, 22]. The majority of patients in the American study had New York Heart Association (NYHA) functional Class II disease at PAH diagnosis, which may account for the higher three-year survival in that study. Additionally, combination PAH therapy is more readily available in America than in Australia, which may partly explain the better survival in America. The NYHA functional class at PAH diagnosis was similar to ours in the French study. Mortality rates in the literature vary depending on whether cohorts include patients with incident disease only or a combination of those with incident and prevalent disease, with the potential of underreporting mortality in cohorts with prevalent disease due to survival bias. To our knowledge, this is the first paper to quantify YLL associated with SSc-PAH.

Of concern in our cohort, was that despite annual screening for PAH, the majority of patients were in WHO functional Class III at PAH diagnosis. This may be because our screening algorithm missed patients with early or mild PAH without a markedly elevated RVSP, which may help to explain the relatively advanced stages of PAH observed in our study. It is becoming increasingly recognised that WHO functional class is an independent predictor of mortality [13, 23], as was shown in our cohort. The 6MWD was not associated with mortality in our study despite previous Australian data showing an association [11], suggesting that 6MWD is a nonspecific outcome measure for PAH, and affected by the other complications of SSc.

Another independent predictor of mortality in our cohort included older age at PAH diagnosis, which has been reported in the literature to be a predictor of poor survival, with one study indicating that patients

**Table 4** Impact of PAH-specific therapy and anticoagulation on health-related quality of life scores in SSc-PAH determined through mixed effects linear regression modeling

| Variables | Coefficient (95% CI) | P value |
| --- | --- | --- |
| Determinants of SF-36 physical component score | | |
| Female gender | 0.4 (−3.9, 4.7) | 0.85 |
| Age at PAH diagnosis, years | 0.1 (−0.1, 0.2) | 0.29 |
| Diffuse disease subtype | −0.3 (−3.8, 3.2) | 0.87 |
| Combination therapy | 1.7 (−1.5, 5.0) | 0.29 |
| Anticoagulation therapy | −3.7 (−7.1, −0.3) | 0.03 |
| GIT involvement[a] | 4.7 (0.9, 8.6) | 0.01 |
| Digital ulcers[a] | −3.7 (−7.2, −0.1) | 0.04 |
| Determinants of SF-36 mental component score | | |
| Female gender | −3.5 (−8.6, 1.6) | 0.18 |
| Age at PAH diagnosis, years | −0.1 (−0.2, 0.1) | 0.67 |
| Diffuse disease subtype | −1.1 (−5.2, 3.0) | 0.59 |
| Combination therapy | 5.2 (1.3, 9.1) | 0.01 |
| Anticoagulation therapy | −2.5 (−6.6, 1.6) | 0.22 |
| GIT involvement[a] | −1.6 (−6.2, 2.9) | 0.48 |
| Digital ulcers[a] | 2.8 (−1.5, 7.1) | 0.19 |
| Determinants of SHAQ score | | |
| Female gender | 0.3 (−0.5, 0.9) | 0.46 |
| Age at PAH diagnosis, years | −0.1 (−0.1, −0.1) | 0.02 |
| Diffuse disease subtype | −0.5 (−1.1, 0.2) | 0.13 |
| Combination therapy | −0.3 (−0.8, 0.3) | 0.38 |
| Anticoagulation therapy | 0.3 (−0.3, 0.9) | 0.28 |
| GIT involvement[a] | 0.7 (0.1, 1.3) | 0.03 |
| Digital ulcers[a] | −0.1 (−0.7, 0.5) | 0.79 |

*Abbreviations: SSc* systemic sclerosis, *PAH* pulmonary arterial hypertension, *GIT* gastrointestinal involvement, *SHAQ* scleroderma health assessment questionnaire
[a]Disease manifestations present if present at PAH diagnosis or at any follow-up visit following PAH diagnosis

diagnosed with PAH over the age of 60 years had three-fold higher mortality risk than those diagnosed under 60 years of age [22].

Certain clinical manifestations such as the presence of digital ulcers, calcinosis and telangiectasia have been reported to predict those patients at a higher risk of developing PAH [24–26]. In our study, the presence of digital ulcers was associated with greater mortality in SSc-PAH, which may represent a common underlying pathogenic mechanism involving endothelial dysfunction. Alternatively, it may be an indicator of recurrent infections or perhaps it identifies patients with a more severe vascular phenotype with obliterative vasculopathy involving the macrovasculature and microvasculature, manifesting in PAH, digital ischaemia, ulcers and amputation.

The presence of moderate or severe ILD is in itself a risk factor for death in SSc [27, 28]. In our cohort of patients, we excluded those with severe ILD defined as FVC <60% and HRCT showing ILD, in whom PAH may have occurred secondary to ILD. However, we included patients with Group 1 PAH and co-existent mild ILD defined by FVC > 60% and mild abnormalities or no abnormalities on HRCT. Mild ILD was present in 51 patients (38.6%) in our cohort and was predictive of death in SSc-PAH. We postulate that the co-existence of these two clinical manifestations could be due to shared underlying pathogenic mechanisms leading to a more severe clinical phenotype or that the occurrence in the lung of two independent pathologic conditions increases the risk of death.

There is evolving evidence to suggest that compared with monotherapy, the treatment of PAH with combination therapy is associated with improved survival in PAH. In small randomised trials and observational studies, combination therapy by means of "add-on" PAH therapy has consistently shown a survival benefit in PAH [11, 29, 30]. More recently, the treatment of PAH with upfront combination therapy compared with monotherapy showed not only a survival benefit, but also reduced hospitalisation for worsening PAH and disease progression [9].

Anticoagulation in PAH remains controversial despite some observational studies showing a survival benefit [1, 10]. The survival benefit is particularly apparent in patients with iPAH as shown in the COMPERA study [31], Interestingly, this study did not show a survival benefit with anticoagulation in the non-idiopathic PAH group, which included patients with PAH secondary to CTD, congenital heart disease and porto-pulmonary hypertension. This may be due to the inclusion of these subgroups all within one category [31]. Furthermore, the REVEAL study showed no significant survival advantage in iPAH or SSc-PAH with the addition of anticoagulation [12]. Therefore, we

believe that further research is required to assess the role of anticoagulation in PAH specifically associated with SSc.

Australian data collected between 2002 and 2009 identified a survival advantage with warfarin therapy in patients with CTD-PAH, the majority of whom had SSc [11]. In our study survival was similar if not worse than in patients diagnosed and treated between 2002 and 2009. Two reasons may explain this. First, our study included only patients with incident PAH whereas the previous study included both prevalent and incident cases, thus increasing potential survival bias. Second, survival in SSc-PAH is worse than that in CTD-PAH due to other autoimmune rheumatic diseases such as systemic lupus erythematosus and rheumatoid arthritis, so the overall survival may have been increased due to the inclusion of CTD-PAH "survivors".

There was improved survival in both studies with anticoagulation as an adjunct to PAH therapy compared with PAH therapy in isolation, despite patients on anticoagulation having had more severe PAH at baseline. We propose that the benefit of anticoagulation relates to the prevention of further micro-thrombotic phenomena occurring in the pulmonary vasculature, which likely plays an important role in the underlying pathogenesis of SSc-PAH. The results of our study provide a rationale for a randomised controlled trial evaluating anticoagulation as adjunct therapy in SSc-PAH, which the trial Systemic Sclerosis Pulmonary Hypertension Intervention with Apixaban (SPHInX) (ACTRN12614000418673) aims to resolve.

MMF has been shown to be associated with improved survival in small groups of patients with SSc-PAH [32]. We were not able to replicate these findings as we only had seven patients on MMF in our cohort, which may be explained by the limited availability and expense of MMF in Australia outside of tertiary hospitals until 2015. We were also interested in the relationship between the use of HCQ and survival in SSc-PAH given its anti-platelet effect. Our study identified a trend towards improved survival with HCQ, but this was not statistically significant. With only 12 patients on HCQ in our cohort, our study may not have been sufficiently powered to show such an association.

Not only does SSc-PAH affect survival, it also has a significant impact on patients' functional capacity and HRQoL [15, 16]. Functional limitations, as captured by the SHAQ, were maintained over time with PAH therapy in our cohort, without a significant improvement in any specific domain, which is consistent with the literature [33, 34].

The physical component of HRQoL, as determined by the SF-36 PCS, was also not improved with combination PAH therapy in our cohort. However, combination PAH therapy was associated with a significant improvement in the mental component of HRQoL as measured using the SF-36 MCS. Reduction in mortality with minimal change in HRQoL has been previously reported in patients with CTD-PAH who are on PAH therapy [30, 34, 35]. The lack of improvement in the physical component of HRQoL following PAH treatment may reflect the complex, multifactorial and individual nature of HRQoL, which is impacted upon by a variety of factors that are difficult to measure and adjust for.

We recognise that there are limitations to our study. Lead-time bias may have contributed to the improvement in survival in patients diagnosed as a result of annual screening, with earlier implementation of PAH-specific therapy and anticoagulation. We excluded patients with co-existent PAH and severe ILD to ensure we captured only those patients with Group 1 PAH. Therefore we did not assess whether severe ILD contributed to mortality, although we assume it would, as mild ILD was a predictor of worse survival. In addition, treatment was not randomised; rather, it was prescribed at the individual physician's discretion as there is no standard nationwide protocol for the SSc-PAH treatment.

## Conclusion
Despite advanced therapy, the median survival in SSc-PAH is only 4 years. In our study, the addition of anticoagulation to standard combination therapy was associated with a significant survival advantage, further pointing to mechanisms involving endothelial abnormalities and small vessel thrombosis in the pathogenesis of PAH. Although there was no significant improvement in physical function or in the physical components of HRQoL scores over time, these remained stable with PAH therapy.

## Abbreviations
6MWD: Six-minute walk distance; ABS: Australian Bureau of Statistics; ANA: Anti-nuclear antibodies; APLA: Antiphospholipid antibodies; ASCS: Australian Scleroderma Cohort Study; ASIG: Australian Scleroderma Interest Group; CTD: Connective tissue disease; DLCO: Diffusing lung capacity for carbon monoxide; ENA: Extractable nuclear antigens; ERA: Endothelin receptor antagonists; FVC: Forced vital capacity; GAVE: Gastric antral vascular ectasia; HCQ: Hydroxychloroquine; HRCT: High-resolution computer tomography; HRQoL: Health-related quality of life; HRT: Hormone replacement therapy; ILD: Interstitial lung disease; INR: International normalised ratio; iPAH: Idiopathic pulmonary arterial hypertension; lcSSc: Limited cutaneous systemic sclerosis; Mci: mean cardiac index; MCS: Mental component scores; MMF: Mycophenolate mofetil; mPAP: Mean pulmonary arterial pressure; mRAP: Mean right atrial pressure; NYHA: New York Heart Association; PAH: Pulmonary arterial hypertension; PAWP: Pulmonary arterial wedge pressure; PBS: Pharmaceutical Benefit Scheme; PCS: Physical component scores; PDE5: Phosphodiesterase-5-inhibitors; PFT: Pulmonary function test; PPIs: Proton pump inhibitors; PROs: Patient-reported outcomes; PVR: Pulmonary vascular resistance; RFTs: Respiratory function tests; RHC: Right heart catheterization; RVSP: Right ventricular systolic pressure; SF-36: Medical Outcomes Study Short Form-36; SHAQ: SSc-specific health assessment questionnaire; SMR: Standardised mortality ratio; SSc: Systemic sclerosis/scleroderma; TTE: Transthoracic echocardiogram; V/Q scan: Ventilation-perfusion scan; YLL: Years of life lost

## Acknowledgements
Investigators of the Australian Scleroderma Interest Group (ASIG): we would like to acknowledge all investigators of the ASIG, including Catherine Hill, Adelaide, South Australia; Sue Lester, Adelaide, South Australia; Peter Nash, Sunshine Coast, Queensland; Gian Ngian, Melbourne Victoria; Mandana Nikpour, Melbourne, Victoria; Susanna Proudman, Adelaide, South Australia; Maureen Rischmueller, Adelaide, South Australia; Janet Roddy, Perth, Western Australia; Joanne Sahhar, Melbourne, Victoria; Wendy Stevens, Melbourne, Victoria; Gemma Strickland, Geelong, Victoria; Vivek Thakkar, New South Wales, Jenny Walker, Adelaide, South Australia; Jane Zochling, Hobart, Tasmania.

## Funding
This work was supported by Scleroderma Australia, Arthritis Australia, Actelion Australia, Bayer, CSL Biotherapies, GlaxoSmithKline Australia and Pfizer. Dr Morrisroe holds an NHMRC Scholarship (APP1113954). Dr Nikpour holds an NHMRC Fellowship (APP1071735).

## Authors' contributions
KM: study design, data analysis, interpretation of results and preparation of manuscript. WS: study design, data collection, interpretation of results and preparation of manuscript. MH: data analysis and preparation of manuscript. DP: data collection, interpretation of results and preparation of manuscript. JS: data collection, interpretation of results and preparation of manuscript. GN: data collection, interpretation of results and preparation of manuscript. DC: data collection, interpretation of results and preparation of manuscript. JZ: data collection, interpretation of results and preparation of manuscript. SP: data collection, interpretation of results and preparation of manuscript. MN: study design, data collection, data analysis, interpretation of results and preparation of manuscript. All authors read and approved the final manuscript.

## Competing interests
The authors declare that they have no competing interests. SP, MN and WS have received grants from Actelion Pharmaceutical Auststralia, GlascoSmithKline and Scleorderma Australia. DP reports personal fees and non-financial support from Actelion Australia. The other authors declare that they have no competing interests.

## Ethics approval and consent to participate
All patients provide written informed consent for collection of de-identified data, chart review and storage of serum and DNA for use in research studies including publications. All human research ethics committees of the participating sites have approved the ASCS (Royal Perth Hospital in Western Australia, Royal Adelaide and The Queen Elizabeth Hospitals in South Australia, Sunshine Coast Rheumatology and Prince Charles Hospital in Queensland, John Hunter, Royal Prince Alfred, Royal North Shore and St George Hospitals in New South Wales, Canberra Rheumatology in the Australian Capital territory, St Vincent's Hospital and Monash Medical Centre in Victoria and The Menzies Institute in Tasmania). Ethics Reference HREC-A 02/007.

## Author details
Department of Medicine, The University of Melbourne at St Vincent's Hospital, 41 Victoria Parade, Fitzroy, 3065 Melbourne, Victoria, Australia. [2]Department of Rheumatology St Vincent's Hospital, 41 Victoria Parade, Fitzroy, 3065 Melbourne, Victoria, Australia. [3]Monash University and Monash Health, 246 Clayton Road, Clayton 3168, Victoria, Australia. [4]The University of Sydney at Royal Prince Alfred Hospital, Missenden Road, Camperdown 2050, NSW, Australia. [5]Department of Rheumatology, Menzies Institute for Medical Research, Hobart, Australia. [6]Rheumatology Unit, Royal Adelaide Hospital, North Terrace, Adelaide, SA 5000, Australia. [7]Discipline of Medicine, University of Adelaide, Adelaide, SA 5000, Australia.

## References

1. Chifflot H, Fautrel B, Sordet C, Chatelus E, Sibilia J. Incidence and Prevalence of Systemic Sclerosis: A systematic literature review. Semin Arthritis Rheum. 2008;37(4):223–35.
2. Hao Y, Hudson M, Baron M, Carreira P, Stevens W, Rabusa C, Tatibouet S, Carmona L, Joven BE, Huq M, et al. Early Mortality in a Multinational Systemic Sclerosis Inception Cohort. Arthritis Rheumatol. 2017;69(5):1067–77.
3. Tyndall AJ, Bannert B, Vonk M, Airo P, Cozzi F, Carreira PE, Bancel DF, Allanore Y, Muller-Ladner U, Distler O, et al. Causes and risk factors for death in systemic sclerosis: a study from the EULAR Scleroderma Trials and Research (EUSTAR) database. Ann Rheum Dis. 2010;69(10):1809–15.
4. Hao Y, Thakkar V, Stevens W, Morrisroe K, Prior D, Rabusa C, Youssef P, Gabbay E, Roddy J, Walker J, et al. A comparison of the predictive accuracy of three screening models for pulmonary arterial hypertension in systemic sclerosis. Arthritis Res Ther. 2015;17(1):7.
5. Muangchan C, Baron M, Pope J. The 15% rule in scleroderma: the frequency of severe organ complications in systemic sclerosis. A systematic review. J Rheumatol. 2013;40(9):1545–56.
6. D'Alonzo GE, Barst RJ, Ayres SM, Bergofsky EH, Brundage BH, Detre KM, Fishman AP, Goldring RM, Groves BM, Kernis JT, et al. Survival in patients with primary pulmonary hypertension. Results from a national prospective registry. Ann Intern Med. 1991;115(5):343–9.
7. Galie N, Humbert M, Vachiery JL, Gibbs S, Lang I, Torbicki A, Simonneau G, Peacock A, Vonk Noordegraaf A, Beghetti M, et al. 2015 ESC/ERS guidelines for the diagnosis and treatment of pulmonary hypertension. Revista espanola de cardiologia (English ed). 2016;69(2):177.
8. Barst RJ, Gibbs JS, Ghofrani HA, Hoeper MM, McLaughlin VV, Rubin LJ, Sitbon O, Tapson VF, Galie N. Updated evidence-based treatment algorithm in pulmonary arterial hypertension. J Am Coll Cardiol. 2009;54(1 Suppl):S78–84.
9. Galie N, Barbera JA, Frost AE, Ghofrani HA, Hoeper MM, McLaughlin VV, Peacock AJ, Simonneau G, Vachiery JL, Grunig E, et al. Initial use of ambrisentan plus tadalafil in pulmonary arterial hypertension. N Engl J Med. 2015;373(9):834–44.
10. Said K. Anticoagulation in pulmonary arterial hypertension: Contemporary data from COMPERA registry. Glob Cardiol Sci Pract. 2014;2014(2):48–52.
11. Ngian G, Nikpour M, Byron J, Tran A, Roddy J, Minson R, Hill C, Chow K, Sahhar J, Stevens W, et al. Survival in Australian patients with connective tissue disease-associated pulmonary arterial hypertension. Intern Med J. 2011;41:12.
12. Preston IR, Roberts KE, Miller DP, Sen GP, Selej M, Benton WW, Hill NS, Farber HW. Effect of warfarin treatment on survival of patients with pulmonary arterial hypertension (PAH) in the Registry to Evaluate Early and Long-Term PAH Disease Management (REVEAL). Circulation. 2015;132(25):2403–11.
13. Launay D, Sitbon O, Hachulla E, Mouthon L, Gressin V, Rottat L, Clerson P, Cordier JF, Simonneau G, Humbert M. Survival in systemic sclerosis-associated pulmonary arterial hypertension in the modern management era. Ann Rheum Dis. 2013;72(12):1940–6.
14. Thenappan T, Shah SJ, Rich S, Tian L, Archer SL, Gomberg-Maitland M. Survival in pulmonary arterial hypertension: a reappraisal of the NIH risk stratification equation. Eur Respir J. 2010;35(5):1079–87.
15. Shafazand S, Goldstein MK, Doyle RL, Hlatky MA, Gould MK. Health-related quality of life in patients with pulmonary arterial hypertension. Chest. 2004;126(5):1452–9.
16. Matura LA, McDonough A, Carroll DL. Health-related quality of life and psychological states in patients with pulmonary arterial hypertension. J Cardiovasc Nurs. 2014;29(2):178–84.
17. Preliminary criteria for the classification of systemic sclerosis (scleroderma). Subcommittee for scleroderma criteria of the American Rheumatism Association Diagnostic and Therapeutic Criteria Committee. Arthritis Rheum 1980, 23(5):581–90
18. LeRoy EC, Medsger Jr TA. Criteria for the classification of early systemic sclerosis. J Rheumatol. 2001;28(7):1573–6.
19. Simonneau G, Gatzoulis MA, Adatia I, Celermajer D, Denton C, Ghofrani A, Gomez Sanchez MA, Kumar RK, Landzberg M, Machado RF, et al. Updated clinical classification of pulmonary hypertension. Turk Kardiyol Dern Ars. 2014;42 Suppl 1:45–54.
20. Johnson SR, Glaman DD, Schentag CT, Lee P. Quality of life and functional status in systemic sclerosis compared to other rheumatic diseases. J Rheumatol. 2006;33(6):1117–22.
21. Maglinte GA, Hays RD, Kaplan RM. US general population norms for telephone administration of the SF-36v2. J Clin Epidemiol. 2012;65(5):497–502.
22. Chung L, Domsic RT, Lingala B, Alkassab F, Bolster M, Csuka ME, Derk C, Fischer A, Frech T, Furst DE, et al. Survival and predictors of mortality in systemic sclerosis-associated pulmonary arterial hypertension: outcomes from the pulmonary hypertension assessment and recognition of outcomes in scleroderma registry. Arthritis Care Res (Hoboken). 2014;66(3):489–95.
23. Ngian GS, Stevens W, Prior D, Gabbay E, Roddy J, Tran A, Minson R, Hill C, Chow K, Sahhar J, et al. Predictors of mortality in connective tissue disease-associated pulmonary arterial hypertension: a cohort study. Arthritis Res Ther. 2012;14:R213.
24. Shah AA, Wigley FM, Hummers LK. Telangiectases in scleroderma: a potential clinical marker of pulmonary arterial hypertension. J Rheumatol. 2010;37(1):98–104.
25. Valenzuela A, Chung L. Calcinosis: pathophysiology and management. Curr Opin Rheumatol. 2015;27(6):542–8.
26. Karakulak UNHV, Maharjan N, Kaya EB, Kilic L, Akdoton A, Tokgozotlu L. Predictors of mortality in scleroderma patients with pulmonary hypertension. J Am Coll Cardiol. 2013;62(14):C17.
27. Bussone G, Mouthon L. Interstitial lung disease in systemic sclerosis. Autoimmun Rev. 2011;10(5):248–55.
28. Mathai SC, Hummers LK, Champion HC, Wigley FM, Zaiman A, Hassoun PM, Girgis RE. Survival in pulmonary hypertension associated with the scleroderma spectrum of diseases: impact of interstitial lung disease. Arthritis Rheum. 2009;60(2):569–77.
29. Simonneau G, Rubin LJ, Galie N, Barst RJ, Fleming TR, Frost AE, Engel PJ, Kramer MR, Burgess G, Collings L, et al. Addition of sildenafil to long-term intravenous epoprostenol therapy in patients with pulmonary arterial hypertension: a randomized trial. Ann Intern Med. 2008;149(8):521–30.
30. Ghofrani H-A, Galiè N, Grimminger F, Grünig E, Humbert M, Jing Z-C, Keogh AM, Langleben D, Kilama MO, Fritsch A, et al. Riociguat for the treatment of pulmonary arterial hypertension. N Engl J Med. 2013;369(4):330–40.
31. Olsson KM, Delcroix M, Ghofrani HA, Tiede H, Huscher D, Speich R, Grunig E, Staehler G, Rosenkranz S, Halank M, et al. Anticoagulation and survival in pulmonary arterial hypertension: results from the Comparative, Prospective Registry of Newly Initiated Therapies for Pulmonary Hypertension (COMPERA). Circulation. 2014;129(1):57–65.
32. Virginia S, Aryeh F. Mycophenolate Mofetil Use In Pulmonary Hypertension In Systemic Sclerosis. Observations From The PHAROS Cohort. In: C54 treatment of pulmonary hypertension. Am J Respir Crit Care Med. 2014;189: A4790.
33. Kowal-Bielecka O, Avouac J, Pittrow D, Huscher D, Behrens F, Denton CP, Foeldvari I, Humbert M, Matucci-Cerinic M, Nash P, et al. Analysis of the validation status of quality of life and functional disability measures in pulmonary arterial hypertension related to systemic sclerosis: results of a systematic literature analysis by the expert panel on outcomes measures in pulmonary arterial hypertension related to systemic sclerosis (EPOSS). J Rheumatol. 2011;38(11):2419–27.
34. Denton CP, Pope JE, Peter HH, Gabrielli A, Boonstra A, van den Hoogen FH, Riemekasten G, De Vita S, Morganti A, Dolberg M, et al. Long-term effects of bosentan on quality of life, survival, safety and tolerability in pulmonary arterial hypertension related to connective tissue diseases. Ann Rheum Dis. 2008;67(9):1222–8.
35. Taichman DB, Shin J, Hud L, Archer-Chicko C, Kaplan S, Sager JS, Gallop R, Christie J, Hansen-Flaschen J, Palevsky H. Health-related quality of life in patients with pulmonary arterial hypertension. Respir Res. 2005;6(1):92.

# Limited cutaneous systemic sclerosis skin demonstrates distinct molecular subsets separated by a cardiovascular development gene expression signature

Emma C. Derrett-Smith[1,2], Viktor Martyanov[3], Cecilia B. Chighizola[4], Pia Moinzadeh[5], Corrado Campochiaro[1], Korsa Khan[1], Tammara A. Wood[3], Pier Luigi Meroni[4], David J. Abraham[1], Voon H. Ong[1], Robert Lafyatis[6], Michael L. Whitfield[3] and Christopher P. Denton[1*]

## Abstract

**Background:** Systemic sclerosis (SSc; scleroderma) is an uncommon autoimmune rheumatic disease characterised by autoimmunity, vasculopathy and fibrosis. Gene expression profiling distinguishes scleroderma from normal skin, and can detect different subsets of disease, with potential to identify prognostic biomarkers of organ involvement or response to therapy. We have performed gene expression profiling in skin samples from patients with limited cutaneous SSc (lcSSc).

**Methods:** Total RNA was extracted from clinically uninvolved skin biopsies of 15 patients with lcSSc and 8 healthy controls (HC). Gene expression profiling was performed on a DNA oligonucleotide microarray chip. Differentially expressed genes (DEG) were identified using significance analysis of microarrays (SAM). Functional enrichment analysis of gene signatures was done via g:Profiler.

**Results:** There were 218 DEG between lcSSc and HC samples (false discovery rate <10%): 181/218 DEG were upregulated in lcSSc samples. Hierarchical clustering of DEG suggested the presence of two separate groups of lcSSc samples: "limited 1" and "limited 2". The limited-1 group (13 samples, 10 unique patients) showed upregulation of genes involved in cell adhesion, cardiovascular system (CVS) development, extracellular matrix and immune and inflammatory response. The CVS development signature was of particular interest as its genes showed very strong enrichment in response to wounding, response to transforming growth factor (TGF)-β and kinase cascade. Neither limited-2 samples (six samples, five unique patients) nor HC samples showed functional enrichment. There were no significant differences in demographic or clinical parameters between these two groups. These results were confirmed using a second independent cohort.

**Conclusions:** Our study suggests the presence of molecular subsets in lcSSc based on gene expression profiling of biopsies from uninvolved skin. This may reflect important differences in pathogenesis within these patient groups. We identify differential expression of a subset of genes that relate to CVS and are enriched in fibrotic signalling. This may shed light on mechanisms of vascular disease in SSc. The enrichment in profibrotic profile suggests that dysregulated gene expression may contribute to vasculopathy and fibrosis in different disease subsets.

**Keywords:** Scleroderma, Genetics, Systemic sclerosis, Vasculopathy, Microarray

---

* Correspondence: c.denton@ucl.ac.uk
[1]Centre for Rheumatology and Connective Tissue Diseases, University College London, London, UK
Full list of author information is available at the end of the article

# Background

Systemic sclerosis (SSc; scleroderma) represents a major clinical challenge and offers insight into fundamental processes relating to autoimmunity, fibrosis and vascular injury and pathology. It is an uncommon immune-mediated rheumatic disease with a very high clinical burden, high mortality and limited treatment options [1, 2] and provides a model for more common forms of organ-based fibrosis in the lung, liver and kidney. Recent observational cohort studies have highlighted remarkable clinical diversity in terms of pattern and extent of skin and internal organ involvement, clinical outcome and response to therapy [3–5]. Most current and emerging treatment strategies focus on intensive immunosuppression though greater understanding of the biology of disease outcomes, in particular mechanisms that determine improvement in skin and organ-based disease, may help to personalize treatment strategies more effectively [6].

The limited cutaneous subset of SSc (lcSSc) is characterised by less severe and extensive skin fibrosis but patients can develop major internal organ complications and the vascular manifestations of SSc, particularly pulmonary arterial hypertension and digital ulceration, are prominent in this subset [3]. Detailed gene expression analysis in SSc biopsies has recently been used to define molecular intrinsic subsets of the disease and to provide mechanistic insight into the pathobiology [7–14]. Interestingly, clinically uninvolved skin in the more extensive diffuse cutaneous subset of SSc has closely replicated gene expression signatures compared with biopsies from clinically involved skin [7] and a number of vasoactive genes have been identified in this way in skin from patients with the limited subset, who cluster separately from healthy controls and from patients with diffuse disease [7]. It has been shown that lesional and non-lesional lcSSc biopsies consistently cluster together and show concordance in their deregulated pathways [7, 14]. The numbers of patients with limited disease in those studies are small but the results are consistent. On this basis we sought to develop greater understanding about the gene expression abnormalities in the more prevalent lcSSc subset through detailed transcriptional analysis of skin biopsies taken from uninvolved forearm skin. We hypothesise that this may give valuable insight into the key pathogenetic processes underlying the disease and also provide potential for defining and characterising molecular subsets of lcSSc. Since the molecular subsets of SSc may also inform clinical decision-making and treatment selection, there may be additional value from extending this concept more broadly into lcSSc.

In this study, we demonstrate differential gene expression in a cohort of lcSSc patients and healthy controls and describe a distinct lcSSc subgroup not identifiable by clinical or serological assessment showing enrichment in cell adhesion, cardiovascular system (CVS) development and extracellular matrix genes. We confirm our findings in a second independent cohort of samples. The CVS development signature was significantly different between both subgroups of limited patients and a control group.

# Methods

## Inclusion criteria and study participants

Demographic information, clinical history including organ involvement, other diagnoses and extent of skin involvement, autoantibody profiles and treatments were retrieved from medical notes or obtained at the time of skin biopsy. Diagnosis of SSc was made according to the 2013 American College of Rheumatologists (ACR)/European League Against Rheumatism (EULAR) classification criteria and assignment to the limited cutaneous subset reflected the distribution and extent of skin thickening at the time of biopsy together with other typical disease characteristics [15]. Autoantibodies were measured in an accredited institutional autoimmune serology laboratory using validated commercial tests with appropriate quality control and blinded assessment of the results at the time of biopsy. In brief, antinuclear antibody (ANA) pattern was screened by indirect immunofluorescence using an HEp-2 cell substrate and further characterisation of defined extractable nuclear antigen (ENA) was by counterimmunoelectrophoresis for anti-ENA using soluble extracts from human spleen and rabbit thymus acetone powder (Pelfreez Biologicals, Rogers, AR, USA) as antigen. All patients included in this study signed informed consent for their clinical and laboratory data to be used in this clinical research project.

## Sample collection

Forearm 4-mm skin punch biopsies were performed both in patients with lcSSc and in healthy controls, and were stored for extraction in RNAlater$^{TM}$ RNA stabilisation reagent (Ambion, Austin, TX, USA) at 4 °C overnight followed by longer-term storage at -70 °C. To avoid a potential confounding effect of different degrees of skin thickening or fibrosis, biopsy sites were selected from skin that was not clinically involved. There were no changes in pigmentation or dryness.

## Microarray processing

Tissue homogenization was performed using Qiagen TissueLyser II. RNA purification was carried out in a QIAcube with Qiagen RNeasy Fibrous Tissue Mini Kit (Qiagen, Gaithersburg, MD, USA). The Agilent 2100 Bioanalyzer (Agilent, Santa Clara, CA, USA) was used to assess the RNA integrity of samples with numbers >7. RNA concentration was measured with Thermo Scientific NanoDrop 2000 Spectrophotometer (Wilmington, DE,

USA). A measure of 200 ng of total RNA was amplified and labelled with Agilent's Quick-Amp Labelling Kit. Cy3-labelled samples and Cy5-labelled Universal Human Reference RNA (Stratagene, La Jolla, CA, USA) were co-hybridized to Agilent's Human Genome (4 × 44 K) Microarrays (G4112F). Data were log2 lowess-normalised and filtered for probes with intensity ≥1.5-fold over local background in Cy3 or Cy5 channels. Data were multiplied by -1 to convert them to log2(Cy3/Cy5) ratios. Probes with >20% missing data were excluded.

### Gene expression data pre-processing

Expression data were pre-processed using GenePattern [16] modules with default settings unless stated otherwise. Missing values were imputed using the ImputeMissingValuesKNN module. Expression data were collapsed from probes to unique genes using the CollapseDataset module with the Agilent 4 × 44 K chip platform. As microarrays were processed in three separate batches, batch bias was adjusted for using GenePattern implementation of ComBat [17] by means of parametric prior method and information about lcSSc samples and controls as a covariate. Batch bias was assessed before and after ComBat using guided principal component analysis (gPCA) [18]. Expression data were adjusted by median-centering genes in Cluster 3.0 [19].

### Differential expression and functional enrichment analysis

Differentially expressed genes were identified using significance analysis of microarrays (SAM) [20]. Two-class unpaired response type was used for comparing two groups and multiclass response type was used for comparing three groups. The number of permutations was set to 500. Expression data for significantly differentially expressed genes were hierarchically clustered in Cluster 3.0 and visualized in Java TreeView [21], version 1.1.6r4. Functional enrichment analysis of gene signatures was done using g:Profiler [22] with the following settings: maximum size of functional category was set to 3500, default multiple testing correction method (g:SCS significance threshold) was used and regulatory motif and protein-protein interaction databases were excluded from the analyses.

## Results

### Subject selection and clinical characteristics

There were 23 subjects included in the discovery cohort: 15 patients with lcSSc and 8 healthy controls. The study samples were collected and analysed in two stages, first in 10 biopsies from patients with lcSSc and from 5 healthy controls that generated the initial CVS signature, and then in samples from an extended cohort with an additional 6 patients with lcSSc and 3 healthy controls. These later samples were collected independently of the first set of samples.

Demographics, clinical characteristics, organ-based disease and therapies are listed in Table 1. The demographics of the control group were broadly similar to patients in terms of age, sex and ethnicity and these are also representative of the single-centre cohort that included the sample population. All patients had established lcSSc with minimum disease duration of 2 years, and most had had the condition for more than 10 years at the time of biopsy. Patients included in the study retained the subset designation according to their early stage disease and therefore no patients who would previously have been designated as having 'diffuse' SSc or those who had higher skin scores in the past were included. Serological findings were again representative of a cohort of lcSSc patients but kept purposefully broad: six patients had centromere pattern staining on indirect immunofluorescence (IIF) for ANA, and four had scl-70 reactivity. Two patients had overlap Ro antibodies and two were ANA-negative; one had serological features of lupus with high double-stranded (ds) DNA antibodies and low C4. There were 6/15 patients with digital ulcers at the time of biopsy and the majority took therapy for a vascular complication, either for significant Raynaud's phenomenon or for digital ulceration. No patients from this cohort had a diagnosis of pulmonary arterial hypertension and none had had a scleroderma renal crisis or myositis. Four had interstitial lung disease and three (more than may be expected) had an overlap diagnosis of inflammatory arthritis: these two latter diagnoses resulted in the significant use of immunosuppressive medications compared with most cohorts of lcSSc patients. The broad but characteristic range of clinical and serological features demonstrated in this cohort allowed us to identify pathogenic factors that may exist at the gene expression level but that cannot be explained by standard outpatient assessment.

### Overview of gene expression profiles

There were 218 differentially expressed genes (DEG) between lcSSc and healthy control samples (false discovery rate (FDR) <10%). Of these 218 genes, 181 (83%) were upregulated in lcSSc samples and were significantly enriched in several terms related to the extracellular matrix (ECM), e.g. ECM organisation and ECM component and response to growth factor, tissue development and regulation of the serine/threonine kinase signalling pathway. This gene signature included genes previously implicated in the pathogenesis of SSc such as *ANGPT2*, *CD163*, *COMP*, *CTGF* and *TIMP2*, among others (Fig. 1a). The full list of significantly differentially expressed genes is available in Additional file 1.

Even though we specifically asked for genes differentially expressed between lcSSc samples and healthy controls, 6 lcSSc samples (5 unique patients) clustered with controls, whereas the remaining 13 lcSSc samples (10 unique

**Table 1** Demographic, clinical and serological characteristics of lcSSc patients and healthy controls

|  |  | Control subjects ($n = 8$) | All LcSSc patients ($n = 15$) |
|---|---|---|---|
| Age, median (range) years |  | 53 (29–70) | 62 (28–15) |
| Sex, N (%) female |  | 4 (50) | 12 (80) |
| Race, N (%) Caucasian |  | 7 (87.5) | 10 (100) |
| MRSS, median (range) |  |  | 6 (3–10) |
| Disease duration from first non-Raynaud's symptom, median (range) years |  |  | 14 (2–40) |
| ANA primary pattern, N (%) patients | Homogenous |  | 4 (27) |
|  | Speckled |  | 2 (13) |
|  | Centromere |  | 6 (40) |
|  | Nucleolar |  | 1 (7) |
| SSc-specific antibodies | Scl-70 |  | 4 (27) |
|  | RNA pol III |  | 0 |
| Vasculopathy, N (%) patients | Digital ulcers |  | 6 (40) |
|  | PAH |  | 0 |
|  | Renal crisis |  | 0 |
| Interstitial lung disease, N (%) |  |  | 4 (27) |
| Inflammatory arthritis, N (%) |  |  | 3 (20) |
| Vascular therapies, N (%) patients | ARB |  | 10 (66) |
|  | Ca channel antagonist |  | 4 (27) |
|  | Iloprost |  | 4 (27) |
|  | PDE5 inhibitor |  | 3 (20) |
| Immunosuppressive therapies, N (%) patients | PDN |  | 4 (27) |
|  | MMF |  | 3 (20) |
|  | MTX |  | 2 (13) |
|  | AZA |  | 1 (7) |
|  | HCQ |  | 3 (20) |

ANA antinuclear antibodies, SSc systemic sclerosis, MRSS modified Rodnan skin score, PAH pulmonary arterial hypertension, ARB angiotensin receptor blocker, PDE cGMP-regulated phosphodiesterase, MTX methotrexate, HCQ hydroxychloroquine, PDN prednisolone, AZA azathioprine

patients) formed a distinct cluster (Fig. 1b). We designated 13 lcSSc samples as the "limited 1" group and 6 lcSSc samples as the "limited 2" group. The expression of 181 genes significantly upregulated in lcSSc vs. healthy controls was also significantly different in all pairwise comparisons between limited 1, limited 2 and control samples (Fig. 1c). Mean ± standard error of the mean expression values for 181 gene signatures were as follows: $0.23 \pm 0.01$ for limited 1, $-0.02 \pm 0.03$ for limited 2 and $-0.46 \pm 0.03$ for healthy control samples.

Since comparison between lcSSc and controls was suggestive of the presence of two lcSSc groups, we performed multiclass SAM to identify DEG between limited-1, limited-2 and healthy control samples: 807 genes were differentially expressed between these three groups (FDR <10%). Again, limited-2 samples clustered with controls and separately from the limited-1 group (Fig. 2; see Additional file 2 for the full gene list).

Genes with significantly increased expression in either the limited-2 group or in healthy controls were not functionally enriched. Genes with significantly increased expression in samples from the limited-1 group (475/807, 58.9%) displayed very strong enrichment in functional terms related to ECM and vasculature development ($p < 10^{-10}$) and strong enrichment in cell adhesion, response to growth factor, mitogen-activated protein kinase (MAPK) cascade and response to wounding ($p < 10^{-5}$), among others. Enrichment in immune signalling was comparatively weak (e.g. $p = 0.0183$ for immune system process and $p = 0.0208$ for inflammatory response). The entire g:Profiler output is listed in Additional file 3.

For the limited-1 group, the term with the most significant functional enrichment was cardiovascular system development ($p = 3.01 \times 10^{-14}$): 70 out of 475 genes with increased expression in limited-1 samples were involved in this biological process. This set of 70 genes essentially recaptured many of the biological themes observed in the bigger limited-1 gene expression signature. For example, there was very strong enrichment in angiogenesis, response to growth factor and cell proliferation ($p < 10^{-10}$)

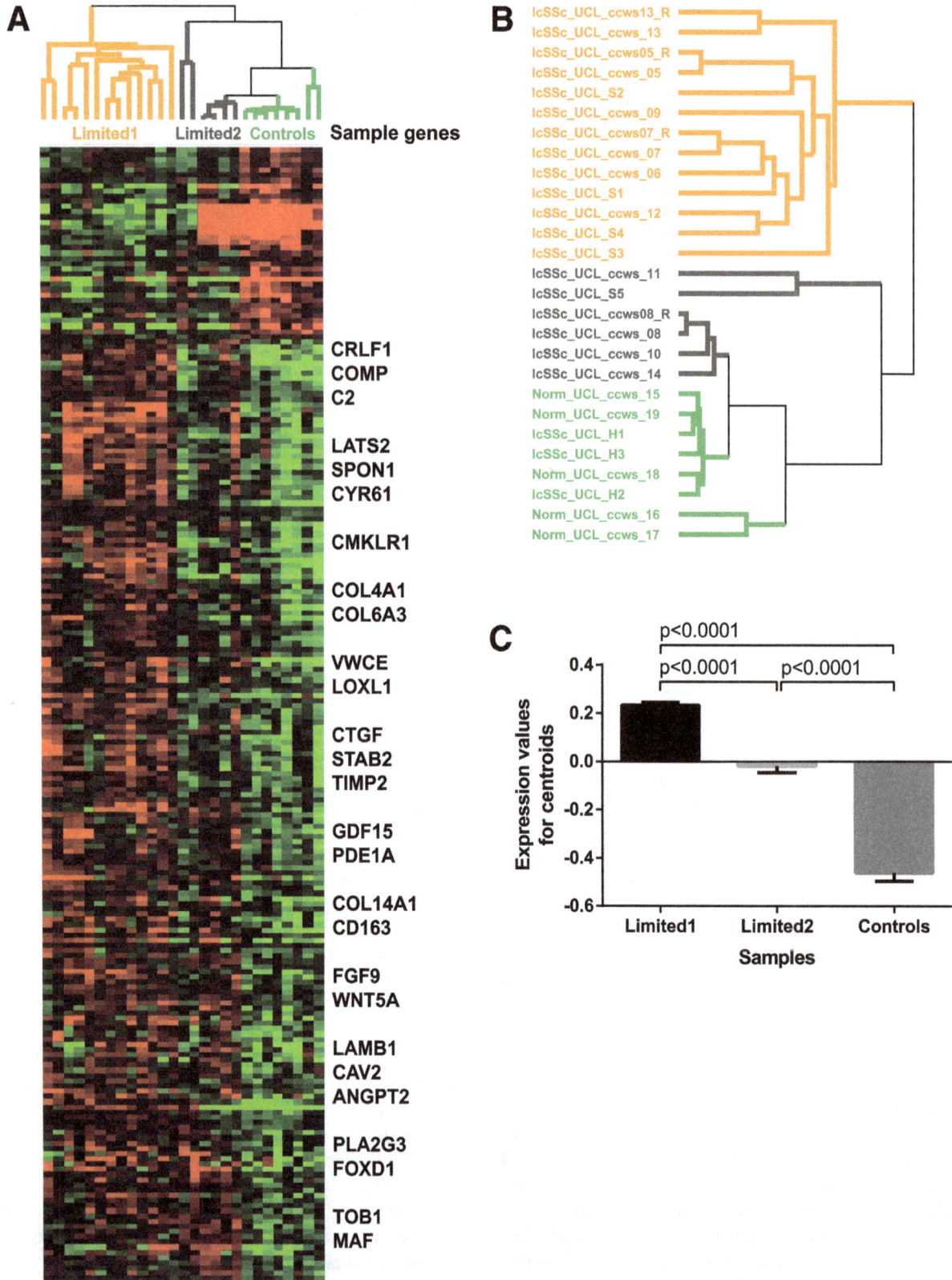

**Fig. 1** (See legend on next page.)

(See figure on previous page.)
**Fig. 1** Gene expression in whole skin samples from patients with limited cutaneous systemic sclerosis (*lcSSc*) and healthy controls (*Controls*). **a** Heatmap: *red* indicates upregulation, *green* indicates downregulation. Gene expression in the *limited 1* subgroup of samples from patients with lcSSc differs markedly from both the *limited 2* subgroup and from healthy controls, which shared similar gene expression patterns. Sample genes of interest are listed. **b** Hierarchical clustering of genes distinguishing lcSSc samples from healthy control samples identifies three distinct clusters, termed limited 1, limited 2 and healthy control. *Norm* Normal. **c** Pairwise comparisons between limited 1, limited 2 and controls. Data are plotted as mean with SEM values. P values were derived from the Kruskal-Wallis test followed by Dunn's multiple comparisons test

and strong enrichment in ECM, cartilage development, MAPK cascade, cell adhesion and response to wounding ($p < 10^{-5}$), among others. It was also strongly enriched in response to transforming growth factor (TGF)-β ($p = 2.87 \times 10^{-7}$, 12/70 genes). Additional file 4 contains the entire g:Profiler output for this analysis. There were no significant differences in demographic, clinical or serological parameters that correlated with limited-1 and limited-2 groups, in particular, the presence of significant microvascular involvement and hallmark antibody reactivities were similar across each group as shown in Table 2 below.

## Validation of microarray gene expression profiles in an independent lcSSc cohort

We applied the same approach described above to validate our findings in an independent cohort of patients with lcSSc derived from an American population (the Boston University cohort), with samples comprising 24 lcSSc and 4 control samples. Similar to this study cohort, analysis of differential expression between lcSSc and control samples suggested the presence of two subgroups of patients with lcSSc (group 1 with 14 lcSSc samples and group 2 with 10 lcSSc samples). We then compared the gene expression of the CVS development gene signature across subgroups of lcSSc patients and controls from the validation study. This gene expression signature was significantly different among both subgroups of patients with LcSSc and a control group (Fig. 3b), paralleling the results from this study (Fig. 3a).

## Discussion

In this study we have assessed molecular heterogeneity in gene expression profiles from skin biopsies taken from uninvolved skin of lcSSc patients compared with matched healthy controls. We have identified two subgroups within the lcSSc patient population in this study, which we termed limited 1 and limited 2. Patients from the limited-2 subgroup correspond to a third of the lcSSc cases and are generally characterised by a subtle alteration in gene expression that resembles but is distinct from the control samples. The majority of lcSSc cases cluster into a limited-1 subgroup associated with a substantial number of genes with significant differential expression, which are involved in multiple functional terms with known or potential relevance to SSc pathogenesis. We have confirmed our findings in a second cohort.

Most compelling is the identification of a cardiovascular system (CVS) development gene expression signature. This is interesting because of the well-recognised vascular abnormalities that are seen in lcSSc [3]. The idea that these pathways may be upregulated or altered in lcSSc even at sites that are not clinically affected is notable and may point towards an inherent susceptibility to vasculopathy that may be a hallmark of SSc. It is plausible that using uninvolved lcSSc skin we were able to minimise the impact of pathways reflecting inflammation and that this may explain the novel findings in our study. It was reassuring to find that several genes identified within this group were well-recognised in scleroderma pathogenesis, including, for instance, *COMP*, *THBS1* and *CTGF*. These have traditionally been considered as pro-fibrotic markers, but all have a role in the regulation of vascular function [23–25]. More traditional "vascular" markers such as *MMP19* and *COL4A1* were also included. It is also attractive to consider that recapitulation of developmental gene expression programmes may be central to susceptibility to development of SSc since it can be envisaged as a disease of perturbed connective tissue repair. There is a strong precedent for the same genetic pathways and programmes that are used in embryonic and post-natal growth and development to be recapitulated in acquired disease [26]. This may also fit with the model of SSc being a susceptibility genotype that we have recently postulated for the key complication of pulmonary arterial hypertension [27].

It is also notable that there were no clear clinical or serological associations with the molecular subgroups of lcSSc. This is relevant since it suggests that gene-expression-based subsets may indeed add to the clinical and serological factors that are already used in the clinic to subgroup patients. This would be analogous to the intrinsic subsets of diffuse cutaneous SSc (dcSSc) that have been reported and that are already of clinical utility [7]. Of note, in the cohort from which the study samples were taken, 40% of patients with limited disease were anti-topoisomerase (Scl-70)-positive and while this is traditionally thought to represent diffuse scleroderma, the patients in this cohort are categorised according to the distribution of skin disease at an early stage of disease and retain that subset over the course of their follow-up period. There were, therefore, no patients included in this study who would have experienced

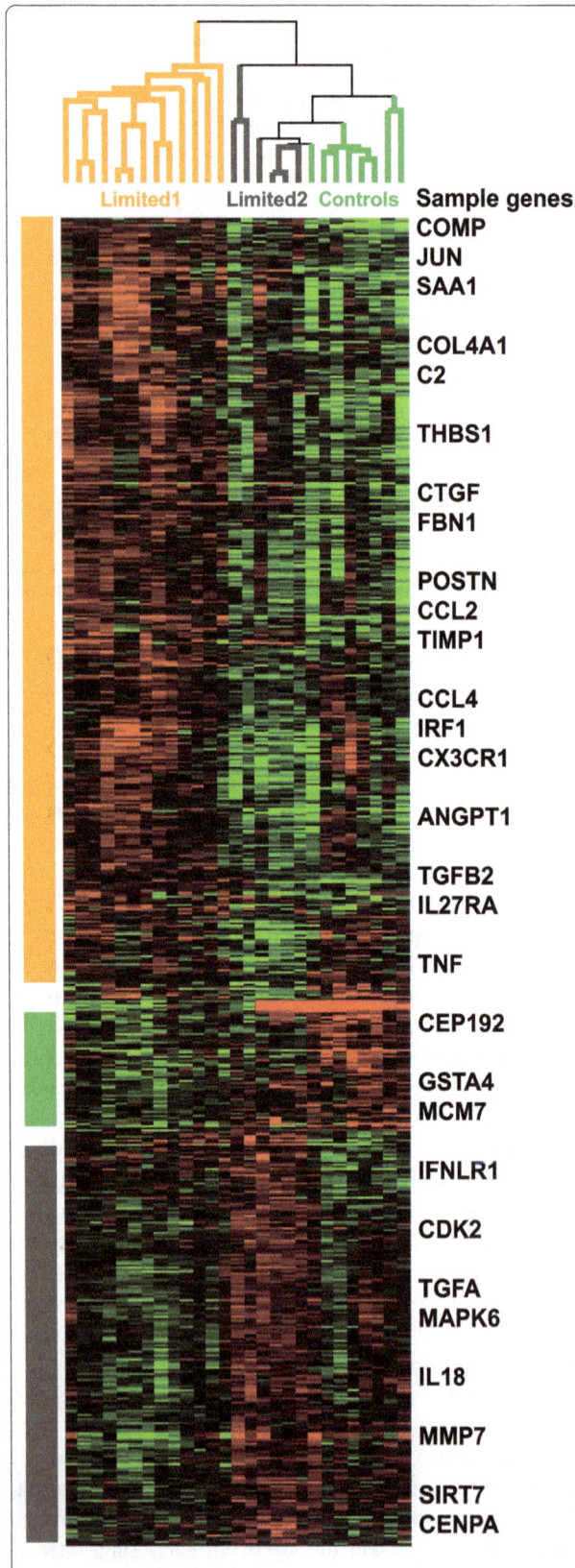

**Fig. 2** Multiclass significance analysis of microarrays (SAM) between the three identified clusters. Multiclass SAM was used to identify 807 differentially expressed genes (false discovery rate <10%) between limited -1, limited -2 and healthy control samples. Sample genes are listed. The majority of differentially expressed genes (475/807, 58.9%) had increased expression in the limited-1 group

remission to a low skin score with previous diffuse or more severe skin disease.

It is striking that many of the genes involved in CVS development are also seen in other relevant pathways such as ECM and response to TGF-β. Not only does this give some key candidate genes and pathways that could be perturbed in SSc but it also is a reminder that these factors that have been focussed on for a role in fibrosis may also have other roles in the biology or the disease. Thus it is plausible that the patterns of gene expression are altered in SSc and that this may have distinct consequences depending upon the stage and subset of disease. Further work will be required to assess whether these differences in expression reflect susceptibility to SSc that depends on genetic or epigenetic factors or whether they are reflective of pathogenetic processes that are occurring within the clinically uninvolved skin in limited SSc.

Strengths of the study include the well-characterised patients from a single centre, which may reduce the variability that can be a hallmark of multicentre cohorts and ensures standard classification and clinical evaluation. In addition, the use of well-established gene expression analysis platforms and semi-automated sample processing minimises technical variation that has been a limitation in some studies. Inclusion of a matched control group of healthy individuals was important to allow reliable interpretation of the "limited" gene expression signature.

Weaknesses of the study are the limitations of a relatively small study cohort that may not allow generalisability of our findings. However, the results are in line with those previously reported for subjects with lcSSc included in earlier gene expression studies [7]. We have validated our results in an independent cohort of patients with consistent findings across all groups. There is also a risk, given the small size of the study that there may be confounding effects on gene expression due to differences in immunosuppressive therapies, as an example. There were no statistically significant differences or strong trends between the limited-1 and limited-2 groups in terms of demographics, clinical history, treatments or serology in our study.

We have not included patients with clinically involved forearm skin in this study. There are no adequately powered studies that confirm concordance between clinically involved and uninvolved skin but previous data do suggest this; these confirmatory studies are required to extend and validate our findings further as part of a

**Table 2** Clinical and laboratory parameters of the limited-1 and limited-2 subgroups

| Clinical feature | | Limited 1 (*n* = 10) | Limited 2 (*n* = 5) |
|---|---|---|---|
| MRSS, median (range) | | 5.5 (3–10) | 6 (5 – 7) |
| Disease duration from first non-Raynaud's symptom, median (range) years | | 16 (4–40) | 6 (2–28) |
| ANA primary pattern, *N* (%) patients | Homogenous | 3 (30) | 1 (20) |
| | Speckled | 1 (10) | 1 (20) |
| | Centromere | 5 (50) | 1 (20) |
| | Nucleolar | 0 | 1 (20) |
| SSc-specific antibodies | Scl-70 | 3 (30) | 1 (10) |
| | RNA pol III | 0 | 0 |
| Vasculopathy, *N* (%) patients | Digital ulcers | 4 (40) | 2 (40) |
| | PAH | 0 | 0 |
| | Renal crisis | 0 | 0 |
| Interstitial lung disease, *N* (%) | | 2 (20) | 2 (40) |
| Inflammatory arthritis, *N* (%) | | 3 (30) | 0 |
| Vascular therapies, *N* (%) patients | ARB | 8 (80) | 2 (40) |
| | Ca channel antagonist | 2 (20) | 2 (40) |
| | Iloprost | 3 (30) | 1 (20) |
| | PDE5 inhibitor | 1 (10) | 2 (40) |
| Immunosuppressive therapies, *N* (%) patients | PDN | 2 (20) | 2 (40) |
| | MMF | 2 (20) | 1 (20) |
| | MTX | 2 (20) | 0 |
| | AZA | 1 (10) | 0 |
| | HCQ | 2 (20) | 1 (20) |

*ANA* antinuclear antibodies, *SSc* systemic sclerosis, *MRSS* modified Rodnan skin score, *PAH* pulmonary arterial hypertension, *ARB* angiotensin receptor blocker, *PDE* cGMP-regulated phosphodiesterase, *MTX* methotrexate, *HCQ* hydroxychloroquine, *PDN* prednisolone, *AZA* azathioprine

larger future study of gene expression in lcSSc. Involved distal skin is not biopsied in our patients due to concerns about wound healing. Finally, both further post-transcriptomic functional studies, and modern techniques that allow structural analysis of mRNA expression most notably to examine the dermal microcirculation and perivascular space would localise gene expression changes and verify that differential gene expression, particularly from the CVS development cluster, are reflected by differential protein expression.

## Conclusions

We showed that gene expression profiling of biopsies from uninvolved skin in lcSSc differentiates two potential

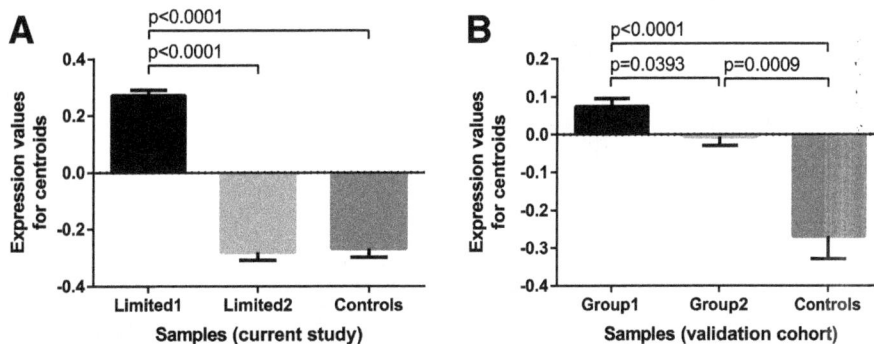

**Fig. 3** Cardiovascular development trends in discovery and validation cohorts. Pairwise comparisons between limited 1, limited 2 and control samples in the discovery cohort (**a**) and an independent validation cohort (**b**). Data are plotted as mean with SEM values. *P* values were derived from the Kruskal-Wallis test followed by Dunn's multiple comparisons test. *CVS* cardiovascular system

subgroups that overlap with other clinical and serological features. This may reflect important differences in pathogenesis within these patient groups. In addition, we identified differential expression of a subset of genes that relate to CVS development. Since the lcSSc subset is characterised by vasculopathy in the skin and internal organs, this may shed light on underlying mechanisms of vascular disease in SSc. The clinical implications of our findings will need to be analysed in future larger studies.

## Additional files

**Additional file 1:** Genes significantly differentially expressed between lcSSc and control groups. Green cells: genes with increased expression in controls. Yellow cells: genes with increased expression in lcSSc samples. (XLSX 16 kb)

**Additional file 2:** Genes significantly differentially expressed between the limited-1, limited-2 and control groups. Orange cells: genes with increased expression in limited 1 group. Green cells: genes with increased expression in controls. Grey cells: genes with increased expression in limited 2 group. (XLSX 38 kb)

**Additional file 3:** g:Profiler output for 475 genes with increased expression in the limited-1 group (multiclass SAM, FDR <10%). Additional files 3 contain the following column headers. Descriptions are as follows: *p* value: significance of enrichment in a given term corrected for multiple hypothesis testing using default g:GOSt method g:SCS. Q&T: overlap between genes in the query (Q) and genes in the genome annotated to a given term (T). t type: term category - Gene Ontology: Biological Process (BP), Molecular Function (MF), Cellular Component (CC); KEGG (keg); Reactome (rea). t name: term name. Q&T list: list of genes forming the overlap between query (Q) and genome lists for a given term (T). (XLSX 25 kb)

**Additional file 4:** g:Profiler output for 70 genes with increased expression in the limited-1 group annotated to cardiovascular system development. Additional file 4 contains the following column headers. Descriptions are as follows: *p* value: significance of enrichment in a given term corrected for multiple hypothesis testing using default g:GOSt method g:SCS. Q&T: overlap between genes in the query (Q) and genes in the genome annotated to a given term (T). t type: term category - Gene Ontology: Biological Process (BP), Molecular Function (MF), Cellular Component (CC); KEGG (keg); Reactome (rea). t name: term name. Q&T list: list of genes forming the overlap between query (Q) and genome lists for a given term (T). (XLSX 29 kb)

## Abbreviations

ANA: Antinuclear antibody; AZA: azathioprine; CVS: Cardiovascular system; dcSSc: Diffuse cutaneous systemic sclerosis; DEG: Differentially expressed genes; ECM: Extracellular matrix; ENA: extractable nuclear antigen; EULAR: European League Against Rheumatism; FDR: False discovery rate; HC: Healthy controls; IIF: Indirect immunofluorescence; lcSSc: Limited cutaneous systemic sclerosis; MAPK: Mitogen-activated protein kinase; MRSS: Modified Rodnan skin score; PDN: prednisolone; SAM: Significance analysis of microarrays; SSc: Systemic sclerosis; TGF: Transforming growth factor

## Acknowledgements
Not applicable.

## Funding
This work was supported by a grant from EULAR Orphan Diseases Programme. The funding body was not involved in design of the study and collection, analysis or interpretation of data or writing the manuscript. In addition, our research activity benefits from support from grants awarded by Arthritis Research UK, Scleroderma & Raynaud's UK and the British Heart Foundation. PM's work was supported by a grant from Koeln Fortune 224/2011, 131/2013 and 155/2014.

## Authors' contributions
CD and MW conceived and designed the study; ED-S, CCh, PM, KK and CCa obtained the data; ED-S, VM, CCh, PM and TW analyzed the data. ED-S, VM, VO, DA, PLM, RL, MW and CD interpreted the data. ED-S, VM, MW and CD drafted the manuscript and CCh, PM, KK, TW, CCa, VO, DA, PLM and RL critically appraised it. All authors read and approved the final manuscript and are accountable.

## Authors' information
Not applicable.

## Competing interests
The authors declare that they have no competing interests.

## Author details
[1]Centre for Rheumatology and Connective Tissue Diseases, University College London, London, UK. [2]University Hospitals Birmingham NHS Foundation Trust, Birmingham, UK. [3]Department of Molecular and Systems Biology, Geisel School of Medicine at Dartmouth, Hanover, NH, USA. [4]Experimental Laboratory of Immunological and Rheumatologic Researches, IRCCS Istituto Auxologico Italiano, University of Milan, Milan, Italy. [5]Department of Dermatology and Venerology, University of Cologne, Cologne, Germany. [6]Division of Rheumatology and Clinical Immunology, University of Pittsburgh Medical Center, Pittsburgh, PA, USA.

## References

1. Denton C and Moinzadeh P. Systemic sclerosis. In: Oxford Textbook of Rheumatology. Fourth Edition. Edited by Richard A. Watts, Philip G. Conaghan, Christopher Denton, Helen Foster, John Isaacs and Ulf Müller-Ladner. Oxford: Oxford University Press; 2013.
2. Varga J. Overview: Pathogenesis Integrated. In: John V, Denton CP, Wigley FM, editors. Scleroderma, from Pathogenesis to Comprehensive Management. New York: Springer; 2012. p. 163–4.
3. Nihtyanova SI, Schreiber BE, Ong VH, Rosenberg D, Moinzadeh P, Coghlan JG, Wells AU, Denton CP. Prediction of pulmonary complications and long term survival in systemic sclerosis. Arthritis Rheum. 2014;66(6):1625–35.
4. Herrick A, Lunt M, Whidby N, Ennis H, Silman A, McHugh N, Denton C. Observational study of treatment outcome in early diffuse cutaneous systemic sclerosis. J Rheumatol. 2010;37:116–24.
5. Villalta D, Imbastaro T, Di Giovanni S, Lauriti C, Gabini M, Turi MC, Bizzaro N. Diagnostic accuracy and predictive value of extended autoantibody profile in systemic sclerosis. Autoimmun Rev. 2012;12:114–20.
6. Chakravarty EF, Martyanov V, Fiorentino D, Wood TA, Haddon DJ, Jarrell JA, Utz PJ, Genovese MC, Whitfield ML, Chung L. Gene expression changes reflect clinical response in a placebo-controlled randomized trial of abatacept in patients with diffuse cutaneous systemic sclerosis. Arthritis Res Ther. 2015;17:159.
7. Milano A, Pendergrass SA, Sargent JL, George LK, McCalmont TH, Connolly MK, Whitfield ML. Molecular subsets in the gene expression signatures of scleroderma skin. PLoS One. 2008;3:e2696.
8. Hinchcliff M, Huang CC, Wood TA, Matthew Mahoney J, Martyanov V, Bhattacharyya S, Tamaki Z, Lee J, Carns M, Podlusky S, Sirajuddin A, Shah SJ, Chang RW, Lafyatis R, Varga J, Whitfield ML. Molecular signatures in skin associated with clinical improvement during mycophenolate treatment in systemic sclerosis. J Invest Dermato. 2013;133:1979–89.
9. Gardner H, Shearstone JR, Bandaru R, Crowell T, Lynes M, Trojanowska M, Pannu J, Smith E, Jablonska S, Blaszczyk M, Tan FK, Mayes MD. Gene profiling of scleroderma skin reveals robust signatures of disease that are imperfectly reflected in the transcript profiles of explanted fibroblasts. Arthritis Rheum. 2006;54:1961–73.
10. Rice LM, Stifano G, Ziemek J, Lafyatis R. Local skin gene expression reflects both local and systemic skin disease in patients with systemic sclerosis. Rheumatology (Oxford). 2016;55(2):377–9.
11. Rice LM, Ziemek J, Stratton EA, McLaughlin SR, Padilla CM, Mathes AL, Christmann RB, Stifano G, Browning JL, Whitfield ML, Spiera RF, Gordon JK, Simms RW, Zhang Y, Lafyatis R. A longitudinal biomarker for the extent of skin disease in patients with diffuse cutaneous systemic sclerosis. Arthritis Rheumatol. 2015;67(11):3004–15.

12. Assassi S, Swindell WR, Wu M, Tan FD, Khanna D, Furst DE, Tashkin DP, Jahan-Tigh RR, Mayes MD, Gudjonsson JE, Chang JT. Dissecting the heterogeneity of skin gene expression patterns in systemic sclerosis. Arthritis Rheumatol. 2015;67(11):3016–26.

13. Farina G, Lafyatis D, Lemaire R, Lafyatis R. A four-gene biomarker predicts skin disease in patients with diffuse cutaneous systemic sclerosis. Arthritis Rheum. 2010;62:580–8.

14. Johnson ME, Mahoney JM, Taroni J, Sargent JL, Marmarelis E, Wu MR, Varga J, Hinchcliff ME, Whitfield ML. Experimentally-derived fibroblast gene signatures identify molecular pathways associated with distinct subsets of systemic sclerosis patients in three independent cohorts. PLoS One. 2015;10(1):e0114017.

15. van den Hoogen F, Khanna D, Fransen J, Johnson SR, Baron M, Tyndall A, Matucci-Cerinic M, Naden RP, Medsger Jr TA, Carreira PE, Riemekasten G, Clements PJ, Denton CP, Distler O, Allanore Y, Furst DE, Gabrielli A, Mayes MD, van Laar JM, Seibold JR, Czirjak L, Steen VD, Inanc M, Kowal-Bielecka O, Müller-Ladner U, Valentini G, Veale DJ, Vonk MC, Walker UA, Chung L, Collier DH, Csuka ME, Fessler BJ, Guiducci S, Herrick A, Hsu VM, Jimenez S, Kahaleh B, Merkel PA, Sierakowski S, Silver RM, Simms RW, Varga J, Pope JE. 2013 classification criteria for systemic sclerosis: an American College of Rheumatology/European League against Rheumatism collaborative initiative. Arthritis Rheum. 2013;65:2737–47.

16. Reich M, Liefeld T, Gould J, Lerner J, Tamayo P, Mesirov JP. GenePattern 2.0. Nat Genet. 2006;38(5):500–1.

17. Johnson WE, Li C, Rabinovic A. Adjusting batch effects in microarray expression data using empirical Bayes methods. Biostatistics. 2007;8(1):118–27.

18. Reese SE, Archer KJ, Therneau TM, Atkinson EJ, Vachon CM, de Andrade M, Kocher JP, Eckel-Passow JE. A new statistic for identifying batch effects in high-throughput genomic data that uses guided principal component analysis. Bioinformatics. 2013;29(22):2877–83.

19. de Hoon MJ, Imoto S, Nolan J, Miyano S. Open source clustering software. Bioinformatics. 2004;20(9):1453–4.

20. Tusher VG, Tibshirani R, Chu G. Significance analysis of microarrays applied to the ionizing radiation response. Proc Natl Acad Sci U S A. 2001;98(9):5116–21.

21. Saldanha AJ. Java Treeview – extensible visualization of microarray data. Bioinformatics. 2004;20(17):3246–8.

22. Reimand J, Kull M, Peterson H, Hansen J, Vilo J. g:Profiler–a web-based toolset for functional profiling of gene lists from large-scale experiments. Nucleic Acids Res. 2007;35(Web Server issue):W193–200.

23. Fu Y, Kong W. Cartilage Oligomeric Matrix Protein: Matricellular and Matricrine Signaling in Cardiovascular Homeostasis and Disease. Curr Vasc Pharmacol. 2017 [epub ahead of print].

24. Lawler PR, Lawler J. Molecular basis for the regulation of angiogenesis by thrombospondin-1 and -2. Cold Spring Harb Perspect Med. 2012;2:a006627.

25. Sonnylal S, Shi-Wen X, Leoni P, Naff K, Van Pelt CS, Nakamura H, Leask A, Abraham D, Bou-Gharios G, de Crombrugghe B. Selective expression of connective tissue growth factor in fibroblasts in vivo promotes systemic tissue fibrosis. Arthritis Rheum. 2010;62(5):1523–32.

26. Rayner KJ, Liu PP. Long Noncoding RNAs in the Heart: The regulatory roadmap of cardiovascular development and disease. Circ Cardiovasc Genet. 2016;9(2):101–3.

27. Gilbane AJ, Derrett-Smith E, Trinder SL, Good RB, Pearce A, Denton CP, Holmes AM. Impaired bone morphogenetic protein receptor II signaling in a transforming growth factor-β-dependent mouse model of pulmonary hypertension and in systemic sclerosis. Am J Respir Crit Care Med. 2015;191(6):665–77.

# Sustained benefit from combined plasmapheresis and allogeneic mesenchymal stem cells transplantation therapy in systemic sclerosis

Huayong Zhang[†], Jun Liang[†], Xiaojun Tang, Dandan Wang, Xuebing Feng, Fan Wang, Bingzhu Hua, Hong Wang and Lingyun Sun[*]

## Abstract

**Background:** Systemic sclerosis (SSc) is an autoimmune disease involving the skin and several internal organs. Most therapies available for this disease are symptomatic. Given the difficulty in treating SSc, we conducted this study to investigate the effect of combined plasmapheresis (PE) and allogeneic mesenchymal stem cells transplantation (MSCT) therapy on SSc.

**Methods:** Fourteen patients underwent three repeated PE treatments with subsequent pulse cyclophosphamide on days 1, 3 and 5. Patients received a single MSCT ($1 \times 10^6$ cells/kg of body weight) on day 8. During follow up, evaluations performed included complete physical examination, serologic testing, and organ function.

**Results:** The mean modified Rodnan skin score (MRSS) improved from $20.1 \pm 3.1$ to $13.8 \pm 10.2$ ($P < 0.001$) at 12 months of follow up. Three patients had interstitial lung disease, all had improvement of lung function and improved computed tomography (CT) images after 12 months of combined therapy. This combined treatment also significantly decreased the anti-Scl70 autoantibody titer and serum transforming growth factor-β and vascular endothelial growth factor levels during follow up.

**Conclusion:** The results indicate that PE combined with MSCT is a feasible treatment associated with possible clinical benefit for SSc patients.

**Keywords:** Systemic sclerosis (SSc), Plasmapheresis (PE), Mesenchymal stem cells (MSCs)

## Background

Systemic sclerosis (SSc) is a rare chronic autoimmune disease characterized by increased synthesis and deposition of extra-cellular matrix in skin and various internal organs. Skin involvement, important in diagnosis and classification of SSc, is an almost universal feature of SSc [1]. Depending on the extent of skin fibrosis, SSc can be classified as two main subtypes, the limited cutaneous form (lcSSc) and the diffuse cutaneous form (dcSSc). The extensive degree of skin involvement coincides with future severe internal organ manifestations, poor prognosis and mortality, at least in the early phase of dcSSc [2]. Although skin disease does not directly threaten life, the thick skin can lead to psychological stress and thus worsens the quality of life.

Many inflammatory cytokines and growth factors are associated with the onset and progression of fibrosis, such as transforming growth factor (TGF)-β, endothelin-1, interleukin (IL)-17, IL-23 and tumor necrosis factor (TNF)-α [3–6]. In general, skin disease in SSc patients is treated with immunosuppressive agents such as methotrexate (MTX) or mycophenolate mofetil (MMF) [7, 8], but are not acceptable to all Chinese patients in terms of

* Correspondence: lingyunsun@nju.edu.cn
[†]Equal contributors
Department of Rheumatology and Immunology, The Affiliated Drum Tower Hospital of Nanjing University Medical School, 321 Zhongshan Road, Nanjing 210008, China

side effects and cost. There are also various novel therapies focusing on skin disease, including anti-inflammatory immunosuppressive agents such as imatinib or rituximab, and extracorporeal shock waves [9–12]. However, assessment of their effects remains inconclusive. A few studies on plasmapheresis (PE) for treatment of SSc have demonstrated improvement in the modified Rodnan Skin Score (MRSS), decreased level of cytokines, soluble adhesion molecules and immunolaboratory markers after treatment [13–15]. However, patients often received three repeated PE treatments every 2–3 months in these studies as a high frequency of PE would increase the risk of infection due to allogeneic blood transfusion. Thus, newer therapies are needed with enhanced efficacy and less toxicity in the treatment of skin disease in SSc.

Mesenchymal stem cells (MSCs) are a subset of multipotent adult somatic stem cells that have the ability to undergo self-renewal, proliferation and pluripotent differentiation. They can be obtained from different sources such as bone marrow, umbilical cord, and adipose tissue in the human body [16–19]. Besides their multi-lineage differentiation potential [20–22], MSCs also harbor immunosuppressive activities owing to their paracrine effects and interaction with different immune cells [23–26], and limited immunogenicity with low human leukocyte antigen (HLA) I and no HLA II expression [27]. These properties of MSCs have offered a new strategy in the treatment of numerous autoimmune inflammatory diseases and demonstrated promising results in safety and efficacy. To date, MSC transplantation (MSCT) has been proved in our center to be effective in the treatment of refractory systemic lupus erythematosus, rheumatoid arthritis and inflammatory bowel disease [28–31].

Recently studies have shown deficiency of MSCs in SSc patients. Compared with healthy controls, bone marrow MSCs (BM-MSCs) isolated from SSc patients display a more mature and myofibroblast-like phenotype, which re-programs these cells toward pro-angiogenic behavior [32]. MSCs from SSc patients also exhibit abnormal functional activities, such as increased expression of TGF-β and vascular endothelial growth factor (VEGF), and impairment of endothelial cell differentiation, which may play critical roles during the development of fibrosis in SSc [33, 34]. Based on these findings, allogeneic MSCT appears a promising therapy for SSc. Indeed, one animal experiment has shown that MSCT results in lower expression of fibrotic markers in both skin and lung, and decreased levels of anti-topoisomerase (anti-scl70) autoantibodies, suggesting systemic effect of MSCs [35]. Our previous pilot study in five SSc patients also showed that MSCT results in decreased antinuclear antibody (ANA) titer, and improvement in the MRSS and Health Assessment Questionnaire (HAQ) [36]. Thus, we aimed to evaluate the effectiveness and

safety of combination therapy with PE and MSCT for treatment of SSc on the basis of their different mechanisms in treating SSc patients.

## Methods

### Patient eligibility

Fourteen patients were recruited after approval by the Ethics Committee of Drum Tower Hospital. All patients provided signed, written, informed consent. Inclusion criteria were age 18–70 years, diagnosed as dcSSc according to 1980 American College of Rheumatology and/or the LeRoy and Medsger criteria. Exclusion criteria were: (1) pregnancy and lactation period; (2) heart failure and ventricular arrhythmia; (3) human immunodeficiency virus or hepatitis C virus seropositivity; (4) serum hepatitis B virus DNA of more than 10,000 copies/ml in patients with positive hepatitis B surface antigen; (5) presence of active untreated infectious disease; (6) presence of hepatic, portal or splenic vein thrombosis on ultrasonography; (7) presence of severe comorbid diseases (e.g., severe respiratory or cardiac disease), or presence of any type of malignancy.

### MSC culturing

The MSCs were obtained from the umbilical cord (UC). The UC-derived MSCs were prepared by the Stem Cell Center of Jiangsu Province (Jiangsu Beike Bio-Technology, Taizhou, Jiangsu). Fresh UCs was obtained from informed healthy mothers in a local maternity hospital after normal deliveries. The UCs were rinsed twice in PBS consisting of penicillin and streptomycin to remove the cord blood. Then the washed cords were cut into 1-$mm^2$ pieces and floated in low-glucose DMEM containing FBS (Stemcell, Vancouver, Canada). The pieces of cord were subsequently incubated at 37 °C in a humidified atmosphere consisting of 5% $CO_2$ in air. Non-adherent cells were removed by washing. The medium was replaced every 3 days after the initial plating. When well-developed colonies of fibroblast-like cells appeared after 10 days, the cultures were trypsinized and passaged into a new flask for further expansion. Flow cytometric analysis confirmed the cells expressed CD106, CD105, CD90, CD71, CD44, CD29, but not CD34, CD14, CD3 or CD45. The capacity of MSCs to differentiate along adipogenic and osteogenic lineages was evaluated as previously described [25]. MSCs at passage 3 with a purity of more than 95% were used.

### PE and MSCT

Patients received three repeated PE treatments every two days on days 1, 3 and 5, with the removal and reinfusion of 800–1000 ml plasma at each time. Patients received an intravenous cyclophosphamide (CTX) regimen to inhibit B cell proliferation triggered by rapidly decreased autoantibodies and circulating immune complex. The total amount of CTX (1.0 g/m² body surface area) was divided to use on the following day after each PE (0.4–0.6 g each time). On day 8, patients received single MSC infusion ($1 \times 10^6$ cells/kg of body weight). Patients were discharged after at least 48 hours of observation post MSCT.

### Follow up and outcome measurements

After MSCT, each patient returned for follow up at 1, 3, 6 and 12 months. At each follow-up visit, complete physical examination, serologic testing and organ function were performed. Skin thickening was measured using the MRSS score, which was performed by at least one experienced attending physician. Serum levels of anti-scl70 IgG and the changes in TGF-β, VEGF, interferon (IFN)-γ, IL-4 and IL-10 were measured by ELISA (R&D, USA).

### Statistical analysis

GraphPad Prism 5.0 software was used for statistical analyses. Results were expressed as median (range). The paired or unpaired $t$ test was used for statistical comparison of variables before and after treatment by GraphPad Prism 5.0 software. A level of $P < 0.05$ was considered statistically significant.

## Results

### Demographic findings

Fourteen patients with SSc underwent allogeneic MSCT; all of those were classified as having the diffuse cutaneous subsets of the disease. Their average age was 37.4 years (range 19–67). The average disease duration was 27 months (range 6–84). Table 1 displays patients' demographics and drug regimens received at the time of MSCT. The mean follow-up period was $15.6 \pm 4.3$ months (range 7–21). Twelve patients were followed up for more than 12 months.

### Modified Rodnan skin score

There was a significant improvement in the MRSS over the course of 1 year following the treatment. At 12 months of treatment, the mean MRSS improved from $20.1 \pm 3.1$ to $13.8 \pm 10.2$ ($P < 0.0001$) and the mean difference in MRSS was −6.2 points (95% CI −3.1 to −9.3). This change was not seen after 1 month of treatment, but was evident at 3 months, with a mean improvement of −3.3 points (−0.3 to −6.3; $P < 0.5$) and at 6 months with a mean improvement of −4.7 points (−1.7 to −7.7; $P < 0.001$) (Fig. 1).

### Non-skin fibrosis-related manifestations

Three of fourteen patients had interstitial lung disease (ILD); all patients had improvement in lung function after 12 months of combined therapy, with increased

**Table 1** Clinical and demographic characteristics of the patients enrolled in the study

| Case | Age (years) | Sex | Duration (mo) | MRSS baseline | Organ involvement | Previous treatments | Maintain treatments | Infectious AE |
|---|---|---|---|---|---|---|---|---|
| 1 | 26 | M | 17 | 26 | | P 15 mg/d + MTX 10 mg/w | P 5 mg/d + MTX 10 mg/w | Minor respiratory tract infection |
| 2 | 21 | F | 24 | 23 | | P10mg/d + penicillamine 0.375/d | No treatment | |
| 3 | 25 | M | 6 | 19 | | no treatment | No treatment | |
| 4 | 35 | F | 30 | 17 | | P 5 mg/d + penicillamine 0.375/d | No treatment | |
| 5 | 28 | F | 84 | 21 | ILD acral ulcers | P 20 mg/d + CTX 0.4/2 w | P 10 mg/d + CTX 0.6/2 mo | Minor respiratory tract infection |
| 6 | 43 | F | 60 | 20 | | Penicillamine 0.375/d | No treatment | |
| 7 | 19 | F | 36 | 19 | | P 10 mg/d + AZA100 mg/d | P 5 mg/d + AZA50 mg/d | Minor respiratory tract infection |
| 8 | 56 | M | 40 | 15 | ILD | P 15 mg/d CTX 0.4/2 w | P 5 mg/d CTX 0.4/mo | Minor respiratory tract infection |
| 9 | 46 | F | 7 | 21 | | P 10 mg/d + GTW | GTW | |
| 10 | 30 | F | 42 | 18 | | P10mg/d + MMF 0.75 BID | No treatment | Minor respiratory tract infection |
| 11 | 38 | F | 12 | 20 | ILD dysphagia | P 20 mg/d + CTX 0.1 QD + GTW | P10mg + CTX 0.4/2 w + GTW | |
| 12 | 67 | F | 6 | 25 | | P 10 mg/d + AZA 100 mg/d | P 5 mg/d + AZA 50 mg/d | Diarrhea |
| 13 | 53 | F | 6 | 17 | | P 5 mg/d + MMF 0.75 BID | P 5 mg/d | |
| 14 | 36 | F | 6 | 21 | | No treatment | No treatment | |

Duration was from the first symptom of disease to the time receiving plasmapheresis (PE) + mesenchymal stem cell transplantation (MSCT). Skin *MRSS* modified Rodnan skin score, *AE* adverse events, *ILD* interstitial lung disease, *P* prednisone, *CTX* cyclophasphomide, *MTX* methotrexate, *AZA* azathioprine, *GTW* glycosides of *Tripterygium wilfordi*, *MMF* mycophenolate mofetil, *BID* twice daily

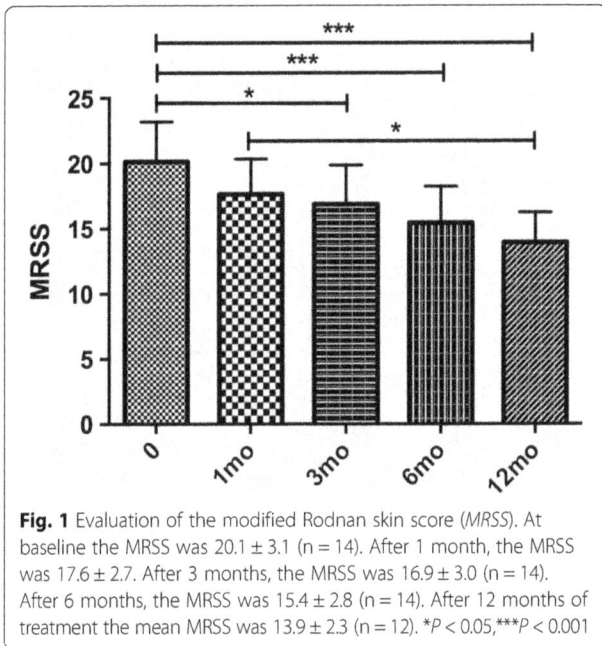

**Fig. 1** Evaluation of the modified Rodnan skin score (*MRSS*). At baseline the MRSS was 20.1 ± 3.1 (n = 14). After 1 month, the MRSS was 17.6 ± 2.7. After 3 months, the MRSS was 16.9 ± 3.0 (n = 14). After 6 months, the MRSS was 15.4 ± 2.8 (n = 14). After 12 months of treatment the mean MRSS was 13.9 ± 2.3 (n = 12). *$P < 0.05$,***$P < 0.001$

CO diffusing capacities (DLco) and forced vital capacity (FVC) (Fig. 2). Improved computed tomography (CT) images were also observed in these patients (Fig. 3). One of fourteen patients had an acral ulcer. Pain from the skin ulcer improved 1 month after combined therapy

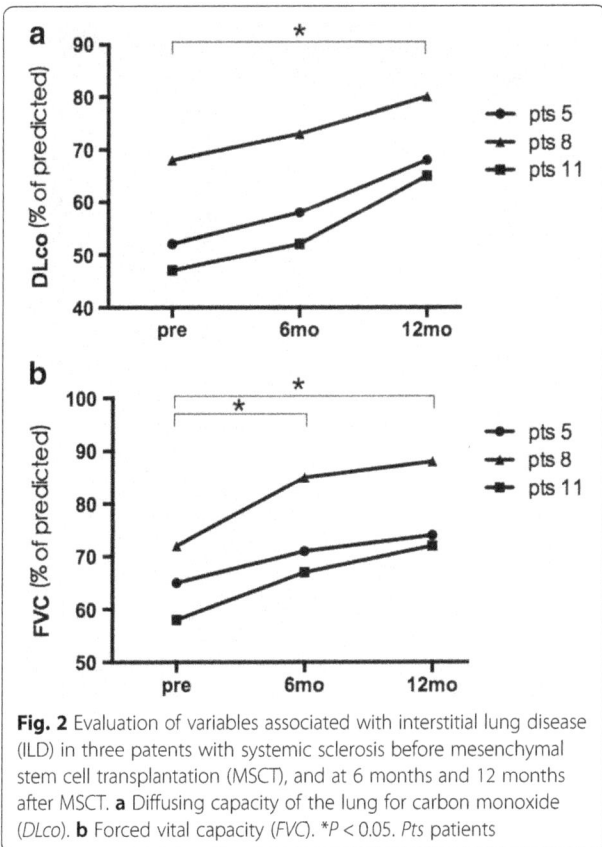

**Fig. 2** Evaluation of variables associated with interstitial lung disease (ILD) in three patents with systemic sclerosis before mesenchymal stem cell transplantation (MSCT), and at 6 months and 12 months after MSCT. **a** Diffusing capacity of the lung for carbon monoxide (*DLco*). **b** Forced vital capacity (*FVC*). *$P < 0.05$. *Pts* patients

and the lesion size was reduced and healed 3 months after the treatment and did not recur till the last follow up. One of fourteen patients had dysphagia, which responded to the combined treatment during the whole follow up.

### Serology changes

This combined therapy significantly decreased serum anti-Scl70 autoantibody titer, TGF-β and VEGF levels (Fig. 4) during the follow up. There were no changes in the levels of IFN-γ, IL-4 or IL-10. The anti-Scl70 auto-antibody titers decreased from 125.98 ± 91.13 RU/ml at baseline to 98.77 ± 88.46 RU/ml ($P = 0.66$, n = 7) at 1-month follow up; the titers were reduced to 66.91 ± 74.69 RU/ml (3-month follow up, $P < 0.05$, n = 7), 50.98 ± 71.39 RU/ml (6-month follow up, $P < 0.05$, n = 7) and 61.32 ± 52.68 RU/ml (12-month follow up, $P < 0.01$, n = 7), respectively. The serum TGF-β levels were decreased from 148.94 ± 79.85 ng/ml at baseline to 52.47 ± 21.98 ng/ml (1-month follow up, $P < 0.05$, n = 9), 45.94 ± 22.33 ng/ml (3-month follow up, $P < 0.01$, n = 9), 57.25 ± 40.56 ng/ml (6-month follow up, $P < 0.05$, n = 9) and 71.64 ± 58.20 ng/ml (12-month follow up, $P = 0.0547$, n = 9), respectively. The serum VEGF levels were decreased from 275.71 ± 108.15 pg/ml at baseline to 101.54 ± 69.88 pg/ml (1-month follow up, $P < 0.01$, n = 9), 75.84 ± 42.58 pg/ml (3-month follow up, $P < 0.01$, n = 9), 104.64 ± 56.6 pg/ml (6-month follow up, $P < 0.01$, n = 9) and 145.89 ± 88.20 pg/ml (12-month follow up, $P = 0.1125$, n = 9), respectively.

### Adverse events

No serious adverse events were observed during or imme-diately after PE and MSCT in any of the 14 patients. None of these patients developed graft versus host disease (GvHD) during follow up. Adverse events noted were upper respiratory tract infections reported by five patients and diarrhea reported by one patient during follow-up visits (Table 1). No serious infections occurred.

### Discussion

Skin involvement is the hallmark of SSc; improvement in skin thickening may be useful as a surrogate for im-provement in survival in clinical trials [37]. Therefore, the treating skin symptoms have been the focus of inves-tigation in many clinical trials. Recent studies have assessed different options for the treatment of skin thickness; however, most of these therapies did not show significant efficacy [38]. Herein, we proposed allogeneic MSCT combined with PE as a potential therapy for the diffuse cutaneous form of SSc. In this study, of the total of 14 patients, 11 only had diffuse sclerosis and thicken-ing of the skin without internal organ involvement, in-cluding two newly diagnosed patients who were not

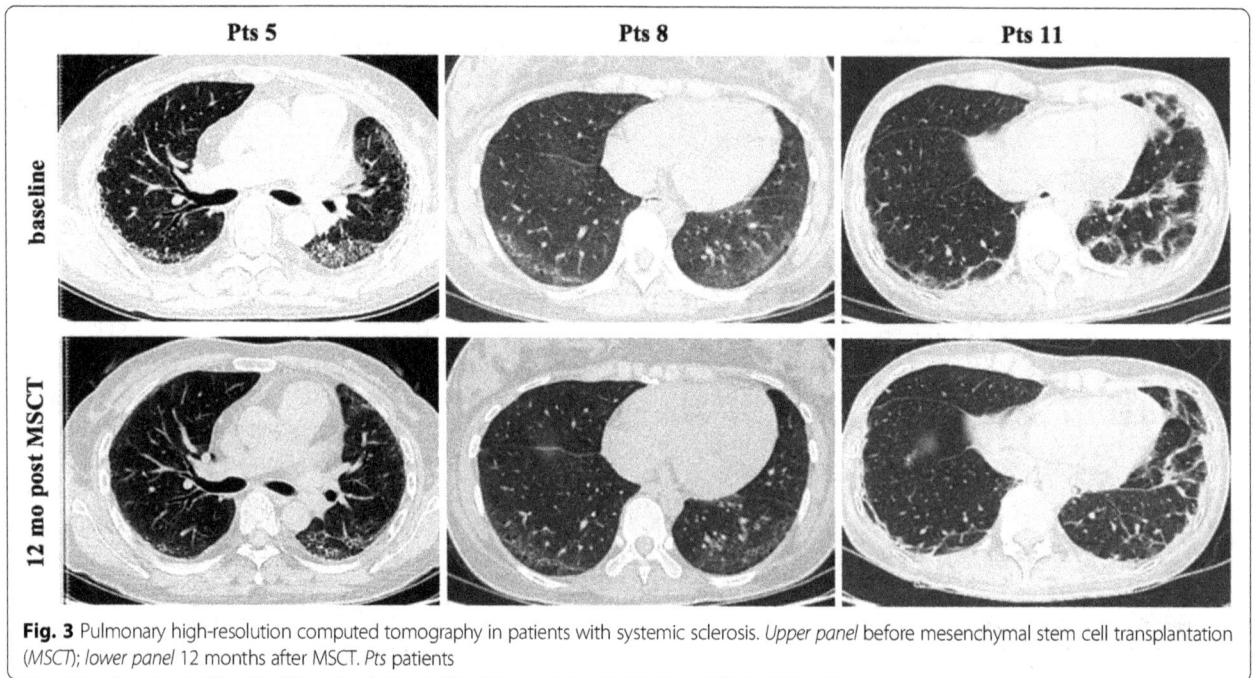

**Fig. 3** Pulmonary high-resolution computed tomography in patients with systemic sclerosis. *Upper panel* before mesenchymal stem cell transplantation (*MSCT*); *lower panel* 12 months after MSCT. *Pts* patients

receiving any treatment before and after PE + MSCT; the other 9 patients received small doses of glucocorticoid in combination with immunosuppresive agents such as MTX or MMF, etc., which 3 patients gradually stopped taking after the combined therapy, and the other 6 cases also had reduced dosage of glucocorticoids and immunosuppressants. The results indicate this combined therapy has a possible benefit in improving MRSS and reducing inflammatory markers including anti-Scl70 autoantibody titer, TGF-β and VEGF levels.

Fibrosis is the final step and is the basis of most prominent clinical manifestations in SSc patients, including skin thickness and tightness [39]. Two fundamental biological processes contribute to the development of skin fibrosis, including vasculopathy with perivascular inflammation and coagulation activation, and fibroblast activation with the excess accumulation of extracellular matrix components. Multiple factors and signaling pathways are involved in the development or persistence of skin involvement in SSc, such as TGF-β, IL-4, IL-6, platelet-derived growth factor (PDGF), IL-1, IL-13, IL-17, IL-5, monocyte chemoattractant protein (MCP)-1, VEGF and connective tissue growth factor (CTGF) [6]. Recently, some experimental studies have revealed MSC deficiency in SSc. MSCs in SSc have a different phenotype from healthy controls [32]. BM-MSCs isolated from SSc patients have upregulation of α-smooth muscle actin (SMA) and smooth muscle (SM)22α genes and reduced proliferative activity, displaying a more mature and myofibroblast-like phenotype. Cipriani P et al. have observed that BM-MSCs from SSc patients have increased senescence biomarkers, through increased activation of the IL-6 pathway

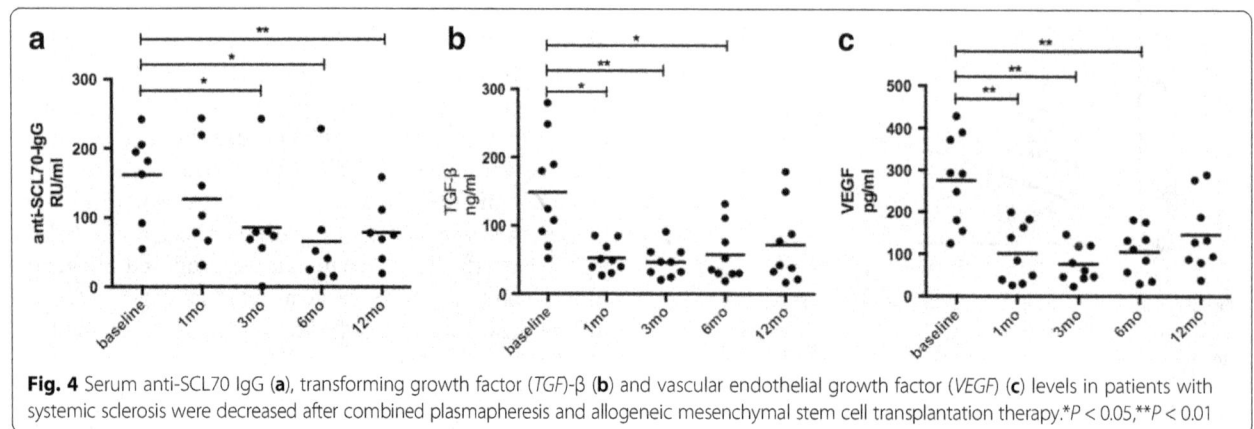

**Fig. 4** Serum anti-SCL70 IgG (**a**), transforming growth factor (*TGF*)-β (**b**) and vascular endothelial growth factor (*VEGF*) (**c**) levels in patients with systemic sclerosis were decreased after combined plasmapheresis and allogeneic mesenchymal stem cell transplantation therapy.*$P < 0.05$,**$P < 0.01$

[40]. Furthermore, MSCs have been proved to not only have the properties of reduced inflammatory and fibrotic processes, but also have the ability to differentiate into endothelial cells [41]. These findings supported the hypothesis that MSCs from SSc patients are structurally and functionally defective, and provide basis for allogeneic MSCT as a potential therapy for SSc patients. Our results showed that MSCT combined with PE downregulated serum levels of TGF-β, which is a major cytokine involved in early angiogenesis and latent collagen production leading to fibrosis [42]. In addition, the combined therapy was shown to reduce the levels of VEGF, which was elevated in SSc patients and could stimulate angiogenesis [6]. We also noted lower levels of anti-Scl70 antibodies after the combined treatment, suggesting reduced B cell activation.

Some studies have suggested that MSCs can exhibit a protective effect on skin tightness and thickness [36, 43]. PE is also reported to be able to improve the Rodnan skin score in small case series of SSc patients [13]. These two therapies were taken into account for combination in view of their seemingly complementary characteristics. PE could quickly remove serum pro-inflammatory substances such as inflammatory cytokines, antibodies, immunoglobulins and complements, which play major roles in the immune responses against normal skin and fibrosis. MSC could secrete anti-inflammatory cytokines, anti-fibrotic factors and trophic molecules, and differentiate into epithelial cells, which will all promote regeneration of skin. Moreover, the self-renewal capacity of MSCs would make the therapeutic effects last a long time. However, it is difficult to tell which treatment is important in the resulting clinical and laboratory test improvements. Future randomized clinical trials with larger sample sizes and long-term follow up are required to further verify the results of this study.

In addition to improving the skin lesions, the data also suggest that the combined therapy can improve internal function in these patients. ILD is a common visceral lesion in SSc patients. For more than 15 years, CTX has commonly been used in the treatment of SSc-ILD. CTX is a cytotoxic immunosuppressive agent that suppresses lymphokine production and modulates lymphocyte function. In a landmark study, the Scleroderma Lung Study Research Group noted that CTX achieved a modest but significant beneficial effect on lung function and patients' quality of life. After 12 months of therapy, FVC increased in 49.3% of the patients who received the CTX treatment. However, unfortunately, it also provoked a serious adverse event [44]. In our study, there were three patients with different degrees of ILD, all of whom had received glucocorticoids and CTX for at least 3 ~ 6 months before the combined therapy, but without improvement in the pulmonary symptoms. However, lung function and CT images in these three patients all improved significantly, after 12 months of combined therapy, FVC increased from 65.0 ± 7.0% to 81.7 ± 8.5%. We have gradually reduced the dosage of glucocorticoids and CTX to maintaining treatment. Compared with glucocorticoids and immunosuppressive agents, this combined therapy has shown a low side reaction and good safety; only a few patients had mild upper respiratory tract infections and diarrhea.

Our study has limitations. First, we were aware of the limitation of the small sample size of this study population, thus this is an exploratory analysis. The adequacy of sample size is important to clinical trials but depends on the availability of patients. A lower prevalence of SSc explained the sample size in this trial to some extent. Second, the uncontrolled study design (automatically also not blinded) may result in a substantial overestimation of therapeutic effect.

## Conclusions

This study indicates that MSCT combined with PE is a feasible treatment associated with possible clinical benefit in SSc patients. The true value and safety will require much more robust data from a controlled trial and longer-term follow up in many more SSc patients.

**Abbreviations**
ANA: Anti-nuclear antibody; BM-MSCs: Bone marrow mesenchymal stem cells; CT: Computed tomography; CTGF: Connective tissue growth factor; CTX: Cyclophosphamide; dcSSc: Diffuse cutaneous systemic sclerosis; DLco: Diffusing capacity of the lung for carbon monoxide; DMEM: Dulbecco's modified Eagle's medium; ELISA: Enzyme-linked immunosorbent assay; FBS: Fetal bovine serum; FVC: Forced vital capacity; GvHD: Graft versus host disease; HAQ: Health Assessment Questionnaire; HLA: Human leukocyte antigen; IL: Interleukin; ILD: Interstitial lung disease; IFN: Interferon; lcSSc: Limited cutaneous systemic sclerosis; MCP: Monocyte chemoattractant protein; MMF: Mycophenolate mofetil; MRSS: Modified Rodnan skin score; MSCs: Mesenchymal stem cells; MSCT: Mesenchymal stem cell transplantation; MTX: Methotrexate; PBS: Phosphate-buffered saline; PDGF: Platelet-derived growth factor; PE: Plasmapheresis; scl70: Topoisomerase; SM: Smooth muscle; SMA: Smooth muscle actin; SSc: Systemic sclerosis; TGF: Transforming growth factor; TNF: Tumor necrosis factor; UC: Umbilical cord; VEGF: Vascular endothelial growth factor

**Acknowledgements**
We thank all the patients participating in this study.

**Funding**
This work was supported by the National Natural Science Foundation of China (number 81671608, 81202350, 81571586 and 81302559), Jiangsu Six Talent Peaks Project (2015-WSN-074), Jiangsu 333 High Level Talents Project, Jiangsu Government Scholarship for Overseas Studies, Jiangsu Health International Exchange Program sponsorship, Nanjing Young Medical Talents Project, Nanjing Health Bureau Key Project (ZKX15018) and Jiangsu Provincial Special Program of Medical Science (BE2015602).

**Authors' contributions**
HZ, JL and LS contributed to study design, data acquisition, data interpretation and drafting the manuscript. XT and DW analyzed the data and revised the manuscript. XF, FW, BH and HW recruited patients and revised the manuscript. All authors read and approved the final manuscript.

**Competing interests**
The authors declare that they have no competing interests.

**References**
1. Czirjak L, Foeldvari I, Muller-Ladner U. Skin involvement in systemic sclerosis. Rheumatology (Oxford). 2008;47 Suppl 5:v44–5.
2. Domsic RT, Rodriguez-Reyna T, Lucas M, Fertig N, Medsger Jr TA. Skin thickness progression rate: a predictor of mortality and early internal organ involvement in diffuse scleroderma. Ann Rheum Dis. 2011;70:104–9.
3. Cipriani P, Di Benedetto P, Ruscitti P, Verzella D, Fischietti M, Zazzeroni F, et al. Macitentan inhibits the transforming growth factor-beta profibrotic action, blocking the signaling mediated by the ETR/TbetaRI complex in systemic sclerosis dermal fibroblasts. Arthritis Res Ther. 2015;17:247.
4. Arnett FC, Gourh P, Shete S, Ahn CW, Honey RE, Agarwal SK, et al. Major histocompatibility complex (MHC) class II alleles, haplotypes and epitopes which confer susceptibility or protection in systemic sclerosis: analyses in 1300 Caucasian, African-American and Hispanic cases and 1000 controls. Ann Rheum Dis. 2010;69:822–7.
5. Czeslick EG, Simm A, Grond S, Silber RE, Sablotzki A. Inhibition of intracellular tumour necrosis factor (TNF)-alpha and interleukin (IL)-6 production in human monocytes by iloprost. Eur J Clin Invest. 2003;33: 1013–7.
6. Pattanaik D, Brown M, Postlethwaite BC, Postlethwaite AE. Pathogenesis of systemic sclerosis. Front Immunol. 2015;6:272.
7. Johnson SR, Feldman BM, Pope JE, Tomlinson GA. Shifting our thinking about uncommon disease trials: the case of methotrexate in scleroderma. J Rheumatol. 2009;36:323–9.
8. Walker KM, Pope J, participating members of the Scleroderma Clinical Trials C, Canadian Scleroderma Research G. Treatment of systemic sclerosis complications: what to use when first-line treatment fails – a consensus of systemic sclerosis experts. Semin Arthritis Rheum. 2012;42:42–55.
9. Quillinan NP, McIntosh D, Vernes J, Haq S, Denton CP. Treatment of diffuse systemic sclerosis with hyperimmune caprine serum (AIMSPRO): a phase II double-blind placebo-controlled trial. Ann Rheum Dis. 2014;73:56–61.
10. Bosello SL, De Luca G, Rucco M, Berardi G, Falcione M, Danza FM, et al. Long-term efficacy of B cell depletion therapy on lung and skin involvement in diffuse systemic sclerosis. Semin Arthritis Rheum. 2015;44: 428–36.
11. Khanna D, Saggar R, Mayes MD, Abtin F, Clements PJ, Maranian P, et al. A one-year, phase I/IIa, open-label pilot trial of imatinib mesylate in the treatment of systemic sclerosis-associated active interstitial lung disease. Arthritis Rheum. 2011;63:3540–6.
12. Tinazzi E, Amelio E, Marangoni E, Guerra C, Puccetti A, Codella OM, et al. Effects of shock wave therapy in the skin of patients with progressive systemic sclerosis: a pilot study. Rheumatol Int. 2011;31:651–6.
13. Szucs G, Szamosi S, Aleksza M, Veres K, Soltesz P. Plasmapheresis therapy in systemic sclerosis. Orv Hetil. 2003;144:2213–7.
14. Dau PC, Callahan JP. Immune modulation during treatment of systemic sclerosis with plasmapheresis and immunosuppressive drugs. Clin Immunol Immunopathol. 1994;70:159–65.
15. Szekanecz Z, Aleksza M, Antal-Szalmas P, Soltesz P, Veres K, Szanto S, et al. Combined plasmapheresis and high-dose intravenous immunoglobulin treatment in systemic sclerosis for 12 months: follow-up of immunopathological and clinical effects. Clin Rheumatol. 2009;28:347–50.
16. Guillot PV, Gotherstrom C, Chan J, Kurata H, Fisk NM. Human first-trimester fetal MSC express pluripotency markers and grow faster and have longer telomeres than adult MSC. Stem Cells. 2007;25:646–54.
17. in t Anker PS, Noort WA, Scherjon SA, Kleijburg-van der Keur C, Kruisselbrink AB, van Bezooijen RL, et al. Mesenchymal stem cells in human second-trimester bone marrow, liver, lung, and spleen exhibit a similar immunophenotype but a heterogeneous multilineage differentiation potential. Haematologica. 2003;88:845–52.
18. Chen PM, Yen ML, Liu KJ, Sytwu HK, Yen BL. Immunomodulatory properties of human adult and fetal multipotent mesenchymal stem cells. J Biomed Sci. 2011;18:49.
19. Trivanovic D, Kocic J, Mojsilovic S, Krstic A, Ilic V, Djordjevic IO, et al. Mesenchymal stem cells isolated from peripheral blood and umbilical cord Wharton's jelly. Srp Arh Celok Lek. 2013;141:178–86.
20. Jiang Y, Jahagirdar BN, Reinhardt RL, Schwartz RE, Keene CD, Ortiz-Gonzalez XR, et al. Pluripotency of mesenchymal stem cells derived from adult marrow. Nature. 2002;418:41–9.
21. Paul D, Samuel SM, Maulik N. Mesenchymal stem cell: present challenges and prospective cellular cardiomyoplasty approaches for myocardial regeneration. Antioxid Redox Signal. 2009;11:1841–55.
22. Ju S, Teng GJ, Lu H, Jin J, Zhang Y, Zhang A, et al. In vivo differentiation of magnetically labeled mesenchymal stem cells into hepatocytes for cell therapy to repair damaged liver. Invest Radiol. 2010;45:625–33.
23. Nauta AJ, Fibbe WE. Immunomodulatory properties of mesenchymal stromal cells. Blood. 2007;110:3499–506.
24. Sotiropoulou PA, Perez SA, Gritzapis AD, Baxevanis CN, Papamichail M. Interactions between human mesenchymal stem cells and natural killer cells. Stem Cells. 2006;24:74–85.
25. Tse WT, Pendleton JD, Beyer WM, Egalka MC, Guinan EC. Suppression of allogeneic T-cell proliferation by human marrow stromal cells: implications in transplantation. Transplantation. 2003;75:389–97.
26. Ooi YY, Dheen ST, Tay SS. Paracrine effects of mesenchymal stem cells-conditioned medium on microglial cytokines expression and nitric oxide production. Neuroimmunomodulation. 2015;22:233–42.
27. Le Blanc K, Mougiakakos D. Multipotent mesenchymal stromal cells and the innate immune system. Nat Rev Immunol. 2012;12:383–96.
28. Liang J, Zhang H, Hua B, Wang H, Lu L, Shi S, et al. Allogenic mesenchymal stem cells transplantation in refractory systemic lupus erythematosus: a pilot clinical study. Ann Rheum Dis. 2010;69:1423–9.
29. Liang J, Li X, Zhang H, Wang D, Feng X, Wang H, et al. Allogeneic mesenchymal stem cells transplantation in patients with refractory RA. Clin Rheumatol. 2012;31:157–61.
30. Xu J, Wang D, Liu D, Fan Z, Zhang H, Liu O, et al. Allogeneic mesenchymal stem cell treatment alleviates experimental and clinical Sjogren syndrome. Blood. 2012;120:3142–51.
31. Liang J, Zhang H, Wang D, Feng X, Wang H, Hua B, et al. Allogeneic mesenchymal stem cell transplantation in seven patients with refractory inflammatory bowel disease. Gut. 2012;61:468–9.
32. Cipriani P, Marrelli A, Benedetto PD, Liakouli V, Carubbi F, Ruscitti P, et al. Scleroderma Mesenchymal Stem Cells display a different phenotype from healthy controls; implications for regenerative medicine. Angiogenesis. 2013;16:595–607.
33. Vanneaux V, Farge-Bancel D, Lecourt S, Baraut J, Cras A, Jean-Louis F, et al. Expression of transforming growth factor beta receptor II in mesenchymal stem cells from systemic sclerosis patients. BMJ Open. 2013;3(1). doi: 10. 1136/bmjopen-2012-001890.
34. Guiducci S, Manetti M, Romano E, Mazzanti B, Ceccarelli C, Dal Pozzo S, et al. Bone marrow-derived mesenchymal stem cells from early diffuse systemic sclerosis exhibit a paracrine machinery and stimulate angiogenesis in vitro. Ann Rheum Dis. 2011;70:2011–21.
35. Maria AT, Toupet K, Bony C, Pirot N, Vozenin MC, Petit B, et al. Antifibrotic, antioxidant, and immunomodulatory effects of mesenchymal stem cells in HOCl-induced systemic sclerosis. Arthritis Rheumatol. 2016;68:1013–25.
36. Akiyama K, Chen C, Wang D, Xu X, Qu C, Yamaza T, et al. Mesenchymal-stem-cell-induced immunoregulation involves FAS-ligand-/FAS-mediated T cell apoptosis. Cell Stem Cell. 2012;10:544–55.
37. Steen VD, Medsger Jr TA. Improvement in skin thickening in systemic sclerosis associated with improved survival. Arthritis Rheum. 2001;44: 2828–35.
38. Khanna D, Denton CP. Evidence-based management of rapidly progressing systemic sclerosis. Best Pract Res Clin Rheumatol. 2010;24:387–400.
39. Carrai V, Miniati I, Guiducci S, Capaccioli G, Alterini R, Saccardi R, et al. Evidence for reduced angiogenesis in bone marrow in SSc: immunohistochemistry and multiparametric computerized imaging analysis. Rheumatology (Oxford). 2012;51:1042–8.
40. Cipriani P, Di Benedetto P, Liakouli V, Del Papa B, Di Padova M, Di Ianni M, et al. Mesenchymal stem cells (MSCs) from scleroderma patients (SSc) preserve their immunomodulatory properties although senescent and normally induce T regulatory cells (Tregs) with a functional phenotype: implications for cellular-based therapy. Clin Exp Immunol. 2013;173:195–206.
41. Doan CC, Le TL, Hoang NS, Doan NT, Le VD, Do MS. Differentiation of umbilical cord lining membrane-derived mesenchymal stem cells into endothelial-like cells. Iran Biomed J. 2014;18:67–75.

# Systemic sclerosis associated interstitial lung disease - individualized immunosuppressive therapy and course of lung function: results of the EUSTAR group

Sabine Adler[1*], Dörte Huscher[2,3], Elise Siegert[3], Yannick Allanore[4], László Czirják[5], Francesco DelGaldo[6], Christopher P. Denton[7], Oliver Distler[8], Marc Frerix[9], Marco Matucci-Cerinic[10], Ulf Mueller-Ladner[9], Ingo-Helmut Tarner[9], Gabriele Valentini[11], Ulrich A. Walker[12], Peter M. Villiger[1], Gabriela Riemekasten[13] and EUSTAR co-workers on behalf of the DeSScipher project research group within the EUSTAR network

## Abstract

**Background:** Interstitial lung disease in systemic sclerosis (SSc-ILD) is a major cause of SSc-related death. Imunosuppressive treatment (IS) is used in patients with SSc for various organ manifestations mainly to ameliorate progression of SSc-ILD. Data on everyday IS prescription patterns and clinical courses of lung function during and after therapy are scarce.

**Methods:** We analysed patients fulfilling American College of Rheumatology (ACR)/European League against Rheumatism (EULAR) 2013 criteria for SSc-ILD and at least one report of IS. Types of IS, pulmonary function tests (PFT) and PFT courses during IS treatment were evaluated.

**Results:** EUSTAR contains 3778/11,496 patients with SSc-ILD (33%), with IS in 2681/3,778 (71%). Glucocorticoid (GC) monotherapy was prescribed in 30.6% patients with GC combinations plus cyclophosphamide (CYC) (11.9%), azathioprine (AZA) (9.2%), methotrexate (MTX) (8.7%), or mycophenolate mofetil (MMF) (7.3%). Intensive IS (MMF + GC, CYC or CYC + GC) was started in patients with the worst PFTs and ground glass opacifications on imaging. Patients without IS showed slightly less worsening in forced vital capacity (FVC) when starting with FVC 50–75% or >75%. GC showed negative trends when starting with FVC <50%. Regarding diffusing capacity for carbon monoxide (DLCO), negative DLCO trends were found in patients with MMF.

**Conclusions:** IS is broadly prescribed in SSc-ILD. Clusters of clinical and functional characteristics guide individualised treatment. Data favour distinguished decision-making, pointing to either watchful waiting and close monitoring in the early stages or start of immunosuppressive treatment in moderately impaired lung function. Advantages of specific IS are difficult to depict due to confounding by indication. Data do not support liberal use of GC in SSc-ILD.

**Keywords:** Systemic sclerosis, Interstitial lung disease, Immunosuppressants, Follow up, Lung function

* Correspondence: sabine.adler@insel.ch
Sabine Adler and Dörte Huscher contributed equally to this work
Peter M. Villiger and Gabriela Riemekasten contributed equally to this work
[1]Department of Rheumatology, Immunology and Allergology, University Hospital and University of Bern, Freiburgstrasse 4, 3010 Bern, Switzerland
Full list of author information is available at the end of the article

## Background

Interstitial lung disease (ILD) in systemic sclerosis (SSc-ILD) is caused by alveolitis-induced fibrosis of the intra-alveolar tissue, leading to progressive decline in lung function [1]. It is the most frequent cause of SSc-associated death [2]. Current treatment options aim at reducing pulmonary interstitial inflammation in order to prevent progression of fibrosis and consecutive deterioration of lung function.

Cyclophosphamide (CYC) is widely used in the treatment of SSc-ILD, especially in induction therapy as reflected by the European League Against Rheumatism (EULAR) recommendations for SSc-ILD treatment [3]. Unfortunately, the toxicity of CYC makes it unsuitable for long-term use. Furthermore, within the first scleroderma lung study, the effect of CYC waned a few months after cessation [4]. Mycophenolate mofetil (MMF) has been suggested as an alternative for induction and maintenance IS [5] and has been shown to stabilise lung function in two studies [6, 7]. There are recent data from the scleroderma lung study II on the risks and benefits of a 2-year course of MMF versus a 1-year course of oral CYC. Herein, MMF displayed a better safety profile and a 1-year course of CYC improved skin and lung function to a comparable extent [8]. Azathioprine (AZA) reflects the common practice of introducing a steroid-sparing anti-rheumatic agent in patients with idiopathic pulmonary fibrosis yet might be rather harmful [9]. In SSc-ILD, the evidence for AZA is inconclusive [10–12]. Methotrexate (MTX) is recommended for treatment of skin manifestations in early diffuse cutaneous SSc (dcSSc) [13]. Its use in SSc-ILD remains controversial as lung fibrosis is a rare but potentially severe side effect [14] and evidence for anti-fibrotic efficacy in the lungs is lacking. As skin and lung involvement may appear simultaneously, MTX is sometimes prescribed in SSc-ILD. Rituximab (RTX) is among the most frequently used biological agents in SSc with a recent case-control study and an observational study suggesting beneficial effects on lung function [15]. As elevated interleukin-6 (IL-6) in SSc-patients has been associated with higher incidence of progressive pulmonary decline, tocilizumab (TCZ) was recently introduced as a therapeutic strategy within the faSScinate study [16, 17]. This randomised controlled trial demonstrated a benefit from TCZ, with a significantly smaller decline in forced vital capacity (FVC); unfortunately, this effect waned at 48 weeks. Low-dose glucocorticoids (GCs) used to be the standard treatment for SSc-ILD. This is remarkable as GCs have never been shown to improve ILD outcomes and are suspected to dose-dependently increase the risk of SSc renal crisis [18]. GCs are variously prescribed at least initially in combination therapy in severe and progressive ILD [13, 19]. Overall, current evidence does not allow convincing recommendations on the use of IS in ILD. The updated EULAR/European League against Rheumatism Scleroderma Trial and Research (EUSTAR) guidelines will be in line with this conclusion [20].

The EUSTAR database offers a unique opportunity to analyse IS therapy in SSc-ILD. The aims of this study were (1) to analyse current use of IS drugs, (2) to test correlation between drug use and lung function tests and (3) to define specific treatments for defined disease characteristics.

## Methods

We included patients aged ≥ 18 years fulfilling the American College of Rheumatology (ACR) 1980 or ACR/EULAR 2013 classification criteria for SSc [21] with signs of ILD on pulmonary high resolution computed tomography (HRCT) and/or chest x-ray and at least one report on IS.

Data analysis comprised first EUSTAR documentation from 2004 until 6 May 2014. The entire observation period of each patient since initial diagnosis of ILD was considered. In order to receive comprehensive overviews of IS in SSc-ILD we referred to all documented visits at which IS was used. Missing IS information was counted as "never IS" if at least one item from the list of immunosuppressive therapies was answered. Patients with IS therapy ("ever IS") at any time were compared to patients who had never received IS ("never IS"). For our analysis of "never IS" versus "ever IS" patients were included at the visit when IS was documented for the first time or time of first ILD documentation for "never IS". For comparison of the features of patients receiving different IS we selected patients with at least one follow up since the documentation of ILD. We then grouped patients according to forced vital capacity (FVC) and diffusing capacity of the lung for carbon monoxide (DLCO) at the initiation of therapy, mimicking the classification by Steen [22] in order to generate three groups with different SSc-ILD severity: "mild" for DLCO >60% and FVC >85%, "moderate" for DLCO 51–60% and FVC 80–85% and "severe" for DLCO <51% and FVC <80%.

Standard EUSTAR documentation comprises current history, past medical history, medications, physical examination including modified Rodnan skin score (mRSS), laboratory results, lung and heart function tests, radiological imaging and capillaroscopy [23]. Disease duration is calculated from the time since first non-Raynaud's symptom. Yearly follow-up documentation is recommended. As a EUSTAR rule, each participating centre must obtain an ethics vote from their respective ethics committee. Afterwards, participating patients need to sign an individual consent form prior to inclusion into EUSTAR analysis.

## Statistics

Continuous parameters were compared by the Mann-Whitney test, frequencies by the $chi^2$ or Fisher exact test; $p$ values <0.05 were considered significant. No adjustment for multiple testing was done. Course of lung function under treatment was evaluated by linear regression analysis of change in DLCO and FVC from treatment start to at least one follow-up measurement. Patients were grouped by ranges of starting values (<50%, 50–75% and >75% predicted). Due to small numbers of cases for many treatment combinations, no individual combinations could be considered. Instead, additive and multiplicative effects of single drugs on the overall group trend were tested within each stratum: with additive effects indicating patients were taking that drug over the same overall time trend, but at a higher or lower level, meaning better or worse initial lung function, but afterwards the same course of DLCO or FVC; and with multiplicative effects signalling a steeper slope of the trend for patients using that drug, meaning either a better or worse course than the overall trend. We adjusted for the potential confounders of sex, age, extent of skin involvement, disease duration and initial DLCO or FVC values, respectively. Statistical analyses were performed using IBM SPSS Statistics, version 19.

## Results

### Patients on IS have more severe and active ILD compared to those without IS

Epidemiological data are shown in Table 1. Overall, IS was used in 2681/3778 (71%) patients with SSc-ILD, but only in 39.8% of patients with SSc without ILD ($p < 0.05$, data not shown).

### IS is used in a wide variety of monotherapy or combination therapy

Frequencies of immunosuppressants ever used and highest therapy combinations ever used per patient are shown in Fig. 1. Of the patients taking GC therapy, the average prednisone dosage was > 10 mg/day in 17%, and > 20 mg/day in 5.3% of patients.

Individual treatment regimens are shown in Fig. 2, with more than 3 immunosuppressive drugs being exceptions ($n = 17$ patients, not shown).

### Intensive IS is reserved for patients with severe and active ILD

Patient characteristics at the start of the most frequent monotherapy and combination therapy are described in Table 2.

Compared to patients in the never IS group, patients receiving GC monotherapy had significantly higher prevalence of SSc-related organ complications except for pulmonary hypertension and renal crisis. Within the "ever IS" group, patients receiving GC monotherapy were the oldest and had the longest disease duration. Patients who took MTX were only slightly different from patients in the never IS group. Patients who took MTX/GC had significantly worse DLCO, forced expiratory volume in one second (FEV-1) and modified Rodnan skin score (mRSS), indicating more severe disease and possibly also concomitant obstructive pulmonary disease. Patients who took AZA had significant impairment in FVC and DLCO, but no differences in New York Heart Association (NYHA) class. Interestingly, they had lower mRSS values than the never IS group. AZA/GC was used in patients with a more prominent reduction in DLCO and FVC values and with more patients in NYHA III and IV than in AZA monotherapy. Patients who took MMF had severe impairment of FVC and DLCO, which was even more pronounced when GC was added to MMF. Values for DLCO and FVC were lower and severe NYHA classification more frequent than in MMF monotherapy. Patients who took CYC had the most severely impaired lung function and highest rate of restrictive lung disease. Patients receiving MTX monotherapy had the best values for DLCO, FVC ($p < 0.001$) and total lung capacity (TLC), lowest prevalence of pulmonary hypertension ($p < 0.05$) and shortest disease duration. In contrast, patients who took CYC monotherapy had worst impairment in lung function and the highest rates of ground glass opacifications on imaging, plus the most severe skin fibrosis and highest mRSS values.

### A cluster of lung function parameters is associated with specific choices of IS

Sorting different therapy arms by average impairment in FVC and DLCO revealed clusters of ranges of lung function. Consequently, we grouped patients based on mean FVC and DLCO according to the classification of Steen [22]. Group I (mild impairment) had FVC of 86.9% and DLCO of 60.8%; group II (moderate impairment) had FVC of 83.4% and DLCO of 56.7%; and group III (severe impairment) had FVC of 76.6% and DLCO of 49.6%. Next we assessed whether other parameters were associated with specific choices of IS (Fig. 3).

Patients in group III had the worst FVC and DLCO, highest mRSS values, worst NYHA class and the highest rates of ground glass opacifications and restrictive defects. Compared to patients in the never IS group, patients in all three groups had significantly worse FVC, DLCO and TLC and more frequent ground glass opacifications. Patients in groups II and III had more severe NYHA class (both $p < 0.001$).

Compared to patients in the never IS group, the rate of ground glass opacification rates (24.4%) was twice that in groups I and II (43.9% and 40.2%, respectively), and even more often in group III (54.3%, all treatment

**Table 1** Characteristics of patients with SSc-ILD never or ever using immunosuppressive therapy

| | Total | Never used IS therapy | Ever used IS therapy | P value |
|---|---|---|---|---|
| Number of patients | 3778 | 1097 (29%) | 2681 (71%) | |
| Age (mean, SD) | 55.5 ± 13.4 | 59.0 ± 13.6 | 54.0 ± 13.0 | <0.001 |
| Female | 83.6% | 86.5% | 82.4% | 0.002 |
| BMI (mean, SD) (n = 1901) | 24.6 ± 4.7 | 24.5 ± 5.1 | 24.7 ± 4.6 | n.s. |
| Duration of SSc, years (mean, SD) | 8.5 ± 7.9 | 10.8 ± 9.2 | 7.6 ± 7.1 | <0.001 |
| (median (IQR)) | 6.2 (2.8; 11.9) | 8.4 (4.3; 15.0) | 5.4 (2.4; 10.8) | |
| mRSS (n = 3515) | | | | |
| (mean, SD) | 10.6 ± 8.7 | 8.9 ± 7.6 | 11.3 ± 9.0 | <0.001 |
| (median (IQR)) | 8.0 (4.0; 17.0) | 7.0 (4.0; 17.0) | 9.0 (4.0; 17.0) | |
| Extent of skin involvement (n = 3713) | | | | |
| diffuse | 44.4% | 29.4% | 50.3% | |
| limited | 46.9% | 60.9% | 41.3% | <0.001 |
| sclerodactyly only | 7.5% | 7.4% | 7.6% | |
| none | 1.2% | 2.4% | 0.8% | |
| Present scleroderma pattern (n = 1081) | 92.6% | 92.3% | 92.7% | n.s. |
| active | 40.7% | 41.5% | 40.4% | |
| early | 21.1% | 25.3% | 19.4% | 0.076 |
| late | 38.2% | 33.2% | 40.2% | |
| SSc activity index ≥3 (n = 3557) | 20.0% | 12.8% | 22.9% | <0.001 |
| DLCO, % predicted (mean, SD) (n = 2909) | 62.0 ± 20.2 | 67.4 ± 19.8 | 59.9 ± 20.0 | <0.001 |
| FVC, % predicted (mean, SD) (n = 2239) | 87.5 ± 21.8 | 94.9 ± 20.9 | 84.4 ± 21.5 | <0.001 |
| FVC:DLCO ratio (n = 2072) | 1.5 ± 0.5 | 1.5 ± 0.5 | 1.5 ± 0.5 | n.s. |
| FEV-1, % predicted (mean, SD) (n = 2239) | 86.2 ± 19.9 | 90.7 ± 19.0 | 84.2 ± 20.0 | <0.001 |
| TLC, % predicted (mean, SD) (n = 2239) | 85.0 ± 20.5 | 90.6 ± 20.1 | 82.6 ± 20.2 | <0.001 |
| History (n = 3755) | | | | |
| worsening of skin | 18.2% | 12.5% | 20.6% | <0.001 |
| worsening of fingers | 22.7% | 20.7% | 23.6% | n.s. |
| esophageal symptoms | 66.2% | 65.0% | 66.6% | n.s. |
| stomach symptoms | 25.9% | 22.1% | 27.5% | <0.001 |
| intestinal symptoms | 24.9% | 24.2% | 25.2% | n.s. |
| arterial hypertension | 23.2% | 23.7% | 23.0% | n.s. |
| renal crisis | 2.0% | 1.7% | 2.1% | n.s. |
| dyspnoea | 17.3% | 12.2% | 19.4% | <0.001 |
| worsening of cardiopulmonary manifestations | 19.1% | 14.8% | 20.9% | <0.001 |
| palpitations | 27.9% | 23.8% | 29.5% | <0.001 |
| Raynaud's present | 96.7% | 96.1% | 97.0% | n.s. |
| NYHA class (n = 2426) | | | | |
| I | 44.0% | 49.9% | 41.6% | |
| II | 38.7% | 37.8% | 39.0% | <0.001 |
| III | 15.2% | 10.1% | 17.3% | |
| IV | 2.1% | 2.1% | 2.1% | |
| Laboratory measures (n = 1346 –,648) | | | | |
| ANA+ | 94.9% | 95.6% | 94.6% | n.s. |
| ACA+ | 21.9% | 38.6% | 15.1% | <0.001 |

**Table 1** Characteristics of patients with SSc-ILD never or ever using immunosuppressive therapy *(Continued)*

| | Total | Never used IS therapy | Ever used IS therapy | P value |
|---|---|---|---|---|
| SCL70+ | 48.8% | 36.4% | 53.8% | <0.001 |
| U1 RNP+ | 6.4% | 2.9% | 7.9% | <0.001 |
| RNA+ | 4.5% | 4.1% | 4.7% | n.s. |
| PM-Scl+ | 4.5% | 3.7% | 4.9% | n.s. |
| CRP elevation | 27.5% | 18.5% | 31.3% | <0.001 |
| CK elevation | 9.3% | 5.8% | 10.7% | <0.001 |
| Proteinuria | 6.4% | 5.7% | 6.7% | n.s. |
| Hypocomplementemia | 6.0% | 4.9% | 6.4% | n.s. |
| ESR mm/h (mean, SD) | $25.8 \pm 20.7$ | $23.7 \pm 17.6$ | $26.7 \pm 21.7$ | 0.048 |
| Conduction blocks ($n = 3451$) | 14.1% | 12.8% | 14.6% | n.s. |
| Pulmonary hypertension ($n = 3451$) | 23.2% | 22.7% | 23.3% | n.s. |
| Diastolic function abnormal ($n = 3363$) | 24.3% | 21.1% | 25.5% | 0.008 |
| Pericardial effusion ($n = 2227$) | 12.6% | 13.2% | 12.4% | n.s. |
| Ground glass opacification ($n = 2014$) | 41.1% | 30.3% | 45.5% | <0.001 |
| PFT restrictive defect ($n = 3457$) | 45.9% | 35.6% | 49.9% | <0.001 |
| Echo | | | | |
| LVEF (%) ($n = 2095$) | $61.4 \pm 6.2$ | $62 \pm 6.6$ | $61.8 \pm 6.5$ | 0.005 |
| PAPsys (mmHg) ($n = 1835$) | $33 \pm 14.9$ | $32.4 \pm 12.7$ | $32.6 \pm 13.4$ | n.s. |
| Right heart catheter | | | | |
| RVSP (mmHg) ($n = 96$) | $46.8 \pm 21.9$ | $40.5 \pm 17.9$ | $42.5 \pm 19.3$ | n.s. |
| PAPmean (mmHg) ($n = 146$) | $36.2 \pm 15.4$ | $28.5 \pm 12.0$ | $30.8 \pm 13.5$ | 0.003 |
| PVR (dyn · sec · cm-5) ($n = 94$) | $541.5 \pm 498$ | $213.5 \pm 258.1$ | $328.6 \pm 391.2$ | 0.001 |
| PWP (mmHg) ($n = 113$) | $12.1 \pm 7.0$ | $12.2 \pm 9.6$ | $12.2 \pm 9.0$ | n.s. |
| CI (l/min/m2) ($n = 100$) | $2.8 \pm 0.6$ | $3.3 \pm 1.1$ | $3.1 \pm 1.0$ | 0.021 |
| 6 MWD | | | | |
| 6 MWD (m) ($n = 551$) | $444.9 \pm 129.6$ | $421.3 \pm 123.8$ | $428.1 \pm 125.9$ | 0.021 |
| O2 saturation at rest ($n = 457$) | $96 \pm 6.3$ | $95.9 \pm 4.3$ | $96.0 \pm 5.0$ | n.s. |
| O2 saturation at exercise ($n = 389$) | $92.9 \pm 8.0$ | $92.2 \pm 8.0$ | $92.4 \pm 8.0$ | n.s. |

*BMI* body mass index, *mRSS* modified Rodnan skin score, *DLCO* diffusing capacity of the lung for carbon monoxide, *FVC* forced vital capacity, *FEV-1* forced expiratory volume in one second, *TLC* total lung capacity, *NYHA* New York Heart Association, *ANA* anti-nuclear antibodies, *ACA* anti-centromere antibodies, *SCL70* anti-topoisomerase I antibody, *U1 RNP* U1-small nuclear ribonucloprotein particle, *RNA* ribonucleic acid antibody, *PM SCL* polymyositis scleroderma antibody, *CRP* C-reactive protein, *CK* creatin kinase, *ESR* erythrocyte sedimentation rate, *PFT* pulmonary function test, *LVEF* left ventricular ejection fraction, *PAPsys* systolic pulmonary arterial pressure, *RVSP* right ventricular systolic pressure, *PAPmean* mean pulmonary arterial pressure, *PVR* pulmonary vascular resistance, *PWP* pulmonary wedge pressure, *CI* cardiac index, *6 MWD* 6 minute walk distance, *n.s.* not significant

groups $p < 0.001$). The same trend was seen in the frequency of restrictive defects with the lowest rates in patients in the never IS group (36%) and an increasing frequency of 46.3% in group II and 61.0% in group III (both $p < 0.001$).

### Specific types of IS display minimal influence on the course of lung function

Follow-up documentation ranging from 1 month to 13 years was available in 73.6% of patients with SSc-ILD. Change in lung function over time was analysed in the respective subgroups of patients with <50%, 50–75% and >75% of FVC or DLCO predicted at treatment initiation and are shown in Fig. 4.

The group starting with < 50% of predicted FVC had the steepest decline in FVC (Fig. 4a). Here, GCs had negative multiplicative effects (Fig. 4c), thus there was even worse deterioration. In comparison, the group starting between 50 and 75% of predicted FVC had a less steep decline (Fig. 4a), with a positive additive effect in ACA-positive patients (Fig. 4b), but at the same time a negative multiplicative effect, meaning they started at higher FVC levels but had a steeper decline. Here, in patients in the never IS group a positive multiplicative effect was seen, indicating a less steep decline. The group starting with > 75% of predicted FVC had only a slight decline in FVC (Fig. 4a, b) with a negative additive effect in Scl70-positive patients but at the same time a positive multiplicative effect

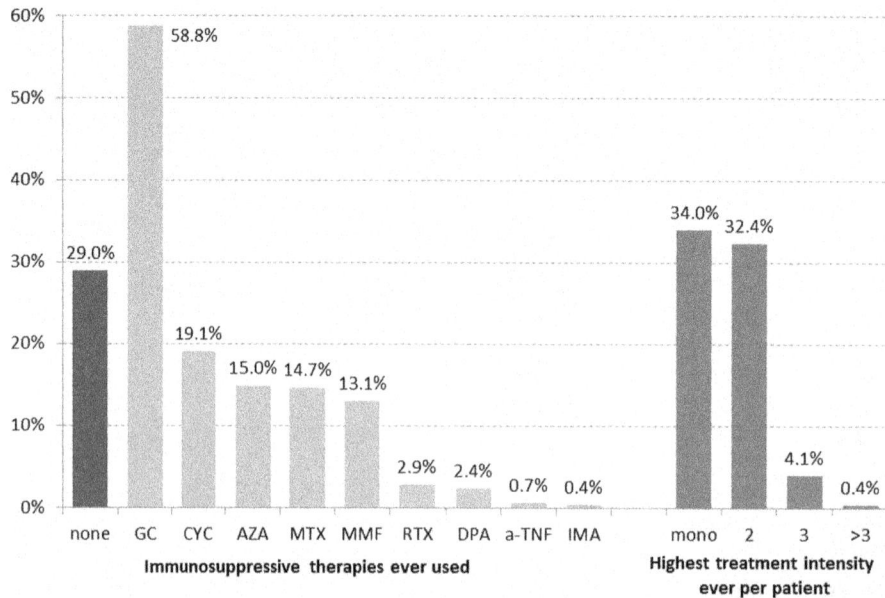

**Fig. 1** Frequencies of immunosuppressants ever used and highest therapy combination ever used per patient. *GC* glucocorticoids, *CYC* cyclophosphamide, *AZA* azathioprine, *MTX* methotrexate, *MMF* mycophenolate mofetil, *RTX* rituximab, *DPA* D-penicillamine, *a-TNF* anti-tumour necrosis factor, *IMA* imatinib

(Fig. 4c), meaning they started at lower FVC levels but had a flatter rate of decline. Here again, there were positive multiplicative effects in patients in the never IS group or in those receiving GCs, indicating less or no decline or even slight improvement.

Within the group starting with < 50% of predicted DLCO the overall course was represented by a slightly improving slope (Fig. 4b). Compared to that general trend, CYC and MMF had negative additive effects, meaning their course was following the same slope, but on a lower level, while ACA positivity had a positive additive effect, hence the course was on a higher level (Fig. 4d). In patients starting with DLCO values between 50 and 75% of predicted the overall trend was of slight

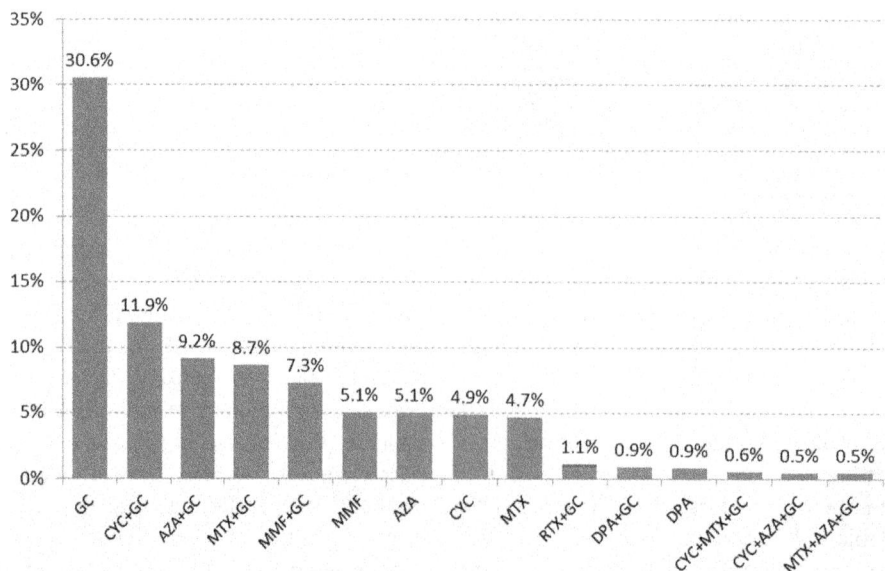

**Fig. 2** Monotherapies (Mono) and combinations of immunosuppressants ever used, percentages are based on the number of patients. Treatment regimens with frequencies <0.5% were omitted. *GC* glucocorticoids, *CYC* cyclophosphamide, *AZA* azathioprine, *MTX* methotrexate, *MMF* mycophenolate mofetil, *RTX* rituximab, *DPA* D-penicillamine, *a-TNF* anti-tumour necrosis factor, *IMA* imatinib

**Table 2** Characteristics of patients with dSSc or lSSc at the start of specific therapy

| | Never used IS | | AZA | | CYC | | MMF | | MTX | | GC | | AZA + GC | | CYC + GC | | MMF + GC | | MTX + GC | |
|---|---|---|---|---|---|---|---|---|---|---|---|---|---|---|---|---|---|---|---|---|
| | n | % | n | % | n | % | n | % | n | % | n | % | n | % | n | % | n | % | n | % |
| **Sex** | | | | | | | | | | | | | | | | | | | | |
| male | 103 | 14.4 | 14 | 10.6 | 18 | 24.0 | 22 | 20.4 | 18 | 17.8 | 108 | 15.2 | 42 | 18.5 | 35 | 21.0 | 47 | 24.2 | 29 | 14.9 |
| female | 612 | 85.6 | 118 | 89.4 | 57 | 76.0 | 86 | 79.6 | 83 | 82.2 | 604 | 84.8 | 185 | 81.5 | 132 | 79.0 | 147 | 75.8 | 165 | 85.1 |
| total | 715 | 100.0 | 132 | 100.0 | 75 | 100.0 | 108 | 100.0 | 101 | 100.0 | 712 | 100.0 | 227 | 100.0 | 167 | 100.0 | 194 | 100.0 | 194 | 100.0 |
| **Extent of skin involvement** | | | | | | | | | | | | | | | | | | | | |
| diffuse | 278 | 38.9 | 74 | 56.1 | 46 | 61.3 | 79 | 73.1 | 71 | 70.3 | 389 | 54.6 | 132 | 58.1 | 96 | 57.5 | 137 | 70.6 | 119 | 61.3 |
| limited | 437 | 61.1 | 58 | 43.9 | 29 | 38.7 | 29 | 26.9 | 30 | 29.7 | 323 | 45.4 | 95 | 41.9 | 71 | 42.5 | 57 | 29.4 | 75 | 38.7 |
| total | 715 | 100.0 | 132 | 100.0 | 75 | 100.0 | 108 | 100.0 | 101 | 100.0 | 712 | 100.0 | 227 | 100.0 | 167 | 100.0 | 194 | 100.0 | 194 | 100.0 |
| **NYHA** | | | | | | | | | | | | | | | | | | | | |
| I | 200 | 53.2 | 63 | 50.0 | 21 | 30.9 | 43 | 45.3 | 47 | 52.2 | 260 | 39.4 | 80 | 37.6 | 45 | 27.8 | 64 | 36.4 | 82 | 46.6 |
| II | 128 | 34.0 | 50 | 39.7 | 26 | 38.2 | 34 | 35.8 | 34 | 37.8 | 254 | 38.5 | 82 | 38.5 | 69 | 42.6 | 66 | 37.5 | 78 | 44.3 |
| III | 40 | 10.6 | 10 | 7.9 | 19 | 27.9 | 17 | 17.9 | 9 | 10.0 | 118 | 17.9 | 39 | 18.3 | 42 | 25.9 | 38 | 21.6 | 15 | 8.5 |
| IV | 8 | 2.1 | 3 | 2.4 | 2 | 2.9 | 1 | 1.1 | 0 | .0 | 28 | 4.2 | 12 | 5.6 | 6 | 3.7 | 8 | 4.5 | 1 | .6 |
| total | 376 | 100.0 | 126 | 100.0 | 68 | 100.0 | 95 | 100.0 | 90 | 100.0 | 660 | 100.0 | 213 | 100.0 | 162 | 100.0 | 176 | 100.0 | 176 | 100.0 |
| | of N | % | of N | % | of N | % | of N | % | of N | % | of N | % | of N | % | of N | % | of N | % | of n | % |
| ACA+ | 662 | 36.7 | 101 | 12.9 | 56 | 12.5 | 89 | 11.2 | 81 | 9.9 | 614 | 18.9 | 191 | 9.4 | 153 | 5.9 | 149 | 9.4 | 165 | 17.0 |
| SCL70+ | 665 | 38.2 | 106 | 64.2 | 59 | 62.7 | 92 | 56.5 | 85 | 64.7 | 617 | 53.3 | 197 | 57.4 | 155 | 64.5 | 157 | 64.3 | 167 | 59.3 |
| Pulmonary hypertension | 657 | 22.5 | 111 | 13.5 | 55 | 34.5 | 93 | 23.7 | 83 | 14.5 | 588 | 23.1 | 195 | 25.1 | 151 | 29.1 | 156 | 28.8 | 166 | 16.3 |
| Ground glass opacification | 315 | 24.4 | 67 | 53.7 | 51 | 54.9 | 68 | 61.8 | 49 | 42.9 | 435 | 36.3 | 138 | 42.0 | 121 | 59.5 | 117 | 48.7 | 105 | 38.1 |
| PFT restrictive defect | 666 | 36.6 | 102 | 48.0 | 56 | 62.5 | 78 | 60.3 | 82 | 37.8 | 574 | 42.9 | 191 | 50.8 | 151 | 59.6 | 144 | 61.8 | 161 | 41.0 |
| | mean | std | mean | std | Mean | std | mean | std | mean | std | mean | std | mean | std | mean | std | mean | std | mean | std |
| Age (years) | 58.6 | 14.0 | 56.5 | 11.5 | 55.7 | 12.4 | 55.4 | 12.4 | 54.8 | 12.0 | 58.9 | 12.7 | 54.1 | 12.3 | 53.9 | 13.1 | 53.7 | 12.7 | 56.9 | 12.9 |
| Body mass index | 24.4 | 5.0 | 25.3 | 4.9 | 25.3 | 4.1 | 25.1 | 5.1 | 25.0 | 5.0 | 25.0 | 4.7 | 25.3 | 4.8 | 24.5 | 3.5 | 26.2 | 5.1 | 24.7 | 5.4 |
| Disease duration (years) | 10.4 | 8.5 | 10.4 | 7.3 | 9.4 | 6.6 | 10.6 | 7.3 | 8.2 | 4.8 | 11.9 | 7.6 | 10.1 | 6.8 | 8.6 | 6.2 | 9.8 | 7.0 | 10.0 | 7.4 |
| mRSS | 9.6 | 7.6 | 6.8 | 5.7 | 11.6 | 7.4 | 9.9 | 8.2 | 10.4 | 8.5 | 8.9 | 8.0 | 8.2 | 7.1 | 10.2 | 8.1 | 10.3 | 8.4 | 11.0 | 7.9 |
| DLCO (% pred.) | 68.0 | 19.7 | 59.8 | 17.2 | 46.3 | 18.8 | 55.7 | 16.7 | 64.1 | 17.8 | 57.3 | 19.8 | 55.5 | 19.6 | 49.6 | 18.2 | 50.7 | 16.4 | 60.0 | 18.2 |
| FVC (% pred.) | 95.7 | 20.6 | 86.6 | 18.9 | 73.6 | 20.4 | 81.8 | 20.9 | 89.9 | 19.6 | 85.0 | 22.6 | 79.9 | 19.4 | 77.3 | 20.3 | 77.0 | 22.1 | 85.8 | 20.2 |
| FVC:DLCO ratio | 1.5 | .5 | 1.6 | .5 | 1.8 | .6 | 1.7 | .7 | 1.4 | .4 | 1.6 | .5 | 1.6 | .5 | 1.7 | .6 | 1.7 | .6 | 1.5 | .5 |
| FEV-1 (% pred.) | 93.5 | 18.8 | 84.0 | 17.1 | 77.5 | 21.4 | 80.5 | 18.6 | 91.2 | 17.7 | 84.9 | 21.8 | 81.4 | 18.4 | 79.9 | 21.9 | 76.8 | 22.5 | 85.3 | 18.8 |
| TLC (% pred.) | 89.1 | 20.5 | 81.2 | 18.8 | 70.0 | 16.5 | 75.9 | 18.1 | 92.5 | 18.5 | 80.0 | 19.3 | 75.4 | 21.1 | 72.5 | 16.7 | 74.0 | 17.8 | 84.9 | 20.1 |

Only therapy regimens with frequencies of at least 5% are displayed (for patients on immunosuppressive therapy, only therapy episodes started during follow up were included to exclude possibly long-lasting therapy episodes documented at baseline). dSSc diffuse cutaneous systemic sclerosis, lSSc limited systemic sclerosis, IS immunosuppression, AZA azathioprine, CYC cyclophosphamide, MMF mycophenolate mofetil, MTX methotrexate, GC glucocorticoid, NYHA New York Heart Association, ACA anti-centromere antibodies, SCL70 anti-topoisomerase I antibody, PFT pulmonary function test, mRSS modified Rodnan skin score, DLCO diffusing capacity of the lung for carbon monoxide, FVC forced vital capacity, FEV-1 forced expiratory volume in one second, TLC total lung capacity, pred. predicted, N number of patients within this specific group of medication

| | never IS | MTX | MTX +GC | AZA | GC | MMF | AZA +GC | MMF +GC | CYC +GC | CYC |
|---|---|---|---|---|---|---|---|---|---|---|
| FVC (% pred.), mean | 95.7 | 89.5 | 85.8 | 86.6 | 84.8 | 81.8 | 80.0 | 77.0 | 77.2 | 73.8 |
| | | | 86.9 | | | 83.4 | | | 76.6 | |
| DLCO/SB (% pred.), mean | 68.0 | 63.9 | 59.9 | 59.8 | 57.2 | 55.7 | 55.4 | 50.7 | 49.6 | 46.4 |
| | | | 60.8 | | | 56.7 | | | 49.6 | |
| FVC and DLCO/SB reduction | "reference" | group I "mild" | | | group II "moderate" | | | group III "severe" | | |

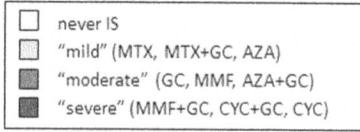

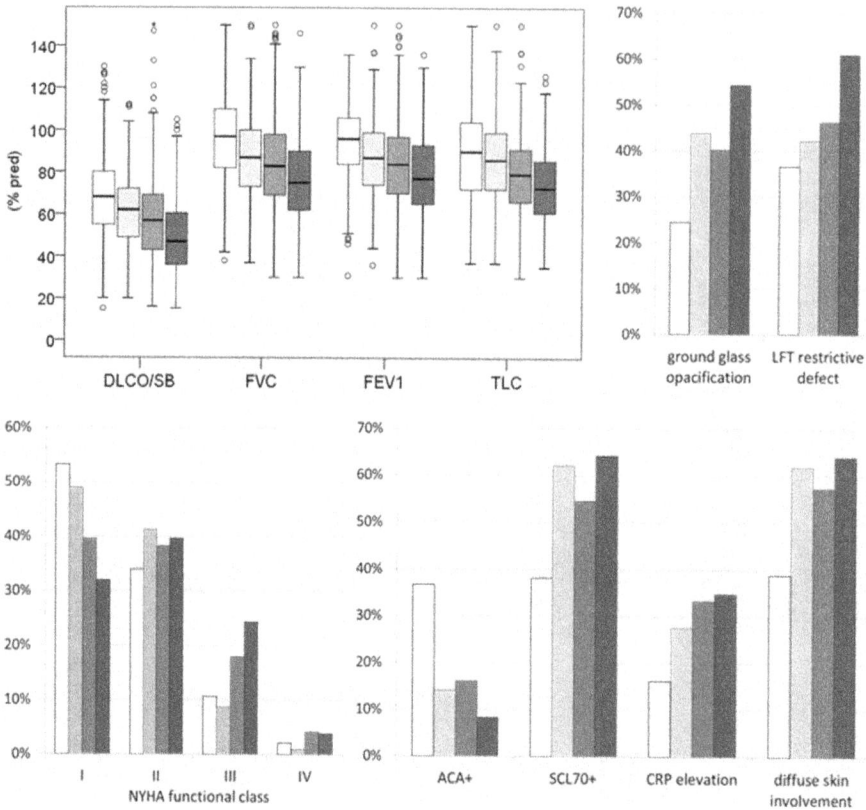

**Fig. 3** Patients grouped according to severity of lung function combined with the respective immunosuppression (IS) and clinical parameters. *never IS* patients who had never taken immunosuppressant drugs, *FVC* forced vital capacity, *DLCO* diffusing capacity of the lung for carbon monoxide, *SB* single breath, *MTX* methotrexate, *GC* glucocorticoid, *AZA* azathioprine, *MMF* mycophenolate mofetil, *CYC* cyclophosphamide, *PFT* pulmonary function test, *NYHA* New York Heart Association, *ACA* anti-centromere antibodies, *SCL70* anti-topoisomerase I antibody, *CRP* C-reactive protein

deterioration (Fig. 4b), with a negative additive effect of TNF inhibitors, again meaning it already started at a lower level but had the same gradient of deterioration. Here, ACA had a slightly negative multiplicative effect, meaning DLCO courses had a steeper decrease than the general trend, while in patients in the never IS group a positive multiplicative effect was seen, meaning a flatter decrease (Fig. 4b, d), with a positive additive effect of Scl70 positivity and a negative additive effect of GCs. There was a negative multiplicative effect of MMF, meaning an even steeper decrease than the general

trend, while there was a positive multiplicative effect in patients in the never IS group (Fig. 4d), meaning less decline or even slight improvement compared to the overall trend.

Adjusted for potential confounders and initial FVC or DLCO value no other medications than GCs, MMF, or "never IS" showed multiplicative effects on the course of lung function divergent from the general trend of the entire patient population. CYC and TNF inhibitors had only additive effects, pointing toward lower initial DLCO or FVC values in these

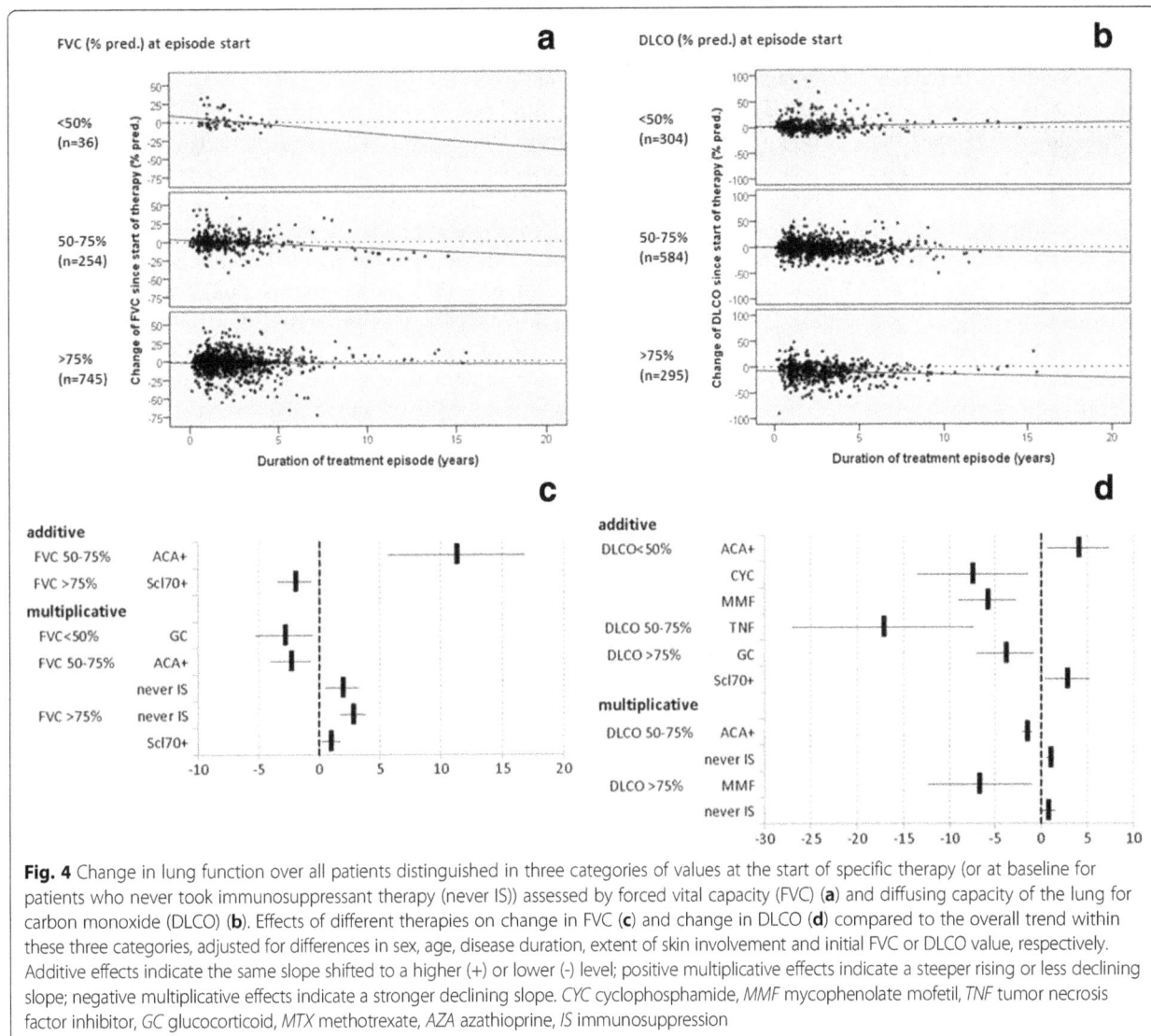

**Fig. 4** Change in lung function over all patients distinguished in three categories of values at the start of specific therapy (or at baseline for patients who never took immunosuppressant therapy (never IS)) assessed by forced vital capacity (FVC) (**a**) and diffusing capacity of the lung for carbon monoxide (DLCO) (**b**). Effects of different therapies on change in FVC (**c**) and change in DLCO (**d**) compared to the overall trend within these three categories, adjusted for differences in sex, age, disease duration, extent of skin involvement and initial FVC or DLCO value, respectively. Additive effects indicate the same slope shifted to a higher (+) or lower (-) level; positive multiplicative effects indicate a steeper rising or less declining slope; negative multiplicative effects indicate a stronger declining slope. *CYC* cyclophosphamide, *MMF* mycophenolate mofetil, *TNF* tumor necrosis factor inhibitor, *GC* glucocorticoid, *MTX* methotrexate, *AZA* azathioprine, *IS* immunosuppression

patients, but no differing time trends compared to patients on other treatments.

## Discussion

Our analysis of observational data describes current IS strategies in patients with SSc-ILD from the EUSTAR cohort. It shows clusters of clinical characteristics correlated with IS choices and identifies factors that might influence future IS decisions.

A large proportion of patients with SSc-ILD did not receive IS despite having dcSSc (34% of patients), active scleroderma pattern on nail fold capillaroscopy (40% of patients) and Valentini disease activity index (VDAI) ≥3 (12% of patients). On average these patients have longer disease duration and show fewer signs of alveolitis on HRCT. These characteristics may suggest that the greatest decline in lung function has already happened and stabilisation of lung function in the absence of active

inflammation is expected without any further IS medication [22], or they might represent patients with overall benign disease courses. In our analysis, positive trends in lung function over time - especially in patients starting with 50–75% of predicted FVC - support this notion. It contrasts with a scleroderma lung study showing a mild 12-month decline in FVC of 4.2%, and in DLCO of 8.2%, irrespective of disease duration [1]. On the other hand our data are in agreement with a study documenting that FVC values within the first 3 years after disease onset strongly predict SSc-ILD outcome [24].

GCs were used most frequently in 58% of the patients in high proportions and even at dosages >10 mg/day and >20 mg/day. This comes as a surprise and has to be questioned, as the effect of GCs on lung function was marginal at best and only slightly positive in patients with > 75% of predicted FVC who might as well continue without any IS at all. Furthermore, it is well-established that this treatment regimen is associated with higher rates of infection and scleroderma renal crisis [25]. Of note, patients receive combinations of GC with MTX, AZA, MMF or CYC regardless of lung function parameters or NYHA class. Collectively our data show that combining GCs with another IS therapy reflects the standard of care in many centres worldwide.

The second most frequently used therapy was CYC, as recommended by the EUSTAR guidelines for patients with severe and progressive SSc-ILD. Two meta-analyses failed to show a significant benefit of CYC on SSc-ILD on lung function tests [26]. However, a statistically non-relevant improvement might still represent a patient-relevant effect on quality of life as reflected by the Short Form-36 (SF-36) data evaluated within the first scleroderma lung study [4]. In our analysis, patients treated with CYC monotherapy or CYC/GC started with the worst DLCO values, worst NYHA class, highest frequencies of restrictive defects and PH, and the highest mRSS. More than 60% of these patients showed signs of active inflammation reflected by high ESR, CRP elevation or ground glass opacifications on HRCT. Stratification of these patients by their starting values did not result in differences in the slope of DLCO or FVC values compared to all other patients. Interestingly, Becker et al. describe the highest SSc-ILD response rates assessed by FVC and DLCO in patients with low FVC values prior to CYC therapy [27] indicating a potential for reversal of fibrosis.

MMF, often regarded as potential maintenance therapy in SSc-ILD, was used as monotherapy in moderate or - combined with GC - severe lung impairment, in our analysis. A prospective open-label trial on MMF describes early and significant improvement in DLCO, non-significant improvement in FVC and reduction in ground glass opacifications in five patients with disease duration between 1.5 and 3 years [28]. A meta-analysis argues along these lines, suggesting that MMF may stabilise lung function [29]; however, the superiority of MMF compared to CYC was not verified [7]. The very recent randomized controlled, double-blind, parallel group trial comparing MMF with oral CYC shows significant improvement in pre-specified measures of lung function over 2 years. It did not reach its primary endpoint, i.e. MMF to be more effective than CYC; however, MMF had a better side-effect profile [8].

An uncontrolled study of AZA maintenance therapy after 1-year induction with CYC showed stabilising effects of AZA in SSc-ILD, but involved only 13 patients [30]. Retrospective data on 36 patients with SSc-ILD comparing oral CYC with AZA shows significant effects of AZA on DLCO and FVC, yet no effects of CYC [12]. Our data cannot confirm this as AZA had only a very

slightly positive effect on DLCO in patients starting with DLCO >75%, thus being almost equal to the effect of "never IS".

Studies analyzing the effects of MTX on SSc-ILD are rare. This might be due to the fact that ILD is one of the possible side effects of MTX and hence physicians might be hesitant to prescribe it to patients with SSc-ILD. Indeed, there is one study showing no effects of MTX on lung function despite trends towards positive effects on the mRSS [31]. However, this study was small ($n = 29$) and covered a relatively short timeframe (24 weeks). A study with 11 patients taking MTX describes subjective improvement in dyspnoea in 5 patients, no change in another 5 and worsening in 1 patient [32]. In our data, MTX was used in patients that resembled those of the never IS group except for higher mRSS and more frequent ground glass opacifications. Comparing MTX + GC to MTX alone displayed significant differences in mRSS, DLCO, FVC, FEV-1 and rates of ground glass opacifications. Nevertheless, its effect on the course of PFTs was negligible.

Overall, our data describe treatment patterns in patients with SSc-ILD that are used across European centres yet are only partially in accordance with EUSTAR recommendations. Most clinicians chose intensive IS in active lung disease. Common choices were not only CYC+/-GC as recommended by current guidelines, but also MMF + GC. None of the specific types of IS was clearly superior to another in influencing the course of lung function in any DLCO or FVC group. The only positive trends seen were in patients in the never IS group and patients taking GC, starting with > 75% of predicted FVC, and in the never IS group, patients taking AZA and MTX starting with > 75% of predicted DLCO all had a reduced rate of deterioration over time. Thus, if carefully monitored for changes in lung function, patients with SSc-ILD with only small PFT impairment might benefit from on-demand IS instead of ongoing IS.

Our study has some limitations: The retrospective design leaves us with some missing data, reducing the large number of patients within this data set to small groups when addressing specific questions of immunosuppressive treatment. Furthermore, changes in the prescription pattern might be missed, and data on when and why the immunosuppressive treatment was changed are lacking. Additional prospective data are urgently warranted. The prospective observational trial of the Seventh Framework Programme (FP7) project "DeSScipher" (a study to decipher the optimal management of systemic sclerosis) launched in 2012 will allow assessment of the dynamics of SSc-ILD-related treatment patterns in terms of escalation and de-escalation and to evaluate their efficacy.

## Conclusions

IS is broadly prescribed in SSc-ILD. Clusters of clinical and functional characteristics guide individualised treatment. The data favour differential decision-making pointing either to watchful waiting and close monitoring in the early stages or start of immunosuppressive treatment in patients with SSc-ILD and moderately impaired lung function. Advantages of specific IS are difficult to depict due to confounding by indication. Data do not support liberal use of GC in SSc-ILD.

### Abbreviations

6MWD: Six minute walk distance; ACA: Anti-centromere antibodies; ACR: American College of Rheumatology; ANA: Anti-nuclear antibodies; a-TNF: Anti-tumour necrosis factor; AZA: Azathioprine; BMI: Body mass index; CI: Cardiac index; CK: Creatin kinase; CRP: C-Reactive protein; CYC: Cyclophosphamide; dcSSc: Diffuse cutaneous systemic sclerosis; DeSScipher: Study to decipher the optimal management of systemic sclerosis; DLCO: Diffusing capacity for carbon monoxide; D-PA: D-penicillamine; ESR: Erythrocyte sedimentation rate; EULAR: European League against Rheumatism; EUSTAR: European League against Rheumatism Scleroderma Trial and Research; FEV-1: Forced expiratory volume in one second; FP7: Seventh Framework Programme; FVC: Forced vital capacity; GC: Glucocorticoids; HRCT: High resolution computed tomography; ILD: Interstitial lung disease; IMA: Imatinib; IS: Immunosuppressive treatment; lSSc: Limited systemic sclerosis; LVEF: Left ventricular ejection fraction; MMF: Mycophenolate mofetil; mRSS: Modified Rodnan skin score; MTX: Methotrexate; NYHA: New York Heart Association; O2: Oxygen; PAPmean: Mean pulmonary arterial pressure; PAPsys: Systolic pulmonary arterial pressure; PFT: Pulmonary function test; PM SCL: Polymyositis scleroderma antibody; PVR: Pulmonary vascular resistance; PWP: Pulmonary wedge pressure; RNA: Ribonucleic acid antibody; RTX: Rituximab; RVSP: Right ventricular systolic pressure; SCL 70: Anti-topoisomerase I; SSc: Systemic sclerosis; TCZ: Tocilizumab; TLC: Total lung capacity; U1RNP: U1-small nuclear ribonucloprotein particle; VDAI: Valentini disease activity index

### Acknowledgements

We appreciate the work of all members of the participating EUSTAR centres represented by the list of co-workers on behalf of the DeSScipher project research group within the EUSTAR network, which is provided as Additional file 1.

### Funding

This work was funded by the EU research grant HEALTH-F5-2012-305495 and by the research funds of the Department of Rheumatology, Immunology and Allergology, University of Bern, Switzerland.

### Authors' contributions

SA and DH extracted and analysed the data and drafted and edited the manuscript. ES analysed the data and edited the manuscript, YA, LZ, FDG, CD, OD; MF, MMC, UML, IT, GV and UW were involved in analysis and interpretation of the data and revised the manuscript. PV analysed and interpreted the data and drafted and edited the manuscript. GR designed the study, analysed and interpreted the data and edited the manuscript. All authors agreed to be accountable for all aspects of the work in ensuring that questions related to the accuracy or integrity of any part of the work are appropriately investigated and resolved, and gave final approval of the version to be published.

### Competing interests

The authors declare that they have no competing interests.

### Author details

[1]Department of Rheumatology, Immunology and Allergology, University Hospital and University of Bern, Freiburgstrasse 4, 3010 Bern, Switzerland. [2]German Rheumatism Research Center, A Leibniz Institute, Berlin, Germany. [3]Department of Rheumatology and Clinical Immunology, Charité University Hospital, Berlin, Germany. [4]Department of Rheumatology A, Descartes University, APHP, Cochin Hospital, Paris, France. [5]Department of Rheumatology and Immunology, University of Pecs, Pecs, Hungary. [6]University of Leeds, Leeds, UK. [7]UCL Division of Medicine, Centre for Rheumatology, Royal Free Hospital, London, UK. [8]Department of Rheumatology, University Hospital Zurich, Zurich, Switzerland. [9]Department of Rheumatology and Clinical Immunology, Osteology and Physical Therapy, Justus-Liebig-University Giessen, Kerckhoff Klinik, Bad Nauheim, Germany. [10]Department Experimental and Clinical Medicine, Division of Rheumatology AOUC, University of Florence, Florence, Italy. [11]Department of Rheumatology, Second University of Naples, Naples, Italy. [12]Department of Rheumatology, University of Basel, Basel, Switzerland. [13]Department of Rheumatology, University Medical Center Schleswig-Holstein, Kiel, Germany.

### References

1. Khanna D, Tseng CH, Farmani N, Steen V, Furst DE, Clements PJ, et al. Clinical course of lung physiology in patients with scleroderma and interstitial lung disease: analysis of the Scleroderma Lung Study Placebo Group. Arthritis Rheum. 2011;63(10):3078–85.
2. Steen VD, Medsger TA. Changes in causes of death in systemic sclerosis, 1972-2002. Ann Rheum Dis. 2007;66(7):940–4.
3. Kowal-Bielecka O, Landewe R, Avouac J, Chwiesko S, Miniati I, Czirjak L, et al. EULAR recommendations for the treatment of systemic sclerosis: a report from the EULAR Scleroderma Trials and Research group (EUSTAR). Ann Rheum Dis. 2009;68(5):620–8.
4. Tashkin DP, Elashoff R, Clements PJ, Roth MD, Furst DE, Silver RM, et al. Effects of 1-year treatment with cyclophosphamide on outcomes at 2 years in scleroderma lung disease. Am J Respir Crit Care Med. 2007; 176(10):1026–34.
5. Nihtyanova SI, Brough GM, Black CM, Denton CP. Mycophenolate mofetil in diffuse cutaneous systemic sclerosis – a retrospective analysis. Rheumatology (Oxford). 2007;46(3):442–5.
6. Koutroumpas A, Ziogas A, Alexiou I, Barouta G, Sakkas LI. Mycophenolate mofetil in systemic sclerosis-associated interstitial lung disease. Clin Rheumatol. 2010;29(10):1167–8.
7. Panopoulos ST, Bournia VK, Trakada G, Giavri I, Kostopoulos C, Sfikakis PP. Mycophenolate versus cyclophosphamide for progressive interstitial lung disease associated with systemic sclerosis: a 2-year case control study. Lung. 2013;191(5):483–9.
8. Tashkin DP, Roth MD, Clements PJ, Furst DE, Khanna D, Kleerup EC, et al. Mycophenolate mofetil versus oral cyclophosphamide in scleroderma-related interstitial lung disease (SLS II): a randomised controlled, double-blind, parallel group trial. Lancet Respir Med. 2016; 4(9):708–19.
9. Raghu G, Depaso WJ, Cain K, Hammar SP, Wetzel CE, Dreis DF, et al. Azathioprine combined with prednisone in the treatment of idiopathic pulmonary fibrosis: a prospective double-blind, randomized, placebo-controlled clinical trial. Am Rev Respir Dis. 1991;144(2):291–6.
10. Poormoghim H, Rezaei N, Sheidaie Z, Almasi AR, Moradi-Lakeh M, Almasi S, et al. Systemic sclerosis: comparison of efficacy of oral cyclophosphamide and azathioprine on skin score and pulmonary involvement-a retrospective study. Rheumatol Int. 2014;34(12):1691-9.
11. Nadashkevich O, Davis P, Fritzler M, Kovalenko W. A randomized unblinded trial of cyclophosphamide versus azathioprine in the treatment of systemic sclerosis. Clin Rheumatol. 2006;25(2):205–12.
12. Hoyles RK, Ellis RW, Wellsbury J, Lees B, Newlands P, Goh NS, et al. A multicenter, prospective, randomized, double-blind, placebo-controlled trial of corticosteroids and intravenous cyclophosphamide followed by oral azathioprine for the treatment of pulmonary fibrosis in scleroderma. Arthritis Rheum. 2006;54(12):3962–70.

13. Walker KM, Pope J, participating members of the Scleroderma Clinical Trials C, Canadian Scleroderma Research G. Treatment of systemic sclerosis complications: what to use when first-line treatment fails–a consensus of systemic sclerosis experts. Semin Arthritis Rheum. 2012;42(1):42–55.

14. Arakawa H, Yamasaki M, Kurihara Y, Yamada H, Nakajima Y. Methotrexate-induced pulmonary injury: serial CT findings. J Thorac Imaging. 2003;18(4):231–6.

15. Lepri G, Avouac J, Airo P, Anguita Santos F, Bellando-Randone S, Blagojevic J, et al. Effects of rituximab in connective tissue disorders related interstitial lung disease. Clin Exp Rheumatol. 2016;34 Suppl 100(5):181–5.

16. De Lauretis A, Sestini P, Pantelidis P, Hoyles R, Hansell DM, Goh NS, et al. Serum interleukin 6 is predictive of early functional decline and mortality in interstitial lung disease associated with systemic sclerosis. J Rheumatol. 2013;40(4):435–46.

17. Khanna D, Denton CP, Jahreis A, van Laar JM, Frech TM, Anderson ME, et al. Safety and efficacy of subcutaneous tocilizumab in adults with systemic sclerosis (faSScinate): a phase 2, randomised, controlled trial. Lancet. 2016;387(10038):2630–40.

18. Steen VD, Medsger Jr TA. Case-control study of corticosteroids and other drugs that either precipitate or protect from the development of scleroderma renal crisis. Arthritis Rheum. 1998;41(9):1613–9.

19. Mouthon L, Berezne A, Guillevin L, Valeyre D. Therapeutic options for systemic sclerosis related interstitial lung diseases. Respir Med. 2010;104 Suppl 1:S59–69.

20. Kowal-Bielecka O, Fransen J, Avouac J, Becker M, Kulak A, et al. Update of EULAR recommendations for the treatment of systemic sclerosis. Ann Rheum Dis. 2017;76(8):1327–1339.

21. Rodnan GP, Medsger TA, Altman RD, D'Angelo WA, Fries JF, LeRoy EC, Kirsner AB, MacKensie AH, MacShane DJ, Myers AR, Sharp GC. Preliminary criteria for the classification of systemic sclerosis (scleroderma). Subcommittee for scleroderma criteria of the American Rheumatism Association Diagnostic and Therapeutic Criteria Committee. Arthritis Rheum. 1980;23(5):581-90.

22. Steen VD, Conte C, Owens GR, Medsger Jr TA. Severe restrictive lung disease in systemic sclerosis. Arthritis Rheum. 1994;37(9):1283–9.

23. Walker UA, Tyndall A, Czirjak L, Denton C, Farge-Bancel D, Kowal-Bielecka O, et al. Clinical risk assessment of organ manifestations in systemic sclerosis: a report from the EULAR Scleroderma Trials And Research group database. Ann Rheum Dis. 2007;66(6):754–63.

24. Morgan C, Knight C, Lunt M, Black CM, Silman AJ. Predictors of end stage lung disease in a cohort of patients with scleroderma. Ann Rheum Dis. 2003;62(2):146–50.

25. Iudici M, van der Goes MC, Valentini G, Bijlsma JW. Glucocorticoids in systemic sclerosis: weighing the benefits and risks - a systematic review. Clin Exp Rheumatol. 2013;31(2 Suppl 76):157–65.

26. Nannini C, West CP, Erwin PJ, Matteson EL. Effects of cyclophosphamide on pulmonary function in patients with scleroderma and interstitial lung disease: a systematic review and meta-analysis of randomized controlled trials and observational prospective cohort studies. Arthritis Res Ther. 2008;10(5):R124.

27. Becker MO, Schohe A, Weinert K, Huscher D, Schneider U, Burmester GR, et al. Responders to cyclophosphamide: results of a single-centre analysis among systemic sclerosis patients. Ann Rheum Dis. 2012;71(12):2061–2.

28. Liossis SN, Bounas A, Andonopoulos AP. Mycophenolate mofetil as first-line treatment improves clinically evident early scleroderma lung disease. Rheumatology (Oxford). 2006;45(8):1005–8.

29. Tzouvelekis A, Galanopoulos N, Bouros E, Kolios G, Zacharis G, Ntolios P, et al. Effect and safety of mycophenolate mofetil or sodium in systemic sclerosis-associated interstitial lung disease: a meta-analysis. Pulm Med. 2012;2012:143637.

30. Paone C, Chiarolanza I, Cuomo G, Ruocco L, Vettori S, Menegozzo M, et al. Twelve-month azathioprine as maintenance therapy in early diffuse systemic sclerosis patients treated for 1-year with low dose cyclophosphamide pulse therapy. Clin Exp Rheumatol. 2007;25(4):613–6.

31. van den Hoogen FH, Boerbooms AM, Swaak AJ, Rasker JJ, van Lier HJ, van de Putte LB. Comparison of methotrexate with placebo in the treatment of systemic sclerosis: a 24 week randomized double-blind trial, followed by a 24 week observational trial. Br J Rheumatol. 1996;35(4):364–72.

32. Krishna Sumanth M, Sharma VK, Khaitan BK, Kapoor A, Tejasvi T. Evaluation of oral methotrexate in the treatment of systemic sclerosis. Int J Dermatol. 2007;46(2):218–23.

# Characterization of inflammatory cell infiltrate of scleroderma skin: B cells and skin score progression

Silvia Bosello[1,2†], Cristiana Angelucci[3†], Gina Lama[3], Stefano Alivernini[1,2], Gabriella Proietti[3], Barbara Tolusso[1,2], Gigliola Sica[3], Elisa Gremese[1,2] and Gianfranco Ferraccioli[1,2*]

## Abstract

**Background:** The purpose of this study was to investigate the frequency and the distribution of inflammatory cell infiltrate in two sets of cutaneous biopsies derived from clinically affected and unaffected skin in patients with systemic sclerosis (SSc) and to test correlation between the cell infiltrate and the progression of skin involvement.

**Methods:** Skin was immunohistochemically assessed to identify CD68, CD3, CD20 and CD138-positive (+) cells in clinically affected and unaffected skin in 28 patients with SSc. Patients were followed for 6 months and the characteristics of the infiltrate were analyzed according to disease duration, clinical features and skin involvement progression.

**Results:** In all SSc cutaneous specimens, cellular infiltrates were found in a perivascular location predominantly in the mid and deeper portions of the dermis. All the analyzed biopsies showed a $CD3^+$ and $CD68^+$ cell infiltrate and the mean number of $CD3^+$ and of $CD68^+$ cells was higher in clinically involved skin ($CD3^+$, 71.7 ± 34.6 and $CD68^+$, 26.3 ± 8.4, respectively) than in clinically uninvolved skin ($CD3^+$, 45.7 ± 36.0 and $CD68^+$, 13.6 ± 6.1, respectively) ($p < 0.001$ for both comparisons). $CD20^+$ cells were found in 17 (60.7%) patients and in these patients the mean number of $CD20^+$ cells was higher in clinically involved (4.7 ± 5.9) than in uninvolved skin (1.9 ± 2.9), ($p = 0.04$). There was a greater number of $CD20^+$ cells in patients with early SSc compared with patients with long-standing disease. $CD138^+$ cells were found in 100% of biopsies of clinically involved skin and in 89.3% of biopsies of uninvolved skin. The mean number of $CD138^+$ cells was higher in clinically involved skin (3.6 ± 2.3) than in clinically uninvolved skin (1.9 ± 1.7), ($p < 0.001$). Seven patients experienced more than 20% worsening in the skin score after 6 months of follow up; all of them had a $CD20^+$ skin infiltrate on biopsy of clinically involved skin.

**Conclusions:** Our results confirm that mononuclear cells are present in the skin of all patients with SSc, underlining the role of inflammatory cell infiltrates in skin involvement in SSc. B cells in the skin seem to characterize patients with early diffuse skin disease and to correlate with skin progression.

**Keywords:** Systemic sclerosis, T cells, B cells, Macrophages, Skin involvement

* Correspondence: gianfranco.ferraccioli@unicatt.it; gff1990@gmail.com
†Equal contributors
Unità Operativa Complessa di Reumatologia, Istituto di Reumatologia e
Scienze Affini, Università Cattolica del Sacro Cuore, Rome, Italy
1Fondazione Policlinico Universitario Agostino Gemelli, Via G. Moscati,
31-00168 Rome, Italy
Full list of author information is available at the end of the article

## Background

Progressive systemic sclerosis (SSc) or scleroderma is a chronic connective tissue disorder characterized by vascular and cellular abnormalities that predominate in the early stages of disease and eventually lead to extensive cutaneous and visceral fibrosis, which is most prominent in the later stages [1–3]. The pathologic phenotype of the disease is complex and, consequently, its etiology and the effective therapies to prevent its progression remain elusive.

Cutaneous mononuclear cells are a frequent histopathological finding in SSc. Previous studies have recorded an increase in the number of mast cells [4, 5], macrophages [3, 6–11] and T lymphocytes [3, 6, 8–12], in particular in the early stages of SSc. Furthermore, microarray analysis in the lungs and in the skin of patients with scleroderma indicates overexpression of macrophage marker genes [13–16]. In vitro studies have demonstrated that all these cells can produce several cytokines and stimulate fibroblasts [1].

To date, although there have been various reports of studies of the B cell infiltrate in SSc [3, 6, 8–10, 13, 17–19], its characterization in skin affected by scleroderma is still incomplete. Recently, some encouraging results suggested a possible use of an anti-CD20 monoclonal antibody (rituximab) for the treatment of early, progressive and diffuse scleroderma, suggesting a role for B cells in the pathogenesis of the disease in the early stage [17–23]. In fact, it has been shown that patients with SSc present with autoantibody production [24], hyper-γ-globulinemia, polyclonal B cell hyperactivity [25] and abnormalities in the B cell compartments, characterized by an increase in naïve cells and a decrease in activated memory B cells [26]. In addition, in scleroderma there is markedly increased expression of CD19, a signal transduction molecule of B cells that regulates production of autoantibodies, in both memory and naïve B cells [26, 27]. In patients with diffuse SSc (dSSc), analysis of DNA microarrays of cutaneous biopsies have demonstrated higher expression of clusters of genes of $CD20^+$ cells and of plasma cells [13].

In an attempt to further clarify the characteristics of the cellular infiltrate, and mostly the possible role of B cells in skin fibrosis, we investigated the frequency and the distribution of mononuclear cells in two sets of cutaneous biopsies derived from clinically affected and unaffected skin from patients with SSc. The characteristics of the infiltrate were also analyzed according to disease duration, clinical features of the patients and skin score modification after 6 months.

## Methods

### Patients

Patients with SSc (n = 28 (24 female and 4 male)) attending the outpatient clinic of the Division of Rheumatology of our institution agreed to undergo skin biopsies on both clinically affected and unaffected skin and were included in the study. All patients fulfilled the old and the new classification criteria for scleroderma proposed by the European League Against Rheumatism (EULAR) and the American College of Rheumatology (ACR) [28, 29]. Informed signed consent to undergo biopsies and to provide skin samples and clinical data for research purposes was provided by all the patients. This research has been performed in accordance with the Declaration of Helsinki and it was approved by our institutional ethics committee (Comitato Etico Università Cattolica del Sacro Cuore 1883/12).

Demographic and clinical characteristics were collected in all patients with SSc enrolled in the study. Patients were grouped according to the classification proposed by LeRoy in patients with limited SSc (lSSc) or diffuse SSc (dSSc) [30]. The extent of skin involvement was evaluated by the Rodnan skin score, performed by two assessors (always the same at every evaluation) whose results were averaged [31], at the time of skin biopsy and after a mean follow-up time of 6.5 ± 0.8 months. A modification of skin score higher than 20% was considered clinically significant progression [32, 33]. Antinuclear antibodies (ANA) were determined by indirect immunofluorescence using Hep-2 cells as substrates and autoantibody specificities were further assessed by ELISA (Shield, Dundee, UK).

Cutaneous specimens were taken from patients with SSc, by surgical excision with a 6-mm punch from the distal forearm for the clinically involved skin (skin score >1 at this site) and from the buttock for clinically uninvolved skin (skin score = 0 at this site). The presence of mononuclear inflammatory cells was investigated in all skin specimens, in particular CD3 as a marker of T lymphocytes, CD20 as a marker of B-lymphocytes (local mature B cells and memory B cells), CD138 as a marker of plasma cells and CD68 as a marker of residential macrophages.

At the time of the skin biopsies, the activity index [34] and the severity index [35] were assessed and Global Health (GH) status and Health Assessment Questionnaires (HAQ) were administered to patients to evaluate the influence of the disease on daily functions.

All 28 patients continued to receive iloprost (an infusion of 0.5–2 ng/kg body weight/min for 5 days every 2 months), calcium channel blockers (nifedipine 20–40 mg/day) and acetylsalicylic-acid from the moment of diagnosis. Patients receiving corticosteroids or immunosuppressive drugs at the time of skin biopsy were excluded from the study. During the follow-up period, 12 patients were treated with anti-CD20 monoclonal antibody (rituximab) with or without cyclophosphamide for skin disease progression and/or lung involvement, while the other 16 patients did not receive immunosuppressive drugs.

Internal organ involvement was evaluated no longer than one month before or after the skin biopsies. All patients with SSc underwent pulmonary function tests (PFTs) to define forced vital capacity (FVC) and diffusing capacity for carbon monoxide (DLCO), and high resolution computed tomography (HRCT) was performed to assess lung involvement [36]. Renal involvement was defined as a scleroderma crisis or as the presence of proteinuria or elevation in creatinine serum level. Electrocardiography (ECG) and echocardiography were also performed in all patients: cardiac involvement was defined as the presence of conduction disturbance, left ventricular ejection fraction (LVEF) and <50%, pulmonary artery systolic pressure (PASP) >35 mmHg on echocardiography. Gastro-intestinal involvement was defined as the presence of gastroesophageal reflux symptoms or the evidence of gastrointestinal motility disturbance.

Four female healthy subjects (age range 36–55 years) gave their informed consent to undergo forearm skin biopsy, as controls.

### Immunohistochemical analysis

Immunohistochemical analysis was carried out on 5-μm thick tissue sections on polylysine-coated slides. After deparaffinization and rehydration, antigen retrieval was performed. Slide-mounted sections were heated in a microwave oven at 700 watt two times for 4 min in 10 mmol/L sodium citrate buffer (pH 6.0). Quenching of endogenous peroxidase activity was performed with Tris-buffered saline (TBS) (pH 7.6) containing 2% hydrogen peroxide ($H_2O_2$) for 10 min at room temperature (RT). To prevent non-specific binding, blocking was performed with Super block (UCS Diagnostics, Rome, Italy) for 8 min at RT. Sections were incubated with anti-CD3 mouse monoclonal antibodies (mAb) (1:50 dilution; Clone PS1, Abcam, Cambridge, MA, USA) or anti-CD20 mouse mAb (1:100 dilution; Clone L26; Novus Biologicals, Littleton, CO, USA) or human anti-CD138 (Syndecan-1) rabbit polyclonal antibodies (Ab) (1:25 dilution; Spring Bioscience, CA, USA). Tissues were then incubated with the Super Picture HRP Polymer Conjugated Broad Spectrum (Invitrogen, Carlsbad, CA, USA) for 30 min at RT and the chromogenic reaction was developed with 3,3′-diaminobenzidine tetrahydrochloride solution (Zymed Laboratories, South San Francisco, CA, USA). The nuclei were lightly counterstained with hematoxylin. Negative controls without primary Abs were performed for all reactions. Human tonsil specimens were used as positive controls. CD68 was immunohistochemically assessed using an autostainer (BOND MAX III, Leica Biosystems, Newcastle, UK), according to the manufacturer's standard protocol, using an anti-CD68 mouse anti-human mAb (ready to use; clone 514H12, Leica Biosystems) [37].

Cellular infiltrates were studied in the dermis and/or subcutaneous tissue and were classified as either perivascular or diffuse. Positive cells were counted by two independent observers in a total of six randomly selected fields (total area 7.38 mm$^2$) for each section at ×400 magnification, under a light microscope (Axioskop 2 plus, Zeiss). The total number of positive cells was calculated and reported as mean ± SD, median and range.

### Statistical analysis

All analyses were carried out using SPSS 15.0 (Chicago, IL, USA). Categorical variables were expressed as numbers, and quantitative variables as mean ± SD if normally distributed, and as median plus range if not. Categorical variables were analyzed using the chi-square ($X^2$) test or Fisher's test, depending on sample size restrictions. Non-normally distributed continuous data were compared using the Mann-Whitney test and the Wilcoxon test (for paired data). A value of $p < 0.05$ was considered statistically significant. Correlation was tested using Spearman's rank order correlation for non-normally distributed interval data.

## Results

### Demographic, clinical and immunological characteristics of enrolled patients with SSc

Demographic and clinical characteristics of patients with SSc enrolled in the study are shown in Table 1.

The mean age (± SD) of the patients with SSc was 44.6 ± 15.4 years and the median disease duration was 16.0 (range 3.0–360.0) months. There were 19 patients (67.9%) with early disease, defined as diagnosis up to 3 years after the occurrence of Raynaud's phenomenon; the remaining 9 patients (32.1%) had long-standing disease. There were 20 patients (71.4%) with dSSc. The baseline mean modified Rodnan skin score was 15.8 ± 11.3 (range 2.0–43.0). Anti-topoisomerase antibodies (anti-Scl-70 Abs) were present in 21 (75.0%) patients and anti-centromere Abs (ACA) in 3 patients (10.7%). One patient presented with RNA polymerase III autoantibody positivity; the other three patients were ANA positive only (one with a nucleolar pattern and two with a homogeneous pattern) (Additional file 1: Table S1).

### Skin CD20$^+$ B-cells and CD138$^+$ plasma cell infiltrates characterize patients with SSc based on disease duration and subset

In all 56 cutaneous specimens from patients with SSc, mononuclear cell infiltrates were found in a perivascular location, predominantly in the mid and deeper portions of the dermis. CD20$^+$ cells were found in 17 (60.7%) out of the 28 patients with SSc: 9 of these patients (52.9%) had CD20$^+$ cells in either clinically involved or uninvolved skin, 7 (41.2%) had CD20$^+$ cells only in the

**Table 1** Demographic and clinical characteristics of patients with SSc enrolled in the study

| Characteristic | Value |
| --- | --- |
| Age (years), mean (SD) | 44.6 (15.4) |
| Age (years), median (range) | 46.0 (20.0–67.0) |
| Female, number (%) | 24 (85.7) |
| Male, number (%) | 4 (14.3) |
| Disease duration (months), mean (SD) | 44.7 (71.5) |
| Disease duration (months), median (range) | 16.00 (3–360) |
| Early disease, number (%) | 19 (67.9) |
| Long-standing disease, number (%) | 9 (32.1) |
| Anti-Scl-70 positivity, number (%) | 21 (75.0) |
| ACA positivity, number (%) | 3 (10.7) |
| RNA polymerase III positivity, number (%) | 1 (3.6) |
| ANA positivity[a], number (%) | 3 (10.7) |
| dSSc, number (%) | 20 (71.4) |
| lSSc, number (%) | 8 (28.6) |
| Skin score, mean (SD) | 15.8 (11.3) |
| Skin score, median (range) | 14.0 (2.0–43.0) |
| Activity index, mean (SD) | 4.4 (2.0) |
| Activity index, median (range) | 4.2 (1.0–8.5) |
| Severity index, mean (SD) | 8.0 (2.6) |
| Severity index, median (range) | 7.5 (4.0–14.0) |
| FVC (%), mean (SD) | 87.8 ± 22.1 |
| FVC (%), median (range) | 94.0 (41.0–123.0) |
| DLCO (%), mean (SD) | 57.3 ± 18.4 |
| DLCO (%), median (range) | 57.0 (26.0–93.0) |
| HRCT interstitial score, mean (SD) | 7.6 (2.3) |
| HRCT interstitial score, median (range) | 7.0 (4.0–14.0) |
| HRCT alveolar score, mean (SD) | 6.7 (5.0) |
| HRCT alveolar score, median (range) | 6.0 (0.0–16) |
| ESR, mm/h, mean (SD) | 20.4 (20.3) |
| ESR, median (range) | 12.0 (2.0–84.0) |

The values are indicated as the mean (SD) and median (range) or number (percentage)

ANA antinuclear antibodies, ACA anticentromere antibodies, anti-Scl-70 anti-topoisomerase antibodies, dSSc diffuse skin disease, lSSc limited skin disease, FVC forced vital capacity, DLCO diffusion lung carbon monoxide, ESR erythrocyte sedimentation rate

[a]ANA positivity: two patients who were ANA-positive presented with a homogeneous pattern, and one patient presented with a nucleolar pattern

involved skin and one patient with diffuse skin disease and anti-Scl-70 Abs had CD20$^+$ cells only in clinically uninvolved skin. Importantly no CD20$^+$ cells were found in biopsy specimens from healthy volunteers.

In the subgroup that had CD20$^+$ staining, the mean number of CD20$^+$ cells was higher in involved (4.7 ± 5.9) than in uninvolved skin (1.9 ± 2.9), ($p$ = 0.04, Table 2). Among the 17 patients with CD20$^+$ cells on skin biopsy,

12 patients (70.6%) had early disease, 14 (82.3%) had diffuse skin involvement and 12 (70.6%) had anti-Scl-70 Ab positivity. Patients with early SSc had higher numbers of CD20$^+$ cells (6.3 ± 6.5) than patients with long-standing disease (1.2 ± 0.9, ($p$ = 0.009)) in involved skin. In clinically involved skin, patients with dSSc had numbers of CD20$^+$ cells (4.9 ± 6.4) comparable to patients with lSSc (4.3 ± 4.0), but interestingly all patients with CD20$^+$ cells in the clinically uninvolved skin had diffuse disease (Fig. 1).

All patients with B cells in clinically uninvolved skin had anti-Scl-70 Abs, RNA polymerase III autoantibody positivity or ANA positivity; none of the patients with ACA positivity had a B cell aggregate in uninvolved skin.

The 17 patients with CD20$^+$ cells in their skin had shorter disease duration (33.2 ± 36.8 months), compared to patients without B cell aggregate in skin biopsies (61.9 ± 104.6 months), but this difference was not statistically significant, and there was no significant correlation between the number of CD20$^+$ cells and disease duration. No association emerged between the presence of CD20$^+$ cells and restrictive lung involvement or heart or gastrointestinal disease.

The number of CD20$^+$ cells in involved skin cells directly correlated with the number of CD20$^+$ cells in uninvolved skin ($r$ = 0.62, $p$ < 0.001) and with the number of CD3$^+$ cells in involved skin ($r$ = 0.4, $p$ = 0.03). Furthermore, CD20$^+$ cells in involved skin were inversely correlated with DLCO values ($r$ = − 0.5, $p$ = 0.01) and with FVC values ($r$ = − 0.5, $p$ = 0.003).

CD138$^+$ cells were found in 100% of involved skin biopsies and in 89.3% of clinically uninvolved skin samples (Table 2), but none of the healthy controls had plasma cells in the skin.

The mean number of CD138$^+$ cells was higher in clinically involved skin (3.6 ± 2.3) than in uninvolved skin (1.9 ± 1.7 ($p$ < 0.001)) (Fig. 2). Although in patients with early disease the number of CD138$^+$ cells in involved skin (4.2 ± 2.6) and in uninvolved skin (2.1 ± 1.9) was higher than in longstanding disease (involved skin 2.6 ± 1.4, uninvolved skin 1.7 ± 1.1), this difference was not statistically significant. Furthermore, no statistically significant difference was found in the mean number of CD138$^+$ in patients with diffuse skin disease either in involved (4.1 ± 2.6) or uninvolved (2.1 ± 1.9) skin compared to patients with lSSc (involved skin 2.5 ± 1.0, uninvolved skin 1.7 ± 1.0). No differences were observed in plasma cell infiltrates in patients with different autoantibodies specificities or in patients with different organ involvement.

In involved skin, the number of CD138$^+$ cells directly correlated with the number of CD20$^+$ cells ($r$ = 0.6, $p$ = 0.01) and with the number of CD3$^+$ cells ($r$ = 0.5, $p$ = 0.01), whereas there was no significant correlation on analysis of the non-affected skin samples.

**Table 2** CD68[+], CD3[+], CD20[+] and CD138[+] cell counts on paired skin specimens in the 28 patients with SSc

| | Clinically involved skin | Clinically uninvolved skin | P |
|---|---|---|---|
| CD68[+] mean (SD) | 26.3 (8.3)[a] | 13.6 (6.1)[a] | 0.001 |
| CD68[+] median (range) | 24.5 (12.0–40.0) | 12.5 (3.0–25.0) | |
| CD3[+] mean (SD) | 71.7 (34.6)[a] | 45.7 (36.0)[a] | 0.001 |
| CD3[+] median (range) | 70.0 (7.0–146.0) | 29.8 (1.0–130.0) | |
| CD20[+] mean (SD)* | 4.7 (5.9)[b] | 1.9 (2.9)[b] | 0.04 |
| CD20[+] median (range) | 2.0 (0.0–25.0) | 1.0 (0.0–11.5) | |
| CD138[+] mean (SD) | 3.6 (2.3)[a] | 1.9 (1.7)[c] | < 0.001 |
| CD138[+] median (range) | 3.0 (0.5–11.5) | 1.5 (0.0–9.0) | |

The values are the mean (SD) and median (range)

[a]Mean (SD) and median (range) of CD68[+], CD3[+], CD138[+] in clinically involved skin (forearm) and of CD68[+] *and* CD3[+] in clinically uninvolved skin (buttock) refers to the duplicate skin samples from patients

[b]Mean (SD) and median (range) of CD20[+] was calculated considering only the 17 patients (60.7%) that had almost one CD20+ cell in clinically involved skin or in clinically uninvolved skin

[c]Mean (SD) and median (range) of CD138[+] in clinically uninvolved skin was calculated considering 25 out of 28 (89.3%) patients with CD138 + cells in uninvolved skin specimens

## Skin CD3[+] T-lymphocyte infiltrates are differentially presented in patients with SSc based on the skin compartment and autoantibody positivity

CD3[+] cells were found in all skin biopsies of both healthy subjects and patients with SSc. In healthy subjects, CD3[+] cell number was significantly smaller (8.0 ± 2.0) compared to that in involved (71.7 ± 34.6, ($p < 0.001$)) or uninvolved (45.7 ± 36.0, ($p < 0.001$)) skin from patients with SSc.

The mean number of CD3[+] cells was higher in clinically involved skin than clinically uninvolved skin, ($p = 0.001$) (Table 2, Fig. 3). No statistically significant difference in the mean number of CD3[+] cells was found in skin from patients with early compared to long-standing SSc, either in involved or uninvolved skin (Table 2).

The mean number of CD3[+] cells in involved skin was higher in patients with dSSc (75.1 ± 35.8) than in patients with lSSc (63.2 ± 31.7), but this difference was not statistically significant, probably due to the wide variation in cell numbers.

The number of CD3[+] cells was comparable in involved skin from patients with SSc regardless to anti-Scl-70 Ab positivity. In clinically uninvolved skin biopsies, patients with anti-Scl-70 Abs had a greater number of T lymphocytes (51. 7 ± 38.7) than anti-Scl-70 Ab-negative patients (27.7 ± 18.8, ($p = 0.05$)). It is worth mentioning that the small group of patients with ACA positivity had a smaller number of CD3[+] cells in both affected and unaffected skin. The number of CD3[+] cells in involved skin directly correlated with the number of CD3[+] cells in uninvolved skin ($r = 0.5$, $p = 0.009$) and inversely correlated with DLCO ($r = - 0.4$, $p = 0.002$), but there was no correlation with the Rodnan skin score, disease activity or severity scores.

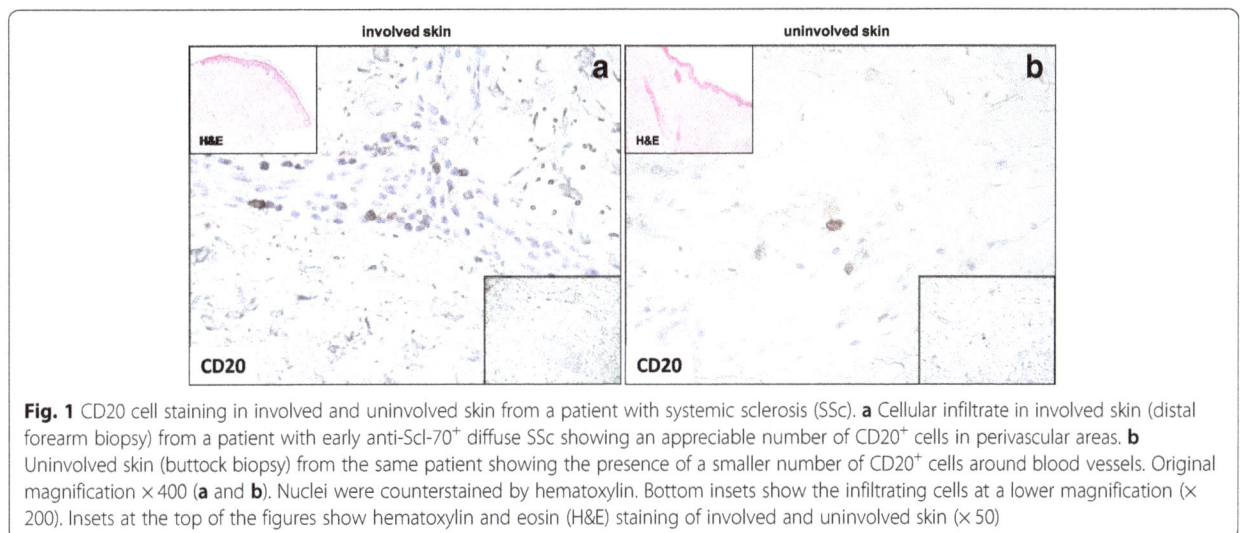

**Fig. 1** CD20 cell staining in involved and uninvolved skin from a patient with systemic sclerosis (SSc). **a** Cellular infiltrate in involved skin (distal forearm biopsy) from a patient with early anti-Scl-70[+] diffuse SSc showing an appreciable number of CD20[+] cells in perivascular areas. **b** Uninvolved skin (buttock biopsy) from the same patient showing the presence of a smaller number of CD20[+] cells around blood vessels. Original magnification × 400 (**a** and **b**). Nuclei were counterstained by hematoxylin. Bottom insets show the infiltrating cells at a lower magnification (× 200). Insets at the top of the figures show hematoxylin and eosin (H&E) staining of involved and uninvolved skin (× 50)

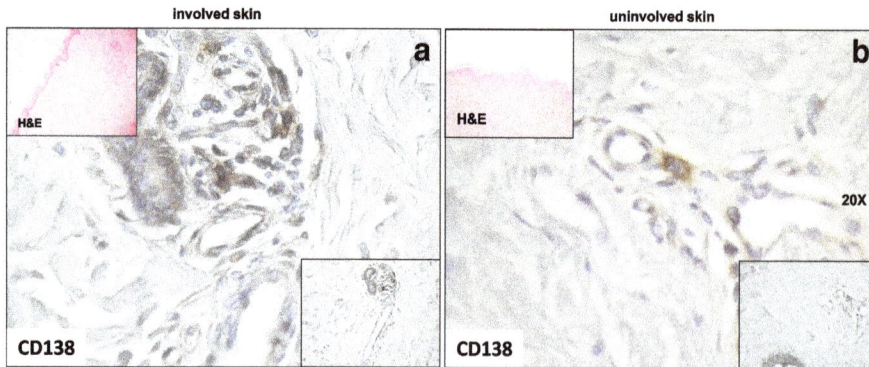

**Fig. 2** CD138 cell staining in involved and uninvolved skin from a patient with systemic sclerosis (SSc). **a** Involved skin (distal forearm biopsy) from a patient with an early anti-Scl-70$^+$ diffuse SSc showing an appreciable number of CD138$^+$ cells in perivascular areas. **b** Uninvolved skin (buttock biopsy) of the same patient showing the presence of a smaller number of CD138$^+$ cells around blood vessels. Original magnification $\times$ 400 (**a** and **b**). Nuclei were counterstained by hematoxylin. Bottom insets show the infiltrating cells at a lower magnification ($\times$ 200). Insets at the top of the figures show hematoxylin and eosin (H&E) staining of involved and uninvolved skin ($\times$ 50)

## Skin CD68$^+$ macrophage infiltrates are differentially presented in patients with SSc based on the skin compartment

Using paired skin samples, CD68$^+$ cell count was significantly higher in clinically involved (26.3 $\pm$ 8.3) compared to uninvolved skin from patients with SSc (13.6 $\pm$ 6.1) ($p$ = 0.001) (Fig. 4), the CD68$^+$ cells having a preferential perivascular distribution within the dermis.

Grouping patients with SSc according to the disease subset, we found that CD68$^+$ cell count was significantly higher in clinically uninvolved skin from patients with SSc with a diffuse phenotype (14.8 $\pm$ 5.8) compared to patients with SSc with limited disease (8.3 $\pm$ 4.7) ($p$ = 0.05), whereas there was no difference in macrophage infiltrate when comparing involved skin samples from patients with dSSc (27.2 $\pm$ 7.8) to skin samples from patients with lSSc (22.3 $\pm$ 11.7) ($p$ = 0.78). The number of CD68$^+$ cells was comparable in involved skin from patients with SSc

despite anti-Scl-70 Ab positivity. In clinically uninvolved skin, patients with anti-Scl-70 Abs had a greater number of CD68$^+$ cells (15.0 $\pm$ 5.1) than patients with SSc without anti-Scl-70 Abs (4.0 $\pm$ 1.4) ($p$ = 0.02, Table 2).

## Cell infiltrate and skin score progression: the role of B cells

During follow up 12 patients were treated with rituximab with or without cyclophosphamide because of the progression of skin disease, while 16 patients did not receive any treatments because no progression of skin score was present at the time of biopsy (Table 3). At study entry, patients with SSc had comparable immunohistological findings in terms of CD68, CD3, CD20 and CD138 cells in clinically affected and unaffected skin samples after treatment stratification. However, treated patients had a decrease in skin score during follow up from 21.1 $\pm$ 10.9 to 11.2 $\pm$ 6.2 ($p$ = 0.03), and all but one

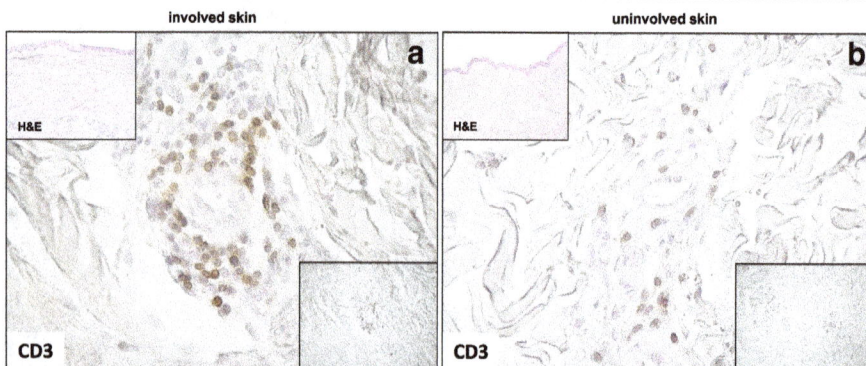

**Fig. 3** CD3 cell staining in involved and uninvolved skin from a patient with systemic sclerosis (SSc). **a** Involved skin (distal forearm biopsy) from a patient with early anti-Scl-70$^+$ diffuse SSc showed massive infiltration with CD3$^+$ cells in perivascular areas. **b** Uninvolved skin (buttock biopsy) from the same patient showing the presence of a smaller number of CD3$^+$ cells around blood vessels. Original magnification $\times$ 400 (**a** and **b**). Nuclei were counterstained by hematoxylin. Bottom insets show the infiltrating cells at a lower magnification ($\times$ 200). Insets at the top of the figures show hematoxylin and eosin (H&E) staining of involved and uninvolved skin ($\times$ 50)

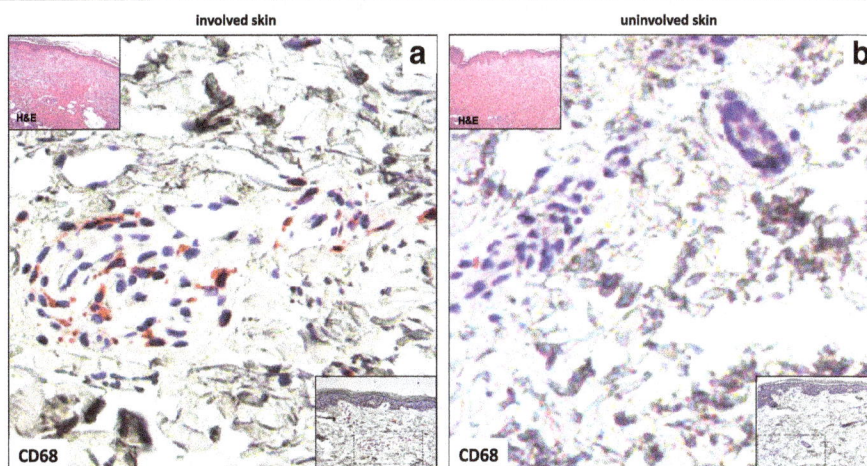

**Fig. 4** CD68 cell staining in involved and uninvolved skin from a patient with systemic sclerosis (SSc). **a** Involved skin (distal forearm biopsy) from a patient with early anti-Scl-70+ diffuse SSc showed an infiltrate of CD68+ cells (red) in perivascular areas. **b** Uninvolved skin (buttock biopsy) from the same patient showing the presence of a smaller number of CD68+ cells around blood vessels. Original magnification ×400 (**a** and **b**). Nuclei were counterstained by hematoxylin. Insets at the bottom of the figures show the infiltrating cells at a lower magnification (×200). Insets at the top of the figures show hematoxylin and eosin (H&E) staining of involved and uninvolved skin (×50)

experienced a response >20% in the skin score. The clinical response in term of skin score improvement was not associated with the rate of baseline cell infiltrate.

Among the 16 patients that did not receive immunosuppressive therapy during the follow up, 9 patients had a stable skin score or worsening of the score was less than 20% after 6.5 ± 0.8 months, while 7 patients (43.7%) had more than 20% worsening of the skin score. The baseline and follow-up skin score in the latter patients were respectively 11.9 ± 10.6 and 15.7 ± 10.3 ($p$ = 0.02). Among the 17 patients with B cell skin infiltrate at baseline, 8 patients were treated due to progressive skin involvement and 7 untreated patients had worsening during follow up. In the remaining two untreated patients with baseline B cell skin infiltrate, the skin score remained stable during the follow up.

In the 16 untreated patients, 9 patients with scleroderma (56.2%) had CD20+ cell skin infiltrate at baseline: 7 of them (77.8%) experienced worsening of the skin score, while none of the patients without CD20+ cells in the skin specimens experienced worsening of the skin score (Fisher's test, $p$ = 0.03). The mean number of CD20+ cells in involved skin from the seven patients with worsening of the skin score was higher than that in patients without worsening, but the difference was not statistically significant. Furthermore, the mean number of baseline CD138+ cells in involved skin (4.6 ± 3.6) and uninvolved (2.6 ± 1.1) skin biopsies was slightly higher in patients with skin progression compared to patients without skin worsening (involved skin 2.7 ± 1.1, uninvolved skin 1.7 ± 1.3), ($p$ value not significant).

The mean number of baseline CD3+ cells in affected and unaffected skin of patients with a worsening of skin score (involved skin 79.3 ± 48.3, uninvolved skin 44.8 ± 37.0) was comparable to the mean number of CD3+ cells in patients with stable skin score (involved skin 78.6 ± 20.0, uninvolved skin 50.3 ± 31.9), ($p$ value not significant in both comparisons).

Comparable results were obtained for CD68 staining; in fact, the mean number of baseline CD68+ cells in affected and unaffected skin in patients with skin progression (involved skin 31.3 ± 9.1, uninvolved skin 10.3 ± 4.7) was similar to the mean number of CD68+ cells in patients with a stable skin score (involved skin 24.7 ± 4.5, uninvolved skin 14.3 ± 9.3), ($p$ value not significant in both comparisons).

## Discussion

A cutaneous cellular infiltrate is a frequent histopathologic finding in SSc [3, 6, 7, 10]. Cutaneous mononuclear cell infiltrates [3–12] may play a major role in starting and to mediating dermal sclerosis through their effects on fibroblasts [1].

In our study, T lymphocytes and macrophages were found in all cutaneous specimens from patients with SSc that were analyzed, predominantly in a perivascular location in the mid and/or deeper portion of the dermis. In previous studies, mononuclear cell infiltrates, including macrophages [3, 6–9] and T lymphocytes [3, 6, 8–12], with an increased number also of mast cells [3, 5, 6], were reported in SSc skin biopsies, above all in the early phases of the disease. In particular, Fleischmajer and co-workers [6] found that only 49% of patients with SSc had diffuse or perivascular cellular infiltrates in the dermis or subcutaneous tissue; the cells were identified as lymphocytes, plasma cells and macrophages. In this

**Table 3** Clinical and histological characteristics according to immunosuppressive/immunomodulatory treatment and clinical outcome in the 28 patients with SSc

| | Immunosuppressive treatment (12 patients) | No immunosuppressive treatment (16 patients) | P |
|---|---|---|---|
| Age (years), mean (SD) | 39.3 (13.9) | 48.6 (16.2) | ns |
| Female/male, number | 10/2 | 14/2 | ns |
| Disease duration (months), mean (SD) | 42.8 (100.3) | 45.8 (41.5) | ns |
| Early/longstanding disease, number | 10/2 | 9/7 | ns |
| dSSc/lSSc number | 11/1 | 9/7 | 0.05 |
| Skin score baseline, mean (SD) | 21.1 (10.9) | 11.9 (10.6) | 0.03 |
| Anti-scl-70 antibodies positivity, number (%) | 10 | 11 | ns |
| ACA positivity, number | 0 | 3 | |
| ANA positivity, number | 2 | 2 | |
| Presence of CD20+ cell in skin biopsy, number (%)[a] | 8 (66.7) | 9 (56.3) | ns |
| CD20+ in clinically involved skin, mean (SD) | 2.3 (3.1) | 3.4 (6.3) | ns |
| CD20+ in clinically uninvolved skin, mean (SD) | 1.5 (3.3) | 0.9 (1.6) | ns |
| CD138+ in clinically involved skin, mean (SD) | 3.5 (1.5) | 3.8 (2.9) | ns |
| CD138+ in clinically uninvolved skin, mean (SD) | 1.7 (1.8) | 2.2 (2.1) | ns |
| CD3+ in clinically involved skin, mean (SD) | 62.0 (28.9) | 78.9 (37.4) | ns |
| CD3+ in clinically uninvolved skin, mean (SD) | 43.7 (40.2) | 47.2 (33.9) | ns |
| CD68+ in clinically involved skin, mean (SD) | 25.3 (9.1) | 38.0 (7.4) | ns |
| CD68+ in clinically uninvolved skin, mean (SD) | 14.4 (5.7) | 12.3 (6.9) | ns |
| Skin score after 6-month follow up, mean (SD) | 11.3 (6.9) | 13.0 (10.9) | ns |
| Patients with decrease >20% of skin score after 6-month follow up[b] | 11 (91.7) | 3 (18.7) | 0.01 |
| Patients with worsening >20% of skin score after 6-month follow up | 0 (0.0) | 7 (56.3) | 0.01 |
| *Patients with CD20 + cells on skin biopsy* | 0 (0.0) | 7 (77.8) | |
| *Patients without CD20+ cells on skin biopsy* | 0 (0.0) | 0 (0.0) | |

The values are indicated as the mean (SD) or number (percentage) according to the data distribution

*SSc* systemic sclerosis, *ANA* antinuclear antibodies, *ACA* anticentromere antibodies, *anti-Scl-70* anti-topoisomerase antibodies, *dSSc* diffuse skin disease, *lSSc* limited skin disease, *ns* not significant

[a]Presence of at least one CD20+ cell in involved or uninvolved skin biopsy

[b]In this subgroup, six patients had CD20+ cells in uninvolved skin and were treated with immunosuppressive drug, while none of the untreated patients had CD20+ cells ($p = 0.002$)

cohort, about 40% of the patients had early SSc and we did not find any associations with disease duration or immunological characteristics.

Evidence of cellular skin infiltrate has been reported previously in another study [10], in which up to 50% of the biopsies had relevant dermal mononuclear infiltration, but low/mild infiltrate was found in the other specimens [10]. The patients with relevant infiltrate frequently presented with diffuse disease, shorter disease duration [10, 11] and a higher skin thickening score [10]. The majority of T cells present in the skin infiltrate were activated T lymphocytes [10, 11], suggesting that early CD69+ T cells may actively participate in cell-cell contact with fibroblasts to induce fibrosis in skin lesions [11]. In our study, all specimens had relevant mononuclear infiltration. This discrepancy between the results of the previous studies [10] and our data may be due to differences in disease duration or in the area of the body from which the specimens were

taken. Furthermore, genome-wide gene expression profiling studies of SSc skin biopsies have demonstrated wide heterogeneity, which can be quantitatively measured by DNA microarrays [13, 38–40]. Four specific gene expression signatures in both lesional and non-lesional skin biopsies have been identified in scleroderma compared to healthy controls [39].

Interestingly, in our study, the inflammatory cell infiltration was also present in the clinical uninvolved cutaneous specimens, in which the skin apparently did not have any clinical signs of thickness and sclerosis. This finding is in agreement with the indistinguishable pattern of gene expression found in clinically affected and clinically unaffected tissue from patients with SSc, which was clearly different from the gene expression in healthy subjects [13]. Our immunohistochemical data indicated that in patients with SSc the skin, even when considered as clinically uninvolved, is affected by an inflammatory process, suggesting that pathological changes can be detected even before the onset of skin sclerosis. Gene expression profiling studies have confirmed an altered signature in unaffected skin in patients with systemic sclerosis [13, 16], highlighting the truly systemic inflammatory nature of the disease. Interestingly, in our study, the number of CD68+, CD3+, CD20+ and CD138+ cells was higher in involved skin than in uninvolved skin, suggesting a local role for these cells in accelerating the fibrogenic processes, that lead to clinical skin modifications. The role of macrophages in different target organs in patients with SSc has been recently demonstrated [15, 41] and confirmed in multiple cohorts with skin disease, showing that the gene expression of several activated macrophage markers are elevated in the skin in SSc [14]. Activated macrophages likely play a pivotal role in the pathogenesis of SSc by activating fibroblasts, but as these cells are plastic and readily modulated by the local tissue microenvironment, the cytokine milieu determined also by the presence of B and T lymphocytes, dendritic cells, endothelial cells and fibroblasts might play a role in the pathogenesis of the fibrotic process in the skin [41].

The role of T cells in SSc is already accepted [42]. In this regard, all SSc specimens examined in our study had significant CD3+ cell infiltrate mainly in clinically involved but also in uninvolved skin, supporting the concept that the dermal T lymphocytes play a key role in local pathogenic events in SSc by cytokine production and that lymphocyte/fibroblast interaction in the skin is important in the pathophysiology of SSc. However, the main clue to the specific importance of the immune cell infiltrates did arise from the longitudinal assessment of the course of the skin involvement. The mechanistic exploration of the pathogenic infiltrate still needs to be defined. The positive response to rituximab in a subgroup of patients with SSc, regardless of the baseline presence of B cell skin infiltrates, indirectly supports the notion that there might be a complex relationship among all mononuclear cells in determining clinical modification and fibrosis in scleroderma and probably the T and B cell crosstalk can have a role in promoting the fibrotic process.

Even though a recent analysis of DNA microarrays of cutaneous biopsies from patients with dSSc demonstrated higher expression of clusters of genes in CD20+ cells [13], in some immunohistochemical studies the B cells were rare or absent [3, 8–10]. Recently, the analysis of B cell infiltrate performed in skin biopsies from patients treated with anti-CD20 therapy demonstrated improvement in the skin score and stabilization of FVC, DLCO and clinical symptoms [17–21, 23]. In our study, B cell infiltrate seems to be characteristic of the skin in scleroderma, in fact CD20+ and CD138+ cells were absent in all specimens from healthy subjects. B lymphocytes were detected in up

to 61% of patients with SSc and the mean number of CD20+ and CD138+ cells was lower than the number of CD3+ and CD68+ cells. Fifty percent of these patients had B cells both in involved and in uninvolved skin, while the other 50% had B cells only in involved skin, while plasma cells were present in all involved skin and in all but three samples of clinically uninvolved skin. The presence of plasma cells suggests that specific chemotaxis or local maturation of memory B cells had occurred. The wide variability in the identification of B cells in skin biopsies in our study and in other studies could be related to the different cell signatures previously reported [39]. Certainly, the clinical effects seem not to depend upon the cell numbers found in the skin biopsy samples.

The great majority of patients with SSc who had CD20+ cells on skin biopsies had anti-Scl-70 Ab positivity or early disease or diffuse skin involvement. Patients with early disease had a greater number of CD20+ cells in involved skin compared with patients with long-standing disease, and the presence of CD20+ cells in uninvolved skin seems to be characteristic of patients with dSSc. Our sample size was not large enough to draw definite conclusions, but our data suggest that B cells are associated with the classical negative prognostic factor of scleroderma such as diffuse phenotype and antiscl-70 Ab positivity. Among the various immune cells, B cells appear to be the only ones linked to progression of skin involvement over time.

Albeit the number of patients enrolled in this study was limited, the worsening of skin involvement in the group of patients with CD20+ cells on skin biopsy after 6-month follow up suggests a possible prognostic value of B cell presence in the progression of skin involvement. No prognostic role was evident for plasma cells, suggesting that very likely they were already there, and that the arrival of the new B cells was the most important event for the diseased skin. The presence of B cells in the majority, but not in all patients, indicates an important, though not essential role for cutaneous B cells in more aggressive scleroderma disease, above all during the earliest phases when the inflammatory process and cell-cell interactions very likely play an essential role in the development of fibrosis over time. B cells in the skin may be involved in the initiation and expansion of the SSc inflammatory process. Of interest, even plasma cells were present either in the involved or the uninvolved skin and in 10 patients in this cohort on analysis of the peripheral blood B cell subsets, we found that the number of CD20+ and CD138+ cells in the skin specimens correlated directly with the percentage of circulating CD27+CD38+ plasmablasts (unpublished data). Either resident and circulating B cells can determine, with their multiple functions as Ab-producing cells, antigen presenting cells and profibrotic and proinflammatory cytokine (IL-6, IL-4, transforming growth factor (TGF)-β)-secreting cells [1, 43], an autoimmune milieu that could be of great impact in the development of fibrosis. B cells directly stimulate fibroblasts by a direct contact-based mechanism [44] and a plethora of soluble factors present in the inflammatory skin condition contributes to the commitment of B cells in autoantibody-producing plasma cells, which, again, can directly stimulate fibroblasts.

The limited number of patients with scleroderma and of healthy controls in this study did not allow us to infer robust correlation with disease phenotype and organ involvement, but further studies on sequential biopsies after therapy could allow us to investigate temporal associations with different types of cell infiltrates, and to test correlation with the characteristics of inflammatory infiltrate with fibrotic involvement, such as the collagen score and myofibroblast score.

## Conclusions

These results highlight that a subgroup of patients with SSc exhibit an imbalance in B cell infiltrate and that cutaneous mononuclear cells of the innate and adaptive immune system may play a role in mediating dermal fibrosis in different stages of scleroderma disease and in patients with diffuse skin involvement. Therapeutic approaches decreasing the numbers of cutaneous lymphocytes, in particular B cells, and/or interfering with their functions might prove useful in the management of cutaneous involvement in SSc from the earliest phases of the disease.

## Abbreviations

Abs: Antibodies; ACA: Anti-centromere antibodies; ANA: Antinuclear antibodies; anti-Scl-70 Abs: Anti-topoisomerase antibodies; DLCO: diffusing capacity for carbon monoxide; dSSc: Diffuse systemic sclerosis; ELISA: Enzyme-linked immunosorbent assay; ESR: Erythrocyte sedimentation rate; FVC: Forced vital capacity; GH: Global Health; $H_2O_2$: Hydrogen peroxide; HAQ: Health Assessment Questionnaire; HRCT: High resolution computed tomography; IL: Interleukin; lSSc: Limited systemic sclerosis; LVEF: Left ventricular ejection fraction; mAb: monoclonal antibodies; PASP: Pulmonary artery systolic pressure; PFT: Pulmonary function test; RT: Room temperature; SD: Standard deviation; SSc: Systemic sclerosis; TBS: Tris-buffered saline

## Acknowledgements
None.

## Funding
The GILS supported the study.

## Authors' contributions
SB conceived and designed the study, collected clinical data and biopsies and analyzed and interpreted data, wrote the manuscript and gave final approval of the version to be published. CA designed the experiments, analyzed immunohistochemical results, participated in data analyses and in the writing of the manuscript, revised the manuscript and gave final approval of the version to be published. SA collected clinical data and biopsies, performed immunohistochemistry, interpreted data, revised the manuscript critically for important intellectual content and gave final approval of the version to be published. GL gave technical support and conceptual advice in immunohistochemistry, revised the manuscript critically and gave final approval of the version to be published. GP gave technical support and conceptual advice in immunohistochemistry, revised the manuscript critically and gave final approval of the version to be published. BT collected clinical data, analyzed data, revised the manuscript critically for important intellectual content, and gave final approval of the version to be published. GS provided a critical interpretation of the experimental data, revised the manuscript critically for important intellectual content and gave final approval of the version to be published. EG collected clinical data, analyzed data, critically revised the manuscript and gave final approval of the version to be published. GF conceived and designed the study, interpreted data, revised the manuscript critically for important intellectual content and gave final approval of the version to be published. All authors read and approved the final manuscript.

## Competing interests
The authors declare that they have no competing interests.

## Author details
[1]Unità Operativa Complessa di Reumatologia, Istituto di Reumatologia e Scienze Affini, Università Cattolica del Sacro Cuore, Rome, Italy. [2]Fondazione Policlinico Universitario Agostino Gemelli, Via G. Moscati, 31-00168 Rome, Italy. [3]Istituto di Istologia ed Embriologia, Università Cattolica del Sacro Cuore, Rome, Italy.

## References
1. Gu YS, Kong J, Cheema GS, Keen CL, Wick G, Gershwin ME. The immunobiology of systemic sclerosis. Semin Arthritis Rheum. 2008;38:132–60.
2. Derk CT, Jimenez SA. Systemic sclerosis: current views of its pathogenesis. Autoimmun Rev. 2003;2:181–91.
3. Prescott R, Freemont A, Jones C, Hoyland J, Fielding P. Sequential dermal microvascular and perivascular changes in the development of scleroderma. J Pathol. 1992;166:255–63.
4. Nishioka K, Kobayashi Y, Katayama I, Takijiri C. Mast cells in diffuse scleroderma. Arch Dermatol. 1987;123:205–8.
5. Hawkins RA, Claman HN, Clark RAF, Steigerwald JC. Increased dermal mast cell populations in progressive systemic sclerosis: a link in chronic fibrosis? Ann Intern Med. 1985;102:182–6.
6. Fleischmajer R, Perlish JS, Reeves JRT. Cellular infiltrates in scleroderma skin. Arthritis Rheum. 1977;20:975–84.
7. Ishikawa O, Ishikawa H. Macrophages infiltration in the skin of patients with systemic sclerosis. J Rheumatol. 1992;19:1202–6.
8. Hussein MR, Hassan HI, Hofny ER, Elkholy M, Fatehy NA, Abd Elmoniem AE, et al. Alterations of mononuclear inflammatory cells, CD4/CD8+ cells, interleukin-1β, and tumor necrosis factor-α in the bronchoalveolar lavage fluid, peripheral blood, and skin of patients with systemic sclerosis. J Clin Pathol. 2005;58:178–84.
9. Krailing BM, Maul G, Jimenez SA. Mononuclear cellular infiltrates in clinically involved skin from patients with systemic sclerosis of recent onset predominantly consist of monocytes/macrophages. Pathobiology. 1995;63:48–56.
10. Roumm A, Whiteside TL, Medseger T, Rodnan G. Lymphocytes in the skin of patients with progressive systemic sclerosis. Arthritis Rheum. 1984;27:645–53.
11. Kalogerou A, Gelou E, Mountantonakis S, Settas L, Zaforiou E, Sakkas L. Early activation in the skin from patients with systemic sclerosis. Ann Rheum Dis. 2005;64:1233–5.
12. Antiga E, Quaglino P, Bellandi S, Volpi W, Del Bianco E, Comessatti A, et al. Regulatory T cells in the skin lesions and blood of patients with systemic sclerosis and morphoea. Br J Dermatol. 2010;162:1056–63.
13. Whitfield ML, Finlay DR, Murray JI, Troyanskaya OG, Chi JT, Pergamenschikov A, et al. Systemic and cell type-specific gene expression patterns in scleroderma skin. Proc Natl Acad Sci USA. 2003;100:12319–24.

14. Taroni JN, Greene CS, Martyanov V, Wood TA, Christmann RB, Farber HW, et al. A novel multinetwork approach reveals tissue-specific cellular modulators of fibrosis in systemic sclerosis Genome Med. 2017;9(1):27.

15. Assassi S, Swindell WR, Wu M, Tan FD, Khanna D, Furst DE, et al. Dissecting the heterogeneity of skin gene expression patterns in systemic sclerosis. Arthritis Rheumatol. 2015;67:3016–26.

16. Johnson ME, Pioli PA, Whitfield ML. Gene expression profiling offers insights into the role of innate immune signaling in SSc. Semin Immunopathol. 2015;37:501–9.

17. Lafyatis R, Kissin E, York M, Farina G, Viger K, Fritzler MJ, et al. B cell depletion with rituximab in patients with diffuse cutaneous systemic sclerosis. Arthritis Rheum. 2009;60:578–83.

18. Smith V, Van Praet JT, Vandooren B, Van der Cruyssen B, Naeyaert JM, Decuman S, et al. Rituximab in diffuse cutaneous systemic sclerosis: an open-label clinical and histopathological study. Ann Rheum Dis. 2008;69: 193–7.

19. Bosello S, De Santis M, Lama G, Spanò C, Angelucci C, Tolusso B, et al. B cell depletion in diffuse progressive systemic sclerosis: safety, skin score modification and IL-6 modulation in a thirty-six months follow-up open label trial. Arthritis Res Ther. 2010;12:R 54.

20. Daoussis D, Liossis SN, Tsamandas AC, Kalogeropoulou C, Kazantzi A, Sirinian C, et al. Experience with rituximab in scleroderma: results from a 1-year, proof-of-principle study. Rheumatology. 2010;49:271–80.

21. Bosello SL, De Luca G, Rucco M, Berardi G, Falcione M, Danza FM, et al. G. Long-term efficacy of B cell depletion therapy on lung and skin involvement in diffuse systemic sclerosis. Semin Arthritis Rheum. 2015; 44:428–36.

22. Bosello S, De Luca G, Tolusso B, Lama G, Angelucci C, Sica G, et al. B cells in systemic sclerosis: a possible target for therapy. Autoimmun Rev. 2011;10: 624–30.

23. Jordan S, Distler JH, Maurer B, Huscher D, van Laar JM, Allanore Y, et al. Effects and safety of rituximab in systemic sclerosis: an analysis from the European Scleroderma Trial and Research (EUSTAR) group. Ann Rheum Dis. 2015;74:1188–94.

24. Okano Y. Antinuclear antibody in systemic sclerosis (scleroderma). Rheum Dis Clin N Am. 1996;22:709–35.

25. Famularo G, Giacomelli R, Alesse E, Cifone MG, Morrone S, Boirivant M, et al. Polyclonal B lymphocyte activation in progressive systemic sclerosis. J Clin Lab Immunol. 1989;29:59–63.

26. Sato S, Fujimoto M, Hasegawa M, Takehara K. Altered blood B lymphocyte homeostasis in systemic sclerosis: expanded naive B cells and diminished but activated memory B cells. Arthritis Rheum. 2004;50:1918–27.

27. Sato S, Hasegawa M, Fujimoto M, Tedder TF, Takehara K. Quantitative genetic variation in CD19 expression correlates with autoimmunity. J Immunol. 2000;165:6635–43.

28. Subcommittee for Scleroderma Criteria of the American Rheumatism Association Diagnostic and Therapeutic Criteria Committee. Preliminary criteria for the classification of systemic sclerosis (scleroderma). Arthritis Rheum. 1980;23:581–90.

29. van den Hoogen F, Khanna D, Fransen J, Johnson SR, Baron M, Tyndall A, et al. 2013 classification criteria for systemic sclerosis: an American college of rheumatology/European league against rheumatism collaborative initiative. Ann Rheum Dis. 2013;72:1747–55.

30. LeRoy EC, Black C, Fleischmajer R, Jablonska S, Krieg T, Medsger TA Jr, et al. Scleroderma (systemic sclerosis): classification, subset and pathogenesis. J Rheumatol. 1988;15:202–5.

31. Valentini G, D'Angelo S, Della Rossa A, Bencivelli W, Bombardieri S. European Scleroderma Study Group to define disease activity criteria for systemic sclerosis: IV: assessment of skin thickening by modified Rodnan skin score. Ann Rheum Dis. 2003;62:904–5.

32. Czirják L, Nagy Z, Aringer M, Riemekasten G, Matucci-Cerinic M, Furst DE, EUSTAR. The EUSTAR model for teaching and implementing the modified Rodnan skin score in systemic sclerosis. Ann Rheum Dis. 2007;66:966–9.

33. Clements P, Lachenbruch P, Siebold J, White B, Weiner S, Martin R, et al. Inter- and intraobserver variability of total skin thickness score (modified Rodnan TSS) in systemic sclerosis. J Rheumatol. 1995;22:1281–5.

34. Valentini G, Silman AJ, Veale D. Assessment of disease activity. Clin Exp Rheumatol. 2003;21(Suppl 29):S39–41.

35. Medsger TA Jr, Bombardieri S, Czirjak L, Scorza R, Della Rossa A, Bencivelli W. Assessment of disease severity and prognosis. Clin Exp Rheumatol. 2003; 21(Suppl 29):S42–6.

36. De Santis M, Bosello S, La Torre G, Capuano A, Tolusso B, Pagliari G, et al. Functional, radiological and biological markers of alveolitis and infections of the lower respiratory tract in patients with systemic sclerosis. Respir Res. 2005;6:96–106.

37. Alivernini S, Kurowska-Stolarska M, Tolusso B, Benvenuto R, Elmesmari A, Canestri S, et al. microRNA-155 influences B-cell function in rheumatoid arthritis. Nat Commun. 2016;7:12970.

38. Gardner H, Shearstone JR, Bandaru R, Crowell T, Lynes M, Trojanowska M, et al. Gene profiling of scleroderma skin reveals robust signatures of disease that are imperfectly reflected in the transcript profiles of explanted fibroblasts. Arthritis Rheum. 2006;54:1961–73.

39. Milano A, Pendergrass SA, Sargent JL, George LK, McCalmont TH, Connolly MK, et al. Molecular subsets in the gene expression signatures of scleroderma skin. PLoS One. 2008;3:e2696.

40. Pendergrass SA, Lemaire R, Francis IP, Mahoney JM, Lafyatis R, Whitfield ML. Intrinsic gene expression subsets of diffuse cutaneous systemic sclerosis are stable in serial skin biopsies. J Invest Dermatol. 2012;132:1363–73.

41. Chia JJ, Lu TT. Update on macrophages and innate immunity in scleroderma. Curr Opin Rheumatol. 2015;27:530–6.

42. Sakkas LI, Platsoucas CD. Is systemic sclerosis an antigen-driven T cell disease. Arthritis Rheum. 2004;50:1721–3.

43. Alivernini S, De Santis M, Tolusso B, Mannocci A, Bosello SL, Peluso G, et al. Skin ulcers in systemic sclerosis: determinants of presence and predictive factors of healing. J Am Acad Dermatol. 2009;60:426–35.

44. François A, Chatelus E, Wachsmann D, Sibilia J, Bahram S, Alsaleh G, et al. B lymphocytes and B-cell activating factor promote collagen an profibrotic markers expression by dermal fibroblasts in systemic sclerosis. Arthritis Res Ther. 2013;15:R168.

# The effects of upper and lower limb exercise on the microvascular reactivity in limited cutaneous systemic sclerosis patients

A. Mitropoulos[1], A. Gumber[2], H. Crank[1], M. Akil[3] and M. Klonizakis[1]* (iD)

## Abstract

**Background:** Aerobic exercise in general and high-intensity interval training (HIIT) specifically is known to improve vascular function in a range of clinical conditions. HIIT in particular has demonstrated improvements in clinical outcomes, in conditions that have a strong macroangiopathic component. Nevertheless, the effect of HIIT on microcirculation in systemic sclerosis (SSc) patients is yet to be investigated. Therefore, the purpose of the study was to compare the effects of two HIIT protocols (cycle and arm cranking) on the microcirculation of the digital area in SSc patients.

**Methods:** Thirty-four limited cutaneous SSc patients ($65.3 \pm 11.6$ years old) were randomly allocated in three groups (cycling, arm cranking and control group). The exercise groups underwent a 12- week exercise program twice per week. All patients performed the baseline and post-exercise intervention measurements where physical fitness, functional ability, transcutaneous oxygen tension ($\Delta TcpO_2$), body composition and quality of life were assessed. Endothelial-dependent as well as -independent vasodilation were assessed in the middle and index fingers using LDF and incremental doses of acetylcholine (ACh) and sodium nitroprusside (SNP). Cutaneous flux data were expressed as cutaneous vascular conductance (CVC).

**Results:** Peak oxygen uptake increased in both exercise groups ($p < 0.01$, d = 1.36). $\Delta TcpO_2$ demonstrated an increase in the arm-cranking group only, with a large effect, but not found statistically significant,($p = 0.59$, d = 0.93). Endothelial-dependent vasodilation improvement was greater in the arm-cranking ($p < 0.05$, d = 1.07) in comparison to other groups. Both exercise groups improved life satisfaction ($p < 0.001$) as well as reduced discomfort and pain due to Raynaud's phenomenon ($p < 0.05$). Arm cranking seems to be the preferred mode of exercise for study participants as compared to cycling ($p < 0.05$). No changes were observed in the body composition or the functional ability in both exercise groups.

**Conclusions:** Our results suggest that arm cranking has the potential to improve the microvascular endothelial function in SSc patients. Also notably, our recommended training dose (e.g., a 12-week HIIT program, twice per week), appeared to be sufficient and tolerable for this population. Future research should focus on exploring the feasibility of a combined exercise such as aerobic and resistance training by assessing individual's experience and the quality of life in SSc patients.

**Keywords:** High-intensity interval training, Vascular function, Quality of life

* Correspondence: m.klonizakis@shu.ac.uk
[1]Centre for Sport and Exercise Science, Collegiate Campus, Sheffield Hallam University, Collegiate Crescent, Sheffield S10 2BP, UK
Full list of author information is available at the end of the article

# Background

Systemic sclerosis (SSc) is an idiopathic systemic auto-immune disease characterized by an ongoing cutaneous and visceral fibrosis, fibroproliferative vasculopathy and immunologic abnormalities [1–4]. The vascular element has an important role in the SSc pathophysiology from early onset to late complications (e.g., pulmonary arterial hypertension and kidney disease). SSc can be distinguished in either limited cutaneous scleroderma (lcSSc) with skin involvement mainly limited to the hands and face; or diffuse cutaneous scleroderma (dcSSc) with skin involvement proximal to the elbows and knees [5]. Blood vessels are directly affected by SSc, as manifested by the diverse clinical complications that take place from the initiation to the propagation of the disease, and have important ramifications on the quality of life (QoL) of patients.

Raynaud's phenomenon (RP) precedes other clinical manifestations and is observed in over 95% of SSc patients [6]. Evidently, RP is triggered by endothelial injuries in association with dysregulations in the vascular tone [7]. In addition to the imbalance of vascular tone, RP is also associated with structural vascular alterations in small- and medium-sized arteries leading to luminal narrowing. As a result, the blood vessels are unable to compensate for the impairment of blood flow during severe RP attacks and this leads to the so-called ischaemia-reperfusion reactions. These vascular complications may progress to gangrene and digital amputation [8]. Notably, SSc has the highest case-specific mortality of any rheumatic disease being also associated with substantial morbidity [9].

Pharmacological agents (e.g., nifedipine) are commonly used as first-line approach. Although it can be effective and provide pain-relief to patients, the short-term (e.g., oedema, headaches, heart palpitations, dizziness and constipation) and long-term (e.g., heart dysfunction, increased cardiovascular risk) side effects of the medical treatment should also be considered as well as the financial cost of treatment. Therefore, alternative approaches with less side effects and cost implications are warranted [10, 11], with a view to reducing dependency on medication.

Exercise in general and high-intensity interval training (HIIT) specifically could be a useful adjunct therapy for this population. HIIT has come to prominence over the last few years for its effectiveness in inducing greater improvements in vascular function than moderate-intensity continuous training in a number of clinical populations (e.g., heart failure, metabolic syndrome, obesity) [12]. Nevertheless, due to the variation in HIIT protocols, limited evidence exists to support which protocol would be the most effective in SSc patients, although the options are many, based on evidence from other patient populations. For example, a HIIT protocol with short intervals (30 s exercise/30 s passive recovery) may elicit more favourable patient-reported satisfaction/enjoyment levels compared to other longer duration exercise protocols [13]. In chronic heart failure patients, a short duration HIIT protocol (30 s exercise/30 s passive recovery) has demonstrated to be a well-tolerated, preferred protocol with a low perception of effort, patient comfort and with a longer time spent at higher percentage of peak oxygen uptake ($\dot{V}O_{2peak}$) than a longer duration HIIT protocol with active recovery phases [13]. Recent evidence supports this notion; when enjoyment levels in an overweight/obese cohort were examined after a short HIIT protocol and demonstrated that performing a HIIT protocol on a cycle ergometer present on an average 4.5 rating on a 7-point scale [14].

Although we know the potential of HIIT in improving both the micro-and the macro- vascular function in several clinical populations such as heart failure [15] and cardiometabolic disease [16] by using the treadmill and cycle ergometer as modes of exercise, no evidence exists about the mode of exercise that would be more effective on digital microcirculation where the RP attacks are present, such as in SSc patients. Assumptions could be made that utilising an upper-body exercise would potentially be more beneficial for the digital microcirculation rather than lower-body exercise where the working muscles promote the blood flow in the lower limbs. Hence, the effects that may occur by the upper- and lower-limb exercise on digital microcirculation in SSc patients should be examined.

We will attempt to bridge the knowledge gap by assessing the effects of a supervised and individually-tailored exercise programme based on arm cranking (ACE) and cycle ergometry (CE) on microvascular reactivity, aerobic capacity, exercise tolerance and enjoyment levels, as well as on QoL in SSc patients.

# Methods

## Patients

We recruited 34 patients (31 women, 3 men) with lcSSc, defined as per the American College of Rheumatology and European League Against Rheumatism criteria [17], with disease duration between 1 to 10 years. All participants were able to undertake exercise. Patients with pulmonary arterial hypertension, interstitial lung disease, those diagnosed with another inflammatory condition and/ or presenting myositis with proximal muscle weakness were excluded. Moreover, patients with New York Heart Association class 3 or 4, smokers or people who stopped smoking within 4 weeks of screening and women who were pregnant were also not permitted to participate. Eligible patients were recruited from the Rheumatology Department of the Royal Hallamshire

Hospital in Sheffield. All patients provided written consent to participate. The regional health research ethics committee for clinical studies approved the protocol. Patients were randomly allocated between the ACE ($n$ = 11), CE ($n$ = 11) and control ($n$ = 12) groups. All the pre- and post-intervention tests were performed at the same time of the day to minimize intra-day variability.

## Procedures

Baseline assessments, undertaken at first visit, included $\dot{V}O_{2peak}$, anthropometry, functional ability, microvascular reactivity and QoL. $\dot{V}O_{2peak}$ test was performed either on an arm crank ergometer (ACE group) or on a cycle ergometer (CE and control group). Thereafter, patients were randomly allocated to three groups (ACE, CE and control group). The exercise groups (ACE and CE) performed a 12-week exercise programme and the control group did not perform any type of physical activity. All groups were followed up after a 12-week period performing the same measurements as in the baseline. Figure 1 depicts the study's procedures.

## Anthropometry

The participant's stature was measured using a Hite-Rite Precision Mechanical Stadiometer. Body weight (kg), body mass index (BMI), fat mass (kg) and lean body mass (kg) segmented in upper and lower limbs were assessed by using bio-electrical impedance analysis (In Body 720, Seoul, Korea). Patients' demographic characteristics are illustrated in Table 1.

## Peak oxygen uptake test

During the cardiopulmonary tests gas exchange was collected and analysed by an online breath-by-breath analysis system (Ultima™, Medical Graphics, Gloucester, UK). Heart rate (HR) was continuously monitored using a Polar heart rate monitor (Polar FS1, Polar Electro, Kemple, Finland) and blood pressure was assessed by the researcher using a manual sphygmomanometer (DuraShock DS54, Welch Allyn, Beaverton, OR, USA) and a stethoscope (Littman Classic II, 3 M, Maplewood, MI, USA). Rating of perceived exertion (RPE) was recorded during the last 10 s of every minute during the exercise test until volitional exhaustion using Borg's scale [18] 6–20 point. Peak power output (PPO) and test duration was measured in both tests. $\dot{V}O_{2peak}$ defined as the average oxygen consumption was recorded from expiratory samples during the final 30 s of exercise.

## Arm crank test

The arm crank ergometer (Lode BV, Groningen, Netherlands) was adjusted to ensure alignment between

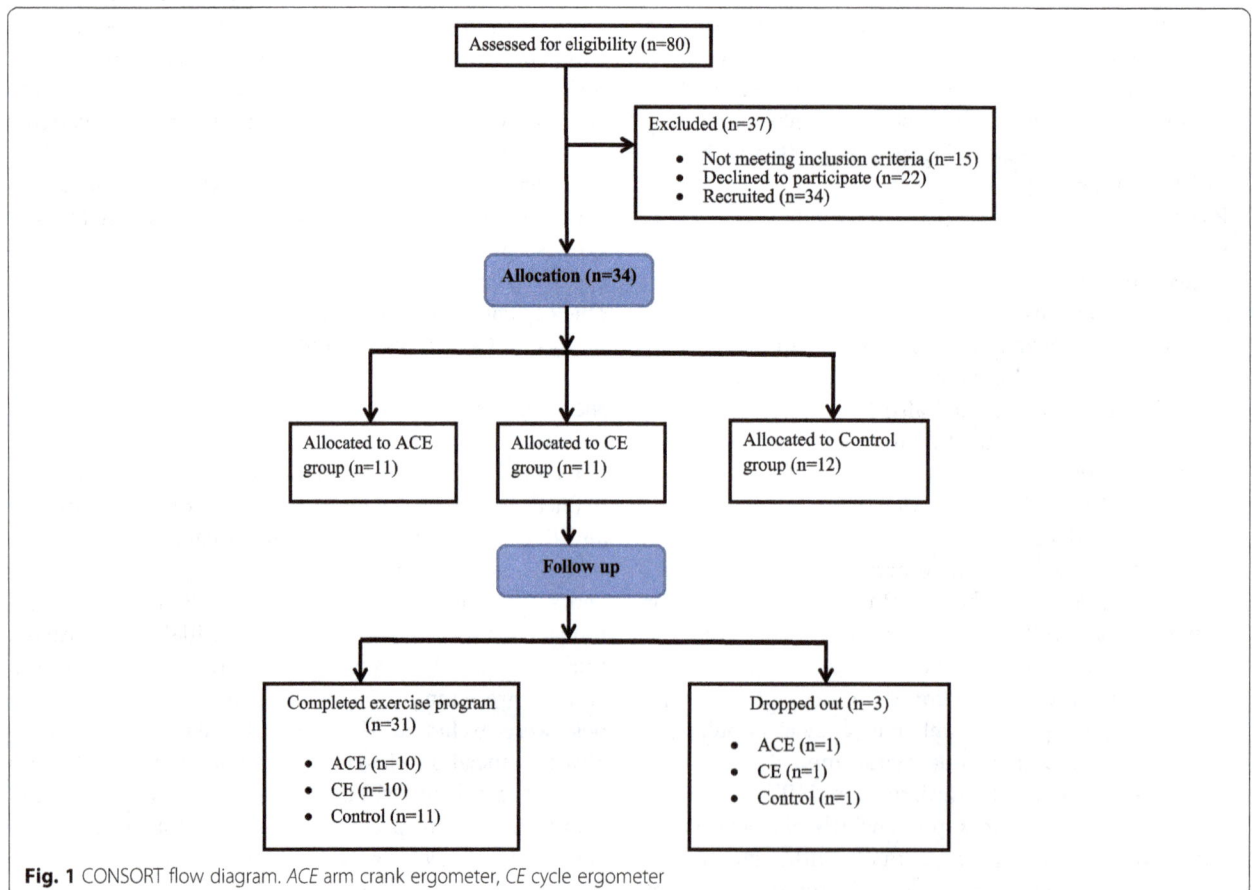

**Fig. 1** CONSORT flow diagram. *ACE* arm crank ergometer, *CE* cycle ergometer

**Table 1** Demographic data (means ± SD)

|  | Baseline ACE | Baseline CE | Baseline Control |
|---|---|---|---|
| Age (years) | 69.1 ± 9.7 | 65.1 ± 10 | 62.2 ± 14.3 |
| Body weight (kg) | 69 ± 15.8 | 66 ± 9.7 | 73.2 ± 14.8 |
| Body mass index (kg/m$^{2)}$ | 25.6 ± 4.8 | 24.5 ± 3.6 | 27.3 ± 4.0 |
| Stature (cm) | 163.7 ± 9.1 | 164.4 ± 7.9 | 163.4 ± 6.7 |
| Disease duration (yrs) | 7.8 ± 2.3 | 7.7 ± 2.1 | 6.3 ± 2.0 |
| Digital ulcers (treatment iloprost infusion) | 0/10 | 0/10 | 4/11 |
| Raynaud's treatment | 6/10 | 5/10 | 8/10 |
| Nifedipine | 4/10 | 4/10 | 4/10 |
| Sildenafil | 2/10 | 1/10 | 4/10 |
| Blood pressure treatment | 6/10 | 4/10 | 4/10 |
| Candesartan | 4/10 | 0/10 | 1/10 |
| Ramipril | 2/10 | 4/10 | 3/10 |

*ACE* arm crank ergometer, *CE* cycle ergometer

the ergometer's crankshaft and the centre of the patient's glenohumeral joint. Patients' sitting position was set up to ensure that the elbows were slightly bent when the arm was outstretched. Patients were instructed to maintain their feet flat on the floor at all times. Due to differences in gender power capabilities, two separate protocols were instructed for men and women. Men commenced at a workload of 30 W and women at 20 W. In both protocols the crank rate was maintained at 70 rev min$^{-1}$ [19, 20] and power requirements increased as a linear ramp at a rate of 10 W/min and 6 W/min for men and women, respectively [20]. The test commenced with 3 min resting and then 3 min of warm-up (unloaded cranking). RPE ≥ 18 and/or inability to maintain a crank rate above 60 rev min$^{-1}$ resulted in the termination of the test. After the exercise termination an unloaded bout of 2–3 min exercise at a crank rate below 50 rev min$^{-1}$ followed allowing for an active recovery period.

### Cycle ergometer test
The cycle ergometer test was performed on an electromagnetic cycle ergometer (Lode Excalibur, Groningen, Netherlands). The test commenced with a 3 min resting period followed by 3 min of unloaded pedalling. Participants were requested to maintain a cycle rate of 60 rev min$^{-1}$ during the exercise test. The starting load and the concomitant increments were individually calculated according to participants' estimated physical fitness and Wasserman's eqs. [21]. RPE ≥ 18 and/or inability to maintain a crank rate above 40–45 rev min$^{-1}$ resulted in the termination of the test. Following the exercise test 2–3 min of unloaded pedalling was performed to allow for an active recovery period.

### Exercise program
Patients undertook twice-weekly supervised exercise sessions at the Centre of Sport and Exercise Science at Sheffield Hallam University. Each session started with a 5 min warm-up on an arm crank or cycle ergometer depending on the group (involving light aerobic exercise and gentle range of motion exercises). This was followed by HIIT for 30 s at 100% of PPO interspersed by 30 s passive recovery for a total of 30 min (Fig. 2). At the end of the session patients undertook a 5 min cool-down period, involving lower- and upper-limb light intensity aerobic exercise and light stretching. Patients were wearing heart rate monitors throughout the exercise sessions. Heart rate and RPE and effect (see below) were assessed at regular intervals throughout the supervised exercise session.

### Functional ability test
The functional ability was assessed through a six-minute walking test (6MWT). Although the 6MWT lacks organ specificity in SSc, it can provide a valuable outcome parameter and thus, is suggested as a regular assessment in this clinical condition [22]. Patients were instructed to walk as far as possible back and forth on a 10 m corridor for 6 min. They were also instructed to slow down, stop and/or rest as necessary if they got out of breath or became exhausted, but to resume walking as soon as they felt able to. The laps and the total walking distance were recorded on a worksheet.

### Microvascular reactivity
Microvascular function was assessed by laser Doppler Fluximtery and Iontophoresis technique in a temperature-controlled room (22–24 °C). Laser Doppler fluximetry (LDF) electrodes were attached to the dorsal aspect of the reference fingers for acetylcholine (ACh)

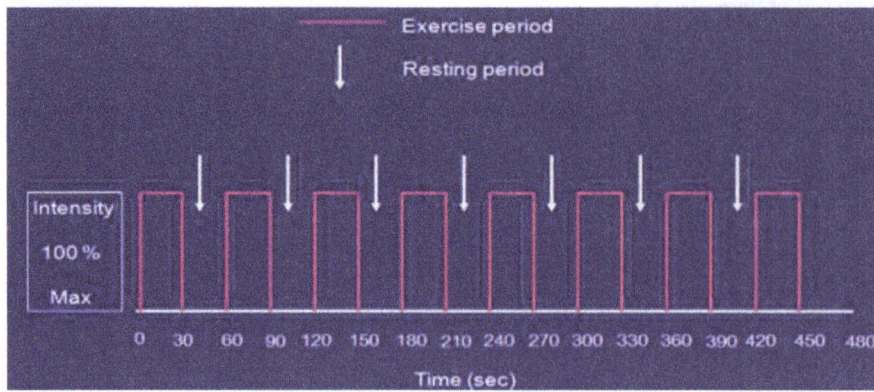

**Fig. 2** Schematic training protocol

and sodium nitroprusside (SNP) administration. These were used as indicators of the changes occurring in the endothelial-dependent and -independent vasodilatory function. Heart rate (Sports Tester, Polar, Finland) and blood pressure of the brachial artery (left arm; Dinamap Dash 2500, GE Healthcare, Chicago, IL, USA) were monitored at 5-min intervals throughout the protocol. The two drug delivery electrodes (PF383; Perimed AB, Jarfalla, Sweden) were positioned over healthy-looking skin, approximately 4 cm apart with one containing 100 μL of 1% ACh (Miochol-E, Novartis, Stein, Switzerland.) and the other 80 μL of 1% SNP (Nitroprussiat, Rottapharm, Monza, Italy). ACh was placed over the middle finger between the distal and proximal interphalangeal joints and SNP was placed over the index finger between the metacarpophalangeal and carpometacarpal joints. The incremental iontophoresis protocol for ACh and SNP delivery is described in Klonizakis et al., [23, 24].

### Transcutaneous oxygen pressure (TcpO$_2$)

TcpO$_2$ measurements were performed during the cardiorespiratory tests using sensors that were non-invasively attached onto the skin and allowed to heat. The sensors induce skin blood capillaries dilatation through heat, which increases the blood flow and results in oxygen diffusion through the skin to the sensor. The sensor measures TcpO$_2$ values inwardly through an electrochemical process.

Measurements were performed using the TINA TCM400 TcpO$_2$ device (Radiometer, Copenhagen, Denmark). The temperature of the probe was set to 44.5 °C to allow maximal skin vasodilation, thereby decreasing the arterial to skin surface oxygen pressure gradient. Before the exercise test 15–20 min were allowed with the probe attached on the skin for stabilisation of TcpO$_2$ value. After the test the TcpO$_2$ values were automatically corrected according to a temperature of 37 °C by the TINA device. The electrode was placed slightly

below the right scapula on the back away from any bone.

Fixation rings were used to hold the probe attached to the skin and this was filled with two small drops of contact fluid before attachment to the sensor. The fluid was then heated causing the subsequent dilatation of the skin. The raw values of the patient's oxygen perfusion, obtained directly from TcpO$_2$ device were defined (Table 2) as previously described in Wasilewski et al. [25].

### Quality of life

The EQ-5D-5 L was the main outcome used to assess the patients' quality of life pre- and post-exercise intervention. The EQ-5D-5 L is a generic measure of health state by considering five key dimensions of daily living (mobility, self-care, ability to undertake usual activities, pain, anxiety/depression) [26]. Participants were asked to describe their level of health on each dimension using one of five levels: no problems, slight problems, moderate problems, severe problems, extreme problems. Patients were also asked about to rate their life satisfaction on a scale of zero to ten as well as to rate the RP pain during the last couple of weeks on one to five ascending grading: not at all, slightly, moderately, severely,

**Table 2** Definitions of TcpO2 quantities

| TcpO2 quantity | Definition |
| --- | --- |
| Baseline | The arithmetic mean of maximum TcpO2 at rest. |
| TcpO2$_{max}$ | The highest TcpO2 value recorded every minute of exercise or at rest. |
| Maximum change from baseline (ΔTcpO2$_{max}$) | The outcome of the subtraction of baseline from TcpO2$_{max}$: e.g. TcpO2$_{max}$ - baseline |
| Changes in transcutaneous oxygen pressure (ΔTcpO2) | The average sum of the change from baseline at rest and exercise period: e.g. $(\Sigma \Delta Y1...n) / n) = \Delta TcpO2$ |

*ΔTcpO$_2$ transcutaneous oxygen tension*

extremely. Digital ulcers and hospitalization for iloprost infusion and amputations were also recorded.

### Exercise tolerance

The exercise tolerance of HIIT was assessed through measures that were interpreted participants' perception regarding the exercise intensity, the effect (Additional file 1), the exercise task self-efficacy (Additional file 2), the intentions (Additional file 3) and the enjoyment (Additional file 4). The above data was collected at the first and last exercise session each month in order to examine several time points during the exercise intervention. Specifically, the questionnaires were repeated at the 1st, 8th, 16th, and 24th exercise sessions. The individual questionnaires and the time points that were incorporated during the exercise session are described in Jung et al. [27].

### Statistical analysis

Data analysis was performed using SPSS software (version 23, IBM SPSS, Armonk, NY, USA) and is presented as mean ± SD. Normal distribution of the data and homogeneity of variances were tested using the Shapiro-Wilk and Levene's test, respectively. The comparison in the anthropometric, physiological and vascular characteristics among the three groups was done through a one-way ANOVA test. Independent t-tests and chi-squared tests were also used to identify the differences between two groups. Effect sizes (Cohen's d) were calculated wherever the results were statistically significant with 0.2, 0.5, and 0.8 representing small, medium, and large effects respectively [28]. To compare the between group differences using a one-way ANOVA we adjusted the ACE values according to the physiological and anthropometrical responses of CE [29]. Statistical significance was set at $p \leq 0.05$.

### Results

#### Compliance and exercise intensity

Compliance to the12-week exercise programme twice weekly was 92% and 88% for the ACE and CE group respectively, with one drop-out for each exercise group. No exercise-related complications were reported. The average percentage peak HR ($\%HR_{peak}$) for each exercise session was 92.1% ± 6.0 for the ACE group and 90.8% ± 7.5 for the CE group. The average rate of perceived exertion (RPE) and effect were 13 ± 1 and + 3 (good) ± 1, respectively, for both exercise groups.

#### Oxygen uptake and pressure

Both ACE (0.86 L min$^{-1}$ d = 0.68) and CE (1.22 ± 0.33 L min$^{-1}$ d = 0.76) $\dot{V}O_{2peak}$ were significantly greater post-exercise intervention compared to baseline ($p < 0.01$). ACE $\dot{V}O_{2peak}$ (21.9 ± 7.1 ml kg$^{-1}$ min$^{-1}$ d = 1.09) improved significantly in comparison to control but not compared to CE group (Table 3).

A tendency to improve was also observed in both ΔTcpO2 ($p = 0.59$, d = 0.93) and transcutaneous oxygen

**Table 3** Physiological and quality of life outcomes

| | ACE (n = 10) | | CE (n = 10) | | Control (n = 11) | |
|---|---|---|---|---|---|---|
| | Pre | Post | Pre | Post | Pre | Post |
| ACh CVC | 0.14 ± 0.06 | 0.19 ± 0.08 | 0.20 ± 0.11 | 0.26 ± 0.1 | 0.20 ± 0.08 | 0.15 ± 0.08 |
| ACh CVC$_{max}$ | 1.28 ± 0.78 | 1.56 ± 0.88* | 1.49 ± 0.99 | 1.26 ± 0.52 | 1.40 ± 0.78 | 0.82 ± 0.47 |
| ACh T$_{max}$ (sec) | 159.4 ± 83 | 104.1 ± 71.8 | 172 ± 57.9 | 119.4 ± 82.9 | 127.9 ± 51.1 | 149.9 ± 70.3 |
| SNP CVC | 0.15 ± 0.08 | 0.24 ± 0.14 | 0.21 ± 0.11 | 0.25 ± 0.08 | 0.20 ± 0.09 | 0.20 ± 0.1 |
| SNP CVC$_{max}$ | 1.73 ± 2.01 | 1.88 ± 1.52 | 1.61 ± 1.21 | 2.38 ± 1.8 | 1.70 ± 1.3 | 1.40 ± 0.56 |
| SNP T$_{max}$ (sec) | 161.2 ± 88.5 | 131.3 ± 77.5 | 167.4 ± 66.3 | 138.8 ± 80.5 | 165.5 ± 56.5 | 166.9 ± 76.4 |
| ΔTcpO2 | 2.5 ± 4.0 | 9.2 ± 12.1 | 1.56 ± 4.8 | 1.56 ± 9.5 | 1.39 ± 3.4 | 0.89 ± 2.6 |
| ΔTcpO2$_{max}$ | 11.5 ± 3.9 | 18.4 ± 16.5 | 11.7 ± 3.6 | 13.6 ± 9.6 | 9.44 ± 7.7 | 8.0 ± 7.0 |
| $\dot{V}O_{2peak}$ (ml kg$^{-1}$ min$^{-1}$) | 17.7 ± 4.7 | 21.9 ± 7.1* | 14.6 ± 2.9 | 18.5 ± 2.8* | 14.3 ± 6.9 | 14.7 ± 6.2 |
| Life satisfaction | 6.5 ± 1.6 | 8.1 ± 1.7*** | 8.4 ± 1.4* | 8.8 ± 1.1*** | 7.5 ± 1.6 | 4.9 ± 1.5 |
| Mobility | 2.4 ± 1.0 | 2.3 ± 0.8 | 1.9 ± 0.9 | 1.7 ± 1.0 | 1.9 ± 0.9 | 2.3 ± 1.2 |
| Self-care | 1.1 ± 0.3 | 1.1 ± 0.3 | 1.2 ± 0.4 | 1.0 ± 0.0 | 1.4 ± 0.9 | 1.7 ± 1.4 |
| Usual activity | 2.3 ± 1.3 | 1.9 ± 1.1 | 1.9 ± 1.0 | 1.6 ± 0.7 | 1.8 ± 1.0 | 2.4 ± 1.2 |
| Pain/ discomfort | 2.4 ± 1.0 | 2.3 ± 1.1 | 2.8 ± 1.1 | 1.8 ± 0.9 | 2.4 ± 0.7 | 2.8 ± 1.2 |
| Anxiety/ depression | 1.7 ± 0.8 | 1.5 ± 0.7 | 1.6 ± 0.7 | 1.2 ± 0.4 | 1.6 ± 0.7 | 1.9 ± 1.4 |
| Raynaud's pain | 2.4 ± 1.4 | 1.8 ± 0.6* | 2.6 ± 1.5 | 1.9 ± 1.2* | 2.4 ± 0.9 | 3.1 ± 1.1 |

Endothelial function presented as cutaneous vascular conductance (CVC). T$_{max}$ is the time taken to reach peak perfusion. *$p < 0.05$ and ***$p < 0.000$ compared to the other groups
*ACE* arm crank ergometer, *SNP* sodium nitroprusside, *ΔTcpO$_2$* transcutaneous oxygen tension *$\dot{V}O_{2peak}$* peak oxygen uptake

tension ($\Delta$TcpO2$_{max}$) ($p = 0.71$, d = 0.80) in ACE group. Although this improvement is not statistically significant the Cohen's d reveals that the effect size of the change is large (> 0.8) both at rest and during provocation (exercise test).

### Cutaneous vascular conductance (CVC)
No statistically significant differences were observed at baseline between the exercise and control groups ($p > 0.05$). Post-exercise intervention improvements were observed in the ACE group, especially over the control group, while values in CE group were slightly decreased (Table 3).

### Feasibility and tolerance of exercise
ACE showed to be the mode of exercise that will more likely ($p < 0.05$) engage SSc patients to physical activity twice per week (6.9 ± 0.3, d = 1.17) compared to the CE group (6.2 ± 0.79). Moreover, ACE demonstrated to be better ($p < 0.05$) regarding participant's confidence to perform two bouts per week (95 ± 7%, d = 0.82) than CE (83 ± 19.5%) but not statistically significant. Both exercise modes aggregated a high score of enjoyment levels > 94 out of 119 with an average effect before, during and after the exercise session of + 3 equals to "good".

### Quality of life and clinical outcomes
The EQ-5D-5 L questionnaire did not demonstrate any significant difference between the groups neither at baseline nor after the completion of the exercise intervention, in any of its five elements. However, both exercise groups reported improved life satisfaction ($p < 0.000$) as well as reduced discomfort and pain of Raynaud's phenomenon ($p < 0.05$) after the exercise intervention compared to the control group (Table 3). We also reported digital ulcers and hospitalization for iloprost infusion for four out of eleven patients (36.3%) in the control group. One of them proceeded to amputation of the distal phalange of the middle finger in one hand.

### Discussion
Overall, this study is the first to demonstrate that upper-limb aerobic exercise may be able to improve microvascular endothelial-dependent function in the digital area in patients with systemic sclerosis experiencing

Raynaud's phenomenon. Cycling indicated that it might have the potential to decelerate the disease progression in the vasculature (ACh) as the endothelial-dependent vasodilation was slightly decreased. On the other hand, the control group showed a decrease in endothelial-dependent function, which might indicate a disease worsening (Table 3). Pearson's correlation coefficient (Table 4) indicated that the endothelial improvement in ACE has a trend to correlate with the soft lean and fat-free mass as well as with skeletal muscle mass. Interestingly, ACh showed that is not correlated with ACE $\dot{V}O_{2peak}$, which does not confirm to previous findings that have shown association of endothelial-dependent function with the improvement in aerobic capacity in patients with rheumatoid arthritis [30]. The correlation between the endothelial-dependent function and the lean muscle is a vital evidence for future exercise prescription for this population. Resistance training is capable to increase muscle mass and to improve microcirculation in obese adults [31]. Thus a combination of the current HIIT protocol with resistance training might increase the chances for further improvement in the endothelial function.

### Endothelial-dependent function
Our results indicate that exercise training may improve the microvascular function in SSc patients. This could be largely attributed to a shear-stress-related mechanism. Shear stress is a mechanical reaction of the blood vessel to accommodate the increased blood flow, which activates the potassium channels and facilitates the calcium influx into the endothelial cells. Endothelial nitric oxide synthase (eNOS) activation and expression are triggered by an increase in intracellular calcium [32], promoting nitric oxide (NO) production and thus vasodilation [33]. It is possible that the recurring induction of NOS activity with exercise training decelerates the degradation of NO by free radicals in these conditions [34] or by reducing directly free radical production [35]. A recent systematic review on exercise training and vascular function [12] supports our findings indicating that the antioxidant status is enhanced after HIIT in patients with cardiometabolic disorders [36–38] and thus, the NO bioavailability is improved. Mitranun et al. [38] assessed the effects of interval aerobic exercise training (three times/week for 12 weeks) on endothelial-

**Table 4** Endothelial-dependent correlations in arm cranking

|  |  | Soft lean mass (kg) | Fat-free mass (kg) | Skeletal muscle mass (kg) | $\dot{V}O_{2peak}$ (L min$^{-1}$) | $\dot{V}O_{2peak}$ (ml kg$^{-1}$ min$^{-1}$) |
|---|---|---|---|---|---|---|
| ACh CVC$_{max}$ | Pearson's r | 0.529 | 0.520 | 0.530 | 0.120 | 0.220 |
|  | sig (2-tailed) | 0.116 | 0.123 | 0.115 | 0.740 | 0.569 |
|  | n = 10 | 10 | 10 | 10 | 10 | 10 |

*Ach* acetylcholine, *CVC* cutaneous vascular conductance

dependent vasodilation in patients with type 2 diabetes mellitus. The vascular outcomes demonstrated reductions in erythrocyte malondialdehyde and serum von Willebrand factor and increases in plasma glutathione peroxidase and nitric oxide (all $p < 0.05$). Therefore, HIIT seems to improve the microvascular function by reducing oxidative stress markers and enhance the antioxidants as well as the vasodilators in cardiometabolic conditions and potentially in connective tissue diseases such as SSc.

### Vascular remodelling, shear stress and exercise training

Evidence for the time course of functional or structural arterial adaptations to exercise training in humans is limited: Short-term effects of exercise improves NO bioavailability, whereas long-term effects induce changes in vascular remodelling [39], an endothelium and NO-dependent outcome [40].

Prior to this study, we hypothesised that upper limb exercise would be more effective to improve microcirculation in the local regions compared to lower limb exercise; however, the existing evidence supported systemic effects occur after exercise training in the lower limbs [12]. Therefore, we proceeded to a comparison between the upper and lower limbs. Interestingly, this systemic effect was not proved with our study, where the microvascular reactivity in the digital area was improved with arm cranking but not with cycling. Similar to our findings, Klonizakis et al., [41] reported that arm exercise did not have any impact on lower limbs microcirculation in post-surgical varicose-vein patients. It seems that systemic effects of exercise training can only affect the vascular function in the large arteries (e.g. brachial artery) but not the conduit and resistance arteries. Moreover, the mass of muscle engaged in exercise training could play an important role in the systemic effects as studies that utilized handgrip training have not demonstrated contralateral limb remodelling [42–44]. The explanation probably relies on the magnitude and pattern of shear stress, which in turn triggers the release of NO and acts as a main determinant for its bioavailability. It is possible that the induced-shear stress by lower limbs is not sufficient to improve the microcirculation in the acral body parts of the upper limbs. Therefore, the volume of blood flow and the magnitude of shear stress induced by HIIT could account for the local effects of exercise training in the smaller arteries [45, 46].

### Clinical outcome

Inadequate blood flow to living tissue is often a painful experience, threatening the life of the tissue involved. Digital tissue loss not only results in disfigurement and functional disability, it is also the clinical manifestation of an underlying systemic disease process [47]. One of the direct consequences of digital ischaemia is the

persistent digital ulcers developing irreversible tissue loss in 30% of patients [48]. In our study four out of eleven patients in the control group developed digital ulcers and required hospitalization for iloprost infusion [49, 50] for a period of 1 to 3 weeks and one patient proceeded to digital amputation of the distal phalange in the middle finger in one hand. Hospitalization is a psychologically-stressful procedure for the patient, which directly affects QoL. The most common side effects of iloprost infusion could be headache, flushing of the skin, nausea, vomiting and sweating. Amputation has been reported to occur in one or more digits due to ischaemia in 20.4% of patients with SSc, 9.2% of which have multiple digit loss [51]. QoL in patients with SSc is adversely affected due to digital ischaemia. Consequently, our protocol has demonstrated that is capable of improving digital ischaemia and preventing disease progression and digital ulcers and thus, improving QoL.

### Transcutaneous oxygen pressure

Although the improvement in oxygen pressure at rest and under provocation (exercise test) was not significant in our study, the effect size of this change was large. This indicates that ACE is able to induce systemic changes in oxygen pressure and vascular function in SSc patients, while the control group showed a slight decrease. It is probable that a higher training load or a larger cohort would have revealed a statistically significant difference between ACE and control group. Evidently, further research is needed to substantiate our findings and explore other training protocols, which will reveal the effects of exercise on skin oxygen pressure, when oxygen demand is higher.

### Quality of life

Both modes of exercise have shown improvement in life satisfaction and reduction in pain or discomfort induced by RP attacks after the exercise training. However, further research is required to confirm the improvement in RP by applying more qualitative measures (e.g. case-specific questionnaires and face-to-face interviews). Exercise tolerance, cardiorespiratory fitness, walking distance, muscle strength and function as well as health-related QoL have been demonstrated to be improved in SSc patients after participation in exercise programmes involving aerobic exercise and aerobic exercise combined with resistance training [52]. Therefore, promoting physical activity for the improvement of QoL in SSc patients should be deemed as one of the priorities for future research.

### Feasibility of HIIT

Our findings demonstrate that HIIT (30 s 100% PPO/ 30 s passive recovery) maintained an average effect of + 3

("Good") throughout the exercise training for both modes of exercise. It is also noteworthy that the patient's effect was similar before, during and after the exercise session which could be explained by the moderate cardiorespiratory stress induced by this protocol. Supportive to this finding is the RPE for both groups which averaged to 13 ("Somewhat hard"), a value which is strongly correlated to anaerobic threshold and low to moderate exercise intensity in a large cohort of adults [53]. Exercise intensity and affective response have presented a negative relationship in inactive and overweight adults and it has been reported that as incremental exercise progresses above the ventilatory threshold, the affective response to exercise becomes more negative [54, 55]. Therefore, a short protocol of HIIT seems to not induce great cardiovascular responses in patients with SSc and that might explain the effect's stability throughout the session.

The intentions regarding engagement to exercise and the task self-efficacy questionnaires as well as the enjoyment levels of the patients could further substantiate whether HIIT is a feasible mode of exercise in SSc patients. Both modes of exercise demonstrated a strong patient's confidence to perform two and three bouts of exercise with arm cranking being slightly higher than cycling. Both modes of exercise were enjoyable for the patients, however, arm cranking was found to be significantly higher in the intentions for engagement in two bouts of exercise per week compared to cycling. HIIT is a feasible protocol to be implemented in patients with SSc and ACE is considered more acceptable than CE potentially, because it is a new mode of exercise for this population and that might increase their interest to perform an alternative type of exercise.

### Limitations

The sample size of the current study could be deemed a limitation for the current study but we need to stress that SSc is not a common condition such as cardiometabolic diseases (e.g. hypertension, obesity, diabetes) and we strictly adhered to the pre-defined eligibility criteria to present a consistent and reproducible outcome. Moreover, the ratio between women and men is uneven, with SSc women to men ratio being estimated to be 5.2:1 in northeast England [56].

TcpO2 is a direct value of vascular function as changes at rest mimic the changes in arterial pO₂ during mild or moderate exercise [57, 58]. However, the time response of these changes is relatively slow (90% time response of TcpO2 being approximately 20 s). Carter and Banham [59] demonstrated that TcpO2 values closely followed those assessed by direct arterial sampling during cardiopulmonary exercise testing with 2 min intervals. We acknowledge that our protocol utilized 1 min intervals

until symptomatic limitation of exercise, which might affect the accuracy of TcpO2, however, we need to stress that the utilization of TcpO2 measurement in our study was more of a research interest aiming to evaluate the improvement in vascular function after an exercise programme rather than accurately depicting hypoxemia levels in the arterial wall.

Our patients were only of limited cutaneous systemic sclerosis, where the change in skin thickness is little over time compared to diffuse cutaneous systemic sclerosis (Khanna et al., 2017). Moreover, it is common practice in the NHS clinics to assess mRSS only in patients with dcSSc. Therefore, we did not include this measurement in our study; however, we believe that this does not affect our results, as the categorisation of the patients is clear. Also the autoantibody specificities for SSc patients are not included in our study as this is not a standard clinical practice in the area of Sheffield.

## Conclusions

- Aerobic exercise in general, and HIIT (30 s 100% PPO/30 s passive recovery) specifically, involving the upper limbs may improve the microvascular reactivity through an enhancement of the endothelial-dependent function. Our results correlated well with the lean muscle mass, which indicates that resistance training could be a complementary training element in inducing further improvements in microcirculation.
- Our protocol appears to reduce digital ischaemia risk, which can be the leading cause for further systemic complications and a major factor affecting the quality of life. Exercise is a non-invasive, adjunct treatment with no adverse effects that is well-tolerable by patients with SSc.
- There is a need for large multi-centre, randomised-controlled studies to further establish the effects of exercise on SSc patients.

### Abbreviations

6MWT: Six-minute walking test; ACE: Arm crank ergometer; Ach: Acetylcholine; BMI: Body mass index; CE: Cycle ergometer; CVC: Cutaneous vascular conductance; dcSSc: Diffuse cutaneous scleroderma; eNOS: Endothelial nitric oxide synthase; HIIT: High-intensity interval training; HR: Heart rate; LDF: Laser Doppler fluximetry; lcSSc: Limited cutaneous scleroderma; NO: Nitric oxide; PPO: Peak power output; QoL: Quality of life; RP: Raynaud's phenomenon; RPE: Rating of perceived exertion; SNP: Sodium nitroprusside; SSc: Systemic sclerosis; V̇E: Minute ventilation; V̇O₂peak: Peak oxygen uptake; VT: Tidal volume; ΔTcpO₂: Transcutaneous oxygen tension

### Acknowledgements

The authors would like to thank the study participants and report no conflicts of interest with this manuscript. The experiments comply with the current UK laws.

**Funding**
The work was supported by the Centre for Sports and Exercise Science, Sheffield Hallam University.

**Authors' contributions**
AM helped to draft the manuscript, designed the exercise intervention, contributed to the study design and critically reviewed and revised the manuscript for important intellectual content. HC developed the qualitative aspects of the study, contributed to the study design and critically reviewed and revised the manuscript for important intellectual content. GA provided statistical and health economics support, contributed to the study design and critically reviewed and revised the manuscript for important intellectual content. MA is the study's clinical lead, contributed to the study design and critically reviewed and revised the manuscript for important intellectual content. MK is the project leader and helped to draft the manuscript, contributed to the study design and critically reviewed and revised the manuscript for important intellectual content. All authors read and approved the final manuscript for publication.

**Competing interests**
The authors declare that they have no competing interests.

**Author details**
[1]Centre for Sport and Exercise Science, Collegiate Campus, Sheffield Hallam University, Collegiate Crescent, Sheffield S10 2BP, UK. [2]Centre for Health and Social Care Research, Sheffield Hallam University, Sheffield, UK. [3]Rheumatology Department, Royal Hallamshire Hospital, Sheffield, UK.

**References**
1. Gabrielli A, Avvedimento EV, Krieg T. Scleroderma. N Engl J Med. 2009;36: 1989–2003.
2. Bolster MBSR. Clinical features of systemic sclerosis. In: Hochberg MC, Silman AJ, Smolen JS, Weinblatt ME, Weisman MH, editors. Rheumatology. 6th ed. Philadelphia: Mosby Elsevier; 2008. p. 1375–85.
3. Jimenez SA, Derk CT. Following the molecular pathways toward an understanding of the pathogenesis of systemic sclerosis. Ann Intern Med. 2004;140:37–50.
4. Varga J, Abraham D. Systemic sclerosis: a prototypic multisystem fibrotic disorder. J Clin Invest. 2007;117:557–67.
5. Isenberg DA, Black C. ABC of Rheumatology. Raynaud's phenomenon, scleroderma, and overlap syndromes. BMJ. 1995;310:795–8.
6. Kavian N, Batteux F. Macro- and microvascular disease in systemic sclerosis. Vasc Pharmacol. 2015;71:16–23.
7. Kahaleh B. Progress in research into systemic sclerosis. Lancet. 2004;364: 561–2.
8. Sunderkötter C, Riemekasten G. Pathophysiology and clinical consequences of Raynaud's phenomenon related to systemic sclerosis. Rheumatology (Oxford). 2006;45:33–5.
9. Altman RD, Medsger TA Jr, Bloch DA, Michel BA. Predictors of survival in systemic sclerosis (scleroderma). Arthritis Rheum. 1991;34:403–13.
10. Pope JE. The diagnosis and treatment of Raynaud's phenomenon: a practical approach. Drugs. 2007;67:517–25.
11. Prescribing & Medicines Team Health and Social Care Information Centre. Prescription Cost Analysis for England 2015. 2016. https://digital.nhs.uk/catalogue/PUB20200. Accessed 07 May 2016.
12. Ramos JS, Dalleck LC, Tjonna AE, Beetham KS, Coombes JS. The impact of high-intensity interval training versus moderate-intensity continuous training on vascular function: a systematic review and meta-analysis. Sports Med. 2015;45:679–92.
13. Meyer P, Normandin E, Gayda M, Billon G, Guiraud T, Bosquet L, et al. High-intensity interval exercise in chronic heart failure: protocol optimization. J Card Fail. 2012;18:126–33.
14. Smith-Ryan A. Enjoyment of high-intensity interval training in an overweight/obese cohort: a short report. Clin Physiol Funct Imaging. 2017;37:89–93.
15. Guiraud T, Nigam A, Gremeaux V, Meyer P, Juneau M, Bosquet L. High-intensity interval training in cardiac rehabilitation. Sports Med. 2012;42:587–605.
16. Kessler HS, Sisson SB, Short KR. The potential for high-intensity interval training to reduce cardiometabolic disease risk. Sports Med. 2012;42:489–509.
17. Hoogen F, Khanna D, Fransen J, Johnson SR, Baron M, Tyndall A, et al. 2013 Classification Criteria for Systemic Sclerosis: An American College of Rheumatology/European League Against Rheumatism Collaborative Initiative. Arthritis Rheum. 2013;65:2737–47.
18. Borg GA. Perceived exertion: a note on "history" and methods. Med Sci Sports. 1973;5:90–3.
19. Smith PM, Price MJ, Doherty M. The influence of crank rate on peak oxygen consumption during arm crank ergometry. J Sports Sci. 2001;19:955–60.
20. Smith PM, Doherty M, Price MJ. The effect of crank rate strategy on peak aerobic power and peak physiological responses during arm crank ergometry. J Sports Sci. 2007;25:711–8.
21. Wasserman K. In: Hansen JE, Sue DY, Stringer WW, Sietsema KE, Sun XG, Whipp BJ, editors. Principles of exercise testing and interpretation : including pathophysiology and clinical applications. London: Wolters Kluwer/Lippincott Williams & Wilkins; 2012. p. 141–2.
22. Deuschle K, Weinert K, Becker MO, Backhaus M, Huscher D, Riemekasten G. Six-minute walk distance as a marker for disability and complaints in patients with systemic sclerosis. Clin Exp Rheumatol. 2011;29:S53–9.
23. Klonizakis M, Tew G, Michaels J, Saxton J. Exercise training improves cutaneous microvascular endothelial function in post- surgical varicose vein patients. Microvasc Res. 2009;78:67–70.
24. Klonizakis M, Tew G, Michaels J, Saxton J. Impaired microvascular endothelial function is restored by acute lower-limb exercise in post-surgical varicose vein patients. Microvasc Res. 2009;77:158–62.
25. Wasilewski R, Ubara EO, Klonizakis M. Assessing the effects of a short-term green tea intervention in skin microvascular function and oxygen tension in older and younger adults. Microvasc Res. 2016;107:65–71.
26. Dolan P. Modeling valuations for EuroQol health states. Med Care. 1997;35: 1095–108.
27. Jung ME, Bourne JE, Little JP. Where does HIT fit? An examination of the affective response to high-intensity intervals in comparison to continuous moderate- and continuous vigorous-intensity exercise in the exercise intensity-affect continuum. PLoS One. 2014;9:e114541.
28. Mullineaux DR, Bartlett RM, Bennett S. Research design and statistics in biomechanics and motor control. J Sports Sci. 2001;19:739–60.
29. Mitropoulos A, Gumber A, Crank H, Klonizakis M. Validation of an arm crank ergometer test for use in sedentary adults. J Sports Sci Med. 2017;16:558–64.
30. Metsios GS, Stavropoulos-Kalinoglou A, Veldhuijzen vZ, Nightingale P, Sandoo A, Dimitroulas T, et al. Individualised exercise improves endothelial function in patients with rheumatoid arthritis. Ann Rheum Dis. 2014;73:748.
31. Dias I, Farinatti P, De Souza MG, Manhanini DP, Balthazar E, Dantas DL, et al. Effects of resistance training on obese adolescents. Med Sci Sports Exerc. 2015;47:2636–44.
32. Laughlin M, Newcomer S, Bender S. Importance of hemodynamic forces as signals for exercise-induced changes in endothelial cell phenotype. J Appl Physiol. 2008;104:588.
33. Busse R, Mülsch A. Induction of nitric oxide synthase by cytokines in vascular smooth muscle cells. FEBS Lett. 1990;275:87–90.
34. Fukai T, Siegfried MR, Ushio-Fukai M, Cheng Y, Kojda G, Harrison DG. Regulation of the vascular extracellular superoxide dismutase by nitric oxide and exercise training. J Clin Invest. 2000;105:1631.
35. Adams V, Linke A, Krankel N, Erbs S, Gummert J, Mohr F, et al. Impact of regular physical activity on the expression of angiotensin II receptors and activity of NADPH oxidase in the left mammarial artery of patients with coronary artery disease. Eur Heart J. 2004;25:224.
36. Wisloff PU, Stoylen MA, Loennechen EJ, Bruvold AM, Rognmo JO, Haram LP, et al. Superior cardiovascular effect of aerobic interval-training versus moderate continuous training in elderly heart failure patients. Med Sci Sports Exerc. 2007;39:S32.
37. Tjønna AE, Lee SJ, Rognmo Ø, Stølen TO, Bye A, Haram PM, et al. Aerobic interval training versus continuous moderate exercise as a treatment for the metabolic syndrome: a pilot study. Circulation. 2008;118:346–54.
38. Mitranun W, Deerochanawong C, Tanaka H, Suksom D. Continuous vs interval training on glycemic control and macro- and microvascular reactivity in type 2 diabetic patients. Scand J Med Sci Sports. 2014;24:e69–76.
39. Laughlin MH, Rubin LJ, Rush JW, Price EM, Schrage WG, Woodman CR. Short-term training enhances endothelium-dependent dilation of coronary arteries, not arterioles. J Appl Physiol. 2003;94:234Y44.

40. Tronc F, Wassef M, Esposito B, Henrion D, Glagov S, Tedgui A. Role of NO in flow-induced remodeling of the rabbit common carotid artery. Arterioscler Thromb Vasc Biol. 1996;16:1256–62.

41. Klonizakis M, Winter E. Effects of arm-cranking exercise in cutaneous microcirculation in older, sedentary people. Microvasc Res. 2011;81:331–6.

42. Sinoway LI, Musch TI, Minotti JR, Zelis R. Enhanced maximal metabolic vasodilatation in the dominant forearms of tennis players. J Appl Physiol (1985). 1986;61:673–8.

43. Green DJ, Cable NT, Fox C, Rankin JM, Taylor RR. Modification of forearm resistance vessels by exercise training in young men. J Appl Physiol (Bethesda, MD: 1985). 1994;77:1829.

44. Green DJ, Fowler DT, O'Driscoll JG, Blanksby BA, Taylor RR. Endothelium-derived nitric oxide activity in forearm vessels of tennis players. J Appl Physiol (Bethesda, MD.: 1985). 1996;81:943.

45. Ribeiro F, Alves AJ, Duarte JA, Oliveira J. Is exercise training an effective therapy targeting endothelial dysfunction and vascular wall inflammation? Int J Cardiol. 2010;141:214–21.

46. Liu L, Yu B, Chen J, Tang Z, Zong C, Shen D, et al. Different effects of intermittent and continuous fluid shear stresses on osteogenic differentiation of human mesenchymal stem cells. Biomech Model Mechanobiol. 2012;11:391–401.

47. Mcmahan Z, Wigley F. Raynaud's phenomenon and digital ischemia: a practical approach to risk stratification, diagnosis and management. Int J Clin Rheumatol. 2010;5:355–70.

48. Ingraham KM, Steen VD. Morbidity of digital tip ulcerations in scleroderma. Arth Rheum. 2006;54:P578.

49. Vitielo M, Abuchar A, Santana N, Dehesa L, Kerdel FA. An update on the treatment of the cutaneous manifestations of systemic sclerosis: The dermatologist's point of view. J Clin Aesthet Dermatol. 2012;5:33–43.

50. Pope J, Fenlon D, Thompson A, Shea B, Furst D, Wells GA, et al. Iloprost and cisaprost for Raynaud's phenomenon in progressive systemic sclerosis. Cochrane Database Syst Rev. 2000;2:CD000953.

51. Wigley FM, Wise RA, Miller R, Needleman BW, Spence RJ. Anticentromere antibody as a predictor of digital ischemic loss in patients with systemic sclerosis. Arthritis Rheum. 1992;35:688–93.

52. Oliveira NC, Portes LA, Pettersson H, Alexanderson H, Boström C. Aerobic and resistance exercise in systemic sclerosis: state of the art. Musculoskeletal Care. 2017;15:316–23.

53. Scherr J, Wolfarth B, Christle JW, Pressler A, Wagenpfeil S, Halle M. Associations between Borg's rating of perceived exertion and physiological measures of exercise intensity. Eur J Appl Physiol. 2013;113:147–55.

54. Blanchard CM, Rodgers WM, Spence JC, Courneya KS. Feeling state responses to acute exercise of high and low intensity. J Sci Med Sport. 2001;4:30–8.

55. Parfitt G, Hughes S. The exercise intensity–affect relationship: evidence and implications for exercise behavior. J Exerc Sci Fit. 2009;7:S34–41.

56. Allcock RJ, Forrest I, Corris PA, Crook PR, Griffiths ID. A study of the prevalence of systemic sclerosis in northeast England. Rheumatology (Oxford). 2004;43:596–602.

57. Brudin L, Berg S, Ekberg P, Castenfors J. Is transcutaneous PO2 monitoring during exercise a reliable alternative to arterial PO2 measurements? Clin Physiol. 1994;14:47–52.

58. Planès C, Leroy M, Foray E, Raffestin B. Arterial blood gases during exercise: validity of transcutaneous measurements. Arch Phys Med Rehabil. 2001;82:1686–91.

59. Carter R, Banham SW. Use of transcutaneous oxygen and carbon dioxide tensions for assessing indices of gas exchange during exercise testing. Respir Med. 2000;94:350–5.

# Prospective evaluation of the capillaroscopic skin ulcer risk index in systemic sclerosis patients in clinical practice

Ulrich A. Walker[1*†], Veronika K. Jaeger[1†], Katharina M. Bruppacher[2], Rucsandra Dobrota[3], Lionel Arlettaz[4], Martin Banyai[5], Jörg Beron[6], Carlo Chizzolini[7], Ernst Groechenig[8], Rüdiger B. Mueller[9], François Spertini[10], Peter M. Villiger[11] and Oliver Distler[3]

## Abstract

**Background:** Nailfold capillaroscopy (NC) is an important tool for the diagnosis of systemic sclerosis (SSc). The capillaroscopic skin ulcer risk index (CSURI) was suggested to identify patients at risk of developing digital ulcers (DUs). This study aims to assess the reliability of the CSURI across assessors, the CSURI change during follow-up and the value of the CSURI in predicting new DUs.

**Methods:** This multicentre, longitudinal study included SSc patients with a history of DUs. NC images of all eight fingers were obtained at baseline and follow-up and were separately analysed by two trained assessors.

**Results:** Sixty-one patients were included (median observation time 1.0 year). In about 40% of patients (assessor 1, $n = 24$, 39%; assessor 2, $n = 26$, 43%) no megacapillary was detected in any of the baseline or follow-up images; hence the CSURI could not be calculated.

In those 34 patients in whom CSURI scores were available from both assessors (26% male; median age 57 years) the median baseline CSURI was 5.3 according to assessor 1 (IQR 2.6–16.3), increasing to 5.9 (IQR 1.3–12.0) at follow-up. According to assessor 2, the CSURI diminished from 6.4 (IQR 2.4–12.5) to 5.0 (IQR 1.7–10.0).

The ability of a CSURI ≥ 2.96 category to predict new DUs was low (for both assessors, positive predictive value 38% and negative predictive value 50%) and the inter-assessor agreements for CSURI categories were fair to moderate.

**Conclusions:** In this study, around 40% of patients could not be evaluated with the CSURI due to the absence of megacapillaries. Clinical decisions based on the CSURI should be made with caution.

**Keywords:** Systemic sclerosis, Nailfold capillaroscopy, Capillaroscopic skin ulcer risk index, Inter-rater reliability, Digital ulcer prediction

* Correspondence: ulrich.walker@usb.ch
†Ulrich A Walker and Veronika K Jaeger contributed equally to this work.
[1]Department of Rheumatology, University Hospital Basel, Petersgraben 4, 4032 Basel, Switzerland
Full list of author information is available at the end of the article

## Background

Systemic sclerosis (SSc) is a chronic connective tissue disease characterised by endothelial cell dysfunction and fibrosis of the skin and internal organs [1, 2]. Microangiopathy is one of the main histopathologic features detectable early in the course of the disease [3]. A gradual progression of vascular abnormalities has been observed during SSc progression [4]. Nailfold capillaroscopy (NC) is an imaging technique that detects morphological abnormalities of nailfold microcirculation. Furthermore, NC is an important tool for the classification and diagnosis of SSc in clinical practice [5, 6]. The three NC patterns early, active and late were found to be associated with Raynaud's phenomenon (RP) as well as with the duration of the disease, possibly reflecting SSc evolution [4]. Although the diagnostic value of the NC patterns is well defined [7], different methodologies have been proposed to assess quantitative NC abnormalities in the follow-up of patients with SSc. However, their clinical applicability remains uncertain.

Sebastiani et al. [8] proposed the capillaroscopic skin ulcer risk index (CSURI) in 2009, as a quantitative measure of nailfold capillary damage that predicts the appearance of new digital ulcers (DUs) as well as the persistence of pre-existing DUs [8, 9]. The CSURI is based on the number of capillaries in the distal nailfold capillary row and the number of megacapillaries, as well as the maximum diameter of the megacapillaries on capillaroscopic evaluation [8, 9].

In order to gain better insight into the value of monitoring quantitative NC abnormalities in clinical practice, this multicentre study was designed to describe the reliability of the CSURI across different trained assessors, to describe the change of CSURI during follow-up, to assess the value of the CSURI in predicting new DUs and to assess associations between the CSURI and demographic and disease characteristics.

## Methods

### Study population and design

This multicentre, prospective, observational study was carried out across eight sites in Switzerland between 2011 and 2015. Adult patients fulfilling the 1980 American College of Rheumatology criteria for SSc and with a history of DUs were included [10]. DUs were defined as a painful area with visually discernible depth and a loss of continuity of epithelial coverage which can be denuded or covered by a scab or necrotic tissue and is vascular in origin. Fissures, paronychia, extrusion of calcium or ulcers over the metacarpophalangeal joints or elbows are not regarded as DUs. In order to be included in this analysis, patients were also required to have at least one follow-up visit; if a patient had more than one follow-up visit, the last one was chosen as the follow-up

visit. All inclusion and exclusion criteria are summarised in Additional file 1: Table S1.

This study was approved by the centres' ethic committees and each patient provided written informed consent.

Demographic patient characteristics and routine clinical data were recorded prospectively on a web-based electronic data capture system. Table 1 presents a description of the data collected. Patients underwent NC at baseline and at follow-up visits. Follow-up visits were performed if deemed necessary by the centres' physicians, but were recommended at 3, 6 and 12 months. Regular external monitoring with primary data verification was performed to ensure data quality.

Prior to commencing the study, the study sites' investigators were trained at an investigator meeting to perform NC. The nailfolds of eight fingers (digits 2–5 on both hands) were examined using the same NC device equipped with a 200× lens with LED illumination and an immersion fluid contact adapter (Optilia instruments AB, Sollentuna, Sweden) in all centres. Four images

**Table 1** Description of collected data

| Demographics |
| --- |
| Age (years) |
| Sex (female/male) |
| Smoking habit (never smoker/ex-smoker/current smoker) |
| Disease characteristics |
| Time since RP onset (years) |
| Time since first non-RP manifestation (years) |
| Cutaneous involvement (limited/diffuse) |
| Modified Rodnan skin score (range 0–51) |
| Erectile dysfunction (yes/no; defined as a score below 22 in the International Index for Erectile Dysfunction-5 [19]) |
| Kidney involvement (yes/no; defined as proteinuria) |
| History of renal crisis (yes/no) |
| RP condition score (range 0–10) |
| DUs (yes/no; defined as a painful area with visually discernible depth and a loss of continuity of epithelial coverage, which can be denuded or covered by a scab or necrotic tissue and is vascular in origin; DUs do not include fissures, paronychia, extrusion of calcium or ulcers over the metacarpophalangeal joints or elbows.) |
| Time since first DU (years) |
| Number of DUs |
| Major digital vascular complications (none/soft tissue infection/gangrene/autoamputation) |
| Laboratory (measured according to local standards in the respective centres) |
| Antinuclear autoantibody positivity (yes/no) |
| Anticentromere autoantibody positivity (yes/no) |
| Anti-topoisomerase autoantibody positivity (yes/no) |

*DU* digital ulcer, *RP* Raynaud's phenomenon

across the nailfold quadrants of each finger were obtained. Digital NC images were stored centrally and examined separately at the end of the study by two identically trained central assessors (UAW and OD). The central assessors were blinded for the patients, the temporal sequence of the fingers and the scoring results of the other assessor. In each NC image, the assessors assessed the total number of capillaries in the distal row, the number of megacapillaries and the maximum diameter of the megacapillaries. Additionally, the images were also evaluated locally at the centres (local assessors). The qualitative assessment—that is, the NC pattern (early/active/late)—was performed by one additional central assessor (RD).

The presence of at least one megacapillary is necessary to calculate the CSURI [8, 9]. The CSURI is calculated for only one image per patient per time point; this image is identified based on the lowest number of capillaries in the distal row as the first criterion and subsequently the highest number of megacapillaries as the second criterion [8, 9]. As described in detail elsewhere, the number of megacapillaries is multiplied by the maximum diameter of the megacapillaries and then divided by the square of the number of capillaries to form the CSURI [8, 9]. For part of the analysis, we categorised the CSURI at 2.96, a threshold which was suggested to be predictive for the prospective development of DUs [9].

### Data analysis

Categorical variables were calculated as frequencies and percentages, and continuous variables were calculated as means with standard deviation (SD) or medians with interquartile range (IQR). Chi-square tests/Fisher's exact tests and Mann–Whitney $U$ tests were applied for across-group comparisons. Intraclass correlation coefficients and Cohen's κ were calculated to assess the agreement between the two assessors. Linear regression analysis was applied to evaluate associations between the change in CSURI between baseline and follow-up and demographic or disease characteristics. All statistical analyses were performed with Stata/IC 13.1 (StataCorp., College Station, TX, USA).

### Results

Between 2011 and 2015, 61 patients from eight centres were enrolled. The median observation time was 1.0 year

(IQR 1.0–1.1). Of these 61 patients, 24 patients according to central assessor 1 (39%) and 26 patients according to central assessor 2 (43%) had no megacapillaries present on any assessed finger either at baseline or at the follow-up visit (Table 2). Due to the absence of megacapillaries, the CSURI could not be calculated for those patients. Therefore, for only 34 of the 61 eligible patients (56%) was the CSURI scorable by both central assessors at both time points. This percentage of patients without megacapillaries was similar across all eight centres ($p$ = 0.72).

According to both central assessors, megacapillaries were present in 43 patients at baseline (Table 2); 30% of these showed an early SSc pattern on NC, 44% an active pattern and 26% a late pattern. Of the 18 patients without megacapillaries present at baseline (Table 2), 6% (one patient) had an early pattern, 28% a late pattern and the remaining 66% of patients showed no SSc specific pattern on NC at baseline.

The following analyses are entirely based on the 34 patients with an available CSURI by both central assessors at both time points, named the study population.

The baseline characteristics of the study population are presented in Table 3. The median observation time in this population was also 1.0 year (IQR 1.0–1.1). There were no statistically significant differences between the patients included in the study population and those excluded from further analysis. The included patients were, however, slightly younger (median age 57 years vs 62 years) and nominally more often had diffuse skin involvement (41% vs 33%) than the excluded patients. As many as 24% of the patients had experienced ulcer complications (soft tissue infections and gangrene).

In the study population, central assessor 1 counted a median of five capillaries in the distal row (range 2–10) and a median of one megacapillary (range 1–6) with a median maximum diameter of 62.5 μm (range 50–130 μm). Central assessor 2 counted a median of five capillaries in the distal row (range 2–10) and two megacapillaries (range 1–20) with a median diameter of 75 μm (range 30–180 μm).

The median baseline CSURI scores were 5.3 (IQR 2.6–16.3) as evaluated by central assessor 1 and 6.4 (IQR 2.4–12.5) as evaluated by central assessor 2. The median

**Table 2** Overview of distribution of patients with absent megacapillaries at any of the assessed fingers (i.e. CSURI non-scorability) at baseline and follow-up according to the central assessors

| | SSc patients (out of 61 patients) who had no megacapillaries on any of the assessed fingers | | |
| --- | --- | --- | --- |
| | Central assessor 1 | Central assessor 2 | Both central assessors combined |
| Baseline | 15 patients (25%) | 17 patients (28%) | 18 patients (30%) |
| Follow-up | 15 patients (25%) | 18 patients (30%) | 18 patients (30%) |
| Any of the two time points | 24 patients (39%) | 26 patients (43%) | 27 patients (44%) |

*CSURI* capillaroscopic skin ulcer risk index, *SSc* systemic sclerosis

**Table 3** Comparison of baseline demographics and disease characteristics between patients included in this analysis (scorable CSURI at baseline and follow-up) and those excluded (CSURI not scorable at baseline and follow-up)

| Baseline characteristic of study population | Included | Excluded | p value |
|---|---|---|---|
| N | 34 | 27 | |
| Age (years) | 56.6 (47.8–64.8) | 61.7 (53.6–64.6) | 0.25 |
| Male sex | 26 | 30 | 0.79 |
| Smoking habit | | | |
| Never smoker | 47 | 37 | 0.23 |
| Ex-smoker | 18 | 37 | |
| Current smoker | 35 | 26 | |
| Bosentan at any time during the observation period | 38 | 33 | 0.69 |
| Disease characteristics | | | |
| Time since RP onset (years) | 7.0 (3–15) | 5.0 (2–21) | 0.65 |
| Time since first non-RP manifestation (years) | 4.5 (1–9) | 5.0 (2–12) | 0.44 |
| Cutaneous involvement | | | |
| Limited | 59 | 67 | 0.53 |
| Diffuse | 41 | 33 | |
| Erectile dysfunction | 13 | 44 | 0.29 |
| Kidney involvement | 0 | 4 | 0.45 |
| History of renal crisis | 0 | 0 | – |
| RP condition score [20] | 3.8 (2–7) | 5.0 (2–7) | 0.49 |
| mRSS | 8 (6–13) | 9 (4–18) | 0.63 |
| Time since first DU (years) | 1.5 (0.7–4.2) | 2.3 (1.1–5.0) | 0.42 |
| DU | 76 | 74 | 0.83 |
| Number of DUs (in patients with DUs) | 3.0 (1–7) | 3.5 (1–6) | 0.99 |
| Previous major digital vascular complication | | | |
| None | 76 | 69 | 0.39 |
| Soft tissue infection | 21 | 15 | |
| Gangrene | 3 | 8 | |
| Autoamputation | 0 | 8 | |
| Laboratory parameters | | | |
| ANA positive | 100 | 96 | 0.25 |
| ACA positive | 48 | 45 | 0.83 |
| Scl-70 positive | 34 | 45 | 0.46 |

Data presented as % or median (interquartile range)

*ACA* anticentromere autoantibodies, *ANA* anti-nuclear autoantibodies, *CSURI* capillaroscopic skin ulcer risk index, *DU* digital ulcer, *mRSS* modified Rodnan skin score, *RP* Raynaud's phenomenon, *Scl-70* anti-topoisomerase I autoantibodies

baseline CSURI was 8.2 (IQR 4.5–23.6) according to the local assessors. According to central assessor 1, the median CSURI score increased to 5.9 (IQR 1.3–12.0) at follow-up, whereas the median CSURI as evaluated by central assessor 2 decreased to 5.0 (IQR 1.7–10.0) at follow-up. The correlation coefficient between the baseline CSURI of the two assessors was 0.42, indicating a fair agreement [11]. There was a poor to fair agreement between the CSURI scored by the central assessors and the local assessors (central assessor 1/local assessors 0.45; central assessor 2/local assessors 0.38).

As evaluated by central assessor 1, 35% of patients had a higher CSURI at follow-up compared to 44% when evaluated by central assessor 2. In only 40% of the 34 patients was the change in CSURI between baseline and follow-up in the same direction for both central assessors; that is, an increase as measured by both assessors, a decrease in the measurements of both assessors or no change (Fig. 1).

According to both central assessors, 10 patients (29%) were in the low-risk category (CSURI < 2.96 [9]) at baseline; however, only seven of those 10 patients were

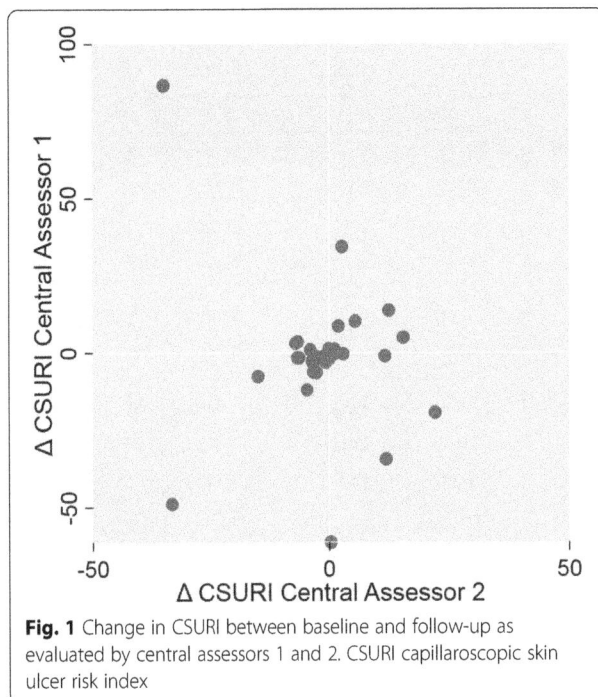

**Fig. 1** Change in CSURI between baseline and follow-up as evaluated by central assessors 1 and 2. CSURI capillaroscopic skin ulcer risk index

concomitantly rated by both assessors as being in the low-risk category. According to the local assessors, five patients (15%) were in the low-risk category; however, only two of those were concomitantly rated by both central assessors into the low-risk category. The inter-assessor agreement of the central assessors for the baseline CSURI risk category was 0.58, indicating a moderate level of agreement [12]. The inter-assessor agreements of the local assessor and central assessor 1 or 2 were both 0.25, indicating a fair agreement.

Central assessor 1 scored 88% of the patients into the same risk category at baseline and at follow-up (i.e. either low–low risk or high–high risk); the remaining 12% were in the low-risk category at follow-up, but in the high-risk category at baseline. According to assessor 2, 73% of patients were in the same risk category at baseline and follow-up, 21% were in the high-risk category at baseline and in the low-risk category at follow-up, and 6% were in the low-risk category at baseline and in the high-risk category at follow-up. The agreement between the two central assessors of this 'change in risk categories' was fair ($\kappa = 0.37$) [12]. There was no agreement between central assessor 1 and central assessor 2 and the local assessors regarding this 'change of risk category' ($\kappa = -0.09$, $\kappa = -0.16$, respectively).

The prevalence of DU at baseline was 76% (Table 3) compared to 59% at follow-up. The ability of CSURI ≥ 2.96 (i.e. the high-risk category) to predict a higher number of DUs at follow-up than at baseline visit was rather low (positive predictive value for both central assessors 38%, for local assessors 48%), as was the ability of CSURI

< 2.96 (i.e. low-risk category) to predict fewer or the same number of DUs at follow-up compared to baseline (negative predictive value for both central assessors 50%, for local assessors 67%). Out of the 34 included patients, 28 patients were classified into the same risk category by both central assessors. The positive and the negative predictive values based on these 28 patients were similarly lower (positive predictive value 38%, negative predictive value 43%) than the predictive values based on all 34 patients. The predictive values in patients who were treated with bosentan at any time during the observation period were similar to those who were not treated with bosentan.

No demographic or disease characteristic was associated with the change in the CSURI between baseline and follow-up simultaneously for both CSURIs, the one scored by assessor 1 and the one scored by assessor 2, in univariate linear regression (Table 4).

## Discussion

This prospective, longitudinal study examined the use of the CSURI in everyday clinical practice and demonstrates that 40% of patients in this multicentre study could not be evaluated with the CSURI at baseline and follow-up visits, mainly due to a normal NC pattern and the lack of any megacapillary as a prerequisite for the calculation of the CSURI [9, 13]. Additionally, the agreement of the CSURI between the two trained and experienced assessors was mediocre at best, as was the agreement between the two central assessors and the local assessors.

Our high percentage of non-scorable patients contrasts with the first CSURI study and the CSURI validation study [8, 9]. In the first study all patients had megacapillaries present, and in the second study only 13 out of an unselected SSc population of 242 patients (5%) were excluded from the study due to the absence of megacapillaries [8, 9]. However, in various other studies that were not applying the CSURI, the percentage of patients without megacapillaries was comparable to our high percentage. For instance, in a study of 188 SSc patients at least one quarter of patients had no megacapillaries [14]. Similarly, in two other studies, 24% and 30% of patients had no megacapillaries in any of the assessed fingers [15, 16]. Our discrepancies with the first CSURI studies are difficult to explain with differences of equipment, given the fact that very similar devices were in use in the first CSURI studies as well as in our study. Our patient population had similar disease duration as the patients consecutively recruited into the first CSURI study [8], but a higher proportion of diffuse SSc patients (41% vs 9%), which may not explain the lower prevalence of megacapillaries in our study.

**Table 4** Univariate linear regression of ΔCSURI (defined as the difference of CSURI between baseline and follow-up) and demographics and disease characteristics ($n = 34$)

| Characteristic of study population | Central assessor 1 | | | Central assessor 2 | | |
|---|---|---|---|---|---|---|
| | β | 95% CI | p value | β | 95% CI | p value |
| Age (years) | −0.095 | −0.75 to 0.56 | 0.77 | 0.222 | −0.08 to 0.53 | 0.15 |
| Male sex | −0.92 | −19.2 to 17.4 | 0.92 | −3.5 | −12.2 to 5.3 | 0.42 |
| Smoking habit | | | | | | |
|   Never smoker | Reference | | | Reference | | |
|   Ex-smoker | 3.61 | −18.7 to 25.9 | 0.74 | −1.4 | − 12.3 to 9.5 | 0.79 |
|   Current smoker | 11.54 | −6.2 to 29.3 | 0.20 | −3.9 | −12.7 to 4.8 | 0.36 |
| Disease characteristics | | | | | | |
|   Time since RP onset (years) | −0.093 | −0.75 to 0.56 | 0.77 | 0.096 | −0.19 to 0.39 | 0.50 |
|   Time since first non-RP manifestation (years) | −1.16 | −2.9 to 0.6 | 0.18 | 0.91 | 0.1 to 1.7 | 0.025 |
|   Time since first DU (years) | −0.81 | −3.0 to 1.4 | 0.46 | 0.90 | 0.0 to 1.8 | 0.046 |
| Previous major digital vascular complication | | | | | | |
|   None | Reference | | | Reference | | |
|   Soft tissue infection | −5.62 | −25.9 to 14.6 | 0.58 | 3.15 | −6.4 to 12.7 | 0.51 |
|   Gangrene | 5.24 | −43.2 to 53.7 | 0.83 | 14.74 | −8.1 to 37.5 | 0.20 |
| Cutaneous involvement | | | | | | |
|   Limited | Reference | | | Reference | | |
|   Diffuse | 4.05 | −12.3 to 20.4 | 0.62 | −3.08 | −10.9 to 4.8 | 0.43 |
| Erectile dysfunction | −7.99 | −14.2 to −1.8 | 0.019 | −7.28 | −21.1 to 6.5 | 0.25 |
| RP condition score [20] at baseline | −0.51 | −2.4 to 1.4 | 0.59 | −0.11 | −1.0 to 0.8 | 0.81 |
| mRSS at baseline | −0.04 | −0.9 to 0.9 | 0.93 | − 0.002 | −0.4 to 0.4 | 0.99 |
| Number of DUs at baseline | 1.05 | −0.8 to 2.9 | 0.25 | 0.55 | −0.3 to 1.4 | 0.21 |
| Laboratory parameters | | | | | | |
|   ACA positive | 6.08 | −10.4 to 22.5 | 0.46 | −0.02 | −8.1 to 8.0 | 0.99 |
|   Scl-70 positive | −16.5 | −34.8 to 1.8 | 0.075 | −2.73 | −12.1 to 6.7 | 0.56 |

*ACA* anticentromere autoantibodies, *CI* confidence interval, *CSURI* capillaroscopic skin ulcer risk index, *DU* digital ulcer, *mRSS* modified Rodnan skin score, *RP* Raynaud's phenomenon, *Scl-70* anti-topoisomerase autoantibodies

In our study, the CSURI had only fair to moderate inter-rater reliability. This contrasts with an 'almost perfect' inter-observer reproducibility reported by Sebastiani et al. [8] in the original CSURI study, with κ = 0.96 based on the CSURI, dichotomised at the 2.96 cut-off value. A slightly lower but still 'almost perfect' inter-rater agreement of 0.85 was found in the validation study [9]. It is unlikely that these discrepancies can be completely explained with a lack of experience or different training, as both central assessors were trained together by authors of the original CSURI publications and used the same digital images and imaging software.

The CSURI was created as a prognostic index to predict the onset of new DUs [8]. In a validation study, Sebastiani et al. [9] demonstrated high predictive values for the development of DUs within 3 months, especially a high negative predictive value of 97%, but also a high positive predictive value of the CSURI of 81% in patients with a history of DUs. However, in another study by

Sebastiani et al. [17] a poorer performance of the CSURI with lower predictive values was also observed in a population of SSc patients treated with bosentan. Differences in DU prediction may therefore be explained by differences in vasoactive medications. When we stratified our patients by bosentan treatment, we did not observe major differences in predictive values. It must, however, also be kept in mind that the predictive values from our study should not be directly compared with the studies by Sebastiani et al. as we assessed the predictive values of a higher number of DUs at follow-up compared to baseline and not 'incident DU' as Sebastiani et al. Additionally, the time between the baseline and the follow-up visit was considerably longer in our study (median time 1 year) than in Sebastiani et al.'s studies (3 months), which could also partly explain the differences in the predictive power of the CSURI.

A recent systematic literature review critically appraising studies reporting the prognostic value of NC in SSc

Prospective evaluation of the capillaroscopic skin ulcer risk index in systemic sclerosis patients...

101

also assessed the predictive value of the CSURI [18]. In line with our study, Paxton and Pauling [18] conclude that it is difficult to draw robust conclusions regarding the prognostic role of the CSURI; the reason for this being high levels of potential biases relating to study confounding as well as the statistical analyses.

It needs to be mentioned that our study has a rather limited sample size, which restricts the power to assess CSURI predictors in terms of demographic and disease characteristics. However, the mediocre performance of the CSURI regarding the inter-rater differences, as well as the high number of patients who could not be included due to the absence of megacapillaries, will not be a result of chance alone, even if a larger sample size would naturally have been beneficial.

## Conclusions

The CSURI was not applicable in a large percentage of patients due to the absence of megacapillaries and demonstrated only fair to moderate inter-rater reliability. Thus, in routine clinical practice, the CSURI should be used with caution for treatment decisions and prediction of incident DUs.

## Abbreviations

CSURI: Capillaroscopic skin ulcer risk index; DU: Digital ulcer; IQR: Interquartile range; NC: Nailfold capillaroscopy; RP: Raynaud's phenomenon; SD: Standard deviation; SSc: Systemic sclerosis

## Funding

This study was sponsored by Actelion Pharma Schweiz AG. The company contributed to the design of the study and was involved in the interpretation of the data and the writing, review and approval of the publication.

## Authors' contributions

UAW, KMB and OD contributed to conception and design. UAW, RD, LA, MB, CC, EG, RBM, FS, PMV and OD contributed to acquisition of data. UAW, VKJ, RD, JB and OD analysed and interpreted data. UAW, VKJ, RD, JB and OD drafted the article. All authors critically revised the manuscript for important intellectual content. All authors read and approved the final manuscript.

## Competing interests

VKJ received travel grant and travel support from Actelion Pharma Schweiz AG. KMB was a former full-time employee of Actelion Pharma Schweiz AG. RD received research funding through an Articulum Fellowship sponsored by Pfizer (2013–2014), a EULAR training bursary and from the FP-7-DeSScipher project, and speaker fees from Actelion. JB is a full-time employee of Actelion Pharma Schweiz AG. CC received travel support and speaker fees from Actelion and Boehringer Ingelheim. OD has a consultancy relationship and/or research funding from AnaMar, Bayer, Boehringer Ingelheim, Catenion, CSL Behring, ChemomAb, Roche, GSK, Inventiva, Italfarmaco, Lilly, medac, Medscape, Mitsubishi Tanabe Pharma, MSD, Novartis, Pfizer, Sanofi and UCB in the area of potential treatments of scleroderma and its complications; in addition, OD has licensed patent mir-29 for the treatment of systemic sclerosis. The remaining authors declare that they have no competing interests.

## Author details

[1]Department of Rheumatology, University Hospital Basel, Petersgraben 4, 4032 Basel, Switzerland. [2]Bellikon, Switzerland. [3]Department of Rheumatology, University Hospital Zurich, Zurich, Switzerland. [4]Institut Central—Hôpital du Valais, Sion, Switzerland. [5]Kantonsspital Luzern, Luzern, Switzerland. [6]Actelion Pharma Schweiz AG, Baden, Switzerland. [7]Immunology & Allergy, University Hospital and School of Medicine, Geneva, Switzerland. [8]Kantonsspital Aarau, Aarau, Switzerland. [9]Kantonsspital St. Gallen, St. Gallen, Switzerland. [10]Division of Immunology and Allergy, Centre Hospitalier Universitaire Vaudois, Lausanne, Switzerland. [11]Department of Rheumatology, Immunology and Allergology, University Hospital and University of Bern, Bern, Switzerland.

## References

1. Gabrielli A, Avvedimento EVEV, Krieg T. Scleroderma. N Engl J Med. 2009; 360(19):1989–2003.
2. Varga J, Trojanowska M, Kuwana M. Pathogenesis of systemic sclerosis: recent insights of molecular and cellular mechanisms and therapeutic opportunities. J Scleroderma Relat Disord. 2017;2(3):137–52.
3. Cutolo M, Sulli A, Smith V. Assessing microvascular changes in systemic sclerosis diagnosis and management. Nat Rev Rheumatol. 2010;6(10):578–87.
4. Cutolo M, Pizzorni C, Secchi ME, Sulli A. Capillaroscopy. Best Pract Res Clin Rheumatol. 2008;22(6):1093–108.
5. van den Hoogen F, Khanna D, Fransen J, Johnson SR, Baron M, Tyndall A, et al. 2013 classification criteria for systemic sclerosis: an American College of Rheumatology/European League against Rheumatism collaborative initiative. Arthritis Rheum. 2013;65(11):2737–47.
6. Smith V, Thevissen K, Trombetta AC, Pizzorni C, Ruaro B, Piette Y, et al. Nailfold capillaroscopy and clinical applications in systemic sclerosis. Microcirculation. 2016;23(5):364–72.
7. Cutolo M, Smith V. Nailfold capillaroscopy. In: Scleroderma. Boston: Springer US; 2012. p. 331–46.
8. Sebastiani M, Manfredi A, Colaci M, D'amico R, Malagoli V, Giuggioli D, et al. Capillaroscopic skin ulcer risk index: a new prognostic tool for digital skin ulcer development in systemic sclerosis patients. Arthritis Rheum. 2009; 61(5):688–94.
9. Sebastiani M, Manfredi A, Vukatana G, Moscatelli S, Riato L, Bocci M, et al. Predictive role of capillaroscopic skin ulcer risk index in systemic sclerosis: a multicentre validation study. Ann Rheum Dis. 2012;71(1):67–70.
10. Masi AT, Rodnan GP, Medsger TA Jr, Altman RD, D'Angelo WA, Fries JF, et al. Preliminary criteria for the classification of systemic sclerosis (scleroderma). Subcommittee for scleroderma criteria of the American Rheumatism Association Diagnostic and Therapeutic Criteria Committee. Arthritis Rheum. 1980;23(5):581–90.
11. Cicchetti DV, D V. Guidelines, criteria, and rules of thumb for evaluating normed and standardized assessment instruments in psychology. Psychol Assess. 1994;6(4):284–90.
12. Landis JR, Koch GG. The measurement of observer agreement for categorical data. Biometrics. 1977;33(1):159–74.
13. Sebastiani M, Manfredi A, Cassone G, Giuggioli D, Ghizzoni C, Ferri C. Measuring microangiopathy abnormalities in systemic sclerosis patients: the role of capillaroscopy-based scoring models. Am J Med Sci. 2014;348(4): 331–6.
14. Pavan TR, Bredemeier M, Hax V, Capobianco KG, da Silva Mendonça Chakr R, Xavier RM. Capillary loss on nailfold capillary microscopy is associated with mortality in systemic sclerosis. Clin Rheumatol. 2018;37(2):475–81.
15. Ruaro B, Sulli A, Alessandri E, Pizzorni C, Ferrari G, Cutolo M, et al. Laser speckle contrast analysis: a new method to evaluate peripheral blood perfusion in systemic sclerosis patients. Ann Rheum Dis. 2014;73(6):1181–5.
16. Lüders S, Friedrich S, Ohrndorf S, Glimm A-M, Burmester G-R, Riemekasten G, et al. Detection of severe digital vasculopathy in systemic sclerosis by colour Doppler sonography is associated with digital ulcers. Rheumatology. 2017;56(11):1865–73.
17. Sebastiani M, Cestelli V, Manfredi A, Praino E, Cannarile F, Spinella A, et al. SAT0621 Validation Study of Predictive Value of Capillaroscopic Skin Ulcer Risk Index (CSURI) in Scleroderma Patients Treated with Bosentan. Ann Rheum Dis. 2015;74(Suppl 2):886.1–886.

# Quantitative videocapillaroscopy correlates with functional respiratory parameters: a clue for vasculopathy as a pathogenic mechanism for lung injury in systemic sclerosis

Alfredo Guillén-Del-Castillo[1], Carmen Pilar Simeón-Aznar[1*], Eduardo L. Callejas-Moraga[2], Carles Tolosa-Vilella[2], Serafín Alonso-Vila[1], Vicente Fonollosa-Pla[1] and Albert Selva-O'Callaghan[1]

## Abstract

**Background:** To determine whether lung involvement is related to microvascular perturbations, nailfold videocapillaroscopy (NVC) was performed in patients with systemic sclerosis (SSc).

**Methods:** A cross-sectional study was consecutively accomplished in 152 SSc patients. NVC, a pulmonary function test and echocardiography were undergone within a 3-month period. Finally, 134 patients with at least eight NVC (200× magnification) images were selected for quantitative and qualitative examinations.

**Results:** Patients with interstitial lung disease presented lower median capillary density (4.86/mm vs 5.88/mm, $p = 0.005$) and higher median of neoangiogenesis (0.56/mm vs 0.31/mm, $p = 0.005$). A higher quantity of neoangiogenesis capillaries was found in patients with pulmonary arterial hypertension (0.70/mm vs 0.33/mm, $p = 0.008$). Multivariate linear regression analysis established a correlation between neoangiogenesis and decreased forced vital capacity (FVC) ($p < 0.001$): for each capillary with neoangiogenesis visualized on average per 1 mm, FVC was 7.3% reduced. In qualitative NVC, a late pattern as defined by Cutolo was also associated with lower FVC ($p = 0.018$). The number of giant capillaries was associated with reduced diffusion capacity of the lung for carbon monoxide (DLCO) ($p = 0.016$); for each giant capillary per 1 mm, DLCO was 11.8% diminished.

**Conclusions:** A good correlation was observed between distinctive quantitative and qualitative NVC features with lung functional parameters such as FVC and DLCO. It is suggested that vasculopathy could play a role in SSc lung involvement.

**Keywords:** Interstitial lung disease, Nailfold videocapillaroscopy, Pulmonary hypertension, Scleroderma, Systemic sclerosis

## Background

Systemic sclerosis (SSc) is a connective tissue disease characterized by microvascular damage. It seems that endothelial activation induces the release of inflammatory mediators, platelet activation and inflammatory cell recruitment [1–3]. Subsequently, intimal and smooth muscle vessel wall proliferation ensues, causing luminal obstruction and activation of myofibroblasts that results in architectural alterations due to an excessive extracellular matrix deposition, reduction in the number of capillaries, tissue hypoxia and dysfunction of vascular regeneration [4].

The lung is one of the most frequently jeopardized organs in SSc; thus interstitial lung disease (ILD) affects around 55–65% of patients subjected to high-resolution computed tomography (HRCT) [5, 6], and pulmonary arterial hypertension (PAH) diagnosed by right heart catheterization (RHC) involves approximately 10% of this population [7, 8]. As a result of its high prevalence

* Correspondence: cpsimeon@vhebron.net
[1]Department of Systemic Autoimmune Diseases, Hospital Universitari Vall d'Hebron, Universitat Autònoma de Barcelona, Passeig Vall d'Hebron 119–129, 08035 Barcelona, Spain
Full list of author information is available at the end of the article

and poor prognosis, pulmonary involvement is nowadays the major cause of SSc-related deaths [9–11]. An exhaustive study of the relation between capillaroscopy features and lung manifestations would facilitate comprehension of the pulmonary pathophysiology.

Capillary microscopy was initially used as a qualitative technique to describe microvascular abnormalities in SSc and other autoimmune-related diseases. Maricq et al. [12] defined the scleroderma pattern as a group of capillaroscopy findings with potential diagnostic value in this disease. Later, these were detailed into active and slow capillaroscopy patterns [13]. More recently, using nailfold videocapillaroscopy (NVC), Cutolo et al. [14] defined a new classification of qualitative capillaroscopy abnormalities into early, active and late scleroderma patterns. The late pattern was related to lower levels of circulating endothelial progenitor cells and higher vascular endothelial growth factor (VEGF), demonstrating that an impairment of vasculogenesis mediates the loss of capillaries [15]. Recently, a sequential quantitative NVC study relating the presence of new incident capillaroscopy features to disease progression has been reported [16]. Nevertheless, no prior studies were focused on extensive quantitative NVC analysis and its correlation with objective lung parameters.

The hypothesis of the present study was that microcirculation damage leads the pathogenesis of the main manifestations in SSc such as ILD and PAH. The main aim of the work was to analyse NVC alterations using a quantitative method and to investigate their correlation with the pulmonary function test (PFT).

## Methods
### Patients
A cross-sectional study was carried out on SSc patients from the Vall d'Hebron Hospital cohort. All patients fulfilled LeRoy et al.'s SSc classification criteria [17], and accomplishment of the 2013 ACR/EULAR classification criteria was also assessed [18]. The study was approved by the Ethics Committee for Clinical Research (PG(AG)4/2015), and all patients provided written informed consent for their participation. NVC was consecutively conducted in 152 patients over a 12-month period. PFTs and echocardiography were performed within a 3-month period. Thirteen patients were excluded with fewer than eight explored nailfold fields, and another five patients for being lung transplant recipients. Finally, 134 SSc patients were selected for the analyses. The disease onset was described as the date of first symptom attributable to SSc including Raynaud's phenomenon (RP). All clinical or parameter data were collected at the time of NVC. Study quality was assessed by the Strengthening the Reporting of Observational Studies in Epidemiology (STROBE) checklist for cross-sectional studies [19].

### Clinical manifestations
Cutaneous subsets were defined as previously [20], according to the extent of skin thickening: limited cutaneous SSc (lcSSc), if skin sclerosis was distal to the elbows and knees or the face; diffuse cutaneous SSc (dcSSc), if skin sclerosis was extended proximally to the elbows or knees; and sine scleroderma SSc (ssSSc), if there was no skin involvement. Manifestations collected included RP, telangiectasias, past or current digital ulcers (DU), calcinosis and past history of scleroderma renal crisis (SRC).

Interstitial lung disease was defined as radiologic evidence of interstitial findings on HRCT examined by an expert thorax radiologist [21]. PAH was defined as mean pulmonary arterial pressure (mPAP) ≥ 25 mmHg with pulmonary artery wedge pressure (PAWP) ≤ 15 mmHg, and pulmonary vascular resistance (PVR) > 3 Wood units in right heart catheterization (RHC) [22, 23]. Cardiac involvement was defined as past or current pericardial effusion, left ventricular ejection fraction (LVEF) < 50%, macrovascular or microvascular ischemic heart disease with no cardiovascular risk factor (CVRF), conduction abnormalities, diastolic dysfunction with no CVRF or mitral regurgitation with no CVRF [24].

Musculoskeletal disease included arthritis, tendon fiction rubs, joint contractures and myositis. Gastrointestinal SSc disease was established if any of the following were present: oesophageal dysmotility, gastric antral vascular ectasia, gastric or bowel dysmotility, intestinal bacterial overgrowth, intestinal pseudo-obstruction or anal sphincter dysfunction.

### Immunology features
Antinuclear antibodies (ANA) were evaluated by indirect immunofluorescence (IIF) assay using HEp-cell line 2. Anticentromere antibodies (ACA) were described by IIF, and anti-topoisomerase I antibodies were determined by enzyme-linked immunosorbent assay. A commercial line blot assay was performed to detect anticentromere proteins A and B, anti-RNA pol III and anti-PM/Scl antibodies (EUROLINE Systemic Sclerosis (Nucleoli) Profile (IgG), Euroimmun, Germany) according to the manufacturer's instructions.

### Pulmonary function test and echocardiography
Complete PFTs including the percentage of the predicted forced vital capacity (FVC) and the percentage of the predicted diffusion capacity of the lung for carbon monoxide (DLCO) were accomplished using MasterLab equipment (MasterLab, Jaegger, Germany), following the ATS/ERS recommendations [25]. Echocardiography was performed by an experienced echocardiographer using a

Vivid E9 system (General Electric Vingmed, Horten, Norway), according to the consensus guidelines [26]. Right ventricular systolic pressure (RVSP), tricuspid regurgitation velocity (TRV) and the presence of other echo pulmonary hypertension (PH) signs were measured. In order to avoid loss of data information about patients with no measurable TRV, the variable 'TRV ≥ 2.9 m/s or other echo PH signs' was created [23].

### Nailfold videocapillaroscopy

Nailfolds were examined using an Optilia Digital Videocapillaroscope (Optilia Instruments AB, Sollentuna, Sweden) with 200× lens magnification and an LED lamp by the same operator (AS-O) who was blinded to clinical patients' conditions. Each patient was acclimatized for at least 20 min at room temperature of 20–24 °C before the examination. NVC was conducted with a contact adapter and immersion oil dropper, studying the middle nailfold from the second to fifth fingers of both hands. Optipix Lite software (Optilia Instruments AB) was used for visualization of consecutive 1-mm-wide images of first-line capillaries. Two images were taken on each finger, although when a finger was not possible to evaluate additional pictures were taken on other fingers. Patients with fewer than eight images were excluded from the study. Quantitative and qualitative analyses of the images were performed blind to clinical data by investigator AS-O. Inter-observer reliability and intra-observer reliability were also explored with a calculated sample size of 45 patients. This sample was randomly selected and blindly assessed once by investigator AG-DC to calculate the inter-observer reproducibility. Afterwards, to estimate the intra-observer repeatability, a second round was independently performed by investigators AS-O and AG-DC with a minimal time interval of 2 weeks between both measurements.

Quantitative NVC was carried out according to previous definitions as follows: capillary density, number of capillaries measured in the distal row following the 90° method [27]; enlarged capillary, an increase in capillary diameter > 20 μm; giant capillary, a capillary dilatation > 50 μm; microhaemorrhage, distal haemosiderin deposits; tortuous, curled capillaries with no cross; and neoangiogenesis, branching, bizarre, bushy, disorganized, ramified or arborized capillaries (Fig. 1) [14, 28, 29].

The mean of each capillaroscopic feature was calculated from the sum of consecutive images for each digit. Subsequently, the average values from eight fingers were added together and divided by the number of studied digits. The resulting value indicated the number of this capillaroscopic feature adjusted by each millimetre of the nailfold.

Qualitative NVC analysis of images was performed following capillaroscopy patterns described by Cutolo et al. (normal, early, active and late) [14].

### Statistical analysis

For the descriptive statistics, qualitative data were expressed as the mean and standard deviation (SD) after approving the normal distribution test; and non-normal qualitative variables were described as the median and interquartile range (IQR). Normal distribution was assessed using the Kolmogorov–Smirnov test. To assess whether there were statistically significant differences between groups of patients, the Mann–Whitney $U$ test was used. Bonferroni correction was applied in multiple comparisons. Associations between NVC and clinical features, PFTs and echocardiography variables were analysed using Spearman's correlation.

In order to analyse inter-observer and intra-observer reliability, a sample size of 45 patients was calculated, based on two observers (AS-O and AG-DC), with a power of 80% to detect that an intra-class coefficient (ICC) of 0.7 was significantly higher than 0.45 [30, 31]. The value of 0.45 was arbitrarily selected as the lowest acceptable limit of reliability. Quantitative NVC features were evaluated as the number per millimetre and determined by the ICC, whereas qualitative NVC features were assessed by Cohen's kappa coefficient. The measurement of observer agreement was defined as described in the literature: < 0.00 = poor; 0.00–0.20 = slight; 0.21–0.40 = fair; 0.41–0.60 = moderate; 0.61–0.80 = substantial; and 0.81–1.00 = almost perfect [32].

Multiple linear regression tests were performed to determine the association with FVC and DLCO. The multivariate models for FVC included NVC features, age at NVC, time elapsed from first symptom to NVC, dcSSc subset, gender, interstitial findings on HRCT, different autoantibodies and DU. For DLCO models, FVC, PAH confirmed by RHC, TRV ≥ 2.9 m/s or other echo PH signs also were introduced. $p < 0.05$ was considered significant. Statistical analysis was conducted with SPSS 20.0 for Windows (SPSS Inc., Chicago, IL, USA).

### Results

#### Population characteristics

Demographic characteristics of the 134 SSc patients are presented in Table 1. The participants were mainly female ($n = 113$, 84.3%) and in the lcSSc subset ($n = 88$, 65.7%). More than 90% of the population fulfilled the 2013 ACR/EULAR classification criteria. ACA were the most common antibodies in 49 (36.6%) patients, followed by anti-topoisomerase I antibodies in 31 (23.1%) patients. Considering major organ involvement, digestive involvement was present in 110 (82.1%) patients, cardiac disease in 103 (76.9%) patients, ILD in 58 (43.3%) patients, musculoskeletal involvement in 40 (29.9%) patients and PAH in 11 (8.2%) patients.

The distribution of different cardiac manifestations was 76.9% of patients presenting cardiac conduction

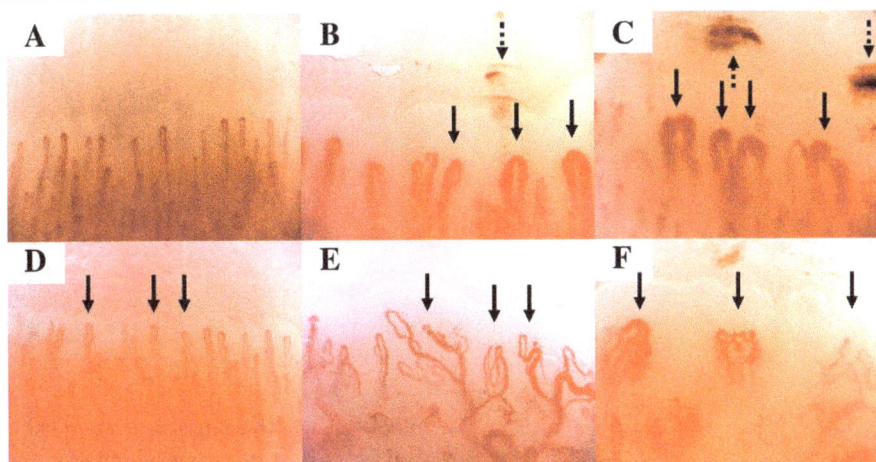

**Fig. 1** Quantitative nailfold videocapillaroscopy: **a** normal capillaries; **b** enlarged capillaries (solid arrows) and microhaemorrhage (dashed arrow); **c** giant capillaries (solid arrows) and microhaemorrhages (dashed arrows); **d** tortuous capillaries (solid arrows); **e** capillaries with neoangiogenesis as ramified capillaries (solid arrows); **f** capillaries with neoangiogenesis as disorganized capillaries (solid arrows)

**Table 1** Demographic, clinical and immunological characteristics of the patients with SSc (n = 134, 100%)

| Variable | Result |
|---|---|
| Age at SSc onset (years) | 38.5 (± 15.7) |
| Age at NVC (years) | 54.7 (± 14.4) |
| Cutaneous subsets, dcSSc/lcSSc/ssSSc | 28 (20.9)/88 (65.7)/18 (13.4) |
| Time elapsed from first symptom to NVC (years) | 16.0 (± 12.6) |
| Time elapsed from first non-RP symptom to NVC (years) | 10.9 (± 9.9) |
| 2013 ACR/EULAR SSc classification criteria fulfilment | 121 (90.2) |
| ACA/ATA/anti-RNA pol III/anti-PM/Scl | 49 (36.6)/31 (23.1)/14 (10.4)/11 (8.2) |
| Raynaud's phenomenon | 132 (98.5) |
| Telangiectasias | 97 (72.4) |
| Digital ulcers | 62 (46.3) |
| Calcinosis | 29 (21.6) |
| Scleroderma renal crisis | 2 (1.5) |
| Interstitial lung disease | 58 (43.3) |
| Pulmonary arterial hypertension | 11 (8.2) |
| Cardiac involvement | 103 (76.9) |
| Musculoskeletal disease | 40 (29.9) |
| Gastrointestinal involvement | 110 (82.1) |
| Overlap features | 19 (14.1) |

Data presented as mean (± standard deviation) for continuous variables and as number (%) for categorical variables

*SSc* systemic sclerosis, *NVC* nailfold videocapillaroscopy, *dcSSc* diffuse cutaneous systemic sclerosis, *lcSSc* limited cutaneous systemic sclerosis, *ssSSc* sine scleroderma systemic sclerosis, *RP* Raynaud's phenomenon, *ACR* American College of Rheumatology, *EULAR* European League Against Rheumatism, *ACA* anticentromere antibodies, *ATA* anti-topoisomerase I

abnormalities, 57.5% mitral regurgitation (with no CVRF), 47% diastolic dysfunction (with no CVRF), 13.4% pericardial effusion, 8.2% microvascular ischemic heart disease (with no CVRF), 3.7% LVEF < 50% and 3% of patients macrovascular ischemic heart disease (with no CVRF). Among all patients, there were 19 (14.1%) with overlap features as follows: nine (6.7%) patients had dermatomyositis, seven (5.2%) patients had Sjögren syndrome and the other three (2.2%) patients had rheumatoid arthritis.

### Pulmonary assessments

PFTs and echocardiography findings are presented in Table 2. The mean predicted FVC (± SD) was 80.8% (± 20.1), with a mean predicted DLCO of 66.2% (± 23.7). Regarding echocardiography, the TRV could be measured in 96 patients with a mean of 2.8 m/s (± 0.3), and no other signs of PH were found in the remaining 38 patients. Among 14 (10.4%) subjects with TRV higher than 2.9 m/s and/or with other echo PH signs, seven patients had been previously diagnosed with PAH by RHC. On the other hand, only 4 out of 120 patients with TRV lower than 2.9 m/s and no other echo PH signs had been formerly diagnosed with PAH by RHC.

### NVC characteristics

A total of 2186 images were analysed from 134 patients, with a mean of 16.3 (± 5.0) images per subject and the median (IQR) of images for each finger was 2 (1–3). The median (IQR) of capillary density adjusted by each millimetre of nailfold was 5.44/mm (4.33–6.74) (Table 3). NVC findings according to the presence of ILD were compared. Median capillary density in ILD patients was 4.86/mm, significantly lower than patients with no ILD whose density was 5.88/mm (p = 0.005). Moreover, the

**Table 2** Pulmonary function test and echocardiography within a 3-month period of nailfold videocapillaroscopy

| Variable | N | Result |
|---|---|---|
| Pulmonary function test | | |
|   FVC, % predicted | 134 | 80.8 (± 20.1) |
|   DLCO, % predicted | 134 | 66.2 (± 23.7) |
|   FVC%/DLCO% | 134 | 1.5 (± 0.4) |
| Echocardiography | | |
|   RVSP (mmHg) | 96 | 30.7 (± 12.0) |
|   TRV (m/s) | 96 | 2.8 (± 0.3) |
|   TRV ≥ 2.9 m/s or other echo PH signs | 134 | 14 (10.4) |

Data presented as mean (± standard deviation) for continuous variables and as number (%) for categorical variables
*FVC* forced vital capacity, *DLCO* diffusion capacity of the lung for carbon monoxide, *RVSP* right ventricular systolic pressure, *TRV* tricuspid regurgitation velocity, *PH* pulmonary hypertension

number of capillaries with neoangiogenesis was higher in ILD patients (0.56/mm vs 0.31/mm, $p = 0.005$). Focusing on PAH, patients with this manifestation also showed greater frequency of capillaries with neoangiogenesis compared with patients with no PAH (0.70/mm vs 0.33/mm, $p = 0.007$). All prior comparisons remained statistically significant after Bonferroni correction ($p < 0.008$).

Concerning qualitative NVC analysis, a late pattern (27.6%) was more prevalent in patients with ILD ($p = 0.006$). In addition, a late pattern showed lower FVC and DLCO values compared with normal, early and active patterns (Table 4).

### Clinical and NVC correlations

Age at NVC was inversely correlated with the number of enlarged capillaries ($\rho = -0.20$, $p = 0.01$) and the quantity of microhaemorrhages ($\rho = -0.25$, $p = 0.003$). The time elapsed from first symptom to NVC was negatively associated with the number of microhaemorrhages ($\rho = -0.25$, $p = 0.003$) and positively with the number of capillaries with neoangiogenesis ($\rho = 0.18$, $p = 0.03$). Higher capillary density was positively correlated with the % DLCO ($\rho = 0.26$, $p = 0.003$) and negatively with the RVSP ($\rho = -0.21$, $p = 0.03$). The number of capillaries with neoangiogenesis was inversely associated with % FVC ($\rho = -0.24$, $p = 0.004$) and % DLCO ($\rho = -0.26$, $p = 0.002$) and was positively associated with RVSP ($\rho = 0.20$, $p = 0.04$).

### Inter-observer and intra-observer reliability

The inter-observer reproducibility for all quantitative NVC features was almost perfect with an ICC higher than 0.80 (Table 5), except for the number of capillaries with neoangiogenesis which displayed a substantial reproducibility (95% CI) of 0.77 (0.58–0.88). Qualitative Cutolo's patterns also showed almost perfect reproducibility with Cohen's $\kappa$ of 0.83 (0.66–1.0), even when each pattern was analysed separately, with the only exception of an early pattern which had a substantial reproducibility with Cohen's $\kappa$ of 0.73 (0.42–1.0).

Regarding intra-observer repeatability, similar results were obtained for quantitative and qualitative variables, with an increment of neoangiogenesis repeatability up to 0.81 (0.56–0.90).

### Multivariate analysis

**Quantitative NVC studies** To elucidate which NVC findings were more strongly associated with pulmonary parameters, a multivariate analysis was conducted using

**Table 3** Nailfold videocapillaroscopy characteristics and comparisons between groups of patients depending on pulmonary involvement

| | ILD comparisons | | p value | PAH comparisons | | p value |
|---|---|---|---|---|---|---|
| | ILD (n = 58) | No ILD (n = 76) | | PAH (n = 11) | No PAH (n = 123) | |
| Quantitative NVC features | | | | | | |
| Capillary density (n) [a] | 4.86 (4.14–5.80) | 5.88 (4.74–6.85) | 0.005* | 5.47 (5.00–5.83) | 5.42 (4.31–6.74) | 0.997 |
| Enlarged capillaries (n) [a] | 0.84 (0.31–1.53) | 0.85 (0.39–1.58) | 0.738 | 0.56 (0.25–0.93) | 0.91 (0.40–1.61) | 0.128 |
| Giant capillaries (n) [a] | 0.26 (0.00–0.64) | 0.30 (0.04–1.07) | 0.362 | 0.06 (0.00–0.40) | 0.29 (0.03–1.02) | 0.167 |
| Microhaemorrhages (n) [a] | 0.12 (0.00–0.38) | 0.13 (0.00–0.42) | 0.735 | 0.06 (0.00–0.22) | 0.14 (0.00–0.40) | 0.101 |
| Tortuous capillaries (n) [a] | 0.45 (0.19–1.31) | 0.72 (0.28–1.49) | 0.216 | 0.63 (0.25–1.71) | 0.59 (0.23–1.43) | 0.773 |
| Neoangiogenesis (n) [a] | 0.56 (0.23–1.28) | 0.31 (0.12–0.62) | 0.005* | 0.70 (0.47–1.80) | 0.33 (0.12–0.78) | 0.007* |
| Qualitative NVC features | | | | | | |
| Cutolo's pattern, early/active/late | 8 (13.8)/23 (39.7)/23 (39.7) | 15 (19.7)/36 (47.4)/14 (18.4) | 0.366/0.373/0.006* | 1 (9.1)/4 (36.4)/6 (54.5) | 21 (17.9)/52 (44.4)/29 (24.8) | 0.688/0.755/0.069 |

Data presented as median (interquartile range) for continuous variables and as number (%) for categorical variables
*ILD* interstitial lung disease, *PAH* pulmonary arterial hypertension, *NVC* nailfold videocapillaroscopy
[a]Adjusted by each millimetre of the nailfold
*Statistically significant comparison after Bonferroni correction ($p < 0.008$)

**Table 4** Association between qualitative nailfold videocapillaroscopy and pulmonary function tests

|  | Cutolo's pattern | | | | |
|---|---|---|---|---|---|
|  | Normal (n = 15) | Early (n = 23) | Active (n = 59) | Late (n = 37) | p value |
| FVC, % predicted | 89.1 (± 20.3) | 82.3 (± 17.2) | 85.3 (± 18.3) | 69.6 (± 20.7)*,** | 0.001 |
| DLCO, % predicted | 77.3 (± 20.8) | 71.4 (± 27.5) | 68.6 (± 20.4) | 54.2 (± 23.3)*,†,‡ | 0.002 |

Data presented as mean (± standard deviation) for continuous variables
FVC forced vital capacity, DLCO diffusion capacity of the lung for carbon monoxide
*$p < 0.01$, late versus normal
**$p = 0.001$, late versus active
†$p < 0.05$, late versus early
‡$p < 0.05$, late versus active

% FVC as a dependent variable. Table 6 presents variables with statistical significance or a tendency to be significant. The number of capillaries with neoangiogenesis in NVC, male gender and ILD on HRCT were associated with a lower % FVC, whereas ACA positivity was identified as a protective factor. The analysis estimated that for each capillary with neoangiogenesis visualized on average per 1-mm nailfold, the FVC would be reduced 7.3%.

A lower % DLCO value was associated with a reduced number of enlarged capillaries and an increased number of giant capillaries, along with ILD on HRCT, lower % FVC, PAH confirmed by RHC, TRV ≥ 2.9 m/s or other echo PH signs on echocardiography. In this way, for each enlarged capillary on average per 1 mm the DLCO would be 7.8% higher; however, for each giant capillary it would be diminished 11.8%.

**Qualitative NVC studies** Multivariate analysis showed an association between late pattern and lower % FVC values. FVC would be diminished 14.3% in a patient with late NVC pattern features (Table 7). None of the NVC patterns were related to DLCO values.

**Table 5** Inter-observer and intra-observer reliability

|  | Inter-observer (95% CI) | Intra-observer (95% CI) |
|---|---|---|
| ICC for quantitative NVC features | | |
| Capillary density | 0.96 (0.93–0.98) | 0.97 (0.93–0.98) |
| Enlarged capillaries | 0.87 (0.77–0.93) | 0.93 (0.83–0.97) |
| Giant capillaries | 0.91 (0.83–0.95) | 0.95 (0.90–0.97) |
| Microhaemorrhages | 0.97 (0.94–0.98) | 0.99 (0.98–0.99) |
| Tortuous capillaries | 0.92 (0.85–0.95) | 0.91 (0.69–0.96) |
| Neoangiogenesis | 0.77 (0.58–0.88) | 0.81 (0.56–0.90) |
| Cohen's κ coefficient for qualitative NVC features | | |
| Cutolo's patterns | 0.83 (0.66–1.0) | 0.81 (0.64–0.97) |
| Normal pattern | 0.92 (0.75–1.0) | 0.83 (0.55–1.0) |
| Early pattern | 0.73 (0.42–1.0) | 0.66 (0.33–0.99) |
| Active pattern | 0.82 (0.65–0.99) | 0.87 (0.71–1.0) |
| Late pattern | 0.87 (0.69–1.0) | 0.81 (0.59–10) |

CI confidence interval, ICC intra-class coefficient, NVC nailfold videocapillaroscopy

## Discussion

This cross-sectional study in an SSc population indicated that the presence of capillaries with neoangiogenesis in NVC was related to lower percentage FVC values independently of other baseline characteristics. According to our results, a patient with one capillary with neoangiogenesis per millimetre on average in NVC would have 7.3% lower FVC percentage regardless of other clinical or capillaroscopic conditions. Concerning qualitative NVC assessments, a late pattern was also associated with lower FVC. We also found a substantial or almost perfect inter-observer and intra-observer reliability of all NVC features.

The median capillary density was similar to that reported previously, but our study included a higher significant number of evaluated images per patient [33, 34]. Prior publications have mainly focused on qualitative NVC, finding correlations between NVC patterns and different variables such as ILD, FVC, DLCO, RVSP, DU

**Table 6** Multiple regression analysis according to quantitative nailfold videocapillaroscopy

|  | B | 95% CI | p value |
|---|---|---|---|
| FVC as dependent variable | | | |
| Male gender | −11.0 | −19.2 to −2.9 | 0.008 |
| Interstitial findings on HRCT | −14.8 | −21.1 to −8.4 | < 0.001 |
| ACA positivity | 7.2 | 0.1 to 14.3 | 0.045 |
| Neoangiogenesis/mm | −7.3 | −11.0 to −3.6 | < 0.001 |
| DLCO as dependent variable | | | |
| Digital ulcers | −6.7 | −13.6 to 0.1 | 0.056 |
| Interstitial findings on HRCT | −9.4 | −16.4 to −2.5 | 0.008 |
| FVC | 0.5 | 0.3 to 0.7 | <0.001 |
| PAH confirmed by RHC | −14.3 | −26.9 to −1.6 | 0.027 |
| TRV ≥ 2.9 m/s or other echo PH signs | −16.4 | −28.3 to −4.6 | 0.007 |
| Enlarged capillaries | 7.8 | 1.1 to 14.4 | 0.021 |
| Giant capillaries | −11.8 | −21.4 to −2.2 | 0.016 |

Only variables with statistical significance or tendency to be significant are presented
B regression coefficient, CI confidence interval, FVC forced vital capacity, HRCT high resolution computed tomography, ACA anticentromere antibodies, DLCO diffusion capacity of the lung for carbon monoxide, PAH pulmonary arterial hypertension, RHC right heart catheterization, TRV tricuspid regurgitation velocity, PH pulmonary hypertension

**Table 7** Multiple regression analysis according to Cutolo's patterns

| | B | 95% CI | p value |
|---|---|---|---|
| FVC as dependent variable | | | |
| Male gender | −12.3 | −21.0 to −3.5 | 0.006 |
| Interstitial findings on HRCT | −13.5 | −20.2 to −6.7 | < 0.001 |
| ACA positivity | 8.6 | −0.1 to 17.4 | 0.051 |
| Cutolo's late pattern | −14.3 | −26.1 to −2.5 | 0.018 |
| DLCO as dependent variable | | | |
| Digital ulcers | −8.3 | −14.8 to −1.8 | 0.013 |
| Interstitial findings on HRCT | −9.8 | −16.8 to −2.8 | 0.006 |
| FVC | 0.5 | 0.3 to 0.7 | < 0.001 |
| PH confirmed by RHC | −14.1 | −26.8 to −1.5 | 0.028 |
| TRV ≥ 2.9 m/s or other echo PH signs | − 14.9 | −26.8 to −3.0 | 0.014 |

Only variables with statistical significance or tendency to be significant are presented

B regression coefficient, CI confidence interval, FVC forced vital capacity, HRCT high resolution computed tomography, ACA anticentromere antibodies, DLCO diffusion capacity of the lung for carbon monoxide, PAH pulmonary arterial hypertension, PH pulmonary hypertension, RHC right heart catheterization, TRV tricuspid regurgitation velocity

or even risk of developing new DU [35–38]. On the other hand, quantitative NVC studies proposed capillaroscopic prognostic tools for the development of new DU or even the progression to SSc [34, 39–41]. We achieved equal or superior intra-observer and inter-observer reliability to previous quantitative NVC studies [27], probably because our work compared the mean of NVC features analysing all images of each patient instead of a single image per patient, which reflects real-life capillaroscopy more. Moreover, qualitative NVC features as Cutolo's patterns were assessed with almost perfect reliability. However, few research projects have concentrated on extensive quantitative analysis and its correlation with clinical variables, specifically with lung parameters.

We found that SSc patients with ILD had a lower capillary density and a higher number of capillaries with neoangiogenesis. These findings support the prior semi-quantitative NVC study, which identified higher mean avascular scores in patients with ground-glass opacities [42]. Similarly, Castellvi et al. [43] described an association between low capillary density defined as < 7 capillaries/mm and lower FVC and DLCO percentages using a semi-quantitative NVC. Smith et al. [37] also found a strong association between NVC patterns and future severe lung involvement at 18–24 months, defined as a punctuation ≥ 2 in lung evaluation on the Medsger severity scale. Nevertheless, the risk of severe ILD or PH was not specified separately [37, 44].

Recently, Avouac et al. [16] published a sequential quantitative NVC study with multivariate Cox analysis revealing that an incident or increased number of giant

capillaries during the follow-up was protective of new DU. Progressive loss of capillaries from baseline predicted overall disease progression, new DU, lung vascular progression defined as new onset of precapillary PH on RHC, skin fibrosis and worsening in the Medsger severity score. Baseline angiogenesis predicted only lung vascular progression. The present study performs a multivariate analysis including clinical, immunological and quantitative/qualitative NVC findings for the investigation of lung parameters at baseline conditions. We identified that the number of capillaries with neoangiogenesis, male gender and the presence of ILD on HRCT were factors independently associated with lower FVC values, while ACA positivity was found to be a protector, which supports Avouac et al.'s work.

Furthermore, regarding qualitative NVC studies, the progression from normal/early/active to a late pattern was related to the development of new DU, lung vascular progression, progression of skin fibrosis and worsening on the Medsger severity scale [16]. According to these findings, the greatest destructive NVC features, as the late pattern, were associated with lower FVC values.

Consequently, it appears that endothelial damage mediates both lung fibrosis and peripheral microvascular changes visualised in NVC. SSc patients with more extensive ILD may also show higher nailfold capillary perturbations, ineffective angiogenesis and vasculogenesis, which reflects a higher frequency of bushy or bizarre capillaries which are denominated as neoangiogenesis [45]. In fact, ILD has already been linked in a multivariate analysis with peripheral vasculopathy in the form of prior/current DU [20].

Recently, a qualitative NVC study has noted the predictive role of NVC and specific autoantibodies in cardiopulmonary involvement [35]. Specifically, active and late NVC patterns were associated with ILD, DLCO < 70% of predicted, reduced maximum oxygen uptake, higher NT pro-BNP and increased systolic pulmonary artery pressure values. However, PH was estimated by indirect measurements and was not confirmed by RHC. In our cohort, the prevalence of PAH confirmed by RHC was 8.2%, similar to previous reports [7, 8]. Surprisingly, we found enlarged capillaries being associated with higher % DLCO values, and giant capillaries were independently correlated with lower DLCO percentage. These findings contrast with a prior publication where new giant or increased giant capillaries during follow-up tended to be protective of lung vascular progression or overall disease progression [16]. This paradoxical association between enlarged capillaries and higher DLCO values could be explained as an adaptive phenomenon. When enlarged capillaries turn into giant capillaries, which means a failure in microvascular adaptation and consequently a severe capillary dysfunction, an impairment of DLCO values occurs. The formation of extremely large capillaries may contribute to gas exchange disturbance in all tissues including the lung, which might result in DLCO decline.

Hofstee et al. [46] found that capillary density was inversely correlated with the mPAP in both SSc-PAH and idiopathic PAH patients. Interestingly, Riccieri et al. [47] demonstrated the existence of greater avascular areas and severe active/late NVC patterns in a group of 12 SSc-PAH patients, and that higher NVC scores and avascular areas scores were correlated with mPAP. Corrado et al. [48] observed capillaroscopic abnormalities in 38.1% of idiopathic PAH patients, with lower capillary density and higher loop width compared to healthy subjects. Furthermore, the authors confirmed a reduced capillary density, and an increased mean capillary width and mean number of capillaries with neoangiogenesis in SSc-PAH patients compared to SSc patients without PAH evidence. Although we also identified a negative correlation of higher capillary density and number of neoangiogenesis capillaries with RVSP values, we did not found an association between those NVC features and PAH defined by RHC in the multivariate analysis, which may be due to the small group of PAH patients.

Limitations of this study included the cross-sectional study, with no follow-up data, which did not allow us to infer whether capillaroscopic findings were linked to a specific outcome of pulmonary disease. However, although an association was observed between microvascular features and functional respiratory parameters, this fact does not prove a causal relationship between them. We cannot exclude that both phenomena would be influenced by an unknown parameter that may lead a parallel change in the first two. Notwithstanding, the present study also had strengths, because all patients had undergone echocardiography and PFTs close to the NVC examination. The images were analysed blind of clinical data by the researchers. For the statistical analysis, patients were excluded with fewer than eight explored fields, either due to technical difficulties or digital amputations. NVC explorations after autologous stem cell transplantation had demonstrated an improvement in vascular damage [49]. Consequently, five lung transplant patients under high immunosuppressive treatment were additionally removed from the study.

## Conclusions

This study describes a lower capillary density and a higher number of capillaries with neoangiogenesis in patients with ILD, and demonstrates a quantitative and qualitative relation between specific NVC abnormalities and lung function tests (both % FVC and % DLCO parameters). It seems that NVC findings are linked to a wide spectrum of clinical variables in SSc, which emphasizes the crucial role of microcirculation damage in this medical condition, especially within the lung.

## Abbreviations
ACA: Anticentromere antibodies; ANA: Antinuclear antibodies; CI: Confidence interval; CVRF: Cardiovascular risk factor; dcSSc: Diffuse cutaneous SSc; DLCO: Diffusion capacity of the lung for carbon monoxide; DU: Digital ulcers; FVC: Forced vital capacity; HRCT: High-resolution computed tomography; ICC: Intra-class coefficient; IIF: Indirect immunofluorescence; ILD: Interstitial lung disease; IQR: Interquartile range; lcSSc: Limited cutaneous SSc; LVEF: Left ventricular ejection fraction; mPAP: Mean pulmonary arterial pressure; NVC: Nailfold videocapillaroscopy; PAH: Pulmonary arterial hypertension; PAWP: Pulmonary artery wedge pressure; PFT: Pulmonary function test; PH: Pulmonary hypertension; PVR: Pulmonary vascular resistance; RHC: Right heart catheterization; RP: Raynaud's phenomenon; RVSP: Right ventricular systolic pressure; SD: Standard deviation; SRC: Scleroderma renal crisis; SSc: Systemic sclerosis; sSSc: Sine scleroderma SSc; STROBE: Strengthening the Reporting of Observational Studies in Epidemiology; TRV: Tricuspid regurgitation velocity; VEGF: Vascular endothelial growth factor

## Acknowledgements
Not applicable.

## Funding
This work was supported by the Instituto de Salud Carlos III and the European Regional Development Fund (ERDF) (grant numbers PI15/02100 and PI16/02088).

## Authors' contributions
AG-DC made substantial contributions to study conception and design, as well as acquisition, analysis and interpretation of data, drafting the article and approval of the final manuscript. CPS-A made substantial contributions to study conception and design, analysis and interpretation of data, revising the manuscript critically for important intellectual content and approval of the final manuscript. ELC-M, CT-V, SA-V and VF-P made substantial contributions to study conception and design, revising the manuscript critically for important intellectual content and approval of the final manuscript. AS-O made substantial contributions to study conception and design, acquisition, analysis and interpretation of data, revising the manuscript critically for important intellectual content and approval of the final manuscript. AG-DC and CPS-A had full access to all of the data in the study and both take responsibility for the integrity and accuracy of the data. Funders had no access to the data and were not involved in study design, acquisition, analysis and interpretation of data or writing the manuscript.

## Competing interests
The authors declare that they have no competing interests.

## Author details
[1]Department of Systemic Autoimmune Diseases, Hospital Universitari Vall d'Hebron, Universitat Autònoma de Barcelona, Passeig Vall d'Hebron 119–129, 08035 Barcelona, Spain. [2]Department of Internal Medicine, Corporació Sanitària Universitària Parc Taulí, Universitat Autònoma de Barcelona, Sabadell, Barcelona, Spain.

## References
1. Denton CP, Ong VH. Targeted therapies for systemic sclerosis. Nat Rev Rheumatol. 2013;9:451–64.
2. Allanore Y, Simms R, Distler O, Trojanowska M, Pope J, Denton CP, et al. Systemic sclerosis. Nat Rev Dis Primers. 2015;1:15002.
3. Denton CP, Khanna D. Systemic sclerosis. Lancet. 2017;390:1685–99.
4. Bhattacharyya S, Wei J, Varga J. Understanding fibrosis in systemic sclerosis: shifting paradigms, emerging opportunities. Nat Rev Rheumatol. 2011;8:42–54.
5. Launay D, Remy-Jardin M, Michon-Pasturel U, Mastora I, Hachulla E, Lambert M, et al. High resolution computed tomography in fibrosing alveolitis associated with systemic sclerosis. J Rheumatol. 2006;33:1789–801.

6.  De Santis M, Bosello S, La Torre G, Capuano A, Tolusso B, Pagliari G, et al. Functional, radiological and biological markers of alveolitis and infections of the lower respiratory tract in patients with systemic sclerosis. Respir Res. 2005;6:96.

7.  Mukerjee D, St George D, Coleiro B, Knight C, Denton CP, Davar J, et al. Prevalence and outcome in systemic sclerosis associated pulmonary arterial hypertension: application of a registry approach. Ann Rheum Dis. 2003;62:1088–93.

8.  Avouac J, Airo P, Meune C, Beretta L, Dieude P, Caramaschi P, et al. Prevalence of pulmonary hypertension in systemic sclerosis in European Caucasians and metaanalysis of 5 studies. J Rheumatol. 2010;37:2290–8.

9.  Steen VD, Medsger TA. Changes in causes of death in systemic sclerosis, 1972-2002. Ann Rheum Dis. 2007;66:940–4.

10. Nihtyanova SI, Schreiber BE, Ong VH, Rosenberg D, Moinzadeh P, Coghlan JG, et al. Prediction of pulmonary complications and long-term survival in systemic sclerosis. Arthritis Rheumatol. 2014;66:1625–35.

11. Simeon-Aznar CP, Fonollosa-Pla V, Tolosa-Vilella C, Espinosa-Garriga G, Campillo-Grau M, Ramos-Casals M, et al. Registry of the Spanish Network for Systemic Sclerosis: Survival, Prognostic Factors, and Causes of Death. Medicine (Baltimore). 2015;94:e1728.

12. Maricq HR, LeRoy EC, D'Angelo WA, Medsger TA Jr, Rodnan GP, Sharp GC, et al. Diagnostic potential of in vivo capillary microscopy in scleroderma and related disorders. Arthritis Rheum. 1980;23:183–9.

13. Maricq HR, Harper FE, Khan MM, Tan EM, LeRoy EC. Microvascular abnormalities as possible predictors of disease subsets in Raynaud phenomenon and early connective tissue disease. Clin Exp Rheumatol. 1983;1:195–205.

14. Cutolo M, Sulli A, Pizzorni C, Accardo S. Nailfold videocapillaroscopy assessment of microvascular damage in systemic sclerosis. J Rheumatol. 2000;27:155–60.

15. Avouac J, Vallucci M, Smith V, Senet P, Ruiz B, Sulli A, et al. Correlations between angiogenic factors and capillaroscopic patterns in systemic sclerosis. Arthritis Res Ther. 2013;15:R55.

16. Avouac J, Lepri G, Smith V, Toniolo E, Hurabielle C, Vallet A, et al. Sequential nailfold videocapillaroscopy examinations have responsiveness to detect organ progression in systemic sclerosis. Semin Arthritis Rheum. 2017;47:86–94.

17. LeRoy EC, Black C, Fleischmajer R, Jablonska S, Krieg T, Medsger TA Jr, et al. Scleroderma (systemic sclerosis): classification, subsets and pathogenesis. J Rheumatol. 1988;15:202–5.

18. van den Hoogen F, Khanna D, Fransen J, Johnson SR, Baron M, Tyndall A, et al. 2013 classification criteria for systemic sclerosis: an American College of Rheumatology/European League Against Rheumatism collaborative initiative. Ann Rheum Dis. 2013;72:1747–55.

19. von Elm E, Altman DG, Egger M, Pocock SJ, Gotzsche PC, Vandenbroucke JP, et al. The Strengthening the Reporting of Observational Studies in Epidemiology (STROBE) statement: guidelines for reporting observational studies. Epidemiology. 2007;18:800–4.

20. Tolosa-Vilella C, Morera-Morales ML, Simeon-Aznar CP, Mari-Alfonso B, Colunga-Arguelles D, Callejas Rubio JL, et al. Digital ulcers and cutaneous subsets of systemic sclerosis: clinical, immunological, nailfold capillaroscopy, and survival differences in the Spanish RESCLE Registry. Semin Arthritis Rheum. 2016;46:200–8.

21. Morales-Cardenas A, Perez-Madrid C, Arias L, Ojeda P, Mahecha MP, Rojas-Villarraga A, et al. Pulmonary involvement in systemic sclerosis. Autoimmun Rev. 2016;15:1094–108.

22. Coghlan JG, Denton CP, Grunig E, Bonderman D, Distler O, Khanna D, et al. Evidence-based detection of pulmonary arterial hypertension in systemic sclerosis: the DETECT study. Ann Rheum Dis. 2014;73:1340–9.

23. Galie N, Humbert M, Vachiery JL, Gibbs S, Lang I, Torbicki A, et al. 2015 ESC/ERS Guidelines for the diagnosis and treatment of pulmonary hypertension: The Joint Task Force for the Diagnosis and Treatment of Pulmonary Hypertension of the European Society of Cardiology (ESC) and the European Respiratory Society (ERS): Endorsed by: Association for European Paediatric and Congenital Cardiology (AEPC), International Society for Heart and Lung Transplantation (ISHLT). Eur Heart J. 2016;37:67–119.

24. Fernandez-Codina A, Simeon-Aznar CP, Pinal-Fernandez I, Rodriguez-Palomares J, Pizzi MN, Hidalgo CE, et al. Cardiac involvement in systemic sclerosis: differences between clinical subsets and influence on survival. Rheumatol Int. 2017;37:75–84. https://doi.org/10.1007/s00296-015-3382-2.

25. Miller MR, Crapo R, Hankinson J, Brusasco V, Burgos F, Casaburi R, et al. General considerations for lung function testing. Eur Respir J. 2005;26:153–61.

26. Lang RM, Badano LP, Mor-Avi V, Afilalo J, Armstrong A, Ernande L, et al. Recommendations for cardiac chamber quantification by echocardiography in adults: an update from the American Society of Echocardiography and the European Association of Cardiovascular Imaging. Eur Heart J Cardiovasc Imaging. 2015;16:233–70.

27. Hofstee HM, Serne EH, Roberts C, Hesselstrand R, Scheja A, Moore TL, et al. A multicentre study on the reliability of qualitative and quantitative nail-fold videocapillaroscopy assessment. Rheumatology (Oxford). 2012;51:749–55.

28. Sulli A, Secchi ME, Pizzorni C, Cutolo M. Scoring the nailfold microvascular changes during the capillaroscopic analysis in systemic sclerosis patients. Ann Rheum Dis. 2008;67:885–7.

29. Maricq HR. Wide-field capillary microscopy. Arthritis Rheum. 1981;24:1159–65.

30. Donner A, Eliasziw M. Sample size requirements for reliability studies. Stat Med. 1987;6:441–8.

31. Walter SD, Eliasziw M, Donner A. Sample size and optimal designs for reliability studies. Stat Med. 1998;17:101–10.

32. Landis JR, Koch GG. The measurement of observer agreement for categorical data. Biometrics. 1977;33:159–74.

33. Morardet L, Avouac J, Sammour M, Baron M, Kahan A, Feydy A, et al. Late nailfold videocapillaroscopy pattern associated with hand calcinosis and acro-osteolysis in systemic sclerosis. Arthritis Care Res (Hoboken). 2016;68:366–73.

34. Cutolo M, Herrick AL, Distler O, Becker MO, Beltran E, Carpentier P, et al. Nailfold videocapillaroscopic features and other clinical risk factors for digital ulcers in systemic sclerosis: a multicenter, prospective cohort study. Arthritis Rheumatol. 2016;68:2527–39.

35. Markusse IM, Meijs J, de Boer B, Bakker JA, Schippers HP, Schouffoer AA, et al. Predicting cardiopulmonary involvement in patients with systemic sclerosis: complementary value of nailfold videocapillaroscopy patterns and disease-specific autoantibodies. Rheumatology (Oxford). 2017;56:1081–88. https://doi.org/10.1093/rheumatology/kew402.

36. Caramaschi P, Canestrini S, Martinelli N, Volpe A, Pieropan S, Ferrari M, et al. Scleroderma patients nailfold videocapillaroscopic patterns are associated with disease subset and disease severity. Rheumatology (Oxford). 2007;46:1566–9.

37. Smith V, Decuman S, Sulli A, Bonroy C, Piettte Y, Deschepper E, et al. Do worsening scleroderma capillaroscopic patterns predict future severe organ involvement? A pilot study. Ann Rheum Dis. 2012;71:1636–9.

38. Silva I, Teixeira A, Oliveira J, Almeida I, Almeida R, Aguas A, et al. Endothelial dysfunction and nailfold videocapillaroscopy pattern as predictors of digital ulcers in systemic sclerosis: a cohort study and review of the literature. Clin Rev Allergy Immunol. 2015;49:240–52.

39. Sebastiani M, Manfredi A, Colaci M, D'Amico R, Malagoli V, Giuggioli D, et al. Capillaroscopic skin ulcer risk index: a new prognostic tool for digital skin ulcer development in systemic sclerosis patients. Arthritis Rheum. 2009;61:688–94.

40. Sebastiani M, Manfredi A, Vukatana G, Moscatelli S, Riato L, Bocci M, et al. Predictive role of capillaroscopic skin ulcer risk index in systemic sclerosis: a multicentre validation study. Ann Rheum Dis. 2012;71:67–70.

41. Trombetta AC, Smith V, Pizzorni C, Meroni M, Paolino S, Cariti C, et al. Quantitative alterations of capillary diameter have a predictive value for development of the capillaroscopic systemic sclerosis pattern. J Rheumatol. 2016;43:599–606.

42. Bredemeier M, Xavier RM, Capobianco KG, Restelli VG, Rohde LE, Pinotti AF, et al. Nailfold capillary microscopy can suggest pulmonary disease activity in systemic sclerosis. J Rheumatol. 2004;31:286–94.

43. Castellvi I, Simeon-Aznar CP, Sarmiento M, Fortuna A, Mayos M, Geli C, et al. Association between nailfold capillaroscopy findings and pulmonary function tests in patients with systemic sclerosis. J Rheumatol. 2015;42:222–7.

44. Medsger TA Jr, Bombardieri S, Czirjak L, Scorza R, Della Rossa A, Bencivelli W. Assessment of disease severity and prognosis. Clin Exp Rheumatol. 2003;21:S42–6.

45. Lambova SN, Muller-Ladner U. Capillaroscopic pattern in systemic sclerosis—an association with dynamics of processes of angio- and vasculogenesis. Microvasc Res. 2010;80:534–9.

# Characterization of the HLA-DRβ1 third hypervariable region amino acid sequence according to charge and parental inheritance in systemic sclerosis

Coline A. Gentil[1*], Hilary S. Gammill[1,2], Christine T. Luu[1], Maureen D. Mayes[3], Dan E. Furst[4] and J. Lee Nelson[1,5]

## Abstract

**Background:** Specific HLA class II alleles are associated with systemic sclerosis (SSc) risk, clinical characteristics, and autoantibodies. HLA nomenclature initially developed with antibodies as typing reagents defining DRB1 allele groups. However, alleles from different DRB1 allele groups encode the same third hypervariable region (3rd HVR) sequence, the primary T-cell recognition site, and 3rd HVR charge differences can affect interactions with T cells. We considered 3rd HVR sequences (amino acids 67–74) irrespective of the allele group and analyzed parental inheritance considered according to the 3rd HVR charge, comparing SSc patients with controls.

**Methods:** In total, 306 families (121 SSc and 185 controls) were HLA genotyped and parental HLA-haplotype origin was determined. Analysis was conducted according to DRβ1 3rd HVR sequence, charge, and parental inheritance.

**Results:** The distribution of 3rd HVR sequences differed in SSc patients versus controls ($p = 0.007$), primarily due to an increase of specific DRB1*11 alleles, in accord with previous observations. The 3rd HVR sequences were next analyzed according to charge and parental inheritance. Paternal transmission of DRB1 alleles encoding a +2 charge 3rd HVR was significantly reduced in SSc patients compared with maternal transmission ($p = 0.0003$, corrected for analysis of four charge categories $p = 0.001$). To a lesser extent, paternal transmission was increased when charge was 0 ($p = 0.021$, corrected for multiple comparisons $p = 0.084$). In contrast, paternal versus maternal inheritance was similar in controls.

**Conclusions:** SSc patients differed from controls when DRB1 alleles were categorized according to 3rd HVR sequences. Skewed parental inheritance was observed in SSc patients but not in controls when the DRβ1 3rd HVR was considered according to charge. These observations suggest that epigenetic modulation of HLA merits investigation in SSc.

**Keywords:** Systemic sclerosis, Human leukocyte antigen, Skewed parental inheritance

## Background

HLA class II genes contribute the largest portion of genetic risk for many autoimmune diseases including systemic sclerosis (SSc) [1]. The HLA DRB1 allele group DRB1*11 has been described consistently in association with SSc in Caucasian adults [1–3]. HLA nomenclature evolved utilizing serological typing reagents resulting in a "language of HLA", with initial groupings based primarily on antibody recognition of the HLA molecule.

However, the β1 chain of the HLA-DR molecule encoded by HLA-DRB1 is characterized by three regions of amino acid sequence hypervariability and the third hypervariable region (3rd HVR) is thought to be the most important site for T-cell recognition [4].

The 3rd HVR comprises amino acids 67–74 on the alpha helix of the HLA β1 chain. Allelic variation of the DRB1 DNA sequence can result in 3rd HVR amino acid sequences that differ for overall 3rd HVR charge and can impact the steric interaction between HLA molecules and T cells. The importance of charge in this region has been well demonstrated in rheumatoid arthritis, where different risk-associated DRβ1 molecules

---

\* Correspondence: cgentil@fredhutch.org
[1]Division of Clinical Research, Fred Hutchinson Cancer Research Center, 1100 Fairview Ave N, Seattle, WA 98109, USA
Full list of author information is available at the end of the article

carry 3rd HVR sequences with a positive charge, whereas a negatively charged 3rd HVR sequence is associated with protection from the disease [5, 6].

In the current study we investigated the DRβ1 3rd HVR, charge, and parental transmission in SSc patients and healthy controls. We sought to examine inheritance according to parental origin because biased HLA transmission has been described in some other autoimmune diseases, including multiple sclerosis, and in some but not all studies of type 1 diabetes [7–9]. The primary purpose of this study was to test the hypothesis that SSc risk is modulated according to whether the mother or the father transmitted an HLA-DRB1 allele and is impacted by DRβ1 3rd HVR charge.

## Methods
### Study participants
A total of 306 unrelated families were studied, 121 in which the proband had SSc and 185 healthy control families. SSc patients were recruited primarily from the Seattle, WA, USA area, with some patients from Alaska, Montana, Oregon and other states and some identified through the SSc family registry based in Houston, TX, USA. Healthy controls were recruited primarily from the Seattle, WA area. The median age at the time of sample collection for HLA genotyping for SSc patients was 43 years (range 18–62) and for controls was 31 years (range 4–73). SSc patients were female and controls were predominantly female (99 female, 22 male). All patients and controls were Caucasian. Study subjects were included providing maternal versus paternal transmission of HLA-DRB1 could be determined by HLA genotyping studies of the patient or control and family members. Eight SSc patients and one control were HLA genotyped but not included in the analysis because parental haplotype transmission could not be determined. All subjects provided written informed consent. The study was approved by the Institutional Review Board of Fred Hutchinson Cancer Research Center.

### HLA genotyping
HLA genotyping was conducted from peripheral blood, buccal swabs, or mouthwash specimens. Genomic DNA was extracted from whole blood or peripheral blood mononuclear cells using the Wizard Genomic DNA Purification Kit (Promega, Madison, WI, USA), from mouthwash specimens using the High Pure PCR Template Preparation Kit (Roche Diagnostics, Indianapolis, IN, USA), or from buccal swabs using the BuccalAmp DNA Extraction Kit (Epicentre Biotechnologies, WI, USA). All subjects were genotyped for HLA-DRB1, as well as for DQA1 and DQB1 loci. DNA-based typing was conducted with the Luminex-based PCR-sequence-specific oligonucleotide probe technique (Luminex; One

Lambda, Canoga Park, CA, USA) with alleles assigned using HLA Fusion™ 3.0 standard analysis software, or Dynal strip detection with sequence-specific oligonucleotide probes (Dynal RELITM SSO, UK) followed by identification of specific alleles by sequencing (Applied Biosystems, Foster city, CA, USA). Amino acid sequences were determined based on the specific alleles and the International Immunogenetics Information System for HLA (IGMT/HLA; www.ebi.ac.uk/ipd/imgt/hla/allele.html).

### HLA-DRβ1 3rd HVR classification
All DRB1 alleles were first categorized according to the encoded 3rd HVR amino acid sequence, from positions 67 through 74 of the HLA-DRβ1 chain (Table 1). Among all possible DRβ1 3rd HVR sequences, 17 were present in at least one study subject with eight sequences present in at least 5% of either patients or controls. Next, 3rd HVR sequences were grouped according to their overall charge: +2, +1, 0, −1, or −2.

In our patient and control populations no subject had a DRB1 allele encoding a 3rd HVR sequence with a −1 charge. Therefore, our study compares four charge groups between SSc and controls.

**Table 1** HLA-DRβ1 categorized according to 3rd HVR sequences, DRB1 alleles encoding each sequence, and associated charges

| 3rd HVR | aa 67–74 | DRB1 alleles | Charge |
|---|---|---|---|
| 1 | LLEQRRAA | 01:01, 01:02, 01:08, 04:04, 04:05, 04:08, 14:02, 14:06, 14:20 | +1 |
| 2 | I–DE— | 01:03, 04:02, 11:02, 13:01, 13:02, 13:04, 13:28 | −2 |
| 3 | —R—— | 10:01 | +2 |
| 4 | I—A— | 15:01, 15:02, 15:03 | 0 |
| 5 | F–D—— | 11:01, 11:04, 12:02, 13:05, 16:01 | 0 |
| 6 | —D—— | 16:02 | 0 |
| 7 | ——K— | 04:01 | +1 |
| 8 | ———————E | 04:03, 04:07 | 0 |
| 9 | I–D–GQ | 07:01 | 0 |
| 10 | F–R—E | 09:01 | +1 |
| 11 | F–D—L | 08:01, 08:02, 08:04, 08:06 | 0 |
| 12 | I–D—L | 08:03 | 0 |
| 13 | F–DE— | 11:03 | −2 |
| 14 | I–D—— | 12:01 | 0 |
| 15 | ——K-GR | 03:01 | +2 |
| 16 | I–DK— | 13:03 | 0 |
| 17 | —R—E | 14:01 | +1 |

Summary is for all 3rd HVR sequences and DRB1 alleles observed in at least one study subject
*3rd HVR* third hypervariable region, *aa* amino acids

## Statistical analysis

After testing the normality of the distribution of continuous variables with the Shapiro–Wilk test, comparisons were made with the Wilcoxon rank-sum test as appropriate. Categorical variables were compared utilizing chi-square tests or, when indicated, Fisher exact tests. The primary outcome analyzed was maternal versus paternal inheritance of the DRβ1 3rd HVR sequence according to charge. In addition, we compared the overall distribution of 3rd HVR sequences and 3rd HVR charge in SSc patients and controls. Analysis was conducted when 5% or more of patients or controls were represented in a category and correction made for multiple comparisons by Bonferroni adjustment of the threshold for significance. Logistic regression was carried out adjusting for sex because some controls were male, but this revealed no differences from the unadjusted associations.

Because a parent of origin effect has not been studied previously in SSc, a precise estimate of statistical power is precluded. However, our available sample size of 121 cases and 185 controls is estimated to provide more than 90% power to detect a two-fold difference in parental origin from an expected 50/50 in controls to 25/75 in cases, assuming $\alpha = 0.05$ and a two-tailed test.

## Results

Among SSc patients, 64% had diffuse SSc and 36% limited SSc (77 and 44 respectively). Antibodies to topoisomerase I (ATA) were positive in 34% of patients (37 of 109 tested) and to centromere (ACA) in 19% of patients (17 of 90 tested). The median age of SSc onset was 37 years, range 16–58.

HLA-DRB1 alleles were classified based on the amino acid sequence of the encoded 3rd HVR (amino acids 67–74) and the overall charge of each unique 3rd HVR sequence was determined (Table 1). Comparing SSc patients with healthy controls, the overall distribution of 3rd HVR sequences was significantly different ($p = 0.007$) (Table 2). The sequence "FLEDRRAA" (sequence category 5 in Table 1) was significantly enriched in SSc patients compared with controls ($p = 0.004$, $p$ value corrected for multiple comparisons $p_c = 0.032$), primarily due to enrichment of DRB1*11:04 among SSc patients, as reported previously [3]. The sequence "FLEDRRAL" (sequence category 11 in Table 1) was also enriched in SSc patients ($p = 0.006$, $p_c = 0.048$) (Table 2), due to some increase of DRB1*08:01 and DRB1*08:02 in SSc patients. These observations are concordant with a previous report of an increase in the motif "FLEDR" in a French population [10]. In contrast to the French study, however, we did not see enrichment of this sequence encoded by DRB5, which instead was decreased in our population (data not shown).

**Table 2** Allele frequencies classified according to the third hypervariable region in controls and SSc patients

| HVR region | Controls n (%) | SSc n (%) | p value | OR (95% CI) |
|---|---|---|---|---|
| 1 | 68 (18.4) | 34 (14.0) | 0.160 | 0.73 (0.46–1.14) |
| 2 | 44 (11.9) | 24 (9.9) | 0.447 | 0.82 (0.48–1.38) |
| 3 | 3 (0.8) | 1 (0.4) | | |
| 4 | 58 (15.7) | 21 (8.7) | 0.012 | 0.51 (0.30–0.87) |
| 5 | 36 (9.7) | 43 (17.8) | 0.004§ | 2.00 (1.25–3.23) |
| 6 | 0 (0.0) | 1 (0.4) | | – |
| 7 | 34 (9.2) | 25 (10.3) | 0.640 | 1.14 (0.66–1.96) |
| 8 | 4 (1.1) | 8 (3.3) | | |
| 9 | 48 (13.0) | 29 (12.0) | 0.718 | 0.91 (0.56–1.49) |
| 10 | 4 (1.1) | 2 (0.8) | | |
| 11 | 8 (2.1) | 16 (6.6) | 0.006# | 3.20 (1.35–7.61) |
| 12 | 1 (0.3) | 0 (0.0) | | – |
| 13 | 5 (1.3) | 6 (2.5) | | |
| 14 | 6 (1.6) | 4 (1.7) | | |
| 15 | 41 (11.1) | 26 (10.7) | 0.896 | 0.97 (0.57–1.63) |
| 16 | 3 (0.8) | 0 (0.0) | | – |
| 17 | 7 (1.9) | 2 (0.8) | | |
| All | 370 | 242 | | |

Third HVR overall distribution, SSc patients versus controls, $p = 0.007$
§$p_c = 0.032$
#$p_c = 0.048$
SSc systemic sclerosis, HVR hypervariable region, OR odds ratio, CI confidence interval, $p_c$ p value corrected for multiple comparisons

Overall, the 3rd HVR charge on SSc haplotypes was similar to that of controls; of the 242 SSc and 370 control haplotypes respectively, 11% and 12% had a +2 charge, 26% and 31% had a +1 charge, 50% and 44% had a charge of 0, and 13% and 13% had a −2 charge. As noted previously, no 3rd HVR sequence represented in our populations carried a −1 charge. Thirty-six percent of SSc patients and 34% of controls carried the same charge on both parental haplotypes. When considering both haplotypes together, 19%, 32%, and 49% of the SSc patients had overall negative, neutral, or positive charge respectively, compared with 20%, 22%, and 58% of healthy controls (Fig. 1).

Analysis was conducted considering maternal or paternal DRB1 allele inheritance according to the charge of the DRβ1 3rd HVR. The overall distribution of inheritance indicated significant skewing among SSc patients ($p < 0.001$). Among SSc patients the father transmitted a 3rd HVR sequence with a +2 charge significantly less often than the mother ($p = 0.0003$). Almost 90% of the time, transmission was maternal rather than paternal (Fig. 1). This skewed parental inheritance remained significant ($p = 0.001$) when corrected for comparing four different categories of charge. The skewed inheritance

**Fig. 1** Distribution of HLA-DRβ1 3rd HVR sequences according to charge and parental inheritance. Colors represent the overall 3rd HVR charge for each (biallelic) individual, considering both maternal and paternal haplotypes; *red*, overall charge was negative; *yellow*, overall charge was neutral; and *green*, overall charge was positive. Among SSc patients there was marked skewing of parental inheritance when the 3rd HVR sequence carried a +2 charge ($p = 0.0003$, $p_c = 0.001$) whereas controls showed a similar frequency of inheritance from either parent, as would be expected. Skewing was also observed, to a lesser extent, among SSc patients when the 3rd HVR sequence carried a 0 charge ($p = 0.021$, $p_c = 0.08$). Columns and rows with a −1 charge are 0 because no study subject had a 3rd HVR sequence with this charge (Color figure online). *SSc* systemic sclerosis

was observed among patients with both diffuse and limited SSc and was not different for those with younger versus older age of SSc onset. Skewed inheritance for overall distribution, and for each charge category, was not observed in the control population in which inheritance was not different from 50–50, as expected. To a lesser extent, 3rd HVR sequences with a 0 charge were inherited more often from the father than the mother among SSc patients ($p = 0.021$, $p_c = 0.084$). Parental transmissions of 3rd HVR sequences with +1 or −2 charge were not significantly skewed (Fig. 1).

While our study was designed to test a hypothesis regarding charge of the DRβ1 3rd HVR sequence and parental inheritance, linkage disequilibrium of DRB1 is very strong with DQA1 and DQB1, and secondary analysis was conducted for these loci. DQβ1 has a similarly located hypervariable region from amino acids 70 through 77. DQB1 alleles represented in our study populations had an overall net charge of +3, +1, 0, −1, or −2 (Table 3). Not surprisingly, the +3 charge for DQβ1 was also significantly decreased for paternal versus maternal

transmission, because DRB1*03:01 (+2 DRβ1 3rd HVR) haplotypes in our populations with few exceptions carried DQB1*02:01, which has a +3 charge. Patterns of linkage disequilibrium did not permit clear separation of the role of DQB1 from DRB1. However, the skewing for DQβ1 with a +3 charge was less pronounced than that described for DRβ1; eight were transmitted paternally versus 31 transmitted maternally. Additionally, DRB1*07:01 haplotypes can carry either DQB1*02:02 (+3) or DQB1*03:03 (0), and there was no suggestion of skewed paternal inheritance for these two haplotypes or an increase in DRB1*07:01–DQB1*02:02 haplotypes in the SSc population overall (Additional file 1: Table S1).

Polymorphisms on DQα1 are distributed somewhat differently from DRβ1 and DQβ1, but considered for amino acids 47–56 the net charge was +4, +2, or +1 for alleles represented in our study population and did not differ due to parental inheritance (Table 4). This result was also consistent with linkage disequilibrium in the HLA class II region, but results for DQA1 could be

**Table 3** DQβ1 hypervariable region and charge, amino acids 70–77[a]

| Allele | Amino acid position | | | | | | | | Overall charge |
|---|---|---|---|---|---|---|---|---|---|
| | 70 | 71 | 72 | 73 | 74 | 75 | 76 | 77 | |
| 05:01/2/3 | G | A | R | A | S | V | D | R | +1 |
| 06:01/4/9/11, 03:01/2/3 | **R** | T | – | – | **E** | – | – | **T** | 0 |
| 06:02/3/11/16 | – | T | – | – | **E** | L | – | **T** | −1 |
| 02:01/2 | **R** | **K** | – | – | A | – | – | – | +3[b] |
| 04:01/2 | **E** | **D** | – | – | – | – | – | **T** | −2 |

[a]Amino acids that differ from the consensus (alleles on the first line) by charge are presented in bold. Sequences encoded by uncommon alleles not present in our study populations are not included
[b]Among SSc patients with DQβ1 + 3 charge, eight were inherited paternally and 31 inherited maternally (*p* corrected = 0.001)

**Table 4** DQα1 hypervariable region and charge, amino acids 47–56[a]

| Allele | Amino acid position | | | | | | | | | | Overall charge[b] |
|---|---|---|---|---|---|---|---|---|---|---|---|
| | 47 | 48 | 49 | 50 | 51 | 52 | 53 | 54 | 55 | 56 | |
| 01:01/2/3/4/5 | R | W | P | E | F | S | K | F | G | G | +1 |
| 02:01 | K | – | – | L | – | H | R | – | R | – | +4 |
| 03:01/2/3 | Q | – | – | L | – | R | R | – | R | R | +4 |
| 04:01 | C | – | – | V | – | R | Q | – | R | – | +2 |
| 05:01/3/5 | C | – | – | V | – | R | Q | – | R | – | +2 |
| 06:01 | C | – | – | V | – | R | Q | – | R | – | +2 |

[a]Amino acids that differ from the consensus (alleles on the first line) by charge are presented in bold. Sequences encoded by uncommon alleles not present in our study populations are not included
[b]Parental inheritance was not skewed according to any DQα1 charge category. Similarly, results were not skewed if alternatively considered to extend to include a polymorphism at DQα1 amino acid 64

distinguished from DRB1 because multiple different DRB1 alleles are on haplotypes with the similar DQA1 alleles and some DQA1 alleles other than DQA1*05:01 also encode a +2 charge.

As expected because of linkage disequilibrium, the DRB1*03:01–DQA1*05:01–DQB1*02:01 haplotype was similarly skewed with three inherited paternally versus 21 inherited maternally ($p_c = 0.001$), although again skewing was somewhat less pronounced than when considered for DRβ1. (Haplotypes that were common in our study population are presented in Additional file 1: Table S1.)

## Discussion

In the current study we investigated patients with SSc and healthy controls, analyzing the DRβ1 3rd HVR according to charge irrespective of specific DRB1 alleles and considered parental inheritance. The importance of the DRβ1 3rd HVR and of charge in this region is well established in another autoimmune disease, rheumatoid arthritis, for which underlying HLA disease susceptibility is believed to be due to amino acid motifs of the DRβ1 3rd HVR that carry a similar charge [5, 6]. Our primary interest was to ask whether SSc patients differed from healthy controls if considered for parental origin of the DRβ1 3rd HVR categorized according to charge. In contrast to healthy individuals among whom parental inheritance was 50–50 as expected, we found significant skewing of parental inheritance in SSc patients. The most striking finding was that the father transmitted a DRB1 allele encoding a +2 charge 3rd HVR significantly less often than the mother in SSc patients. With respect to DRB1 allele frequencies, our study population was similar to prior reports of similar populations [1–3], with the patient population primarily enriched for DRB1*11:04 compared with controls.

Skewed parental inheritance of HLA-DRB1 alleles in SSc strongly suggests a parent-of-origin effect. Parent-of-origin effects are well described for a number of genes and are especially well recognized as important in early development [11]. Skewing from the expected random (50–50) inactivation of maternal versus paternal X-chromosomes has been reported previously in women with SSc, as well as in women with rheumatoid arthritis and some other diseases [12, 13]. A few studies have evaluated parental inheritance of HLA in other auto-immune diseases. In type 1 diabetes, parent-of-origin skewing in HLA inheritance has been described in some, but not all, studies [8, 9]. In patients with multiple sclerosis, HLA transmission was distorted by the parent of origin and by gender of the affected offspring [7]. A differential methylation signal with a peak at HLA-DRB1 was observed in $CD4^+$ T cells of multiple sclerosis patients compared with controls in another study, suggesting a potential explanation for this observation [14].

A number of phenomena can underlie a parent-of-origin effect. The best characterized parent-of-origin effect is that associated with genomic imprinting [11]. Embryonic lethality is one explanation for a parent-of-origin effect and, although skewing was not observed in our healthy population, it is possible that an extreme phenotype could result in loss of embryos destined to develop SSc in later life. The rate of decay for small molecules or epigenetic marks in sperm and ova affecting survival to gametogenesis has also been hypothesized to play a role in distorted haplotype transmission [7]. Additionally, the molecules CCCTC-binding factor (CTCF) and Class II transactivator (CIITA), two units of a transcription complex involved in HLA class II gene transcription, are thought to be subject to epigenetic modifications [15, 16]. The current results are of further interest in light of a recent study that implicated fetal programming in SSc [17] as well as increasing evidence for a role of epigenetic regulation in SSc pathogenesis [18].

There are a number of limitations to our study. SSc patients in our study were all female and it would be of additional interest to know whether males and/or children with SSc differ. Some of our controls were male and younger than the patient population. However, neither would be anticipated to affect the overall study observations because controls had the expected random (50–50) distribution regardless of gender or age. SSc is also a rare disorder offsetting any potential bias due to development of SSc later in life by a younger control. Another limitation is that all of our study subjects were Caucasian because too few patients from other racial/ethnic backgrounds were available for analysis. Also, the number of SSc patients was modest and a larger study would be needed to evaluate potential differences according to clinical and autoantibody characteristics. Another limitation is that alleles carrying a +2 charge other than DRB1*03:01 were uncommon in our population so the skewed inheritance observed could be specific to genes on the DRB1*03:01 haplotype, including DQB1*0201, rather than the DRβ1 3rd HVR +2 charge. It should also be added that some amino acids are subject to posttranslational modification that results in a change of charge [19] and, while this has largely been examined on autoantigens, HLA molecules are themselves also presented as self-peptides by other HLA molecules [20].

## Conclusions

Skewed parental HLA inheritance was observed among SSc patients compared with healthy controls. Paternal transmission was significantly reduced compared with maternal transmission when the HLA-DRB1 allele encoded a 3rd HVR with a +2 charge and to a lesser extent increased when charge was 0, in SSc patients but not in controls. To our knowledge, skewed parental inheritance of HLA-DRB1 alleles has not been reported previously in SSc. Provided our results are replicated, future investigations into the underlying mechanism(s) for a parent-of-origin effect of HLA inheritance in SSc may lead to new insight into the role of HLA molecules in SSc pathogenesis.

## Abbreviations
HLA: Human leukocyte antigen (or allele); HVR: Hypervariable region; SSc: Systemic sclerosis

## Acknowledgements
The authors are grateful to The Scleroderma Family Registry and to all of the patients and family members as well as the healthy controls and their family members for their participation in this study and to Judy Allen MPH and Samantha Bell MPH for study coordination. They thank Alex Forsyth for additional review of HLA alleles and amino acid sequences.

## Funding
This work was supported by NIH grant RO1 AI-41721 and a grant from The Scleroderma Foundation.

## Authors' contribution
CAG and CTL conducted experiments. CAG, HSG, and JLN analyzed and interpreted the data. MDM and DEF contributed patients and clinical assessments and contributed to the summary of results. CAG and JLN primarily wrote the manuscript. JLN conceived the study. All authors approved the final manuscript.

## Competing interests
The authors declare that they have no competing interests.

## Author details
[1]Division of Clinical Research, Fred Hutchinson Cancer Research Center, 1100 Fairview Ave N, Seattle, WA 98109, USA. [2]Department of Obstetrics and Gynecology, University of Washington, Seattle, WA, USA. [3]Division of Rheumatology and Clinical Immunogenetics, University of Texas Health Science Center at Houston, Houston, TX, USA. [4]Division of Rheumatology, University of California, Los Angeles, CA, USA. [5]Division of Rheumatology, University of Washington, Seattle, WA, USA.

## References
1. Mayes MD, Bossini-Castillo L, Gorlova O, Martin JE, Zhou X, Chen WV, et al. Immunochip analysis identifies multiple susceptibility loci for systemic sclerosis. Am J Hum Genet. 2014;94:47–61.
2. Arnett FC, Gourh P, Shete S, Ahn CW, Honey RE, Agarwal SK, et al. Major histocompatibility complex (MHC) class II alleles, haplotypes and epitopes which confer susceptibility or protection in systemic sclerosis: analysis in 1300 Caucasian, African-American and Hispanic cases and 1000 controls. Ann Rheum Dis. 2010;69:822–7.
3. Loubière LS, Lambert NC, Madeleine MM, Porter AJ, Mullarkey ME, Pang JM, et al. HLA allelic variants encoding DR11 in diffuse and limited systemic sclerosis in Caucasian women. Rheumatol Oxf Engl. 2005;44:318–22.
4. Reinsmoen NL, Bach FH. Structural Model for T-cell recognition of HLA class II-associated alloepitopes. Human Immunol. 1990;27(1):51–72.
5. Gregersen PK, Silver J, Winchester RJ. The shared epitope hypothesis. An approach to understanding the molecular genetics of susceptibility to rheumatoid arthritis. Arthritis Rheum. 1987;30(11):1205–13.
6. Reviron D, Perdriger A, Toussirot E, Wendling D, Balandraud N, Guid S, Semana G, Tiberghien P, Mercier P, Roudier J. Influence of shared epitope-negative HLA-DRB1 alleles on genetic susceptibility to rheumatoid arthritis. Arthritis Rheum. 2001;44(3):535–40.
7. Chao MJ, Herrera BM, Ramagopalan SV, Deluca G, Handunetthi L, Orton SM, Lincoln MR, Sadovnick AD, Ebers GC. Parent-of-origin effects at the major histocompatibility complex in multiple sclerosis. Hum Mol Gen. 2010;19(18):3679–89.
8. Sasaki T, Nemoto M, Yamasaki K, Tajima N. Preferential transmission of maternal allele with DQA1*0301-DQB1*0302 haplotype to affected offspring in families with type 1 diabetes. J Hum Genet. 1999;44:318–22.
9. Bronson PG, Ramsay PP, Thomson G, Barcellos LF, and the Type 1 Diabetes Genetics Consortium. Analysis of maternal-offspring HLA compatibility, parent-of-origin and non-inherited maternal effects for the classical HLA loci in type 1 diabetes. Diabetes Obs Metabol. 2009;11 Suppl 1:74–83.
10. Azzouz D, Rak JM, Fajardy I, Allanore Y, Tiev KP, et al. Comparing HLA shared epitopes in French Caucasian patients with Scleroderma. PLoS One. 2012;7(5):e36870.
11. Lawson HA, Cheverud JM, Wolf JB. Genomic imprinting and parent-of-origin effects on complex traits. Nat Rev. 2013;14:609–17.
12. Uz E, Loubiere LS, Gadi VK, Ozbalkan Z, Stewart J, Nelson JL, Ozcelik T. Skewed X-chromosome inactivation in scleroderma. Clin Rev Allergy Immunol. 2008;34(3):352–5.
13. Chabchoub G, Uz E, Maalej A, Mustafa CA, Rebai A, Mnif M, Bahloul Z, Farid NR, Ozcelik T, Ayadi H. Analysis of skewed X-chromosome inactivation in females with rheumatoid arthritis and autoimmune thyroid disease. Arthritis Res Therapy. 2009;11(4):R106.
14. Mc G, Benton M, Lea RA, Boyle M, Tajouri L, Macartney-Coxson D, Scott RJ, Lechner-Scott J. Methylation differences at the HLA-DRB1 locus in CD4+ T-cells are associated with multiple sclerosis. Mult Scler J. 2014;20(8):1033–41.
15. Phillips JE, Corces VG. CTCF: master weaver of the genome. Cell. 2011;137(7):1194–211.
16. Wright KL, Ting JPY. Epigenetic regulation of MHC-II and CIITA genes. Trends Immunol. 2006;27(9):405–12.
17. Donzelli G, Carnesecchi G, Amador C, di Tommaso M, Filippi L, Caporali R, et al. Fetal programming and systemic sclerosis. Am J Obstet Gynecol. 2015;213(6):839.e1–8–8.
18. Altorok N, Almeshal N, Wang Y, Kahaleh B. Epigenetics, the holy grail in the pathogenesis of systemic sclerosis. Rheumatology. 2015;54(10):1759–70.
19. Zavala-Cerna M, Martinez-Garcia E, Torres-Bugarin O, Rubio-Jurado B, Riebeling C, Nava A. The clinical significance of posttranslational modification of autoantigens. Clin Rev Allergy Immunol. 2014;47:73–90.
20. Mohme M, Hotz C, Stevanovic S, Binder T, Lee JH, Okoniewski M, et al. HLA-DR15-derived self-peptides are involved in increased autologous T cell proliferation in multiple sclerosis. Brain. 2013;136:1783–98.

# The association of low complement with disease activity in systemic sclerosis

James Esposito[1,2], Zoe Brown[2], Wendy Stevens[2], Joanne Sahhar[3,4], Candice Rabusa[2], Jane Zochling[5], Janet Roddy[6], Jennifer Walker[7], Susanna M. Proudman[8,9] and Mandana Nikpour[1,2*]

## Abstract

**Background:** In some rheumatic diseases such as systemic lupus erythematosus (SLE), low serum complement ('hypocomplementaemia') is a feature of active disease. However, the role of hypocomplementaemia in systemic sclerosis (SSc) is unknown. We sought to determine the frequency, clinical associations and relationship to disease activity of hypocomplementaemia in SSc.

**Methods:** The study included 1140 patients fulfilling the 2013 American College of Rheumatology criteria for SSc. Demographic, serological and clinical data, obtained prospectively through annual review, were analysed using univariable methods. Linear and logistic regression, together with generalised estimating equations, were used to determine the independent correlates of hypocomplementaemia ever, and at each visit, respectively.

**Results:** At least one episode of hypocomplementaemia (low C3 and/or low C4) occurred in 24.1 % of patients over 1893 visits; these patients were more likely to be seropositive for anti-ribonucleoprotein (OR = 3.8, $p = 0.002$), anti-Ro (OR = 2.2, $p = 0.002$), anti-Smith (OR = 6.3, $p = 0.035$) and anti-phospholipid antibodies (OR = 1.4, $p = 0.021$) and were more likely to display features of overlap connective tissue disease, in particular polymyositis (OR = 16.0, $p = 0.012$). However, no association was found between hypocomplementaemia and either the European Scleroderma Study Group disease activity score or any of its component variables (including erythrocyte sedimentation rate) in univariate analysis. Among patients with SSc overlap disease features, those who were hypocomplementaemic were more likely to have digital ulcers (OR = 1.6, $p = 0.034$), tendon friction rubs (OR = 2.4, $p = 0.037$), forced vital capacity <80 % predicted (OR = 2.9, $p = 0.008$) and lower body mass index (BMI) (OR for BMI = 0.9, $p < 0.0005$) at that visit, all of which are features associated with SSc disease activity and/or severity.

**Conclusions:** While hypocomplementaemia is not associated with disease activity in patients with non-overlap SSc, it is associated with some features of increased SSc disease activity in patients with overlap disease features.

**Keywords:** Systemic sclerosis, Complement, Disease activity

## Background

Systemic sclerosis (SSc) or scleroderma is a systemic autoimmune disorder of unknown aetiology associated with substantial morbidity and mortality [1]. The hallmark pathological features of SSc are vasculopathy, inflammation and progressive perivascular and interstitial fibrosis [2]. Prominent clinical manifestations of SSc include skin thickening, Raynaud's phenomenon, digital ulcers, gut involvement (gastro-oesophageal reflux disease, intestinal hypomotility and pseudo-obstruction), pulmonary arterial hypertension (PAH), interstitial lung disease (ILD) and renal crisis [3]. An 'SSc overlap' syndrome is considered present when a patient with SSc also has clinical and/or serological evidence of one or more of systemic lupus erythematosus (SLE), polymyositis, Sjögren's syndrome or rheumatoid arthritis [2].

* Correspondence: m.nikpour@unimelb.edu.au
[1]Department of Medicine, The University of Melbourne at St Vincent's Hospital (Melbourne), 41 Victoria Parade, Fitzroy, VIC 3065, Australia
[2]Department of Rheumatology, St Vincent's Hospital (Melbourne), 41 Victoria Parade, Fitzroy, VIC 3065, Australia
Full list of author information is available at the end of the article

As in other systemic autoimmune diseases, disease activity leads to irreversible organ damage. Activity reflects features of the disease process that vary over time and are potentially reversible with intervention or spontaneously. Quantifying active disease would assist clinicians in assessment and management of disease activity, which might in turn prevent damage and improve outcomes [4]. Assessing disease activity is necessary for staging the disease and predicting prognosis. It is also useful for distinguishing between those patients requiring aggressive treatment and those for whom symptomatic treatment may be sufficient, as well as for monitoring response to treatment.

In certain rheumatic diseases characterised by distinct episodes of inflammation, such as SLE, validated measures already exist to assist clinicians in the assessment of disease activity [5]. There have been several endeavours to develop disease activity criteria for SSc. The European Scleroderma Study Group (EScSG) activity index was constructed on the basis of evaluation of features of a large multicentre cohort of patients with SSc, compared with a gold standard of disease activity assessment by three experts [6–8]. Univariate analysis of symptoms, signs and laboratory tests was performed to select single items that were significantly associated with the consensus disease activity score. The final index comprised ten components, including clinical features such as arthritis, modified Rodnan skin score (MRSS) and digital ulcers; patient-reported changes in cardiopulmonary, skin and vascular symptoms; and erythrocyte sedimentation rate (ESR) [6, 7]. Hypocomplementaemia was also included [7, 8], but it is not yet known whether low complement is truly a marker of disease activity in SSc.

Various candidate serological markers have been proposed to be related to disease activity in SSc, such as soluble interleukin-2 receptor (sIL-2R), type III procollagen aminopeptide (PIIINP) and von Willebrand factor propeptide [9–11]. However, in patients with SSc, changes in these markers have not been reflected in clinical responses to therapy. For example, chlorambucil administration was followed by normalization of sIL-2R levels but had no effect on disease activity [12]. Similarly, α-interferon administration resulted in a decrease in PIIINP levels without any improvement in disease activity assessed using a validated skin score, grip strength, measurements of digital contractures, Ritchie index, assessment of muscle weakness, and tendon friction rubs [13].

Low serum complement is a candidate serological marker of disease activity in SSc. Aberrant activation of the complement system is implicated in the pathogenesis of a number of systemic autoimmune disorders [14]. For example, in SLE, immune complex formation triggers the complement cascade via the classical pathway, and the resulting low concentrations of complement components C3 and C4 are found in many patients with active and severe SLE [15, 16]. It has been shown that the manifestations of SSc are due to derangements in both innate and adaptive immunity. The association of Toll-like receptor (TLR) signalling variations with SSc suggests that TLR pathways, and hence complement activation and consumption, may play a role in the pathogenesis of SSc [17]. However, unlike SLE, wherein low serum complement is a validated measure of disease activity, the relationship between hypocomplementaemia and disease activity in SSc is less clear.

The aim of this study was to evaluate the frequency of hypocomplementaemia in a cohort of patients with SSc and to evaluate which clinical and serological features are significantly associated with hypocomplementaemia. We hypothesised that hypocomplementaemia is associated with clinical features of disease activity such as arthritis, tendon friction rubs, low body mass index (BMI) (a marker of severe SSc gastrointestinal involvement) and low forced vital capacity (FVC) (a measure of severe ILD).

## Methods

### Patients

Patients were recruited from the Australian Scleroderma Cohort Study, a prospective multi-centre cohort study of risk factors for clinically important outcomes in SSc. All patients fulfilled the 2013 American College of Rheumatology classification criteria for SSc [18]. Patients were recruited from multiple Australian centres that specialize in the care of patients with SSc, which included St Vincent's Hospital and Monash Medical Centre, Victoria; Royal Prince Alfred and St George Hospitals, New South Wales; Sunshine Coast Rheumatology and Prince Charles Hospital, Queensland; Royal Adelaide Hospital, The Queen Elizabeth Hospital and Flinders Medical Centre, South Australia; Royal Perth Hospital, Western Australia; and Menzies Institute for Medical Research, Tasmania. The study was approved by the human research ethics committees of each of the participating centres.

Consent was obtained from all patients prior to the collection of demographic and disease-related data (including clinical and laboratory data) according to a standardized protocol at recruitment and at each subsequent annual review. Patients were included if they had at least one annual visit where complement levels had been recorded, along with demographic, clinical and laboratory data (see below).

### Measurement of complement levels

C3 and C4 levels were measured prospectively at each annual visit in the laboratories of each of the recruiting centres using sera obtained at recruitment and at each subsequent review by performing nephelometry. Complement levels were defined as being either normal or low according to local laboratory standards. Patient visits were then recorded as normocomplementaemic if the patient had a normal C3 and C4 result or hypocomplementaemic if the patient had a low C3 and/or C4.

## Demographic, clinical and laboratory variables
All data were collected prospectively.

### Data collected at recruitment
Demographic data collected at recruitment included age at disease onset and age at recruitment. Disease onset was defined according to the age at which the first non-Raynaud's phenomenon manifestation of SSc occurred. Sex and race were also recorded; race was categorized as white, Asian, Aboriginal or Torres Strait Islander, or other. Disease duration was defined as the time elapsed from disease onset to recruitment, and length of follow-up was defined as the time elapsed from recruitment until the date at which the data were censored for analysis.

Disease-related data gathered included SSc subtype (diffuse or limited) defined according to the LeRoy criteria [19]. The autoantibody status of each patient was determined at recruitment using immunofluorescence for antinuclear antibodies and commercially available assays for antibodies to extractable nuclear antigens Scl-70, Jo-1, ribonucleoprotein (RNP), Ro, La, Smith (Sm), and polymyositis scleroderma (PM-Scl) (enzyme-linked immunosorbent assay [ELISA]; ORGENTEC Diagnostika, Mainz, Germany); antibodies to double-stranded DNA (anti-dsDNA) (Amerlex radioimmunoassay; Trinity Biotech, Bray, Ireland); antibodies to RNA polymerase III (QUANTA Lite RNA Pol III; Inova Diagnostics, San Diego, CA, USA; and MBL Anti-RNA Pol III; MBL International, Woburn, MA, USA); anti-neutrophil cytoplasmic antibodies (ANCA), including proteinase-3 or myeloperoxidase specificity (ELISA; ORGENTEC Diagnostika); rheumatoid factor and anti-phospholipid antibodies, including anti-cardiolipin antibodies (Vital Diagnostics, Bella Vista, Australia); and anti-$\beta_2$-glycoprotein antibodies (ELISA; ORGENTEC Diagnostika).

### Data collected at each annual visit
Disease manifestations were recorded at each visit. Raynaud's phenomenon was defined on the basis of characteristic colour changes in the extremities. The presence of puffy digits (scleroderma), tendon friction rubs, synovitis and muscle atrophy was based on examination findings of the patient's rheumatologist. The MRSS [20] was also calculated and recorded at each visit.

Persistent sicca symptoms were defined as dry eyes or dry mouth at two or more annual visits. Gastrointestinal symptoms, including reflux requiring treatment with proton pump inhibitor, dysphagia, post-prandial bloating, vomiting, diarrhoea (more than three motions per day), constipation (fewer than one motion per day) or anal incontinence (faecal soiling) not due to other causes, were also recorded. Gastric antral vascular ectasia (GAVE) and oesophageal stricture were defined on the basis of endoscopy. Bowel dysmotility was defined on the basis of barium and nuclear medicine studies, antibiotic response and characteristic symptoms. Pseudo-obstruction was defined as the presence of clinical features suggestive of intestinal obstruction in the absence of an anatomical lesion.

Myocardial disease was defined on the basis of endomyocardial biopsy or as the presence of conduction defects, arrhythmias, and right ventricular or left ventricular dysfunction on echocardiography in the absence of other causes. Pericardial effusions were defined on the basis of an echocardiogram showing other than a small (<1-cm thickness), non-significant pericardial effusion.

PAH was defined on the basis of right heart catheterization as a mean pulmonary arterial pressure ≥25 mmHg and a pulmonary arterial wedge pressure ≤15 mmHg. The 6-minute walk distance was also recorded each year as a measure of PAH severity.

ILD was defined on the basis of characteristic changes visualised by chest high-resolution computed tomography. Pulmonary function tests were performed at each annual visit, and forced vital capacity (FVC) and diffusing capacity of the lung for carbon monoxide (DLCO) were recorded as percent predicted values, with FVC used as a measure of ILD activity and/or severity.

Renal crisis was defined as any two of the following three criteria: new-onset severe hypertension (≥180 mmHg systolic and/or ≥100 mmHg diastolic) without an alternate aetiology, microangiopathic haemolytic anaemia, or rising creatinine.

SSc treatment was recorded at each visit as follows: corticosteroids (oral prednisolone), immunosuppressives (leflunomide, methotrexate, azathioprine, penicillamine, hydroxychloroquine, mycophenolate, cyclophosphamide and calcineurin inhibitors), biologic therapies (tumour necrosis factor-α inhibitors, tocilizumab, abatacept, anti-CD20 antibodies and other B-cell modulators) and home oxygen.

## Definition of SSc overlap syndrome
The presence of 'overlap disease' was recorded at each annual visit and was defined as evidence of SSc together with characteristic symptoms or signs of overlap disease, which included persistent sicca symptoms, episodes of inflammatory myositis (muscle weakness together with two or more of elevated serum creatinine kinase, characteristic changes on electromyography and/or magnetic resonance imaging, or muscle biopsy showing typical histopathological changes), or a rheumatologist's report

of overlap with another rheumatic disease, such as rheumatoid arthritis, polymyositis, dermatomyositis, SLE or Sjögren's syndrome.

### European Scleroderma Study Group disease activity score

The EScSG disease activity score and the presence of its ten components were recorded at each visit: scleroderma; digital necrosis; arthritis; MRSS >14; DLCO <80 % predicted; ESR >30 mm/h; hypocomplementaemia (low C3 and/or C4); and patient-reported changes in cardiopulmonary, vascular or skin symptoms in the preceding month. One point is assigned for the presence of each feature, and scores can range from 0 to 10. However, because hypocomplementaemia is one of the ten variables in the EScSG activity score, we calculated a score based on the other nine variables only, in order to avoid overcorrelation in subsequent analysis. Therefore, final scores ranged from 0 to 9, with higher scores indicating higher disease activity.

### Physician global assessment

Physician global assessments of overall health, disease activity and disease damage were also recorded prospectively at each annual visit using a visual analogue scale. Physician global assessments entail the physician's taking note of all the available clinical and laboratory information in order to assign a score that ranges between 0 and 10 for each of overall health, disease activity and disease-related damage. Higher scores represent worse overall health, higher disease activity or greater disease-related damage.

### Statistical analysis

Descriptive statistics (mean ± SD, median [interquartile range], minimum and maximum, and number [percent]) were used to describe the characteristics of the patients and the data set. As there was <5 % missing data for any particular variable, we did not impute missing data.

Univariable comparisons between patients who were persistently normocomplementaemic during follow-up and patients who had experienced at least one episode of hypocomplementaemia during the course of the study were made using the $t$ test for continuous variables, the chi-square test for categorical variables and the Wilcoxon signed-rank test for ordinal variables. In this analysis, disease manifestations were defined as 'present ever'. Additional analyses were performed comparing the two groups described above (persistent normocomplementaemia and at least one episode of hypocomplementaemia) with those who had persistent hypocomplementaemia at every visit during follow-up.

In multivariable analyses, the association between disease features at each visit and hypocomplementaemia at that particular visit was analysed. Here, we used generalised estimating equations (GEEs) to account for the expected correlation that arises when repeated measurements are taken from the same individual at multiple visits over time [21]. Another advantage of this method of analysis is that it overcomes any potential misclassification error that might arise from dividing patients into subgroups based on arbitrary definitions such as hypocomplementaemia ever, persistent hypocomplementaemia and persistent normocomplementaemia. Furthermore, as there is currently no consensus regarding meaningful changes in clinical parameters from one visit to the next, the use of GEEs enables evaluation of the relationship between hypocomplementaemia at a particular visit and actual clinical parameters at that particular visit.

All statistical analyses were performed using STATA 14 software (StataCorp, College Station, TX, USA). All $p$ values were two-tailed, and statistical significance was defined as $p \leq 0.05$. The overall study design and planned analyses are presented in Fig. 1.

## Results

This study included 1140 patients with SSc who had complement levels recorded prospectively at one or more visits.

### Characteristics of cohort and data set

The cohort presented in this study is summarized in Tables 1 and 2. Among the 1140 patients included in this study, the average age of patients was $46.0 \pm 14.1$ years at SSc diagnosis and $57.4 \pm 12.3$ years at recruitment, with a mean follow-up time of $3.4 \pm 1.7$ years. In terms of demographics, 87.2 % of patients were female, 93.3 % were white, 4.7 % were Asian, 1.3 % were Australian Aboriginal or Torres Strait Islander and 0.9 % were of other racial origin. The mean disease duration at recruitment was $11.3 \pm 9.9$ years, with 14.3 % of patients having a disease duration ≤2 years and 31.2 % of patients having a disease duration ≤5 years at recruitment. Diffuse SSc was present in 27.2 % of patients, and 72.8 % of patients had limited SSc.

SSc overlap disease features were present in 23.4 % of patients. The autoantibody profile of patients is summarized in Table 1. Autoantibodies that were found in a significant proportion of the cohort included anti-Scl-70 (15.2 %), anti-centromere (46.2 %), anti-RNA polymerase (13.3 %), anti-dsDNA antibodies (13.3 %), ANCA (12.9 %), rheumatoid factor (27.2 %), anti-phospholipid (25.7 %) and anti-$\beta_2$-glycoprotein (33.0 %) antibodies.

Characteristics of the data set pertaining to complement measurements are summarized in Table 3. Hypocomplementaemia was present at recruitment in 13.2 % of patients and thereafter present ever from recruitment to most recent visit in 24.1 % of patients. The median number of complement measurements per patient was 2,

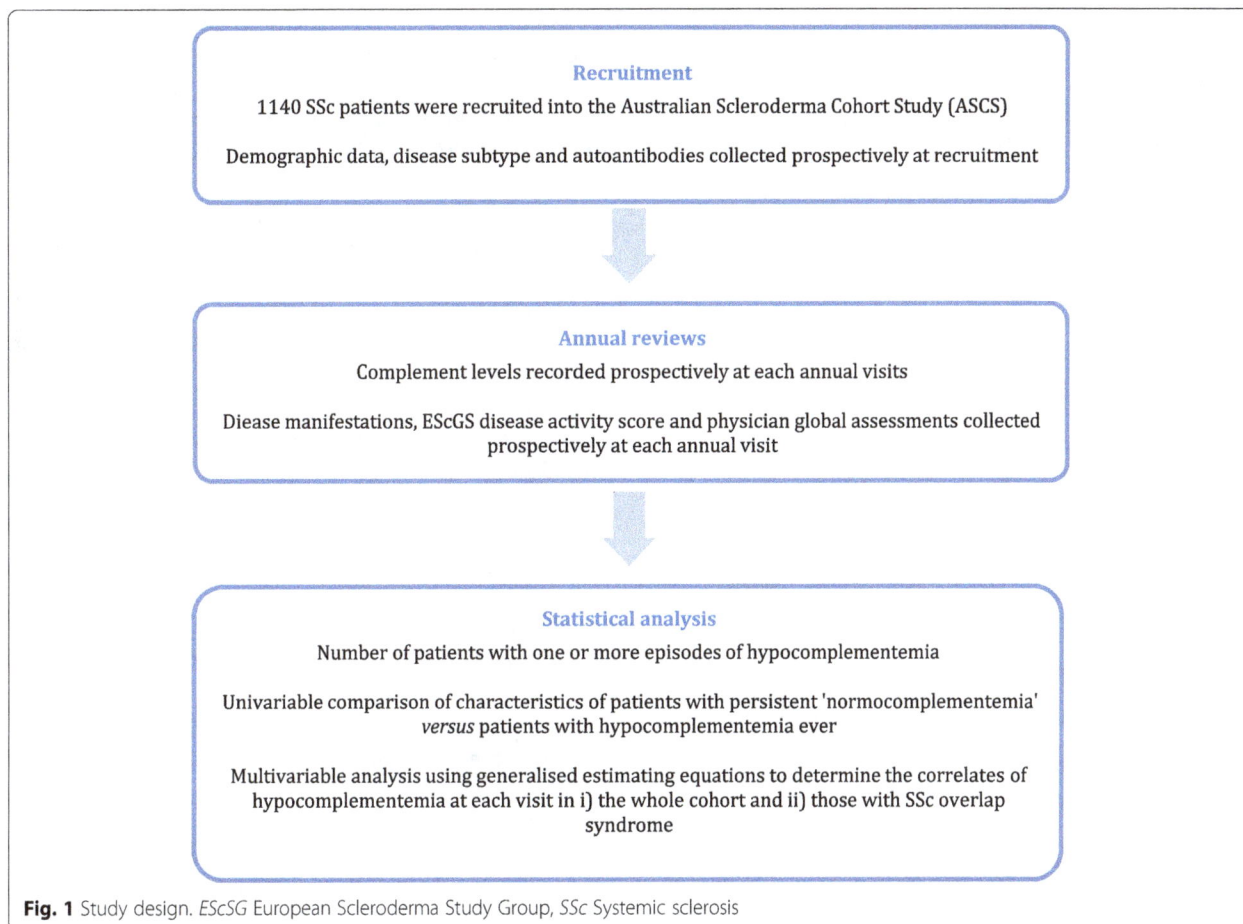

**Recruitment**

1140 SSc patients were recruited into the Australian Scleroderma Cohort Study (ASCS)

Demographic data, disease subtype and autoantibodies collected prospectively at recruitment

**Annual reviews**

Complement levels recorded prospectively at each annual visits

Diease manifestations, EScGS disease activity score and physician global assessments collected prospectively at each annual visit

**Statistical analysis**

Number of patients with one or more episodes of hypocomplementemia

Univariable comparison of characteristics of patients with persistent 'normocomplementemia' *versus* patients with hypocomplementemia ever

Multivariable analysis using generalised estimating equations to determine the correlates of hypocomplementemia at each visit in i) the whole cohort and ii) those with SSc overlap syndrome

**Fig. 1** Study design. *EScSG* European Scleroderma Study Group, *SSc* Systemic sclerosis

with an interquartile range of 1–3. The minimum number of measurements was 1, and the maximum number of measurements was 8. The average time interval between measurements was $1.2 \pm 0.4$ years. A total of 1893 individual visit measurements of complement with corresponding clinical and serological data were available for analysis.

## Univariable analyses

Univariable comparisons between patients who had persistent normocomplementaemia during follow-up and patients who had experienced at least one episode of hypocomplementaemia during the course of the study are summarized in Tables 4 and 5. Patients who had ever been hypocomplementaemic were more likely to have features of overlap disease present (29.5 % vs. 21.5 %, $p = 0.007$), in particular polymyositis (1.8 % vs. 0.1 %, $p = 0.001$). Hypocomplementaemia was also found to be associated with a number of autoantibodies typically associated with other rheumatic diseases, which included anti-RNP (4.5 % vs. 1.2 %, $p = 0.001$), anti-Ro (10.8 % vs. 5.2 %, $p = 0.001$), anti-Sm (1.5 % vs. 0.2 %, $p = 0.016$) and anti-phospholipid (31.3 % vs. 24.0 %, $p = 0.02$) antibodies. Patients with hypocomplementaemia were also more

likely to have a BMI $<20$ kg/m$^2$ (20.5 % vs. 13.0 %, $p = 0.003$), a feature of more active and severe gastrointestinal involvement; scleroderma (72.8 % vs. 66.2 %, $p = 0.044$); and muscle atrophy (23.2 % vs 17.2 %, $p = 0.029$). A significant association with pericardial effusions (9.1 % vs. 5.3 %, $p = 0.023$) was also found.

There was no difference in the mean EScSG disease activity score or physician global assessment score for overall health, disease activity and damage across all visits in patients who were normocomplementaemic compared with those who were hypocomplementaemic. In additional analyses, we found no significant differences between those who had at least one episode of hypocomplementaemia and persistent hypocomplementaemia during follow-up, possibly due to very few patients in the latter group (data not shown).

## Multivariable regression analyses

In the analyses described above, variables were defined as being ever present from disease onset to most recent review. We performed a second series of analyses using GEEs with data gathered at each visit. This set comprised a total of 1893 visits.

**Table 1** Patient characteristics (*n* = 1140)

| Characteristic | *n* (%) or mean ± SD |
|---|---|
| Age at diagnosis, years | 46.0 ± 14.1 |
| Age at recruitment, years | 57.4 ± 12.3 |
| Follow-up duration, years | 3.4 ± 1.7 |
| Sex | |
| Male | 148 (13.0 %) |
| Female | 992 (87.2 %) |
| Race | |
| White | 1012 (93.3 %) |
| Asian | 50 (4.7 %) |
| Australian Aboriginal or Torres Strait Islander | 14 (1.3 %) |
| Other | 9 (0.9 %) |
| Disease duration at recruitment[a] | 11.3 ± 9.9 |
| ≤ 2 years | 163 (14.3 %) |
| ≤ 5 years | 356 (31.2 %) |
| Disease subtype[b] | |
| Diffuse | 310 (27.2 %) |
| Limited | 830 (72.8 %) |
| Overlap disease features present ever[c] | 267 (23.4 %) |
| Rheumatoid arthritis | 22 (1.9 %) |
| Polymyositis | 6 (0.5 %) |
| Dermatomyositis | 1 (0.01 %) |
| Sjögren's syndrome | 21 (1.8 %) |
| SLE | 9 (0.8 %) |
| Serological profile at recruitment | |
| Anti-centromere ANA | 517 (46.2 %) |
| Anti-Scl-70 antibodies | 167 (15.2 %) |
| Anti-RNAP antibodies | 84 (13.3 %) |
| Anti-U1 RNP antibodies | 22 (2.0 %) |
| Anti-Ro antibodies | 72 (6.6 %) |
| Anti-La antibodies | 18 (1.6 %) |
| Anti-Sm antibodies | 6 (0.6 %) |
| Anti-PM-Scl antibodies | 15 (1.4 %) |
| Anti-dsDNA antibodies | 26 (3.1 %) |
| Anti-Jo-1 antibodies | 5 (0.5 %) |
| ANCA | 134 (12.9 %) |
| MPO specificity | 17 (1.6 %) |
| PR-3 specificity | 22 (2.1 %) |
| Rheumatoid factor | 288 (27.2 %) |
| Anti-phospholipid antibodies | 272 (25.7 %) |
| Cardiolipin IgM | 165 (65.0 %) |
| Cardiolipin IgG | 105 (39.3 %) |
| Anti-$\beta_2$-glycoprotein antibody | 84 (33.0 %) |
| Lupus anticoagulant | 26 (3.1 %) |

*Abbreviations: ANA* Anti-nuclear antibody, *Anti-Scl-70* Anti-scleroderma-70 antibodies, *Anti-U1 RNP* Anti-ribonucleoprotein antibodies, *Anti-Sm* Anti-Smith antibodies, *Anti-PM-Scl* Anti-polymyositis scleroderma antibodies, *Anti-dsDNA* Anti-double-stranded DNA antibodies, *Anti-RNAP* Anti-RNA polymerase antibodies, *ANCA* Anti-neutrophil cytoplasmic antibodies, *MPO* Myeloperoxidase, *PR-3* Proteinase-3
[a]Since onset of first non-Raynaud's phenomenon disease manifestation
[b]Disease subtype based on extent of skin involvement, with limited disease being confined to the extremities distal to elbows and knees, as well as the face
[c]Actual overlap disease features specified for only a proportion of patients classified by the treating physician as having 'SSc overlap syndrome'

We analysed data for up to six reviews per patient. We specified an exchangeable working correlation structure to account for the within-individual correlation and computed robust standard errors on the parametric estimates. We ran a univariable model of EScSG disease activity score (with the complement component removed to avoid over-correlation) and a multivariable model containing all of the individual disease activity variables listed in the EScSG disease activity index, with the exception of the complement item, and with some additional disease activity variables (C-reactive protein [CRP] >8 mg/L and BMI) included on the basis of univariable analyses (Table 6). Because scleroderma, muscle atrophy and pericardial effusion, which were statistically significant in univariable analysis, were not statistically significant in multivariable analysis, these variables were removed. Despite lack of significance in a simple univariable comparison, in a multivariable GEE model, FVC <80 % predicted was statistically significant and therefore included in the final model. We ran the multivariable models for (1) the whole cohort (*n* = 886; 1893 visits in total) as well as (2) patients classified as having SSc overlap (*n* = 221; 628 visits in total) and (3) those with non-SSc overlap (*n* = 665; 1265 visits in total) (Table 6).

In the multivariable analysis using the entire cohort, significant correlates of hypocomplementaemia at each visit included a lower BMI (OR for BMI = 0.90, 95 % CI 0.88–0.94, *p* < 0.0005), a lower MRSS (OR for MRSS = 0.98, 95 % CI 0.96–0.99, *p* = 0.013) and a lower ESR (OR for ESR = 0.99, 95 % CI 0.98–0.99, *p* = 0.022). In patients with SSc overlap disease features, significant correlates of hypocomplementaemia at each visit included digital ulcers (OR = 1.62, 95 % CI 1.04–2.51, *p* = 0.034), tendon friction rubs (OR = 2.31, 95 % CI 1.05–5.10, *p* = 0.037), an FVC <80 % predicted (OR = 2.90, 95 % CI 1.32–6.38, *p* = 0.008) and a lower BMI (OR for BMI = 0.90, 95 % CI 0.85–0.95, *p* < 0.0005), all variables that are associated with increased SSc disease activity and/or severity. In patients without overlap disease features, significant correlates of hypocomplementaemia at each visit included a lower BMI (OR for BMI = 0.91, 95 % CI 0.87–0.95, *p* < 0.0005) and a lower ESR (OR for ESR = 0.99, 95 % CI 0.97–0.99, *p* = 0.026).

## Discussion

In this longitudinal cohort study of 1140 patients with SSc, we found that low serum complement occurred at least once in 23.4 % of patients over the study period. We also found that these patients were more likely to have SSc overlap disease features than patients who were normocomplementaemic (29.5 % vs. 21.5 %, *p* = 0.007), in particular polymyositis. We have also demonstrated that hypocomplementaemia is not a measure of disease

**Table 2** Disease manifestations in cohort (n = 1140)

| Characteristics | n (%) or median (25th–75th IQR) |
|---|---|
| Disease manifestation[a] | |
| Raynaud's phenomenon | 1065 (94.0 %) |
| Digital ulcers | 345 (30.5 %) |
| Digital gangrene/amputation | 93 (8.2 %) |
| Telangiectasia | 947 (83.8 %) |
| Calcinosis | 439 (38.9 %) |
| Scleroderma | 763 (67.8 %) |
| Tendon friction rub | 112 (10.0 %) |
| Joint contracture | 431 (38.3 %) |
| Synovitis | 323 (28.7 %) |
| Muscle atrophy | 210 (18.7 %) |
| MRSS score >20 | 207 (18.5 %) |
| Myocardial disease | 87 (7.6 %) |
| Pericardial effusion[b] | 70 (6.2 %) |
| PAH[c] | 298 (26.9 %) |
| ILD[d] | 340 (30.1 %) |
| Gastrointestinal involvement[e] | 638 (56.3 %) |
| GAVE | 113 (10.0 %) |
| Reflux oesophagitis | 958 (84.3 %) |
| Oesophageal stricture | 207 (18.3 %) |
| Oesophageal dysmotility | 457 (40.6 %) |
| Bowel dysmotility | 297 (26.3 %) |
| Pseudo-obstruction | 37 (3.3 %) |
| Renal crises[f] | 44 (3.9 %) |
| eGFR <60 ml/minute | 297 (26.4 %) |
| Myositis[g] | 58 (6.0 %) |
| CRP >8 mg/L | 333 (29.7 %) |
| ESR >30 mm/h | 323 (28.8 %) |
| Blood CK >200 IU/L | 122 (11.0 %) |
| Anaemia[h] | 403 (35.5 %) |
| FVC <80 % predicted | 298 (26.9 %) |
| DLCO <80 % predicted | 832 (79.9 %) |
| EScSG disease activity score[i] | 2.5 (1–4) |
| Treatments[a] | |
| Corticosteroids | 506 (44.4 %) |
| Immunotherapy[j] | 495 (43.4 %) |
| Biological therapy[k] | 16 (1.4 %) |
| Home oxygen | 41 (3.6 %) |

**Table 2** Disease manifestations in cohort (n = 1140) (Continued)

| Physician global assessments[l] | |
|---|---|
| Overall health[m] | 4 (3–6) |
| Activity[n] | 3 (2–5) |
| Damage[n] | 4 (3–6) |

*Abbreviations: MRSS* Modified Rodnan skin score, *EScSG* European Scleroderma Study Group, *PAH* Pulmonary arterial hypertension, *ILD* Interstitial lung disease, *GAVE* Gastric antral vascular ectasia, *eGFR* Estimated glomerular filtration rate, *CRP* C-reactive protein, *ESR* Erythrocyte sedimentation rate, *CK* Creatinine kinase, *FVC* Forced vital capacity, *DLCO* Diffusing capacity of the lung for carbon monoxide corrected for haemoglobin
[a]Ever from disease onset to most recent visit
[b]Pericardial effusion defined by echocardiography
[c]PAH defined by right heart catheterization with a mean pulmonary artery pressure ≥25 mmHg and a pulmonary arterial wedge pressure ≤15 mmHg
[d]Pulmonary fibrosis defined by chest high-resolution computed tomography
[e]Gastrointestinal symptoms defined as the presence of any of reflux, dysphagia, post-prandial bloating, vomiting, constipation, diarrhoea or anal incontinence as defined in text
[f]Renal crisis defined as the presence of at least two of the following: new-onset hypertension, rising creatinine or microangiopathic haemolytic anaemia
[g]Myositis defined as either definite (biopsy), suspected (CK or electromyogram) or possible (magnetic resonance imaging scan)
[h]Anaemia defined as haemoglobin level <135 g/L in males and <120 g/L in females
[i]Calculated without hypocomplementaemia. Final scores range from 0 to 9, with higher scores indicating higher disease activity
[j]Includes leflunomide, methotrexate, azathioprine, penicillamine, hydroxychloroquine, mycophenolate, cyclophosphamide and calcineurin inhibitors
[k]Includes tumour necrosis factor alpha inhibitors, tocilizumab, abatacept, anti-CD20 antibodies and other B-cell modulators
[l]Highest score ever recorded over the study period
[m]Scores range from 0 to 10, with higher scores being indicative of worse overall health
[n]Scores range from 0 to 10, with higher scores being indicative of higher disease activity or damage

**Table 3** Characterisation of complement levels (n = 1140)

| Parameter | n (%) or mean ± SD or median (25th–75th IQR) |
|---|---|
| Hypocomplementaemia[a] | |
| At recruitment | 150 (13.2 %) |
| Ever[b] | 275 (24.1 %) |
| Number of complement measurements per patient | 2 (1–3) |
| 1 | 400 (35.1 %) |
| 2 | 265 (23.3 %) |
| 3 | 196 (17.2 %) |
| 4 | 129 (11.3 %) |
| 5 | 85 (7.5 %) |
| 6 | 50 (4.4 %) |
| 7 | 14 (1.2 %) |
| 8 | 1 (0.1 %) |
| Total number of complement measurements in data set | 1893 |
| Time interval between complement measurements, years | 1.2 ± 0.4 |

[a]A low C3 and/or C4 result
[b]At least one episode of hypocomplementaemia over the study period

**Table 4** Univariable comparison of demographics, disease subtypes and serological profiles in patients with persistent normocomplementaemia and those with at least one episode of hypocomplementaemia

| Characteristic | Persistent normocomplementaemia (n = 865) | At least one episode of hypocomplementaemia (n = 275) | |
|---|---|---|---|
| | n (%) or mean ± SD or median (IQR) | n (%) or mean ± SD or median (IQR) | p Value |
| Age at diagnosis, years | 46.4 ± 0.5 | 44.6 ± 0.8 | 0.071 |
| Sex | | | |
| Male | 113 (13.1 %) | 35 (12.7 %) | 0.89 |
| Female | 752 (86.9 %) | 240 (87.3 %) | 0.89 |
| Disease duration· | 11.3 ± 0.4 | 11.6 ± 0.7 | 0.71 |
| ≤ 2 years | 117 (14.5 %) | 46 (17.5 %) | 0.24 |
| ≤ 5 years | 268 (33.2 %) | 88 (33.5 %) | 0.94 |
| Disease type | | | |
| Diffuse | 238 (27.5 %) | 72 (26.2 %) | 0.67 |
| Limited | 627 (72.5 %) | 203 (73.8 %) | 0.67 |
| Overlap features present[a] | 186 (21.5 %) | 81 (29.5 %) | 0.007 |
| Rheumatoid arthritis | 15 (1.7 %) | 7 (2.6 %) | 0.39 |
| Polymyositis | 1 (0.1 %) | 5 (1.8 %) | 0.001 |
| Dermatomyositis | 0 (0 %) | 1 (0.4 %) | 0.076 |
| Sjögren's syndrome | 14 (1.6 %) | 7 (2.6 %) | 0.32 |
| SLE | 6 (0.7 %) | 3 (1.1 %) | 0.52 |
| Serological profile[a] | | | |
| Anti-centromere ANA | 391 (46.0 %) | 126 (47.0 %) | 0.084 |
| Anti-Scl-70 antibodies | 134 (16.1 %) | 33 (12.3 %) | 0.13 |
| Anti-Jo-1 antibodies | 4 (0.5 %) | 1 (0.4 %) | 0.82 |
| Anti-RNP antibodies | 10 (1.2 %) | 12 (4.5 %) | 0.001 |
| Anti-Ro antibodies | 43 (5.2 %) | 29 (10.8 %) | 0.001 |
| Anti-La antibodies | 12 (1.5 %) | 6 (2.2 %) | 0.38 |
| Anti-Sm antibodies | 2 (0.2 %) | 4 (1.5 %) | 0.016 |
| Anti-PM-Scl antibodies | 10 (1.2 %) | 5 (1.9 %) | 0.43 |
| Anti-dsDNA antibodies | 16 (2.5 %) | 10 (4.9 %) | 0.089 |
| Anti-RNAP antibodies | 61 (13.6 %) | 23 (12.6 %) | 0.74 |
| ANCA | 95 (12.1 %) | 39 (15.2 %) | 0.20 |
| MPO specificity | 14 (1.8 %) | 3 (1.2 %) | 0.50 |
| PR-3 specificity | 14 (1.8 %) | 8 (3.1 %) | 0.20 |
| Rheumatoid factor | 208 (26.1 %) | 80 (31.3 %) | 0.11 |
| Anti-phospholipid antibodies | 192 (24.0 %) | 80 (31.3 %) | 0.02 |
| Cardiolipin IgM | 115 (63.2 %) | 50 (69.4 %) | 0.351 |
| Cardiolipin IgG | 78 (41.5 %) | 27 (34.2 %) | 0.26 |
| β$_2$-glycoprotein | 59 (32.8 %) | 25 (33.3 %) | 0.93 |
| Lupus anti-coagulant | 15 (2.4 %) | 11 (5.0 %) | 0.056 |

*Abbreviations: ANA* Anti-nuclear antibody, *Anti-Scl-70* Anti-scleroderma-70 antibodies, *Anti-RNP* Anti-ribonucleoprotein antibodies, *Anti-Sm* Anti-Smith antibodies, *Anti-PM-Scl* Anti-polymyositis scleroderma antibodies, *Anti-dsDNA* Anti-double-stranded DNA antibodies, *Anti-RNAP* Anti-RNA polymerase antibodies, *ANCA* Anti-neutrophil cytoplasmic antibodies, *MPO* Myeloperoxidase, *PR-3* Proteinase-3, *Ig* Immunoglobulin, *SLE* Systemic lupus erythematosus
[a]Ever from disease onset to most recent visit

activity when applied across the entire cohort of patients with SSc. However, to our knowledge, this is the first study to demonstrate that hypocomplementaemia is a marker of the presence of certain SSc disease features measured at each visit among the subset of patients with overlap disease features. These disease features include digital ulcers, tendon friction rubs, low BMI and low FVC, all of which are clinical features of SSc disease

**Table 5** Univariable associations of hypocomplementaemia with clinical manifestations, treatment, European Scleroderma Study Group disease activity score and physician global assessments

| Characteristic | Persistent normocomplementaemia (n = 859) | At least one episode of hypocomplementaemia (n = 275) | |
|---|---|---|---|
| | n (%) or mean ± SD or median (IQR) | n (%) or mean ± SD or median (IQR) | p Value |
| Disease manifestation[a] | | | |
| Raynaud's phenomenon | 803 (93.5 %) | 262 (95.6 %) | 0.19 |
| BMI <20 kg/m$^2$ | 104 (13.0 %) | 54 (20.5 %) | 0.0030 |
| Digital ulcers | 263 (30.7 %) | 82 (30.0 %) | 0.848 |
| Digital gangrene/amputation | 76 (8.8 %) | 17 (6.2 %) | 0.17 |
| Telangiectasia | 716 (83.6 %) | 231 (84.6 %) | 0.68 |
| Calcinosis | 340 (39.7 %) | 99 (36.3 %) | 0.31 |
| Scleroderma | 565 (66.2 %) | 198 (72.8 %) | 0.044 |
| Tendon friction rub | 88 (10.3 %) | 24 (8.8 %) | 0.47 |
| Joint contracture | 332 (38.9 %) | 99 (36.4 %) | 0.46 |
| Synovitis | 241 (28.3 %) | 82 (30.0 %) | 0.59 |
| Muscle atrophy | 147 (17.2 %) | 63 (23.2 %) | 0.029 |
| MRSS >20 | 158 (18.7 %) | 49 (18.0 %) | 0.81 |
| Myocardial disease | 70 (8.1 %) | 17 (6.2 %) | 0.30 |
| Pericardial effusion | 45 (5.3 %) | 25 (9.1 %) | 0.023 |
| PAH | 90 (10.4 %) | 30 (10.9 %) | 0.82 |
| Pulmonary fibrosis | 263 (30.8 %) | 77 (30.1 %) | 0.40 |
| Gastrointestinal involvement | 493 (57.5 %) | 145 (52.7 %) | 0.17 |
| GAVE | 86 (10.1 %) | 27 (9.9 %) | 0.94 |
| Reflux oesophagitis | 722 (83.8 %) | 236 (85.8 %) | 0.41 |
| Oesophageal stricture | 109 (12.8 %) | 23 (8.4 %) | 0.051 |
| Oesophageal dysmotility | 346 (40.5 %) | 111 (40.8 %) | 0.92 |
| Bowel dysmotility | 226 (26.4 %) | 71 (25.9 %) | 0.88 |
| Pseudo-obstruction | 25 (2.9 %) | 12 (4.4 %) | 0.23 |
| Renal crises | 36 (4.2 %) | 8 (2.9 %) | 0.34 |
| eGFR <60 ml/minute | 229 (22.8 %) | 68 (25.0 %) | 0.55 |
| Myositis | 37 (5.2 %) | 21 (8.5 %) | 0.055 |
| CRP >8 mg/L | 266 (31.1 %) | 67 (24.9 %) | 0.051 |
| ESR >30 mm/h | 252 (29.6 %) | 71 (26.1 %) | 0.27 |
| Blood CK >200 IU/L | 105 (12.1 %) | 44 (16.0 %) | 0.098 |
| Anaemia | 302 (35.1 %) | 101 (36.7 %) | 0.62 |
| FVC <80 % | 225 (26.9 %) | 73 (27.0 %) | 0.97 |
| DLCO <80 % | 631 (80.5 %) | 201 (78.2 %) | 0.43 |
| Treatment[a] | | | |
| Corticosteroids | 380 (43.9 %) | 126 (45.8 %) | 0.58 |
| Immunotherapy | 364 (42.1 %) | 131 (47.6 %) | 0.11 |
| Biologic therapy | 9 (1.0 %) | 7 (2.6 %) | 0.065 |
| Home oxygen | 32 (3.7 %) | 9 (3.3 %) | 0.74 |
| EScSG score[b] | 2.5 (1.4) | 2 (1–4) | 0.16 |
| Physician global assessments[b] | | | |
| Health | 4 (3–6) | 4 (3–6) | 0.25 |
| Activity | 3 (2–5) | 3 (2–5) | 0.076 |
| Damage | 4 (2.5–6) | 4 (3–6) | 0.44 |

*Abbreviations: MRSS* Modified Rodnan skin score, *EScSG* European Scleroderma Study Group, *PAH* Pulmonary arterial hypertension, *ILD* Interstitial lung disease, *GAVE* Gastric antral vascular ectasia, *BMI* Body mass index, *eGFR* Estimated glomerular filtration rate, *CRP* C-reactive protein, *ESR* Erythrocyte sedimentation rate, *CK* Creatinine kinase, *FVC* Forced vital capacity, *DLCO* Diffusing capacity of the lung for carbon monoxide corrected for haemoglobin
[a]Ever from disease onset to most recent visit
[b]Mean score from all visits

**Table 6** Multivariable associations of hypocomplementaemia with features of disease activity at each visit among the whole cohort and analysis subsets determined using generalised estimating equations

| Parameter | Whole cohort (n = 886; 1893 visits) | | SSc with features of overlap disease (n = 221;628 visits) | | SSc without features of overlap disease (n = 665; 1265 visits) | |
|---|---|---|---|---|---|---|
| | Odds ratio (95 % CI) | p Value | Odds ratio (95 % CI) | p Value | Odds ratio (95 % CI) | p Value |
| Self-reported worsening of cardiopulmonary, vascular or skin symptoms[a] | 1.05 (0.57–1.94) | 0.87 | 1.24 (0.48–3.18) | 0.66 | 1.03 (0.45–2.35) | 0.94 |
| Digital ulcers/necrosis[a] | 1.15 (0.84–1.56) | 0.38 | 1.62 (1.04–2.51) | 0.034 | 0.82 (0.53–1.27) | 0.37 |
| Scleroderma[a] | 0.97 (0.76–1.23) | 0.78 | 1.08 (0.75–1.58) | 0.67 | 0.87 (0.63–1.18) | 0.37 |
| Tendon friction rubs[a] | 1.15 (0.64–2.08) | 0.64 | 2.31 (1.05–5.10) | 0.037 | 0.54 (0.19–1.53) | 0.24 |
| Synovitis/arthritis[a] | 0.95 (0.69–1.31) | 0.76 | 1.18 (0.73–1.91) | 0.50 | 0.80 (0.51–1.25) | 0.32 |
| Modified Rodnan skin score >14[a] | 0.98 (0.96–0.99) | 0.013 | 0.97 (0.95–1.01) | 0.087 | 0.98 (0.96–1.01) | 0.16 |
| Erythrocyte sedimentation rate >30 mm/h[a] | 0.98 (0.98–0.99) | 0.022 | 0.99 (0.99–1.01) | 0.97 | 0.99 (0.97–0.99) | 0.026 |
| DLCO <80 % predicted[a] | 0.81 (0.61–1.09) | 0.17 | 1.14 (0.66–1.96) | 0.65 | 0.72 (0.51–1.03) | 0.073 |
| C-reactive protein >8 mg/L[a] | 1.01 (0.99–1.01) | 0.90 | 0.97 (0.93–1.01) | 0.073 | 1.01 (0.99–1.01) | 0.41 |
| BMI[b] | 0.91 (0.88–0.94) | <0.0005 | 0.90 (0.85–0.95) | <0.0005 | 0.91 (0.87–0.95) | <0.0005 |
| FVC <80 % predicted[b] | 1.24 (0.78–1.97) | 0.37 | 2.90 (1.32–6.38) | 0.0080 | 0.87 (0.47–1.61) | 0.65 |

*Abbreviations: BMI* Body mass index, *FVC* forced vital capacity, *DLCO* Diffusing capacity of the lung for carbon monoxide corrected for haemoglobin
All variables listed in the table were included in the final multivariable generalised estimating equation model
[a]Components of European Scleroderma Study Group disease activity index
[b]Additional disease activity variables entered into multivariable regression model on the basis of significance in univariable analysis

activity or severity. This in turn suggests a role for measurement of C3 and C4 in assessment and monitoring of disease activity in patients with overlap SSc.

We found that the prevalence of hypocomplementaemia at recruitment was 13.2 %, which is consistent with previous smaller studies [22, 23]. The finding that hypocomplementaemia is associated with the presence of overlap disease features in SSc is also consistent with trends identified by Hudson et al. in a cohort of 321 Canadian patients with SSc [23]. This suggests that complement consumption plays a significant role in the etiopathogenesis of SSc overlap disease.

Several small studies have cited a role for abnormal complement activation in SSc. Senaldi et al. found that the levels of serum complement fragments Ba, C3d and C4d were higher in patients with diffuse SSc than in patients with limited SSc and that both subtypes had serum complement fragment levels higher than those of normal patients, suggesting that complement consumption occurs in SSc and may also be related to disease activity and/or severity [24]. Batal et al. undertook a study of prognostic factors in systemic sclerosis renal crisis (SRC) in which they retrospectively analysed renal biopsies. They found that peritubular capillary C4d deposition was higher in patients with SRC than in both hypertensive non-SRC and normotensive non-SRC control subjects and suggested a role for immune complex- and antibody-mediated injury in SRC [25]. Whilst in vivo activation of the complement system in SSc remains a possibility, the general consensus is that complement consumption does not play a significant role in the pathophysiology of SSc and that therefore

the presence of hypocomplementaemia in SSc signifies the presence of another overlapping disease. This is consistent with the results of our study, which demonstrated a significant association between hypocomplementaemia and the presence of SSc overlap disease, in particular polymyositis. However, it is intriguing to note that even among patients with overlap disease, low serum complement was associated with disease features classically associated with SSc itself, such as digital ulcers and tendon friction rubs.

Hypocomplementaemia is one of the ten variables listed in the EScSG disease activity index [26, 27]. However, its inclusion has been a point of controversy. In the present study, we were unable to demonstrate a consistent association between hypocomplementaemia and either the EScSG disease activity score (calculated on the basis of nine non-complement variables to avoid over-correlation between independent variables) or any of its component variables in the univariable analysis. In addition, the associations found in the multivariable analysis in the subset of patients with SSc without overlap disease features (non-overlap SSc) suggest that, compared with normo-complementaemic patients, hypocomplementaemic patients have lower EScSG disease activity scores and ESR levels, which is the opposite of what one might expect. This lack of expected correlation with SSc disease activity measures suggests that hypocomplementaemia is not a measure of disease activity in the majority of patients with SSc, which is consistent with the conclusions drawn from previous studies [23]. Only one study suggested the contrary. Cuomo et al. reported the associations between hypocomplementaemia and clinical status in a cohort of 302 Italian patients with SSc and excluded patients with overlap disease features. They found that 16.5 % of their cohort had hypocomplementaemia and that hypocomplementaemia was associated with significantly increased disease activity, significantly increased severity of disease manifestations in the skin, cardiovascular and respiratory systems, and greater functional disability [22]. However, it is unclear whether the results of their study are generalizable to other SSc cohorts, because there was a very high prevalence of patients with anti-Scl-70 and anti-centromere ANA. The latter autoantibodies in particular have been suggested to play a role in complement activation [28].

The lack of association between hypocomplementaemia and other potential markers of disease activity in the EScSG disease activity index may also speak to the latter's not being a very good measure of 'disease activity' per se. A trend toward a significant difference in the physician global assessment of disease activity between the persistently normocomplementaemic and the hypocomplementaemic groups ($p = 0.076$) supports this statement. However, it is also possible that each item in the EScSG disease activity index measures disease activity independently of all other items. Furthermore, it must be noted that functional abnormalities in complement in SSc may occur in the absence of hypocomplementaemia.

To our knowledge, this is the first study to use GEE methods to definitively show that hypocomplementaemia is associated with some features of disease activity in patients with SSc who have overlap disease features. We found that within this subset of patients with SSc, those who were hypocomplementaemic were more likely to manifest digital ulcers, tendon friction rubs, an FVC <80 % predicted and a lower BMI at each visit, all of which are well-established features of disease activity and severity in non-overlap SSc itself. No association was found with either CRP or ESR, possibly because these inflammatory markers generally are not considered to be good measures of disease activity in SSc. In particular, it has been shown that CRP levels are not elevated in most patients with SSc and that CRP levels regress as disease duration increases [29].

This study is not without limitations. As patients had varying lengths of follow-up, some had more annual complement measurements than others, making it possible that there was a low complement reading by chance alone on one or more occasions. However, the use of GEEs for statistical analysis overcomes this issue to a degree because it enables hypocomplementaemia at each visit to be associated with disease features at that particular visit, eliminating the need to divide patients into subgroups based on arbitrary definitions such as hypocomplementaemia ever, persistent hypocomplementaemia and persistent normocomplementaemia.

## Conclusions

In this study, we have shown that hypocomplementaemia in SSc is associated with the presence of SSc overlap features, in particular SSc-polymyositis overlap syndrome. We have also confirmed the results of previous studies by showing that hypocomplementaemia is not a measure of disease activity in non-overlap SSc cohorts. However, to our knowledge, this is the first study to show that hypocomplementaemia is associated with features of disease activity in SSc overlap disease and that, in these patients, the measurement of complement levels is potentially useful for monitoring disease activity and response to treatment.

**Abbreviations**
ANA: Anti-nuclear antibodies; ANCA: Anti-neutrophil cytoplasmic antibodies; Anti-dsDNA: Anti-double-stranded DNA; Anti-PM-Scl: Anti-polymyositis scleroderma antibodies; Anti-RNAP: Anti-RNA polymerase antibodies; Anti-Scl-70: Anti-scleroderma-70 antibodies; Anti-Sm: Anti-Smith; Anti-U1 RNP: Anti-ribonucleoprotein antibodies; BMI: Body mass index; CK: Creatine kinase; CRP: C-reactive protein; DLCO: Diffusing capacity of the lung for carbon monoxide; eGFR: Estimated glomerular filtration rate; ELISA: Enzyme-linked immunosorbent assay; EScSG: European Scleroderma Study Group; ESR: Erythrocyte sedimentation rate; FVC: Forced vital capacity; GAVE: Gastric antral vascular ectasia; GEE: Generalised estimating equation; Ig: Immunoglobulin; ILD: Interstitial lung disease; MPO: Myeloperoxidase; MRSS: Modified Rodnan skin score; PAH: Pulmonary arterial hypertension; PIIINP: Type III procollagen aminopeptide; PR-3: Proteinase-3 specificity; RNA Pol: RNA polymerase; RNP: Ribonucleoprotein; sIL-2R: Soluble interleukin-2 receptor; SLE: Systemic lupus erythematosus; SRC: Systemic sclerosis renal crisis; SSc: Systemic sclerosis; TLR: Toll-like receptor

**Acknowledgements**
We thank Dr Peter Youssef, Dr Alan Sturgess, Dr Fiona Kermeen, Dr Catherine Hill and Dr Peter Nash for contributing data.

**Funding**
MN holds a National Health and Medical Research Council fellowship (APP1071735). This work was supported by Scleroderma Australia, Arthritis Australia, Actelion Pharmaceuticals Australia, Bayer, CSL Behring, GlaxoSmithKline Australia and Pfizer.

**Authors' contributions**
JE designed the study, analysed the data, interpreted the results and prepared the manuscript. WS designed the study, collected data, interpreted the results and prepared the manuscript. ZB, CR, JS, JZ, JR, JW and SMP collected data, interpreted the results and prepared the manuscript. MN designed the study, collected and analysed data, interpreted the results and prepared the manuscript. All authors read and approved the final manuscript.

**Competing interests**
The authors declare that they have no competing interests.

## Author details

[1]Department of Medicine, The University of Melbourne at St Vincent's Hospital (Melbourne), 41 Victoria Parade, Fitzroy, VIC 3065, Australia. [2]Department of Rheumatology, St Vincent's Hospital (Melbourne), 41 Victoria Parade, Fitzroy, VIC 3065, Australia. [3]Department of Rheumatology, Monash Health and Monash University, 246 Clayton Road, Clayton, VIC 3168, Australia. [4]Department of Medicine, Monash Health and Monash University, 246 Clayton Road, Clayton, VIC 3168, Australia. [5]Department of Rheumatology, Menzies Institute for Medical Research, Private Bag 23, Hobart, TAS 7001, Australia. [6]Department of Rheumatology, Royal Perth Hospital, 197 Wellington Street, GPO Box X2213, Perth, WA 6001, Australia. [7]Department of Rheumatology, Flinders Medical Centre, Flinders Drive, Bedford Park, SA 5042, Australia. [8]Rheumatology Unit, Royal Adelaide Hospital, North Terrace, Adelaide, SA 5000, Australia. [9]Discipline of Medicine, University of Adelaide, Adelaide, SA 5000, Australia.

## References

1. Nikpour M, Stevens WM, Herrick AL, Proudman SM. Epidemiology of systemic sclerosis. Best Pract Res Clin Rheumatol. 2010;24(6):857–69.
2. Gabrielli A, Avvedimento EV, Krieg T. Scleroderma. N Engl J Med. 2009; 360(19):1989–2003.
3. Medsger Jr TA. Natural history of systemic sclerosis and the assessment of disease activity, severity, functional status, and psychologic well-being. Rheum Dis Clin North Am. 2003;29(2):255–73.
4. Symmons DPM. Disease assessment indexes: activity, damage and severity. Baillieres Clin Rheumatol. 1995;9(2):267–85.
5. Gladman DD, Ibañez D, Urowitz MB. Systemic Lupus Erythematosus Disease Activity Index 2000. J Rheumatol. 2002;29(2):288–91.
6. Valentini G, Silman AJ, Veale D. Assessment of disease activity. Clin Exp Rheumatol. 2003;21(3 Suppl 29):S39–41.
7. Della Rossa A, Valentini G, Bombardieri S, Bencivelli W, Silman AJ, D'Angelo S, et al. European multicentre study to define disease activity criteria for systemic sclerosis. I. Clinical and epidemiological features of 290 patients from 19 centres. Ann Rheum Dis. 2001;60(6):585–91.
8. Valentini G, Della Rossa A, Bombardieri S, Bencivelli W, Silman AJ, D'Angelo S, et al. European multicentre study to define disease activity criteria for systemic sclerosis. II. Identification of disease activity variables and development of preliminary activity indexes. Ann Rheum Dis. 2001;60(6):592–8.
9. Scheja A, Akesson A, Horslev-Petersen K. Serum levels of aminoterminal type III procollagen peptide and hyaluronan predict mortality in systemic sclerosis. Scand J Rheumatol. 1992;21:5–9.
10. Steen VD, Engel EE, Charley MR, Medsger Jr TA. Soluble serum interleukin 2 receptors in patients with systemic sclerosis. J Rheumatol. 1996;23(4):646–9.
11. Vischer U, Ingerslev J, Wollheim C, Mestries JC, Tsakiris D, Haefeli W, et al. Acute von Willebrand factor secretion from the endothelium in vivo: assessment through plasma propeptide (vWf:AgII) levels. Thromb Haemost. 1997;77:387–93.
12. Clements PJ, Peter JB, Agopian MS, Telian NS, Furst DE. Elevated serum levels of soluble interleukin 2 receptor, interleukin 2 and neopterin in diffuse and limited scleroderma: effects of chlorambucil. J Rheumatol. 1990;17(7):908–10.
13. Stevens W, Vancheeswaran R. Black CM; UK Systemic Sclerosis Study Group. Alpha interferon-2a (Roferon-A) in the treatment of diffuse cutaneous systemic sclerosis: a pilot study. Br J Rheumatol. 1992;31(10):683–9.
14. Chen M, Daha MR, Kallenberg CGM. The complement system in systemic autoimmune disease. J Autoimmun. 2010;34(3):J276–86.
15. Valentijn RM, van Overhagen H, Hazevoet HM, Hermans J, Cats A, Daha MR, et al. The value of complement and immune complex determinations in monitoring disease activity in patients with systemic lupus erythematosus. Arthritis Rheum. 1985;28(8):904–13.
16. Sturfelt G, Sjoholm AG. Complement components, complement activation, and acute phase response in systemic lupus erythematosus. Arthritis Care Res (Hoboken). 1984;75(1):75–83.
17. Bhattacharyya S, Varga J. Emerging roles of innate immune signaling and Toll-like receptors in fibrosis and systemic sclerosis. Curr Rheumatol Rep. 2015;17(1):474.
18. van den Hoogen F, Khanna D, Fransen J, Johnson SR, Baron M, Tyndall A, et al. 2013 classification criteria for systemic sclerosis: an American College of Rheumatology/European League Against Rheumatism collaborative initiative. Arthritis Rheum. 2013;65(11):2737–47.
19. LeRoy EC, Medsger Jr TA. Criteria for the classification of early systemic sclerosis. J Rheumatol. 2001;28(7):1573–6.
20. Clements P, Lachenbruch P, Siebold J, White B, Weiner S, Martin R, et al. Inter and intraobserver variability of total skin thickness score (modified Rodnan TSS) in systemic sclerosis. J Rheumatol. 1995;22(7):1281–5.
21. Ma Y, Mazumdar M, Memtsoudis SG. Beyond repeated-measures analysis of variance: advanced statistical methods for the analysis of longitudinal data in anesthesia research. Reg Anesth Pain Med. 2012;37(1):99–105.
22. Cuomo G, Abignano G, Ruocco L, Vettori S, Valentini G. Hypocomplementemia in systemic sclerosis [in Italian]. Reumatismo. 2008;60(4):268–73.
23. Hudson M, Walker JG, Fritzler M, Taillefer S, Baron M. Hypocomplementemia in systemic sclerosis - clinical and serological correlations. J Rheumatol. 2007;34(11):2218–23.
24. Senaldi G, Lupoli S, Vergani D, Black CM. Activation of the complement system in systemic sclerosis: relationship to clinical severity. Arthritis Rheum. 1989;32(10):1262–7.
25. Batal I, Domsic RT, Shafer A, Medsger Jr TA, Kiss LP, Randhawa P, et al. Renal biopsy findings predicting outcome in scleroderma renal crisis. Hum Pathol. 2009;40(3):332–40.
26. Valentini G, Bencivelli W, Bombardieri S, D'Angelo S, Della Rossa A, Silman AJ, et al. European Scleroderma Study Group to define disease activity criteria for systemic sclerosis. III. Assessment of the construct validity of the preliminary activity criteria. Ann Rheum Dis. 2003;62(9):901–3.
27. Valentini G, D'Angelo S, Della Rossa A, Bencivelli W, Bombardieri S. European Scleroderma Study Group to define disease activity criteria for systemic sclerosis. IV. Assessment of skin thickening by modified Rodnan skin score. Ann Rheum Dis. 2003;62(9):904–5.
28. Yuan J, Chen M, Zhao MH. Complement in antineutrophil cytoplasmic antibody-associated vasculitis. Clin Exp Nephrol. 2013;17(5):642–5.
29. Muangchan C, Harding S, Khimdas S, Bonner A, Group CSR, Baron M, Pope J. Association of C-reactive protein with high disease activity in systemic sclerosis: results from the Canadian Scleroderma Research Group. Arthritis Care Res (Hoboken). 2012;64(9):1405–14.

# Epstein-Barr virus lytic infection promotes activation of Toll-like receptor 8 innate immune response in systemic sclerosis monocytes

Antonella Farina[1,2], Giovanna Peruzzi[3], Valentina Lacconi[1], Stefania Lenna[1], Silvia Quarta[4], Edoardo Rosato[4], Anna Rita Vestri[5], Michael York[1], David H. Dreyfus[6], Alberto Faggioni[2], Stefania Morrone[2], Maria Trojanowska[1] and G. Alessandra Farina[1*] ⓘ

## Abstract

**Background:** Monocytes/macrophages are activated in several autoimmune diseases, including systemic sclerosis (scleroderma; SSc), with increased expression of interferon (IFN)-regulatory genes and inflammatory cytokines, suggesting dysregulation of the innate immune response in autoimmunity. In this study, we investigated whether the lytic form of Epstein-Barr virus (EBV) infection (infectious EBV) is present in scleroderma monocytes and contributes to their activation in SSc.

**Methods:** Monocytes were isolated from peripheral blood mononuclear cells (PBMCs) depleted of the CD19+ cell fraction, using CD14/CD16 negative-depletion. Circulating monocytes from SSc and healthy donors (HDs) were infected with EBV. Gene expression of innate immune mediators were evaluated in EBV-infected monocytes from SSc and HDs. Involvement of Toll-like receptor (TLR)8 in viral-mediated TLR8 response was investigated by comparing the TLR8 expression induced by infectious EBV to the expression stimulated by CL075/TLR8/agonist-ligand in the presence of TLR8 inhibitor in THP-1 cells.

**Results:** Infectious EBV strongly induced TLR8 expression in infected SSc and HD monocytes in vitro. Markers of activated monocytes, such as IFN-regulated genes and chemokines, were upregulated in SSc- and HD-EBV-infected monocytes. Inhibiting TLR8 expression reduced virally induced TLR8 in THP-1 infected cells, demonstrating that innate immune activation by infectious EBV is partially dependent on TLR8. Viral mRNA and proteins were detected in freshly isolated SSc monocytes. Microarray analysis substantiated the evidence of an increased IFN signature and altered level of TLR8 expression in SSc monocytes carrying infectious EBV compared to HD monocytes.

**Conclusion:** This study provides the first evidence of infectious EBV in monocytes from patients with SSc and links EBV to the activation of TLR8 and IFN innate immune response in freshly isolated SSc monocytes. This study provides the first evidence of EBV replication activating the TLR8 molecular pathway in primary monocytes. Immunogenicity of infectious EBV suggests a novel mechanism mediating monocyte inflammation in SSc, by which EBV triggers the innate immune response in infected cells.

**Keywords:** Systemic sclerosis, EBV reactivation, Monocytes, Toll-like receptor 8, Innate immune response, IFN inducible genes

* Correspondence: farina@bu.edu
[1]Rheumatology, Boston University School of Medicine, Arthritis Center, 72 E. Concord Street, E-5, Boston, MA 02118, USA
Full list of author information is available at the end of the article

# Background

Systemic sclerosis (scleroderma; SSc) is a complex auto-immune disease characterized by immune abnormalities, vascular damage, and fibrosis predominantly involving the skin and lungs [1]. An aberrant innate immune response is suspected to activate both immune and non-immune effector cells in SSc, as evidenced by the presence of an interferon (IFN) signature in the affected tissues and the genetic predisposition toward genes linked to the IFN pathways [2, 3].

Monocytes/macrophages are known to play a crucial role in the innate immune process [4]. These cells have been found in SSc tissues, suggesting that monocytes/macrophages might be involved in the pathogenesis of the disease [5, 6]. Abnormalities in monocytes have been documented in SSc [7]. Studies have shown increased expression of several IFN-regulatory genes, including sialic acid-binding Ig-like lectin 1 Siglec1/CD169 (Siglec1), a marker of activated monocytes/macrophages, and numerous monocyte inflammatory cytokines in peripheral blood mononuclear cells (PBMCs) and sera from SSc patients, implicating dysregulation of the innate immune response in the activation of these cells [8–11]. However, what triggers and sustains monocyte activation in SSc remains unclear.

Although innate immunity is classically viewed as a first line of resistance against pathogens, little is known about pathogens as the source of the innate immune activation in SSc [12]. The expression of Epstein-Barr virus (EBV) lytic mRNA and proteins in PBMCs and skin of SSc patients has been associated with aberrant antibody response against EBV lytic antigens [13, 14], suggesting that EBV dysregulation may be more prevalent in SSc patients. The lytic form of EBV infection (infectious EBV) is detected by the host innate immune system. In this regard, monocytes have been shown to detect unmethylated viral genomes by Toll-like receptor (TLR)9 [15], suggesting that these cells participate in the innate immune control of EBV. Given these observations, we sought to investigate whether EBV infection in monocytes might contribute to their activation in SSc. Here, we demonstrate that EBV replicates in primary human monocytes several days post-infection (PI), and viral lytic genes strongly induce TLR8 expression and activation of the innate immune response in healthy donor (HD) and SSc monocytes infected with EBV. The presence of infectious EBV in SSc is substantiated by detecting the expression of EBV lytic mRNA and proteins in freshly isolated SSc monocytes, while it is absent in monocytes from HDs. Using microarray analysis, we show that SSc monocytes carrying infectious EBV exhibit a robust induction of the IFN signature and altered level of TLR8 expression compared to HDs. Our results suggest that monocyte activation in SSc may be a result of aberrantly controlled EBV infection.

# Methods
## Study subjects

All study subjects met the criteria for SSc as defined previously [16]. All subjects gave written informed consent. Subjects selected for this study, diffuse cutaneous SSc (dcSSc) patients ($n = 53$) and normal healthy donors (HD) ($n = 34$), are summarized in Table 1. All the patients and HDs included in the study were positive for EBV serology. All dcSSc patients included in the study were naïve for immunosuppressive therapy (IT) or >6 months free of IT. Due to the variable number of PBMCs and monocytes obtained from the patients and controls, sets of experiments performed on the same subjects are indicated in Table 1.

## PBMC and monocyte isolation

Blood was collected from EBV-seropositive HD and dcSSc patients in CPT tubes designed for one-step cell separation (Becton Dickinson), and PBMCs were isolated as previously described [9]. After positive selection of CD19 cells (CD19+) using magnetic bead isolation (CD19+ selection EasySep, StemCell), monocytes were negatively selected using the Human Monocyte Enrichment Kit without CD16 Depletion (EasySep, StemCell). Purity of the monocyte population was determined by detection of CD163, CD16, and CD19 mRNA expression and using flow cytometry for the surface markers CD14 and CD163 (BD Pharmingen) (Additional file 1: Figure S1A and B).

## Virus preparation and EBV infection of monocytes and THP-1 cells

Viral stocks were obtained from culture supernatants of recombinant EBV-wt B95.8 genomes stably transfected

**Table 1** Clinical and demographic characteristics of the subjects enrolled in the study

|  | dcSSc* | HD |
|---|---|---|
| Number of subjects, n | 53 | 34 |
| Age in years, mean ± SE (range) | 44 ± 1.8 (23–71) | 41 ± 2.7 (23–65) |
| Female, % | 96 | 94 |
| mRSS**, mean ± SE | 17 ± 0.7 | – |
| Monocytes infected with recombinant EBV (qPCR, Western blot and immunofluorescence staining experiments), n | 14 | 8 |
| Monocytes freshly isolated (RT-PCR for DNA, qPCR, Western blot and immunostaining experiments), n | 8 | 6 |
| PBMCs (FACS analysis experiments), n | 13 | 12 |
| Skin biopsies (immunostaining experiments), n | 18 | 8 |

*Inclusion criteria: disease duration <5 years; patients naïve for immunosuppressive therapy (IT) or >6 months free of IT
dcSSc diffuse cutaneous systemic sclerosis, EBV Epstein-Barr virus, HD healthy donor, mRSS modified Rodnan Skin Score, PBMC peripheral blood mononuclear cell, qPCR quantitative polymerase chain reaction, RT-PCR real-time polymerase chain reaction, SE standard error

into 293 cells (293-p2089) as previously described [13]. Before infection, monocytes from SSc patients and HDs were prepared by UV irradiation at 230 mW/cm$^2$, using a Stratalinker XL1500 (Stratagene, Agilent technologies, Santa Clara, CA, USA). Given that human promyelomonocytic THP-1 cells (ATCC TIB-202) are an EBV-negative cell line, UV treatment was not performed on the cells primed for EBV infection. Monocytes and THP-1 cells were seeded at a density of $5 \times 10^4$ cells/well in complete RPMI 1640 medium supplemented with 10% fetal bovine serum (FBS), and infected or mock infected with p2089-wtEBV as previously described [13].

### Cell treatment and reagents

Cells were seeded as indicated above; TLR-agonist stimulation was performed in complete medium with the following ligands (1 µg/ml): R837/imiquimod and CL264/9-benzyl-8-hydroxyadenine (for TLR7), CL075-thiazoloquinoline (for TLR8) (all from Invitrogen, Grand Island, NY, USA), IFNβ (500 U/ml; PBLinterferone), IFNγ (500 U/ml), and tumor necrosis factor (TNF)α (10 ng/ml) (all from R&D Systems). After 24 h of incubation, cells were harvested and stored in RNA lysis buffer for subsequent RNA isolation. When indicated, cells were treated for 24 h with CL075 or infected with EBV in the presence or absence of Bafilomycin-A1 (20 nM) (Sigma-Aldrich, St. Louis, MO, USA). At the indicated times PI or after ligand stimulation, proteins were harvested and analyzed by Western blot analysis.

### Nucleic acid extraction, RNA preparation and real-time polymerase chain reaction

DNA was extracted from monocytes using the Qiagen Extraction Kit (Qiagen, Valencia, CA, USA) and processed as previously described [13].

Total RNA from monocytes and B lymphocytes was extracted using an miRNAsy kit according to the manufacturer's protocol (Quiagen) and processed as previously described [13]. The synthesized cDNAs were used as templates for quantitative real-time polymerase chain reaction (PCR) and primers used as described before [2, 13]. All real-time PCR was carried out using StepOnePlus Sequence Detector (Applied Biosystems, Life Technologies, Grand Island, NY, USA). The change in the relative expression of each gene was calculated using the ΔΔCt formula choosing a healthy human subject [2]. Target and control reactions were run on separate wells of the same quantitative PCR plate [2].

### Quantitative real-time PCR primers

Primers used to detect EBV genes and innate immune mediator genes were designed using Primer Express software (Applied Biosystems) and synthesized by Integrated DNA Technologies. The primers used for quanititative PCR, including 18S endogenous control, are summarized in Additional file 2 (Table S1). Expression of mRNA for the indicated genes was detected using SYBRGreen chemistry amplification (Applied Biosystems) as previously described [13]. To ensure specificity of the primer set, amplicons generated from the PCR reaction were analyzed for specific melting temperatures by using the melting curve software. For MCP1/CCL2, Siglec1, CXCL10, IRF5, IRF7, OAS3, TLR2, TLR3, TLR4, TLR7, TLR9, Myd88, IL-6, CD19, TNFα, LY6E, and 18S TaqMan primers and probe were used (Applied Biosystems).

### Microarray analysis

Microarray analysis of RNA (200 ng) was performed using standard protocols on Affymetrix Human Gene 2.0 ST arrays at the Boston University Microarray Core. All procedures were performed as described in the Affymetrix GeneChip user manual (www.affymetrix.com). CEL files were normalized to produce gene-level expression values using the implementation of the Robust Multiarray Average (RMA) in the affy package (version 1.36.1). Array quality was assessed by computing relative log expression (RLE) and normalized unscaled standard error (NUSE) using the affyPLM package (version 1.34.0). Differential expression was assessed using the moderated (empirical Bayesian) t test implemented in the limma package (version 3.14.4). Correction for multiple hypothesis testing was accomplished using the Benjamini-Hochberg false discovery rate (FDR). All microarray analyses were performed using the R environment for statistical computing (version 2.15.1).

### Western blot analysis

Monocytes were collected and washed with phosphate-buffered saline (PBS). Cell pellets were suspended in 2× SDS-Page buffer. Samples (30 µg) were heat denatured with reducing agent. Cellular extracts and blotted proteins were prepared and probed as previously described [13]. Blotted proteins were probed with each primary monoclonal antibody (mAb) respectively for BFRF1 [17, 18], BFLF2 [19], Zta/Zebra (Argene, bioMérieux, Inc. Durham, NC, USA), phospho-IRF7 (Cell Signaling Technology, Danvers, MA, USA), IRF7 (Abcam, Cambridge, MA, USA), TLR8 (Cell Signaling), and anti-β-actin-antibody (Sigma), and then probed with secondary antibody and visualized using a super signal chemiluminescence kit (Thermo Scientific, Pittsburg, PA, USA).

### Cytofluorimetric analysis

PBMCs were labeled with conjugated mouse mAb against human CD14 (PE-Cy7), CD16 (APC), CD163 (PE), CD169/siglec1 (FITC), and CD19 (APC/FITC) (BD Pharmingen). After incubation with antibodies, the cells were washed and then fixed with 2% formaldehyde. Cytofluorimetric analysis was performed using a BD FACSCanto II flow cytometer (Becton Dickinson, Mountain

View, CA, USA). A total of 50,000 events were acquired for each sample. Data were processed using FlowJo software (Treestar, Inc., USA).

## Immunocytochemistry/immunohistochemistry

Monocytes were stained with mouse monoclonal antibodies against CD14-PE (BD Pharmingen), BFRF1 [18], gp-350-220 [13], rabbit TLR8 (Cell Signaling), and secondary-antibodies-Cy3-conjugated (Jackson IR, West Grove, PA, USA), Alexafluor-350 goat-anti mouse antibody (Invitrogen, Grand Island, NY, USA), or 488-labeling (Zenon kit; Invitrogen). Coverslips were mounted using Vectashield with DAPI (Vector Laboratories, Burlingame, CA, USA) and immunofluorescence staining was examined using a FluoView FV10i confocal microscope system (Olympus, Center Valley, PA, USA) at 488 nm (green), 594 nm (red), and 405 nm (blue). Paraffin sections of skin tissues were stained using mouse mAb against CD163 (AbD Serotec, Raleigh, NC, USA) and Zta/Zebra (Argene, bioMérieux, Inc., Durham, NC, USA) as previously described [13]. Immunohistochemical staining was examined using the Olympus BH2 microscope.

## Statistical analysis

All data are expressed as the mean ± SEM. Statistical comparisons between groups were tested by two-tailed $t$ test. Significance was taken at $P \leq 0.05$.

## Results

### De novo EBV replication occurs in primary cultured monocytes infected with EBV-p2089

Monocytes have been identified as a potential target for EBV infection [15]. The EBV genome has been detected in monocyte/macrophages from patients with several diseases, including rheumatoid arthritis and coronary diseases, supporting the ability of EBV to infect these cells in vivo [20–22]. Based on these observations, we first sought to investigate whether SSc monocytes were also capable of sustaining EBV replication.

Circulating monocytes were isolated from HDs and SSc patients with diffuse cutaneous disease (dcSSc). UV-treated monocytes from 14 SSc patients and 8 HDs were infected with EBV recombinant virus (EBV-p2089). Active EBV infection was detected in monocytes from 11 SSc patients and 5 HD, while it did not occur in 3 SSc patients and 3 HDs 5 days PI (Fig. 1a and b). Specifically, we found that EBV/early-lytic (BFRF1) and EBV/late-lytic (BLLF1) genes were significantly upregulated in EBV-p2089-infected monocytes in the majority of dcSSc ($n = 11$) and HDs ($n = 5$), 5 days PI (Fig. 1a). Since the EBV/early-lytic BFRF1 protein is implicated in nucleo-capsid egress and EBV/late-lytic BLLF1/gp350-220 is expressed on the virion envelope and on EBV producer cells, these results indicate that de novo active viral infection occurs

in monocytes, and that most dcSSc and HD monocytes are able to sustain efficient EBV replication in vitro.

### EBV replication induces TLR8 and innate immune mediators in infected monocytes

Given that EBV replicates in primary cultured monocytes, we next evaluated whether infectious EBV might trigger the innate immune response in EBV-p2089-infected monocytes that were previously UV inactivated. De novo viral replication strongly induced expression of TLR8 mRNA in lytic-infected cells (Fig. 1c), and BFRF1/lytic protein was associated with monocytes expressing high levels of TLR8 (Fig. 1d), suggesting that induction of TLR8 occurs in EBV-infected monocytes. Given that TLR7 together with TLR8 represent the two nucleic acid receptors detecting ssRNA and that TLR3 recognizes dsRNA, we sought to evaluate whether TLR7 and/or TLR3 could also be induced by EBV in infected monocytes. Unexpectedly, EBV-lytic mRNAs did not increase TLR7 expression in the infected cells (Fig. 1e), while TLR3 was only induced in monocytes from two HDs and one dcSSc patient (Additional file 1: Figure S2A). Moreover, we also found that EBV-p2089 induced expression of TLR9 in monocytes from a few HDs and dcSSc patients (Additional file 1: Figure S2B), confirming the previous observation [23]. No significant induction of TLR2 was found in EBV-p2089-infected monocytes (Additional file 1: Figure S2C).

EBV exploits two modes of infection: latent state and lytic replication [24]. Further supporting the linkage between viral replication and activation of the innate immune response, TLR8 or TLR7 expression was not induced in monocytes latently infected by EBV, as confirmed by the lack of infectious EBV in the cells harboring EBV-p2089 DNA (Fig. 1f and g, and h showing one representative dcSSc patient and HD). Notably, the naive EBV genome was expressed in the majority of dcSSc (7/8) and in some (3/6) HD monocytes (Table 2), suggesting that the prevalence of EBV DNA is higher in monocytes from dcSSc patients compared to HDs. Together, these findings suggest that newly lytic EBV mRNA is detected by TLR8 in infected HD and dcSSc monocytes.

To further characterize the TLR8 innate immune response induced by viral/lytic genes, innate immune mediators were examined in EBV-p2089-infected monocytes. MyD88 and IRF7 mRNA, as well as IRF7 protein (phosphorylated and total), expression was induced in the majority of infected monocytes from dcSSc patients and HDs (Fig. 2a and b). Since IRF7 is required to induce the innate antiviral response characterized by IFNs, IFN-regulated genes, and inflammatory cytokines [25], we next determined whether lytic EBV might induce in EBV-p2089 infected monocytes the same inflammatory genes found to be upregulated in dcSSc monocytes. We found that expression of CXCL9, OAS3, Siglec1, and cytokines,

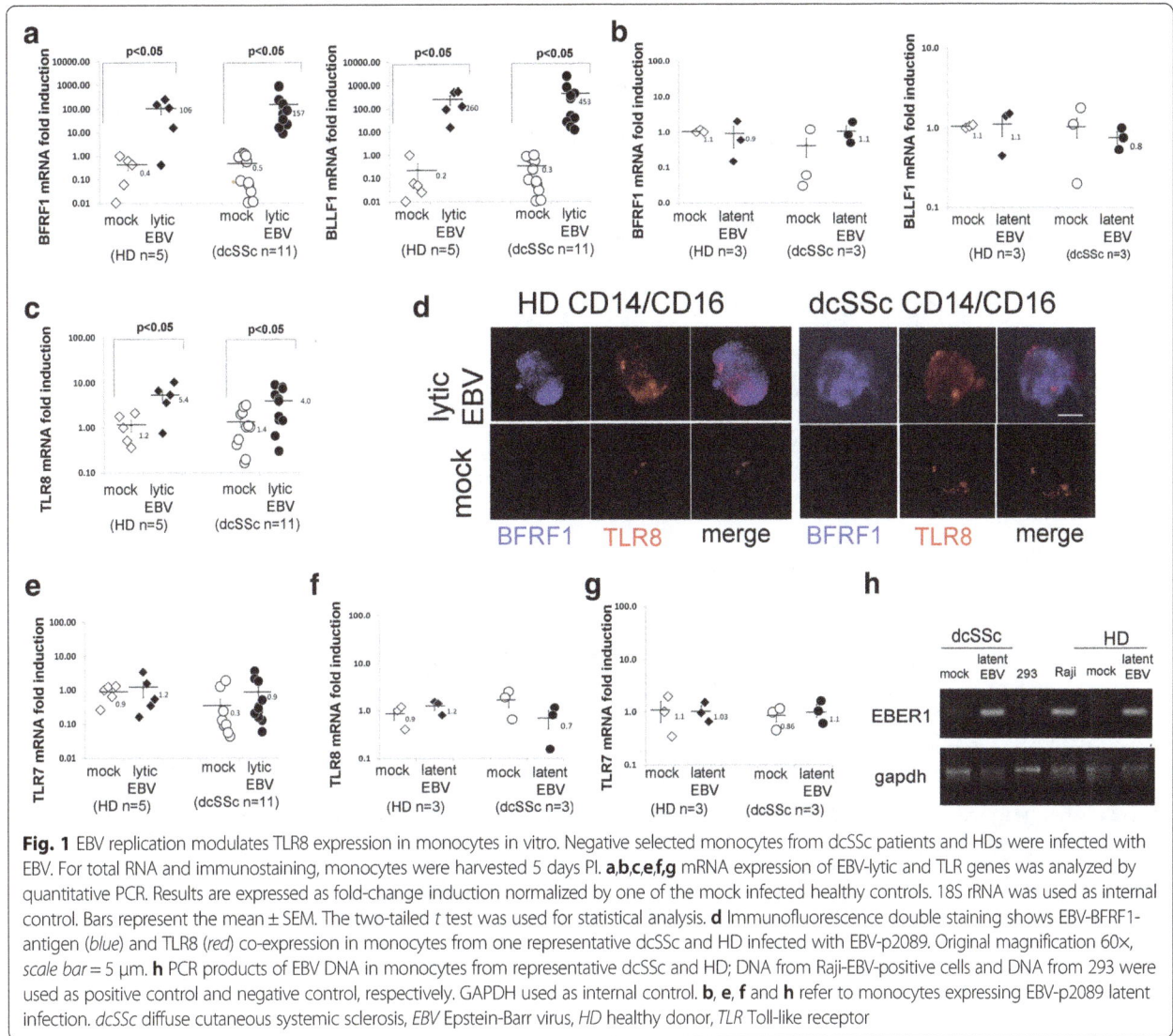

**Fig. 1** EBV replication modulates TLR8 expression in monocytes in vitro. Negative selected monocytes from dcSSc patients and HDs were infected with EBV. For total RNA and immunostaining, monocytes were harvested 5 days PI. **a,b,c,e,f,g** mRNA expression of EBV-lytic and TLR genes was analyzed by quantitative PCR. Results are expressed as fold-change induction normalized by one of the mock infected healthy controls. 18S rRNA was used as internal control. Bars represent the mean ± SEM. The two-tailed *t* test was used for statistical analysis. **d** Immunofluorescence double staining shows EBV-BFRF1-antigen (*blue*) and TLR8 (*red*) co-expression in monocytes from one representative dcSSc and HD infected with EBV-p2089. Original magnification 60×, *scale bar* = 5 μm. **h** PCR products of EBV DNA in monocytes from representative dcSSc and HD; DNA from Raji-EBV-positive cells and DNA from 293 were used as positive control and negative control, respectively. GAPDH used as internal control. **b**, **e**, **f** and **h** refer to monocytes expressing EBV-p2089 latent infection. *dcSSc* diffuse cutaneous systemic sclerosis, *EBV* Epstein-Barr virus, *HD* healthy donor, *TLR* Toll-like receptor

**Table 2** EBV gene expression and DNA in circulating monocytes and in skin macrophages of dcSSc patients

| EBV protein/DNA | Number of dcSSc patients positive/tested | Number of HDs positive/tested |
|---|---|---|
| BFRF1* (monocytes) | 3/8 | 0/6 |
| BFLF2* (monocytes) | 4/8 | 0/6 |
| EBER1 DNA** (monocytes) | 8/8 | 3/6 |
| EBER1 DNA** (B-lymphocytes) | 8/8 | 8/8 |
| BZLF1/Zebra monocytes mRNA *** | 4/8 | 0/6 |
| CD163+/macrophages*** | 6/18 | 0/8 |

*Tested by Western blot
**Tested by real-time polymerase chain reaction
***Tested by immunohistochemistry on skin sections
*dcSSc* diffuse cutaneous systemic sclerosis, *EBV* Epstein-Barr virus, *HD* healthy donor

including CCL2, TNFα, and interleukin (IL)-6, were robustly increased in EBV-p2089-infected monocytes (Fig. 2a). In contrast, no upregulation of innate immune mediators and proinflammatory cytokines was observed in latently infected monocytes (Fig. 2c and Additional file 1: Figure S3). To better appreciate the magnitude of innate immune mediators induced by infectious EBV in infected cells, in a parallel experiment, monocyte fractions not exposed to the virus were stimulated with CL075, a well-established TLR8/ligand positive control [26, 27]. We found that TLR8 ligand stimulation significantly induced the expression of Siglec1 and CCL2 genes in dcSSc and HD monocytes, comparable to the induction observed by infectious EBV in EBV-infected cells (Additional file 1: Figure S4). Statistically, no significant differences were observed in Siglec1 and CCL2 gene induction in TLR8-stimulated and EBV-infected monocytes.

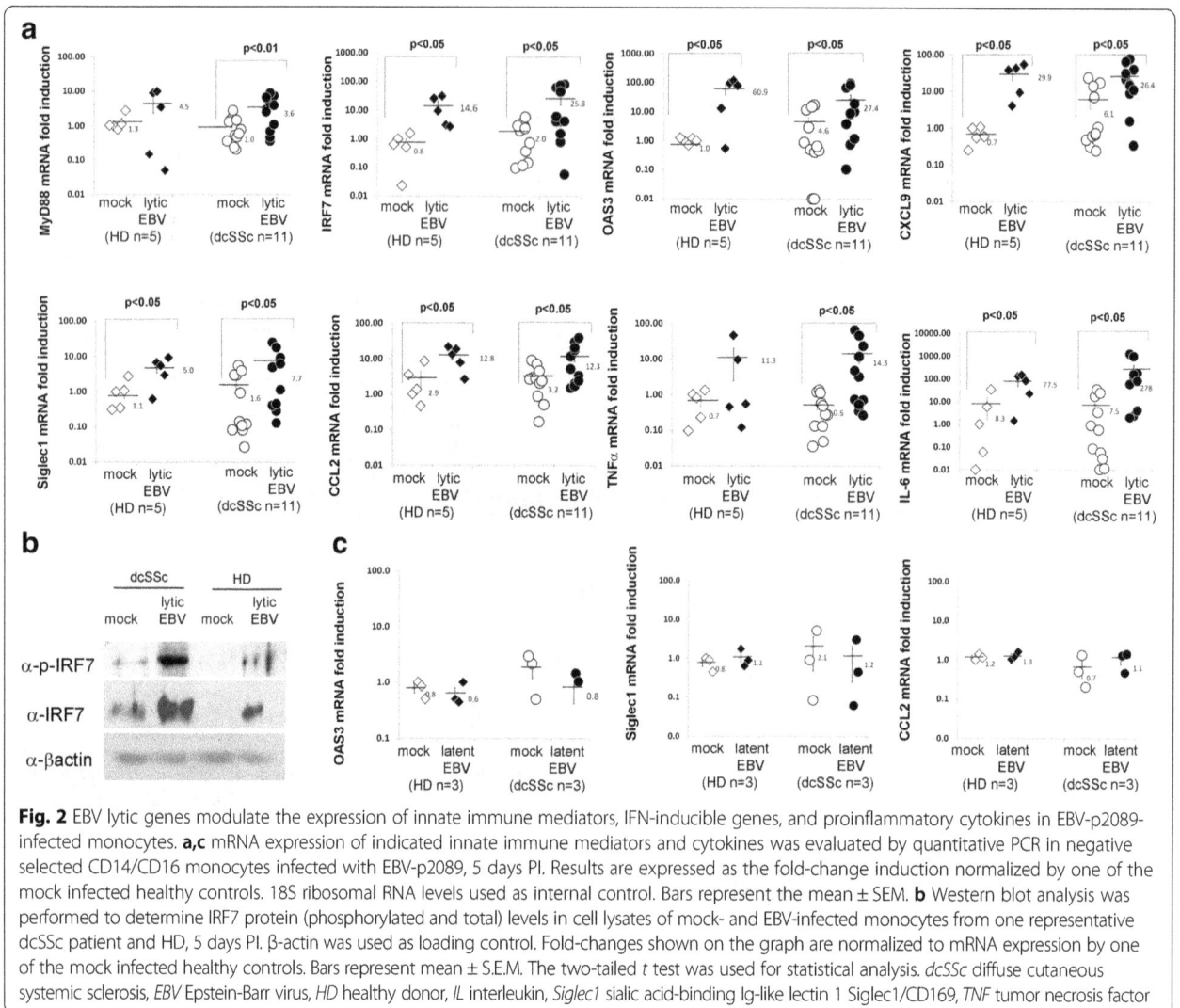

**Fig. 2** EBV lytic genes modulate the expression of innate immune mediators, IFN-inducible genes, and proinflammatory cytokines in EBV-p2089-infected monocytes. **a,c** mRNA expression of indicated innate immune mediators and cytokines was evaluated by quantitative PCR in negative selected CD14/CD16 monocytes infected with EBV-p2089, 5 days PI. Results are expressed as the fold-change induction normalized by one of the mock infected healthy controls. 18S ribosomal RNA levels used as internal control. Bars represent the mean ± SEM. **b** Western blot analysis was performed to determine IRF7 protein (phosphorylated and total) levels in cell lysates of mock- and EBV-infected monocytes from one representative dcSSc patient and HD, 5 days PI. β-actin was used as loading control. Fold-changes shown on the graph are normalized to mRNA expression by one of the mock infected healthy controls. Bars represent mean ± S.E.M. The two-tailed *t* test was used for statistical analysis. *dcSSc* diffuse cutaneous systemic sclerosis, *EBV* Epstein-Barr virus, *HD* healthy donor, *IL* interleukin, *Siglec1* sialic acid-binding Ig-like lectin 1 Siglec1/CD169, *TNF* tumor necrosis factor

Taken together, these results suggest that TLR8 expression and the innate immune inflammatory response are induced by de novo infectious EBV in EBV-infected dcSSc and control monocytes.

### Infectious EBV induces TLR8 protein expression in a TLR8-dependent and TLR8-independent manner in infected THP-1 cells

To elucidate the role of EBV in viral-mediated TLR8 signaling in monocytes, THP-1 monocytic cell line was infected with EBV-p2089. UV treatment did not induce TLR8 mRNA expression in THP-1 UV treated cells (Additional file 1: Figure S5). Given that THP-1 cells are negative for EBV genome expression, UV treatment was not performed on the cells primed for EBV infection. After the exposure to recombinant EBV, 10–20% cell/field of THP-1 cells showed cellular p2089-GFP fluorescence at 1 h PI (Fig. 3a). EBV gp-350/late-lytic proteins were expressed in 2–3% of the cells 1 h PI

(Fig. 3b). Kinetics of EBV infection showed a significant increase of the BFRF1/early-lytic gene over 2–24 h, while the LMP-1/latent gene was significantly induced up 72 h PI (Fig. 3c). Increased expression of TLR8 mRNA was induced in EBV-infected cells by 6 h with maximal induction at 24 h PI (Fig. 4a). In contrast, no induction of TLR8 mRNA was observed in latently infected cells at 72 h PI (Fig. 4a). TLR8 protein expression was also induced in THP-1-EBV-infected cells (Fig. 4b). In conjunction with TLR8, increased expression of IRF7 (phosphorylated and total) was also observed in THP-1-infected cells (Fig. 4b). Intriguingly, we found that IRF7 expression was also induced at 2 h PI, in agreement with the previous studies showing that EBV induces an early innate immune response in monocytes [21, 28].

Viral ssRNA has been identified as a natural agonist of TLR7 and TLR8 [27], and distinct RNA motifs selectively activate TLR7- and/or TLR8-mediated innate immune responses [26]. THP-1 cells were stimulated with TLR

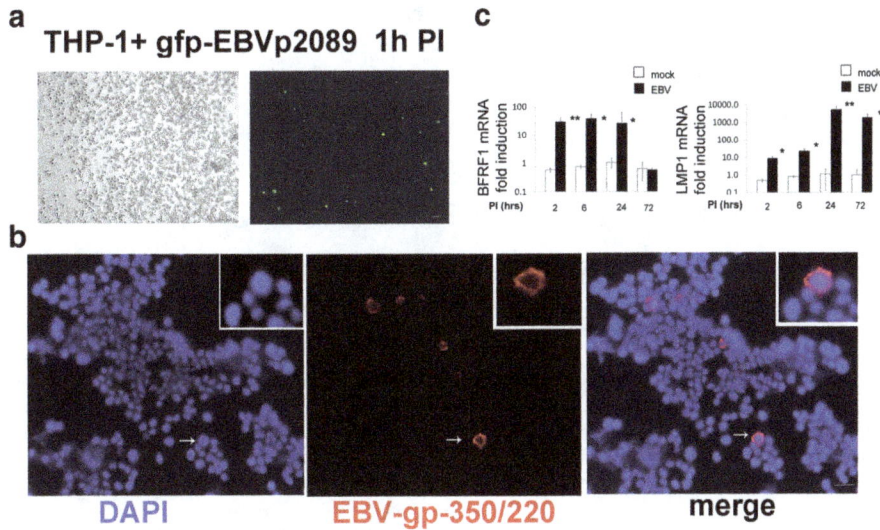

**Fig. 3** EBV lytic genes are expressed in THP-1 cells. THP-1 cells were infected with EBV. Total RNA and proteins were harvested at indicated time points, processed, and analyzed by quantitative PCR and immunofluorescence. **a** Detection of EBV-p2089-GFP in THP-1 after 1 h PI (*left*: phase-contrast light microcopy, *scale bar = 0.1 mm*). **b** Double-indirect immunofluorescence staining of THP-1 cells co-stained with anti-EBV/gp-350 antibodies. Diaminidino-2-phenylindole (*DAPI*) was used as counterstaining for the nuclei. Insert: Higher magnification view for detail (*arrow*) Original magnification 10×; *scale bar = 10 μm*. **c** mRNA expression of indicated genes and proteins in mock-infected and EBV-infected THP-1 cells at indicated time points. Data are expressed as the fold-change normalized to mRNA expression in a mock-infected sample for each time point. Bars represent mean ± SEM from three separate experiments. *P* values calculated using two-tailed *t* test; *\*P < 0.05, \*\*P < 0.01. EBV* Epstein-Barr virus, *PI* post-infection

ligands R837 and CL264 (for TLR7) and CL075 (for TLR8). We found that activation of TLR8 by CL075 induced expression of TLR8 and to a lesser extent IRF7 proteins (Fig. 5a). In contrast, activation of TLR7/agonist ligands failed to induce expression of TLR8 protein (Fig. 5a). IRF7 protein was increased by stimulation of TLR7 ligands (Fig. 5a), IFNβ, IFNγ, and TNFα, and to a lesser extent by TLR8 ligand (Fig. 5b). Moreover, we observed that IFNγ and TNFα also induced TLR8 protein expression in THP-1 cells, although to a lesser extent than selective TLR8 ligand stimulation (Fig. 5b). Consistent with this finding, virally induced TLR8 stimulation was mostly comparable to the induction observed by TLR8/selective agonist/ligand in THP-1 cells (Fig. 6a, Additional file 1: Figure S6A). Notably, the combination of EBV and CL075-TLR8/ligand was more effective in inducing TLR8 (Fig. 6a).

We next investigated whether the TLR8 activation by EBV is mediated in a TLR8-dependent manner in infected THP-1 cells. We found that bafilomycin-A1, an inhibitor of endosomal acidification and autophagy [29], partially decreased TLR8 and IRF7 expression in THP-1 EBV-infected cells, although it strongly reduced TLR8 and IRF7 expression in CL075/TLR8 stimulated cells

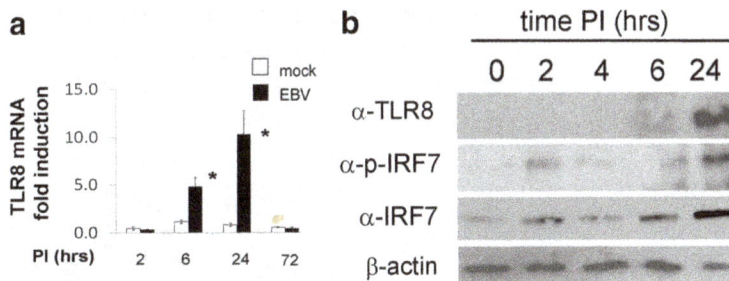

**Fig. 4** TLR8 modulation during EBV infection in THP-1 cells at different time points. THP-1 cells were infected with EBV. Total RNA and proteins were harvested at indicated time points, processed, and analyzed by quantitative PCR and Western blot. **a** TLR8 mRNA expression in mock-infected and EBV-infected THP-1 cells at indicated time points. Data are expressed as the fold-change normalized to mRNA expression in a mock-infected sample for each time point. Bars represent mean ± SEM from three separate experiments. *P* values calculated using two-tailed *t* test; *\*P < 0.05.* **b** Western blot analysis was performed to determine TLR8 and IRF7 protein (phosphorylated and total) levels in cell lysates at indicated time points post-infection (*PI*). β-actin was used as loading control. *EBV* Epstein-Barr virus, *TLR* Toll-like receptor

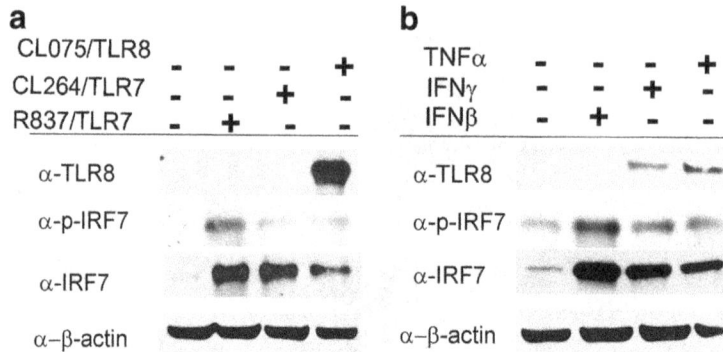

**Fig. 5** CL075/TLR8 synthetic agonist ligand, IFNγ, and TNFα induce TLR8 expression. Cellular lysates from THP-1 cells treated with TLR synthetic ligand: **a** CL264 (adenine analog), R837 (Imiquimod), CL075 (3 M002), or **b** IFNβ, IFNγ, and TNFα or untreated were extracted after 24 h and analyzed by Western blot. Representative immunoblots of TLR8 and IRF7 expression in whole cell lysates. β-actin was used as loading control. *IFN* interferon, *TNF* tumor necrosis factor, *TLR* Toll-like receptor

(Fig. 6b and c, Additional file 1: Figure S6B). Altogether, these results suggest a role on the TLR8 response in mediating EBV active infection.

### IFN-regulated genes and TLR8 are upregulated in freshly purified dcSSc carrying infectious EBV

Consistent with our finding that the newly lytic EBV mRNA possibly activates the TLR8 innate immune response in infected monocytes, we next asked whether viral lytic mRNA would be detected in dcSSc monocytes. Due to the possibility of altering endogenous EBV, UV treatment was not performed on these sets of freshly isolated monocytes. We found expression of BZLF1/EBV-early-lytic-transactivator mRNA in freshly isolated monocytes from four dcSSc patients ($n = 4/8$) (Fig. 7a and Table 2). cDNA sequencing confirmed BZLF1 specificity of the real-time PCR products (data not shown). In contrast, the corresponding B-lymphocyte fraction from dcSSc patients and the monocyte and B-lymphocyte fractions from HDs did not express the BZLF1 gene (Fig. 7a), although EBV DNA was detected in all B lymphocytes and monocytes from dcSSc patients, as well as in B lymphocytes ($n = 6/6$) and in monocytes ($n = 3/6$)

from HDs (Additional file 1: Figure S7, and Table 2). Together, these results suggest that while B lymphocytes carry EBV latent infection, freshly isolated dcSSc monocytes sustain the viral replication.

With the aim of determining whether the innate immune response seen upregulated in EBV-p2089-infected monocytes would also be increased in freshly isolated dcSSc EBV-infected monocytes, the gene expression profile was examined in dcSSc monocytes tested positive for infectious EBV compared to HDs. Remarkably, the microarray analysis revealed that most of the EBV-induced IFN-regulated genes were significantly upregulated (FDR $q < 0.25$) in lytic/EBV-positive dcSSc compared to HD monocytes (Fig. 7b, and Additional file 3: Table S2). To a lesser extent, expression of TLR8, MyD88, IRF7, Siglec1, CXCL10, CCL2, and TNFα was also increased in dcSSc compared to HD monocytes (Fig. 7c). mRNA Affymetrix data (GEO: GSE86984) are available at the public repository Gene Expression Omnibus. Microarray results were confirmed by quantitative PCR in a larger group of dcSSc patients ($n = 8$) and HDs ($n = 6$) (Fig. 7d), further supporting that TLR8 and IFN-regulated genes were significantly increased in dcSSc

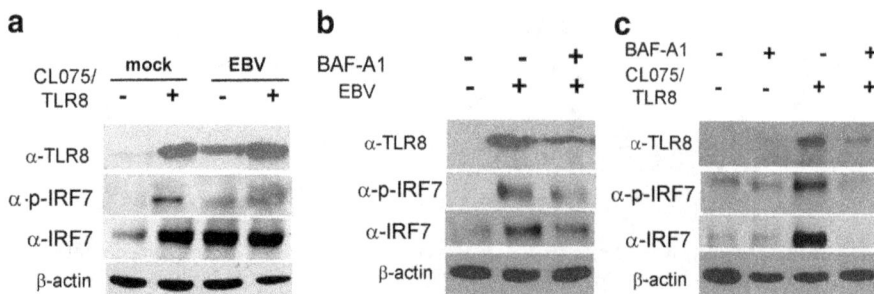

**Fig. 6** EBV-induced TLR8 is partially mediated by TLR8. THP-1 cells were infected with EBV in **a** presence/absence of CL075/TLR8 agonist ligand and **b,c** with/without bafilomycin-A1 (*BAF-A1*). Proteins were assayed 24 h after infection and CL075/TLR8 synthetic ligand stimulation as indicated. Representative immunoblots of TLR8 and IRF7 expression are shown. β-actin was used as loading control. *EBV* Epstein-Barr virus, *TLR* Toll-like receptor

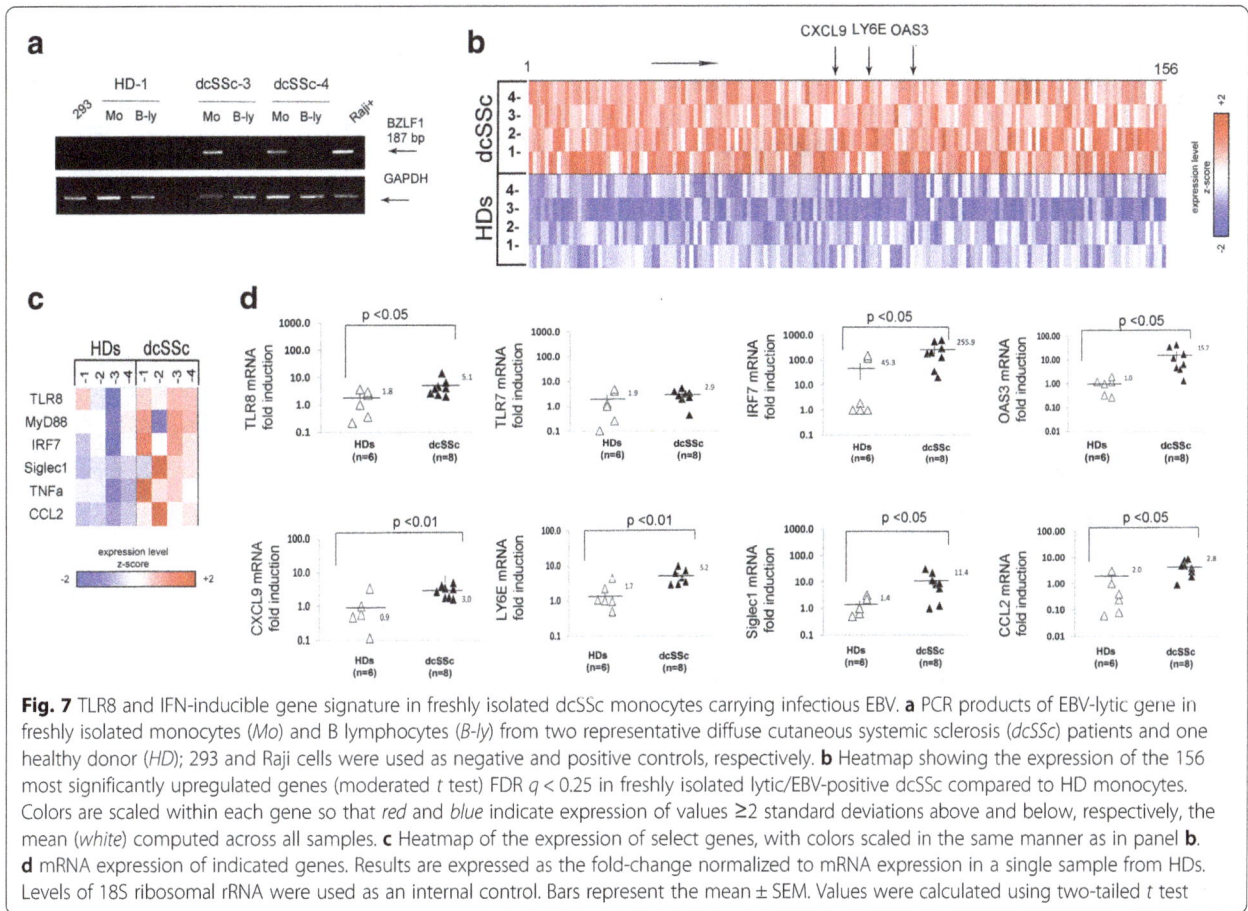

**Fig. 7** TLR8 and IFN-inducible gene signature in freshly isolated dcSSc monocytes carrying infectious EBV. **a** PCR products of EBV-lytic gene in freshly isolated monocytes (*Mo*) and B lymphocytes (*B-ly*) from two representative diffuse cutaneous systemic sclerosis (*dcSSc*) patients and one healthy donor (*HD*); 293 and Raji cells were used as negative and positive controls, respectively. **b** Heatmap showing the expression of the 156 most significantly upregulated genes (moderated *t* test) FDR $q < 0.25$ in freshly isolated lytic/EBV-positive dcSSc compared to HD monocytes. Colors are scaled within each gene so that *red* and *blue* indicate expression of values ≥2 standard deviations above and below, respectively, the mean (*white*) computed across all samples. **c** Heatmap of the expression of select genes, with colors scaled in the same manner as in panel **b**. **d** mRNA expression of indicated genes. Results are expressed as the fold-change normalized to mRNA expression in a single sample from HDs. Levels of 18S ribosomal rRNA were used as an internal control. Bars represent the mean ± SEM. Values were calculated using two-tailed *t* test

compared to HD monocytes. No difference in expression of TLR7, TLR3, and TLR9 was observed in dcSSc compared to HD monocytes (Fig. 7d and data not shown).

These results substantiate the observation that infectious EBV is associated with the activation of TLR8 and IFN proinflammatory response in dcSSc monocytes.

### Segregation of Siglec1 expressing subsets on CD14/CD16 dcSSc monocytes

Circulating monocytes defined by different expression levels of CD14 and CD16 surface markers are known to possess distinct phenotypes and functions [30]. Moreover, altered proportions and conversion of monocyte subsets CD14+/CD16− into CD16+ occur in most autoimmune diseases [31]. Given that EBV lytic infection may occur in a distinct subset of monocytes, which could become positive for the expression of the Siglec1, we next sought to determine whether Siglec1-positive cells might be ascribed to a specific population of ex vivo dcSSc monocytes.

Using FACS analysis, monocytes were identified as previously reported in three subsets: CD14+/CD16− (classical), CD14+/CD16+ (intermediate), and CD14−/CD16+ (non-classical) monocytes (Fig. 8a) [31, 32].

We did not find any significant difference between the percentage of total monocytes or subsets from dcSSc patients compared to HDs (Fig. 8b and c). Interestingly, we found a trend towards an increased number of non-classical monocytes expressing Siglec1 and a slight increase in classical monocytes, but no difference in the intermediate subset (Fig. 8d). These results could suggest that Siglec1-activated monocytes are generally increased in the CD14−/CD16+ non-classical subset and to a lesser extent in the classical subset in dcSSc patients compared to HDs.

### EBV/lytic proteins are present in circulating monocytes and in skin macrophages from patients with dcSSc

To identify whether infectious EBV might be ascribed to a specific population of ex vivo dcSSc monocytes, CD14 and CD16 surface markers were evaluated in freshly isolated EBV-infected cells [30]. EBV/lytic proteins were expressed in a subset of CD14+ and CD16+ monocytes from dcSSc (Fig. 9a and c, arrows; Fig. 9b shows four representative dcSSc patients) (Table 2). In contrast, we did not find any EBV expression in circulating monocytes from six HDs (Fig. 9b shows four representative HDs).

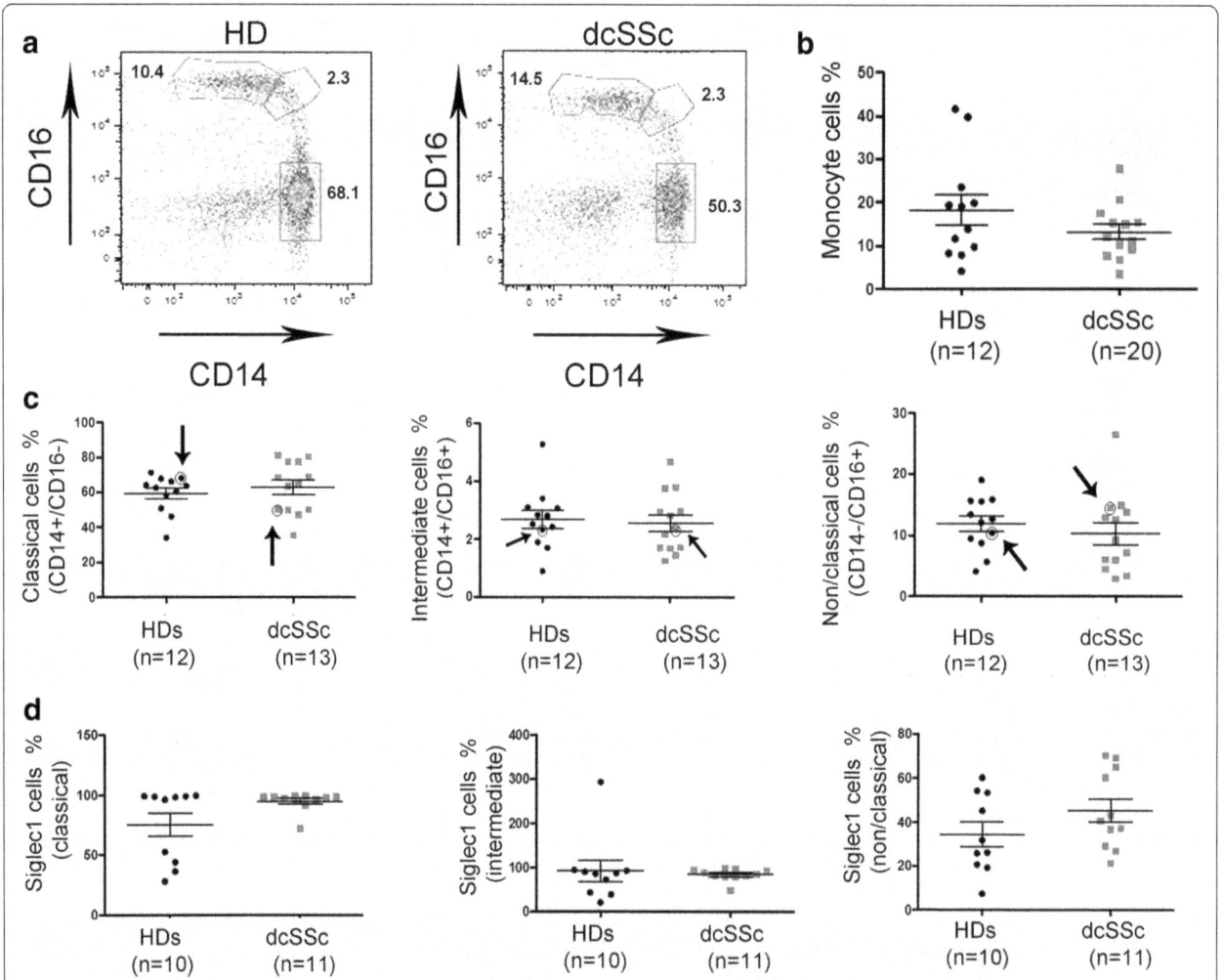

**Fig. 8** Monocyte subsets and Siglec1 expression in dcSSc patients and HD. **a** Representative monocyte subsets from PBMCs of diffuse cutaneous systemic sclerosis (*dcSSc*) patients and healthy donors (*HDs*) defined by the expression of CD14 and CD16 and gating by FACS analysis as CD14+/CD16− (classical, 68% HD), CD14+/CD16+ (intermediate, 2.3% HD), and CD14−/CD16+ (non-classical, 10.4 HD). **b** Number of monocytes (%) in HD compared to dcSSc patients. **c** Frequencies of classical, intermediate, and non-classic monocyte subsets in HD and dcSSc patients. **d** Expression of Siglec1 in the indicated subsets. *P* values calculated using two-tailed *t* test. *Arrows* and *circles* indicate the representative sample for each class of monocytes shown in panel **a**

Given that dcSSc circulating monocytes are carrying infectious EBV, and increased macrophages have been shown in the perivascular areas of SSc skin [8, 33], we next sought to determine whether skin macrophages from dcSSc patients express EBV/lytic proteins. An estimated 2–3% cell/field double positive cells for EBV/nuclear/immediate-early/lytic protein BZLF1/Zebra (Zebra +) and monocyte/macrophage surface/antigen-CD163 (Zebra+/CD163+) were found in 6/18 dcSSc skin biopsies (Fig. 9d, Table 2). As expected, Zebra + staining was found in the nuclei of the infected cells, while CD163 staining was spread around the cell (Fig. 9d, lower panel, high magnification). We did not find any expression of Zebra + or double Zebra+/CD163+ macrophages in the skin from HDs (Fig. 9d). In general, this finding suggests that skin macrophages represent a target of EBV infection in dcSSc patients.

## Discussion

Monocyte/macrophage inflammation and TLR activation have been identified as possible contributors to the pathogenesis of many autoimmune diseases, including SSc. The findings presented here show that activation of TLR8 is induced by EBV/lytic genes in HD and SSc EBV-p2089-infected monocytes and that expression of TLR8 and IFN innate immune mediators is significantly increased in freshly isolated dcSSc monocytes carrying infectious EBV compared to monocytes from HDs. This is the first study that identifies infectious EBV in monocytes from patients with SSc, and mechanistically links EBV with activation of TLR8 and the IFN innate immune response in freshly isolated dcSSc monocytes. These data support a potential role for infectious EBV in contributing to chronic innate immune activation in dcSSc monocytes.

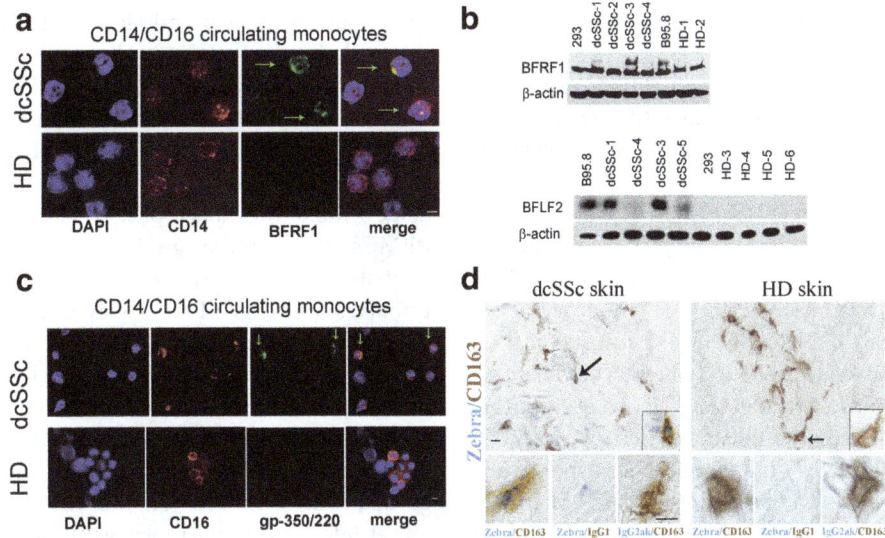

**Fig. 9** EBV-lytic proteins are expressed in dcSSc circulating monocytes and dcSSc skin macrophages. Immunofluorescence and Western blot analysis of CD14/CD16 monocytes freshly purified from PBMCs by negative selection, and immunohistochemistry of skin sections. **a, c** Double immunofluorescence shows the presence of EBV-BFRF1 antigen (*green*) in CD14+ (*red*), and EBV-gp-350-220 (*red*) in CD16+ (*green*) from two representative diffuse cutaneous systemic sclerosis (*dcSSc*) patient and two healthy donors (*HD*). *Green arrows* indicate monocytes expressing EBV/lytic proteins. Original magnification 60×. *Scale bar* = 10 μm. **b** Western blot analysis of EBV-BFRF1 and EBV-BFLF2 lytic proteins in cell lysates of dcSSc and HD monocytes; B95-8/EBV-expressing cells and 293 were used as positive and negative control, respectively. β-actin used as loading control. **d** Representative immunohistologic images of CD163+ macrophages (*brown*) and EBV/lytic protein Zebra + (*blue*) cells in skin sections from dcSSc and HD. Original magnification 2× (*upper panels*) and 10× (*inserts and lower panels*). The *arrows* indicate monocytes represented in the high magnification inserts. *Scale bars* = 5 μm

EBV has been reported to induce an innate immune response characterized by strong release of IL-8 and MCP-1 via TLR9 and TLR2 in monocytes shortly after infection [15, 23]. Likewise, specific viral programs and small non-coding RNA recognized by TLR7, TLR3, and RIG-I have been reported in infected B lymphocytes and plasmacytoid dendritic cells, suggesting that activation of the innate immune response by EBV is dependent on the viral programs carried in the infected cells [15, 34]. In support of these findings, we also observed that TLR9 and TLR3 were increased in a select few monocytes.

One explanation could be that viral replication may not occur simultaneously in all EBV-infected monocytes, and that distinct monocyte populations might also predispose different EBV viral programs in infected cells. Consistent with this observation, we found that monocytes from distinct SSc patients and HDs could be lytically or latently infected after the same exposure time to EBV. Given that the status of EBV infection is dependent on underlying changes within B lymphocytes that permit the stable maintenance of the virus genome or predispose its lytic form [35–39], it is possible that distinct monocyte populations might also influence the establishment of lytic or latent EBV infection.

The key observation that EBV DNA does not induce activation of TLR8 and/or other TLR-inflammatory responses strongly indicates that viral replication might be the prerequisite in activating the innate immune response in the infected cells.

Although immunogenicity of infectious EBV has not yet been taken into account, these findings now lead to the question of which viral-gene mRNA or viral miRNA might specifically interact with TLR8. Further investigation will be required to address this aspect.

An important aspect of this study is that almost all dcSSc and HD monocytes were able to sustain EBV replication in vitro up to 5 days PI. Expression of BZLF1, the EBV immediate early transactivator which promotes the switch from latent to lytic infection, was previously reported as early as 2 h PI with maximum expression at 20 h, suggesting that the EBV replicative cycle occurs very early in infected cells, including monocytes [21, 28, 35, 40–42]. Thus, our data extend this observation to dcSSc monocytes, showing that de novo EBV replication and activation of the IFN innate immune response could be detected up to 5 days PI.

Activation of TLR8 by synthetic ligand mimicked the EBV effects on TLR8, by inducing TLR8 and IRF7 mRNA expression. Intriguingly, selective activation of TLR8 over TLR7 has been shown to inhibit the TLR7-IFNα response, suggesting that the interaction between these two receptors may contribute to the regulation of the innate immune response [43, 44]. Consistent with the observation that TLR8 upregulation inhibits the TLR7-IFNα response, we found that expression of the BFRF1/lytic gene was associated with a trend of TLR7 downregulation in certain infected HD and dcSSc monocytes (Additional file 1: Figure S8), suggesting that activation of TLR8 may be a new strategy employed by EBV to dampen IFNα during lytic replication and control the host innate immune system.

The mechanism for EBV-induced TLR8 expression was in part dependent on the TLR8-activation pathway, since infectious EBV in the presence of bafilomycin did not completely abrogate the signaling resulting in TLR8 and IRF7 upregulation in THP-1 cells. Consistent with our findings that infectious EBV stimulates the production of TNFα mRNA (Fig. 2a) [45], which also upregulates TLR8 protein in THP-1 cells (Fig. 5b), these observations support the idea of EBV using TNFα as a mechanism to synergize with endosomal TLR8 signaling to modulate innate immune responses in infected THP-1 cells. Further investigation will be required to address this aspect.

The relevance of the IFN innate immune response and TLR8 in dcSSc patients has been substantiated by microarray analysis showing the elevated expression levels of IFN-regulated genes, chemokines, and TLR8 mRNA in ex vivo EBV-infected dcSSc monocytes compared to infected HD monocytes. The possible role of TLR8 in autoimmune diseases has been recently considered, since together with TLR7 it is one of the two TLRs expressed on the X chromosome [46]. Because most autoimmune diseases are more prevalent in females, it has been postulated that elevated levels of TLR8, as an X-linked gene, might play a direct role in the pathogenesis of these diseases, including SSc [46]. TLR8 has been implicated in the pathogenesis of arthritis, as its overexpression causes spontaneous inflammatory arthritis in mice [47]. Moreover, a recent study shows that TLR8 agonist stimulation contributes to inflammatory and profibrotic cytokine production in SSc monocytes, further supporting the link between the inflammatory/fibrosis process and TLR8 innate immune activation in the pathogenesis of SSc [48].

Different monocyte subsets may exert specific functions in response to microbes. While CD14+/CD16− classical monocytes produce more proinflammatory cytokines, including IL-6, and production of ROS, CD14−/CD16+, non-classical monocytes selectively produce high levels of TNFα in response to the same trigger [30]. We found EBV lytic proteins in ex vivo CD14+ and/or CD16+ dcSSc monocytes suggesting that EBV might infect more than one monocyte population in SSc. Therefore, it is conceivable that induction of selective cytokines may also be dependent on the monocyte population infected by EBV. In this regard, although EBV-p2089 induced several proinflammatory cytokines in HD and dcSSc monocytes in vitro, the magnitude of the induction was dissimilar among the primary cells (Fig. 2a), possibly reflecting the heterogeneity in the infected monocyte populations. It is also worth mentioning that either the innate immune response or EBV status could be affected by the phenotype of the infected monocytes. Thus, while specific monocyte

subsets may not permit EBV reactivation, other populations may be more permissive to EBV replication when infected. Further studies will be needed to clarify the functional outcomes of EBV infection among distinct monocyte populations.

We show that expression of Siglec1 can be induced by EBV. Previous studies reported increased level of CD169/ Sglec1 monocytes/macrophages in SSc skin, lung, and PBMCs [8, 9, 49], suggesting that CD169+ cells might contribute to the pathogenesis of SSc. While the functional role of Siglec1 in SSc is not entirely clear, it is generally accepted that CD169+ macrophages are involved in cell-cell adhesion as well as cell-pathogen interaction [50, 51]. Consistent with this observation, recent studies have shown that CD169+ macrophages were able to capture several viruses, including HIV, suggesting that sialic acid on the viral envelope facilitates HIV-I infection of macrophages through interacting with Siglec1 [52, 53]. Although the functional role of Siglec1 in EBV infection has not been taken into account, we speculate that EBV might use Siglec1 for cell-to-cell adhesion and viral spread.

Our finding suggests that Siglec1 is inclined to be more induced in SSc non-classical monocytes. This result is in agreement with previous studies which reported increased levels of CD16 and CCL2 in Siglec1-positive monocytes, suggesting that monocytes expressing Siglec1 are more activated to produce cytokines in SSc [8]. While the characterization of the EBV-infected cell population remains to be determined in vivo, it is possible that Siglec1-positive CD14−/CD16+ monocytes might carry active EBV infection. Intriguingly, non-classical monocytes have shown the ability to adhere to the endothelium in vivo and in vitro and to exert specific functions in the response to viruses via TLR7/8 [30, 32]. We speculate that EBV/ Siglec1/CD14−/CD16+ monocytes might facilitate EBV dissemination in SSc tissues by permitting the adhesion of monocytes to the vascular endothelium in vivo.

Our data showed that skin macrophages expressed EBV lytic protein, further suggesting that EBV-infected monocytes might migrate into the skin and facilitate dissemination of EBV to endothelial cells and fibroblasts [13]. Although this is the first report showing the presence of EBV lytic protein in dcSSc skin macrophages, the possibility that monocytes/macrophages might serve as reservoir and/or vehicle for EBV infection in tissue sites is in agreement with a previous study [54].

## Conclusion

This study provides the first evidence of EBV/lytic gene mRNA activating the TLR8 innate immune pathway and suggests a novel mechanism mediating monocyte inflammation in SSc by which EBV triggers the innate immune response in infected cells.

## Additional files

**Additional file 1: Figure S1.** Experimental setup of monocyte purification and monocyte subsets in dcSSc patient and HD groups. (A): a representative cytofluorimetric analysis of CD14 and CD163 expressing monocytes pre- and post- selection from PBMCs. (B): mRNA expression of the indicated genes evaluated in the fraction of CD19+lymphocytes and CD14/CD16 monocytes from dcSSc patients and HDs by qPCR. **Figure S2.** TLRs expression in EBV lytic infected monocytes evaluated by qPCR in negative selected CD14/CD16 monocytes infected with EBV-p2089 5 days post infection (PI). **Figure S3.** Innate immune mediators are not induced in monocytes expressing the latent form of EBV infection in negative selected CD14/CD16 monocytes infected with EBV-p2089, 5 days post infection (PI). **Figure S4.** Increased expression of Siglec1 and CCL2 is equally induced by EBV lytic infection and CL075/TLR8 synthetic ligand in HD and dcSSc EBV-lytic infected monocytes. **Figure S5.** TLR8 mRNA expression in UV radiated THP-1 cells. Bars represent mean ±S.E.M. from 3 separate experiments. **Figure S6.** (A-B) Western Blot analysis of full length of TLR8 and IRF7 expression in EBV-infected/uninfected THP-1 cells. **Figure S7.** PCR products of EBV DNA in monocytes and in B-lymphocytes from representative dcSSc and HD; DNA from Raji-EBV-positive cells and DNA from 293 were used as positive control and negative control, respectively. Gapdh used as internal control. **Figure S8.** The role of BFRF1-lytic gene for selective activation of TLR8 over TLR7 gene expression in EBV-p2089 infected monocytes. mRNA expression of EBV lytic genes and TLR genes was analyzed by q-PCR. Results are expressed as fold induction normalized to each mock-infected control. 18S ribosomal RNA levels were used as internal control. (PDF 527 kb)

**Additional file 2: Table S1.** Real-time PCR primers used for detection of viral and host gene cDNAs. (DOCX 14 kb)

**Additional file 3: Table S2.** Gene expression profile of top induced genes in SSc vs HD monocytes (FDR $q < 0.25$). (DOCX 70 kb)

## Abbreviations
dcSSc: Diffuse cutaneous systemic sclerosis; EBV: Epstein-Barr virus; EBV-p2089: recombinant EBV; FDR: False discovery rate; HD: Healthy donor; IFN: Interferon; IL: Interleukin; IT: Immunosuppressive therapy; PBMC: Peripheral blood mononuclear cell; PCR: Polymerase chain reaction; PI: Post-infection; Siglec1: Sialic acid-binding Ig-like lectin 1 Siglec1/CD169; SSc: Systemic sclerosis; TLR: Toll-like receptor; TNF: Tumor necrosis factor

## Acknowledgements
We thank Yuriy Alekseyev, Ph.D. (Department of Pathology and Laboratory Medicine), and Adam Gower, Ph.D. (Clinical and Translational Science Institute) of Boston University Microarray Resource Core Facility, for supervising all microarray-based experiments and help with data analysis. CTSI award UL1-TR001430.

## Funding
This study was supported by NIH-NIAMS grant R03AR062721-01 and Scleroderma Foundation Established Investigator Grant" to GAF.

## Authors' contributions
All authors participated in the preparation of the manuscript in a significant way. Study design: GAF, AFar, GP, and SM. Acquisition of clinical specimens: ER, SQ, and MY. Experiments performed: AFar, VL, GP, SM, SL, and GAF. Analysis and interpretation of data: AFar, GP, DHD, ER, SQ, MY, ARV, AFag, SM, MT, SL, and GAF. Statistical analysis: ARV and GAF. Manuscript preparation: AFar, GP, SM, SL, MT, and GAF. All authors read the manuscript after revising it critically for relevant scientific content. All authors agreed to be accountable for all aspects of the work in ensuring that questions related to the accuracy or integrity of any part of the work are appropriately investigated and resolved.

## Competing interests
The authors declare that they have no competing interests.

## Authors' information
Not applicable.

## Author details
[1]Rheumatology, Boston University School of Medicine, Arthritis Center, 72 E. Concord Street, E-5, Boston, MA 02118, USA. [2]Department of Experimental Medicine, Sapienza University, Rome, Italy. [3]Istituto Italiano di Tecnologia, CLNS@Sapienza, Rome, Italy. [4]Department of Clinical Medicine, Sapienza University, Rome, Italy. [5]Department of Public Health, Sapienza University, Rome, Italy. [6]Department of Pediatrics, Yale, New Haven, CT, USA.

## References
1. Allanore Y, Distler O. Systemic sclerosis in 2014: advances in cohort enrichment shape future of trial design. Nat Rev Rheumatol. 2015;11(2):72–4.
2. Farina GA, York MR, Di Marzio M, Collins CA, Meller S, Homey B, Rifkin IR, Marshak-Rothstein A, Radstake TR, Lafyatis R. Poly(I:C) drives type I IFN- and TGFbeta-mediated inflammation and dermal fibrosis simulating altered gene expression in systemic sclerosis. J Invest Dermatol. 2010;130(11):2583–93.
3. Broen JC, Radstake TR, Rossato M. The role of genetics and epigenetics in the pathogenesis of systemic sclerosis. Nat Rev Rheumatol. 2014;10(11):671–81.
4. Huang E, Wells CA. The ground state of innate immune responsiveness is determined at the interface of genetic, epigenetic, and environmental influences. J Immunol. 2014;193(1):13–9.
5. Wermuth PJ, Jimenez SA. The significance of macrophage polarization subtypes for animal models of tissue fibrosis and human fibrotic diseases. Clin Transl Med. 2015;4:2.
6. Assassi S, Swindell WR, Wu M, Tan FD, Khanna D, Furst DE, Tashkin DP, Jahan-Tigh RR, Mayes MD, Gudjonsson JE, et al. Dissecting the heterogeneity of skin gene expression patterns in systemic sclerosis. Arthritis Rheumatol. 2015;67(11):3016–26.
7. Duan H, Fleming J, Pritchard DK, Amon LM, Xue J, Arnett HA, Chen G, Breen P, Buckner JH, Molitor JA, et al. Combined analysis of monocyte and lymphocyte messenger RNA expression with serum protein profiles in patients with scleroderma. Arthritis Rheum. 2008;58(5):1465–74.
8. York MR, Nagai T, Mangini AJ, Lemaire R, van Seventer JM, Lafyatis R. A macrophage marker, Siglec-1, is increased on circulating monocytes in patients with systemic sclerosis and induced by type I interferons and toll-like receptor agonists. Arthritis Rheum. 2007;56(3):1010–20.
9. Christmann RB, Hayes E, Pendergrass S, Padilla C, Farina G, Affandi AJ, Whitfield ML, Farber HW, Lafyatis R. Interferon and alternative activation of monocyte/macrophages in systemic sclerosis-associated pulmonary arterial hypertension. Arthritis Rheum. 2011;63(6):1718–28.
10. Brkic Z, van Bon L, Cossu M, van Helden-Meeuwsen CG, Vonk MC, Knaapen H, van den Berg W, Dalm VA, Van Daele PL, Severino A, et al. The interferon type I signature is present in systemic sclerosis before overt fibrosis and might contribute to its pathogenesis through high BAFF gene expression and high collagen synthesis. Ann Rheum Dis. 2016;75(8):1567–73.
11. Liu X, Mayes MD, Tan FK, Wu M, Reveille JD, Harper BE, Draeger HT, Gonzalez EB, Assassi S. Correlation of interferon-inducible chemokine plasma levels with disease severity in systemic sclerosis. Arthritis Rheum. 2013;65(1):226–35.
12. Farina A, Farina GA. Fresh insights into disease etiology and the role of microbial pathogens. Curr Rheumatol Rep. 2015;18(1):1.
13. Farina A, Cirone M, York M, Lenna S, Padilla C, McLaughlin S, Faggioni A, Lafyatis R, Trojanowska M, Farina GA. Epstein-Barr virus infection induces aberrant TLR activation pathway and fibroblast-myofibroblast conversion in scleroderma. J Invest Dermatol. 2014;134(4):954–64.
14. Fattal I, Shental N, Molad Y, Gabrielli A, Pokroy-Shapira E, Oren S, Livneh A, Langevitz P, Pauzner R, Sarig O, et al. Epstein-Barr virus antibodies mark systemic lupus erythematosus and scleroderma patients negative for anti-DNA. Immunology. 2014;141(2):276–85.
15. Lunemann A, Rowe M, Nadal D. Innate immune recognition of EBV. Curr Top Microbiol Immunol. 2015;391:265–87.
16. LeRoy EC, Black C, Fleischmajer R, Jablonska S, Krieg T, Medsger Jr TA, Rowell N, Wollheim F. Scleroderma (systemic sclerosis): classification, subsets and pathogenesis. J Rheumatol. 1988;15(2):202–5.
17. Farina A, Santarelli R, Gonnella R, Bei R, Muraro R, Cardinali G, Uccini S, Ragona G, Frati L, Faggioni A, et al. The BFRF1 gene of Epstein-Barr virus encodes a novel protein. J Virol. 2000;74(7):3235–44.
18. Farina A, Feederle R, Raffa S, Gonnella R, Santarelli R, Frati L, Angeloni A, Torrisi MR, Faggioni A, Delecluse HJ. BFRF1 of Epstein-Barr virus is essential for efficient primary viral envelopment and egress. J Virol. 2005;79(6):3703–12.
19. Gonnella R, Farina A, Santarelli R, Raffa S, Feederle R, Bei R, Granato M, Modesti A, Frati L, Delecluse HJ, et al. Characterization and intracellular

localization of the Epstein-Barr virus protein BFLF2: interactions with BFRF1 and with the nuclear lamina. J Virol. 2005;79(6):3713–27.

20. Schlitt A, Blankenberg S, Weise K, Gartner BC, Mehrer T, Peetz D, Meyer J, Darius H, Rupprecht HJ. Herpesvirus DNA (Epstein-Barr virus, herpes simplex virus, cytomegalovirus) in circulating monocytes of patients with coronary artery disease. Acta Cardiol. 2005;60(6):605–10.

21. Savard M, Gosselin J. Epstein-Barr virus immunossuppression of innate immunity mediated by phagocytes. Virus Res. 2006;119(2):134–45.

22. Lacerte P, Brunet A, Egarnes B, Duchene B, Brown JP, Gosselin J. Overexpression of TLR2 and TLR9 on monocyte subsets of active rheumatoid arthritis patients contributes to enhance responsiveness to TLR agonists. Arthritis Res Ther. 2016;18(1):10.

23. Fiola S, Gosselin D, Takada K, Gosselin J. TLR9 contributes to the recognition of EBV by primary monocytes and plasmacytoid dendritic cells. J Immunol. 2010;185(6):3620–31.

24. McKenzie J, El-Guindy A. Epstein-Barr virus lytic cycle reactivation. Curr Top Microbiol Immunol. 2015;391:237–61.

25. Barnes BJ, Field AE, Pitha-Rowe PM. Virus-induced heterodimer formation between IRF-5 and IRF-7 modulates assembly of the IFNA enhanceosome in vivo and transcriptional activity of IFNA genes. J Biol Chem. 2003;278(19):16630–41.

26. Forsbach A, Samulowitz U, Volp K, Hofmann HP, Noll B, Tluk S, Schmitz C, Wader T, Muller C, Podszuweit A, et al. Dual or triple activation of TLR7, TLR8, and/or TLR9 by single-stranded oligoribonucleotides. Nucleic acid therapeutics. 2011;21(6):423–36.

27. Heil F, Hemmi H, Hochrein H, Ampenberger F, Kirschning C, Akira S, Lipford G, Wagner H, Bauer S. Species-specific recognition of single-stranded RNA via toll-like receptor 7 and 8. Science. 2004;303(5663):1526–9.

28. Savard M, Belanger C, Tardif M, Gourde P, Flamand L, Gosselin J. Infection of primary human monocytes by Epstein-Barr virus. J Virol. 2000;74(6):2612–9.

29. Kuznik A, Bencina M, Svajger U, Jeras M, Rozman B, Jerala R. Mechanism of endosomal TLR inhibition by antimalarial drugs and imidazoquinolines. J Immunol. 2011;186(8):4794–804.

30. Cros J, Cagnard N, Woollard K, Patey N, Zhang SY, Senechal B, Puel A, Biswas SK, Moshous D, Picard C, et al. Human CD14dim monocytes patrol and sense nucleic acids and viruses via TLR7 and TLR8 receptors. Immunity. 2010;33(3):375–86.

31. Burbano C, Vasquez G, Rojas M. Modulatory effects of CD14 + CD16++ monocytes on CD14++CD16– monocytes: a possible explanation of monocyte alterations in systemic lupus erythematosus. Arthritis Rheumatol. 2014;66(12):3371–81.

32. Schmidl C, Renner K, Peter K, Eder R, Lassmann T, Balwierz PJ, Itoh M, Nagao-Sato S, Kawaji H, Carninci P, et al. Transcription and enhancer profiling in human monocyte subsets. Blood. 2014;123(17):e90–9.

33. Higashi-Kuwata N, Jinnin M, Makino T, Fukushima S, Inoue Y, Muchemwa FC, Yonemura Y, Komohara Y, Takeya M, Mitsuya H, et al. Characterization of monocyte/macrophage subsets in the skin and peripheral blood derived from patients with systemic sclerosis. Arthritis Res Ther. 2010;12(4):R128.

34. Martin HJ, Lee JM, Walls D, Hayward SD. Manipulation of the toll-like receptor 7 signaling pathway by Epstein-Barr virus. J Virol. 2007;81(18):9748–58.

35. Hislop AD, Taylor GS, Sauce D, Rickinson AB. Cellular responses to viral infection in humans: lessons from Epstein-Barr virus. Annu Rev Immunol. 2007;25:587–617.

36. Young LS, Arrand JR, Murray PG. EBV gene expression and regulation. In: Human Herpesviruses: Biology, Therapy, and Immunoprophylaxis. Arvin A, Campadelli-Fiume G, Mocarski E, Moore PS, Roizman B, Whitley R, Yamanishi K, editors. Cambridge: Cambridge University Press; 2007.

37. Jones RJ, Smith LJ, Dawson CW, Haigh T, Blake NW, Young LS. Epstein-Barr virus nuclear antigen 1 (EBNA1) induced cytotoxicity in epithelial cells is associated with EBNA1 degradation and processing. Virology. 2003;313(2):663–76.

38. Taylor GS, Long HM, Brooks JM, Rickinson AB, Hislop AD. The immunology of Epstein-Barr virus-induced disease. Annu Rev Immunol. 2015;33:787–821.

39. Knox PG, Li QX, Rickinson AB, Young LS. In vitro production of stable Epstein-Barr virus-positive epithelial cell clones which resemble the virus:cell interaction observed in nasopharyngeal carcinoma. Virology. 1996;215(1):40–50.

40. Kalla M, Hammerschmidt W. Human B cells on their route to latent infection—early but transient expression of lytic genes of Epstein-Barr virus. Eur J Cell Biol. 2012;91(1):65–9.

41. Wu Y, Maruo S, Yajima M, Kanda T, Takada K. Epstein-Barr virus (EBV)-encoded RNA 2 (EBER2) but not EBER1 plays a critical role in EBV-induced B-cell growth transformation. J Virol. 2007;81(20):11236–45.

42. Ladell K, Dorner M, Zauner L, Berger C, Zucol F, Bernasconi M, Niggli FK, Speck RF, Nadal D. Immune activation suppresses initiation of lytic Epstein-Barr virus infection. Cell Microbiol. 2007;9(8):2055–69.

43. Wang J, Shao Y, Bennett TA, Shankar RA, Wightman PD, Reddy LG. The functional effects of physical interactions among Toll-like receptors 7, 8, and 9. J Biol Chem. 2006;281(49):37427–34.

44. Gorden KB, Gorski KS, Gibson SJ, Kedl RM, Kieper WC, Qiu X, Tomai MA, Alkan SS, Vasilakos JP. Synthetic TLR agonists reveal functional differences between human TLR7 and TLR8. J Immunol. 2005;174(3):1259–68.

45. D'Addario M, Ahmad A, Morgan A, Menezes J. Binding of the Epstein-Barr virus major envelope glycoprotein gp350 results in the upregulation of the TNF-alpha gene expression in monocytic cells via NF-kappaB involving PKC, PI3-K and tyrosine kinases. J Mol Biol. 2000;298(5):765–78.

46. Voskuhl R. Sex differences in autoimmune diseases. Biol Sex Differences. 2011;2(1):1.

47. Guiducci C, Gong M, Cepika AM, Xu Z, Tripodo C, Bennett L, Crain C, Quartier P, Cush JJ, Pascual V, et al. RNA recognition by human TLR8 can lead to autoimmune inflammation. J Exp Med. 2013;210(13):2903–19.

48. Ciechomska M, O'Reilly S, Przyborski S, Oakley F, Bogunia-Kubik K, van Laar JM. Histone demethylation and Toll-like Receptor 8-Dependent Cross-Talk in Monocytes Promotes Transdifferentiation of Fibroblasts in Systemic Sclerosis Via Fra-2. Arthritis Rheumatol. 2016;68(6):1493–504. doi:10.1002/art.39602.

49. Farina G, Lafyatis D, Lemaire R, Lafyatis R. A four-gene biomarker predicts skin disease in patients with diffuse cutaneous systemic sclerosis. Arthritis Rheum. 2010;62(2):580–8.

50. Crocker PR, Paulson JC, Varki A. Siglecs and their roles in the immune system. Nat Rev Immunol. 2007;7(4):255–66.

51. Martinez-Pomares L, Gordon S. CD169+ macrophages at the crossroads of antigen presentation. Trends Immunol. 2012;33(2):66–70.

52. Chavez-Galan L, Olleros ML, Vesin D, Garcia I. Much more than M1 and M2 macrophages, there are also CD169(+) and TCR(+) macrophages. Front Immunol. 2015;6:263.

53. Sewald X, Ladinsky MS, Uchil PD, Beloor J, Pi R, Herrmann C, Motamedi N, Murooka TT, Brehm MA, Greiner DL, et al. Retroviruses use CD169-mediated trans-infection of permissive lymphocytes to establish infection. Science. 2015;350(6260):563–7.

54. Tugizov S, Herrera R, Veluppillai P, Greenspan J, Greenspan D, Palefsky JM. Epstein-Barr virus (EBV)-infected monocytes facilitate dissemination of EBV within the oral mucosal epithelium. J Virol. 2007;81(11):5484–96.

# Intestinal dysbiosis is common in systemic sclerosis and associated with gastrointestinal and extraintestinal features of disease

Kristofer Andréasson[1][*] ⓘ, Zaid Alrawi[1], Anita Persson[1], Göran Jönsson[2] and Jan Marsal[3,4,5]

## Abstract

**Background:** Recent evidence suggests a link between autoimmunity and the intestinal microbial composition in several rheumatic diseases including systemic sclerosis (SSc). The objective of this study was to investigate the prevalence of intestinal dysbiosis in SSc and to characterise patients suffering from this potentially immunomodulatory deviation.

**Methods:** This study consisted of 98 consecutive patients subject to in-hospital care. Stool samples were analysed for intestinal microbiota composition using a validated genome-based microbiota test (GA-map™ Dysbiosis Test, Genetic Analysis, Oslo, Norway). Gut microbiota dysbiosis was found present as per this standardised test. Patients were examined regarding gastrointestinal and extraintestinal manifestations of SSc by clinical, laboratory, and radiological measures including esophageal cineradiography, the Malnutrition Universal Screening Tool (MUST), levels of plasma transthyretin (a marker of malnutrition) and faecal (F-) calprotectin (a marker of intestinal inflammation).

**Results:** A majority (75.5%) of the patients exhibited dysbiosis. Dysbiosis was more severe ($r_s = 0.31$, $p = 0.001$) and more common ($p = 0.013$) in patients with esophageal dysmotility. Dysbiosis was also more pronounced in patients with abnormal plasma levels of transthyretin ($p = 0.045$) or micronutrient deficiency ($p = 0.009$). In 19 patients at risk for malnutrition according to the MUST, 18 exhibited dysbiosis. Conversely, of the 24 patients with a negative dysbiosis test, only one was at risk for malnutrition. The mean ± SEM levels of F-calprotectin were 112 ± 14 and 45 ± 8 μg/g in patients with a positive and negative dysbiosis test, respectively. Dysbiosis was more severe in patients with skin telangiectasias ($p = 0.020$), pitting scars ($p = 0.023$), pulmonary fibrosis ($p = 0.009$), and elevated serum markers of inflammation ($p < 0.001$). However, dysbiosis did not correlate with age, disease duration, disease subtype, or extent of skin fibrosis.

**Conclusions:** In this cross-sectional study, intestinal dysbiosis was common in patients with SSc and was associated with gastrointestinal dysfunction, malnutrition and with some inflammatory, fibrotic and vascular extraintestinal features of SSc. Further studies are needed to elucidate the potential causal relationship of intestinal microbe-host interaction in this autoimmune disease.

**Keywords:** Systemic sclerosis, Microbiome, Gastrointestinal, Dysbiosis

* Correspondence: kristofer.andreasson@med.lu.se
[1]Section of Rheumatology, Department of Clinical Sciences, Lund University, Lund, Sweden
Full list of author information is available at the end of the article

## Background

Systemic sclerosis (SSc) is an autoimmune systemic disease of unknown etiology. Genetic factors may only partly explain the pathobiology, and as yet uncharacterised environmental factors have been suggested to have a major influence on the development of SSc [1]. The number of bacteria in the human gastrointestinal (GI) tract has been estimated to $10^{14}$, reaching a biomass of around 2 kg [2]. In both health and disease, these microbiota are in continuous interaction with the epithelium and immune cells of the GI mucosa, and have profound effects on the host's local and systemic immune system [3]. Maintenance of a balanced bidirectional interaction has been suggested to be essential in preventing development and progression of autoimmune diseases [4].

Altered microbiota composition, commonly referred to as dysbiosis, has been shown to induce and modulate systemic inflammation in animal models of rheumatic diseases and other immune-mediated inflammatory diseases (IMIDs) [5–7]. In the field of rheumatology, intestinal dysbiosis has been associated with rheumatoid arthritis (RA), systemic lupus erythematosus, Sjögren's syndrome and ankylosing spondylitis [7–11]. A randomised double-blind placebo-controlled clinical trial in RA patients indicated that disease activity may be sensitive to modulation of gut microbiota through ingestion of probiotics [12]. In contrast, a similar trial did not show any significant differences between probiotics and placebo [13].

In SSc, small intestinal bacterial overgrowth is a well-described complication associated with GI dysmotility, GI discomfort, and malnutrition [14, 15]. Successful treatment of small intestinal bacterial overgrowth in SSc leads to improvement in GI symptoms [14]. Recently, alterations also in the colonic microbial composition in SSc have been reported [16].

Assessment of GI disease in SSc is challenging. Esophageal cineradiography has been suggested as the gold standard in the objective assessment of GI SSc [17]. Others and we have suggested that faecal calprotectin (F-calprotectin) constitutes a feasible tool in the evaluation of GI SSc [15, 18]. Malnutrition is one facet of GI disease that has been linked not only to morbidity and decreased quality of life, but also to increased mortality [19]. The Malnutrition Universal Screening Tool (MUST) is a validated method for identifying SSc patients at risk for malnutrition [20]. Decreased plasma levels of transthyretin, also known as prealbumin, represent a biomarker of malnutrition that also predicts mortality in SSc [19, 21].

The objective of this study was to examine the prevalence of dysbiosis in SSc. Furthermore, we aimed at exploring how intestinal dysbiosis relates to extraintestinal as well as gastrointestinal manifestations of SSc, including malnutrition.

## Methods

### Patients

Consecutive patients fulfilling the American Congress of Rheumatology/European League Against Rheumatism (ACR/EULAR) 2013 classification criteria for SSc and subject to planned in-hospital care due to SSc at the Skane University Hospital in Lund, Sweden between April 2014 and October 2015, were invited to this study. Out of 226 patients, 100 subjects both agreed to participate and were able to provide a fresh stool sample during their in-hospital stay. Patients with inflammatory bowel disease (IBD), intestinal malignancy, and/or colostomy were excluded (n = 2). In total, the study cohort consisted of 98 patients.

### Ethics

The study was approved by the Regional Ethics Review Board, Lund, Sweden, reference number 2011/596. Informed written consent was obtained from all patients before study inclusion and the study conformed to the ethical guidelines of the Declaration of Helsinki.

### Clinical assessment

The following data were collected: age, sex, and disease duration (defined both as years since onset of Raynaud's phenomenon [RP] and years since the first non-RP manifestation). Patients were classified as having either diffuse cutaneous SSc (dcSSc) or limited cutaneous SSc (lcSSc) [22]. Esophageal function was assessed by cineradiography and evaluated by a radiologist, as previously described [23]. The cineradiograms were obtained by recording the swallowing of barium contrast in upright and prone positions using a high-speed camera. Esophageal motility dysfunction was categorised as absent, mild, moderate, or severe. Skin involvement was assessed using the modified Rodnan skin score (mRSS) [24]. The presence or absence of skin telangiectasia and pitting scars were noted. Pulmonary function was evaluated using a body plethysmograph (Erich Jaeger GmbH, Hoechberg, Germany). Lung fibrosis was identified by high-resolution computed tomography. Echocardiography was performed on all patients, and pulmonary arterial hypertension (PAH) was diagnosed by means of right heart catheterisation.

### Assessment of medical records

Medical records were systematically studied. Height and weight were noted as well as weight change during the last 12 months. Individual MUST scores were calculated as previously described [20]. A MUST score of 0 represents low risk for malnutrition, a score of 1 medium risk, and a score of ≥2 high risk. Patients' usage of prescribed drugs including proton pump inhibitors (PPIs), antibiotics, glucocorticoids and immunosuppressive agents were noted.

## Assessment of intestinal symptoms

All patients were systematically questioned regarding the following GI symptoms: heartburn (dyspepsia), dysphagia, diarrhea, and/or constipation. These were recorded as present or not.

## Laboratory examinations

Blood tests included measurements of C-reactive protein (CRP), erythrocyte sedimentation rate (ESR), haptoglobin, orosomucoid, $\alpha_1$-antitrypsin, immunoglobulin (Ig)G, IgM, IgA, vitamin $B_{12}$, folic acid, ferritin, iron, transferrin iron-binding capacity (TIBC) and transthyretin. Subjects with an iron/TIBC ratio < 0.16 were considered to be iron deficient [25]. F-calprotectin was measured using a commercially available enzyme-linked immunosorbent assay (ELISA, Calpro, Lysaker, Norway). The lower limit of the ELISA was 30 μg/g and values below this cutoff were estimated as 20 μg/g. In accordance with published data and recommendations from the manufacturer, we considered F-calprotectin levels < 50 μg/g to be within normal range [26].

## Assessment of gut dysbiosis

The GA-map™ Dysbiosis Test (Genetic Analysis, Oslo, Norway) has been developed and validated in relation to a Scandinavian control population to identify dysbiosis in adults by genetic analysis of a stool sample. The test makes use of 54 bacterial ribosomal RNA probes specific for various intestinal bacterial species or clades to generate genomic data on the intestinal microbiota composition. Using a defined algorithm, these data are subsequently translated into a Dysbiosis Index Score ranging from 1 to 5 (grades 1–2 are defined as eubiosis and 3–5 as dysbiosis). The test has been compared with MiSeq Illumina sequencing-based protocols and proven successful in identifying dysbiosis [6, 27]. In a healthy control population, 84% exhibited eubiosis and 16% dysbiosis [27]. In the current study, gut microbiota eubiosis and dysbiosis were delineated as per the standardised GA-map™ Dysbiosis Test results.

## Statistical analyses

The Mann-Whitney $U$ test was used to compare the degree of dysbiosis and the χ2 test to compare the frequency of dysbiosis in patients with and without various manifestations of SSc. Spearman correlation coefficient ($r_s$) was used to correlate the Dysbiosis Index Score with other continuous variables.

## Results

### Study population characteristics and levels of dysbiosis

Systemic sclerosis patients (n = 98) were examined for an array of characteristics and assessed for intestinal dysbiosis analysing their stools using the GA-map™ Dysbiosis

Test. Patient characteristics are presented in Table 1. A majority (75.5%) of the patients exhibited dysbiosis to some degree (score 3–5), and a significant proportion (24.9%) suffered from severe dysbiosis (score 5, Fig. 1).

### Dysbiosis was associated with gastrointestinal manifestations of systemic sclerosis

A majority of the patients (84%) exhibited esophageal dysfunction, and dysbiosis was significantly more common in this group ($p = 0.013$; Fig. 2). The degree of dysmotility correlated with intestinal dysbiosis (Table 2). Malnutrition was frequent; 53% of the patients exhibited

**Table 1** Patient characteristics

|  | n | (%) |
|---|---|---|
| Systemic sclerosis subtype |  |  |
| limited cutaneous SSc | 77 | (78) |
| diffuse cutaneous SSc | 21 | (22) |
| Autoantibodies |  |  |
| ANA-positive | 87 | (89) |
| ACA-positive | 33 | (34) |
| ARA-positive | 10 | (10) |
| ATA-positive | 11 | (11) |
| Smoking |  |  |
| smoker | 11 | (11) |
| ex-smoker | 43 | (44) |
| non-smoker | 44 | (45) |
| Telangiectasias | 39 | (40) |
| Pulmonary arterial hypertension[a] | 13 | (13) |
| Pitting scars, current | 23 | (23) |
| Lung fibrosis[b] | 35 | (36) |
| Pathological cineradiography | 82 | (84) |
| Regular PPI usage | 78 | (80) |
| Immunosuppressive therapy |  |  |
| mycophenolate mofetil | 23 | (23) |
| methotrexate | 5 | (5) |
| azathioprine | 10 | (10) |
| no immunosuppressive therapy | 60 | (61) |
|  | median | interquartile range |
| Modified Rodnan skin score |  |  |
| limited cutaneous | 2 | (0, 4) |
| diffuse cutaneous | 10 | (4, 22) |
| Disease duration, years[c] | 6 | (2, 16) |
| Prednisolone, daily intake (mg) | 0 | (0, 4) |

*ANA* anti-nuclear antibodies, *ACA* anti-centrome antibodies, *ARA* anti-RNA polymerase III antibodies, *ATA* anti-topoisomerase1 antibodies, *PPI* proton pump inhibitor
[a]As determined by right heart catheterisation
[b]As determined on high-resolution computed tomography
[c]Years since first non-Raynaud's phenomena symptom

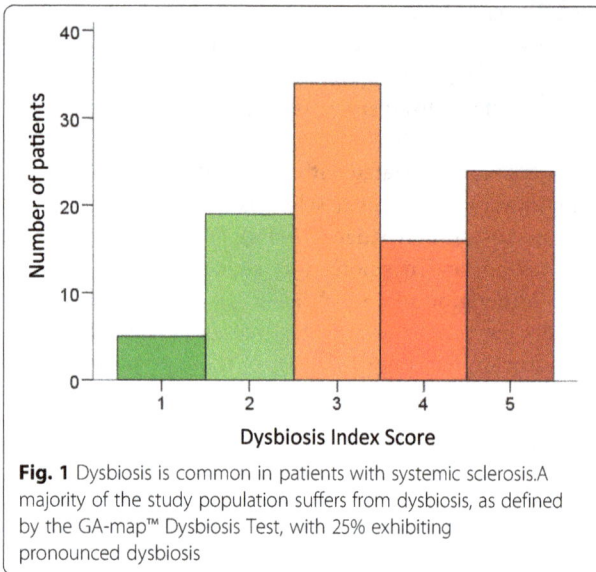

**Fig. 1** Dysbiosis is common in patients with systemic sclerosis. A majority of the study population suffers from dysbiosis, as defined by the GA-map™ Dysbiosis Test, with 25% exhibiting pronounced dysbiosis

deficiency of folic acid, vitamin B12, and/or iron. Nineteen patients had a MUST score of ≥ 1, of which 18 exhibited dysbiosis, and 17 patients had pathological levels of P-transthyretin of which 15 exhibited dysbiosis. Patients with these malnutrition-associated characteristics (any deficiency, MUST ≥ 1, and/or abnormal transthyretin levels) displayed a higher degree of dysbiosis (Fig. 2) compared to the other subjects. Similarly, patients with any self-reported GI symptoms (Fig. 2) and patients using PPIs had a higher degree of dysbiosis compared to the other subjects ($p = 0.019$ and $p = 0.002$, respectively). Subanalysis of different types of self-reported GI symptoms did not reveal any significant associations. A majority of the SSc subjects exhibited abnormal F-calprotectin levels which were associated with the degree of dysbiosis (Fig. 2, Table 2). The mean ± SEM levels of F-calprotectin were $112 ± 14$ and $45 ± 8$ µg/g in patients with a positive and negative dysbiosis test, respectively.

## Dysbiosis was associated with certain extraintestinal manifestations of systemic sclerosis

The degree of dysbiosis was analysed in reference to major fibrotic and vascular extraintestinal manifestations of SSc. Dysbiosis frequencies and severity did not differ between patients with dcSSc and lcSSc (Fig. 2), and the degree of dysbiosis did not correlate with the extent of skin disease (Table 2). However, dysbiosis was more pronounced among patients with pulmonary fibrosis (Fig. 2). We were unable to identify any association between the degree of dysbiosis and vital capacity or carbon monoxide diffusing capacity, ($r_s = -0.126$, $p = 0.216$, n = 98; $r_s = -0.172$, $p = 0.232$, n = 96). Among the 98 patients, 13 (13.3%) suffered from PAH. Dysbiosis was not more common or more severe among these ($p = 0.316$). However, dysbiosis was more severe among the 39 patients exhibiting skin

telangiectasia, and among the 23 patients with pitting scars (Fig. 2). Dysbiosis was not more severe or prevalent among subjects with antibodies against centromere, topoisomerase 1, or RNA polymerase III. The degree of dysbiosis did not correlate with usage of glucocorticoids ($r_s = 0.15$, $p = 0.139$) and was not associated with usage of immunosuppressive therapy or antibiotics ($p = 0.344$ and $p = 0.684$, respectively).

## Dysbiosis was associated with laboratory markers of inflammation

Routine blood tests addressing systemic inflammation were assessed and correlated with the degree of dysbiosis. The grade of dysbiosis correlated with levels of CRP, haptoglobin, orosomucoid, and $\alpha_1$-antitrypsin, but not with the levels of ESR, IgG, IgM or IgA (Table 2). Of note, all three patients with IgA levels above reference levels had a Dysbiosis Index Score of 5 ($p = 0.059$).

## Dysbiosis was common also in patients with early systemic sclerosis

Disease duration was defined by two different measures and subsequently correlated with the degree of dysbiosis. The Dysbiosis Index Score did not correlate either with disease duration defined as years since RP debut or disease duration defined as years since first non-RP symptom or age (Table 2). Dysbiosis was prevalent among patients with less than 2 years since the debut of RP or first non-RP symptom (73% and 72%, respectively), similarly to patients with more long-standing disease (76% and 76%, Fig. 2).

## Analysis of specific bacterial genera

In a secondary analysis, we examined the frequency of specific bacterial genera and species previously associated with SSc, included in the GA-map™ Dysbiosis Test. A large proportion of patients with SSc exhibited low levels of *Faecalibacterium prausnitzii* (66/98; 67.3%) and/or *Clostridiaceae* (25/98; 25.5%) compared to eubiotic individuals. Also, relatively high levels of *Lactobacillus* (31/98; 31.6%) but not *Bifidobacterium* (6/98; 6.1%) were common among our subjects.

## Discussion

In this cross-sectional study encompassing 98 SSc patients we show that intestinal dysbiosis is common in SSc and is related to GI manifestations of disease. Also, we show that dysbiosis is associated with certain extraintestinal SSc features of inflammatory, vascular, and fibrotic type. We present data showing that intestinal dysbiosis is already present early in the course of SSc, indicating that dysbiosis may precede initial signs of fibrosis.

Several IMIDs have been associated with alterations in the microbial composition in the intestine, including

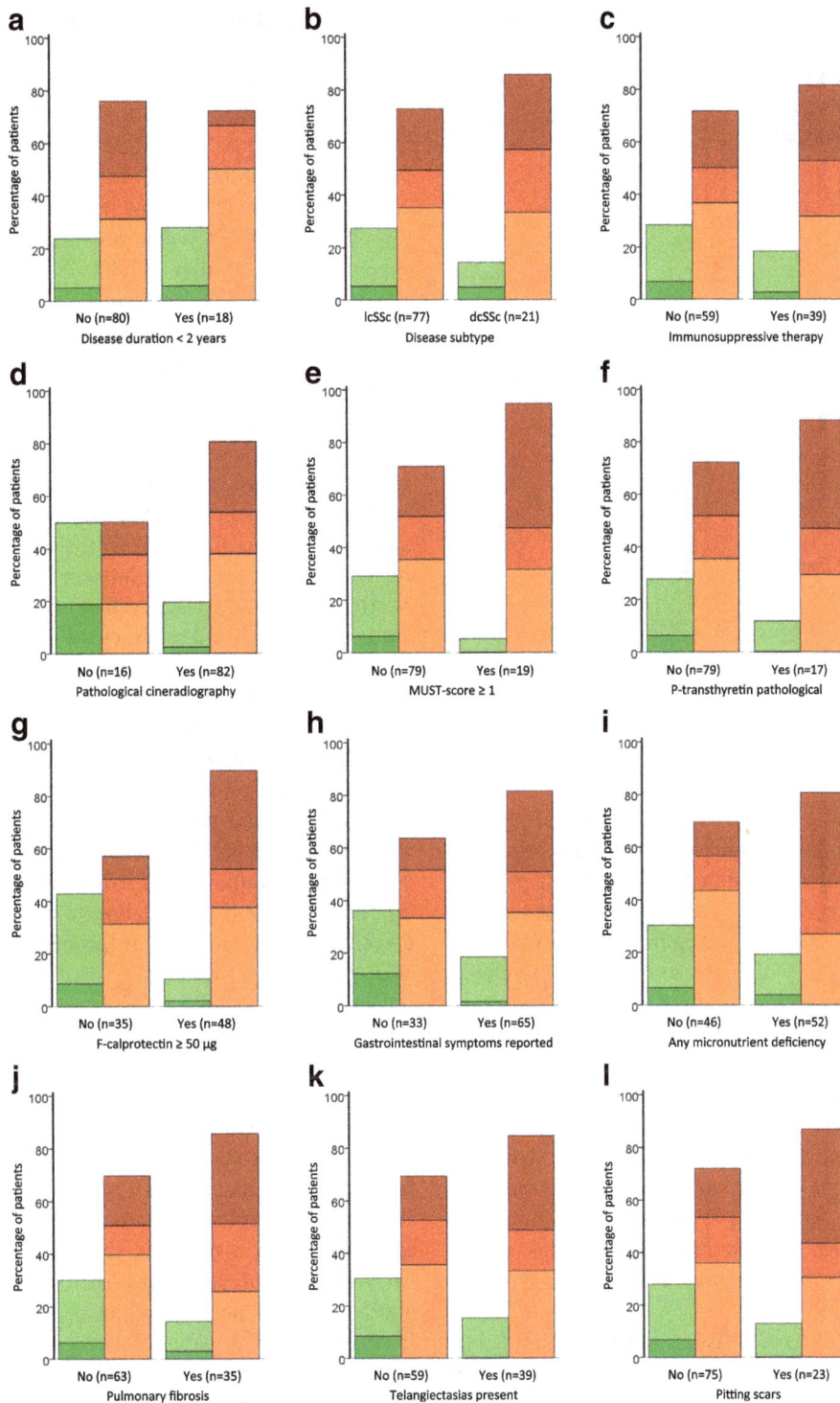

**Fig. 2** Dysbiosis correlates with gastrointestinal and some extraintestinal manifestations of SSc, but not disease subtype or immunosuppressive therapy. Dysbiosis was prevalent in patients with both short and long disease duration (**a**), lcSSc and dcSSc (**b**) as well as in patients with and without immunosuppressive therapy (**c**), with no significant differences between groups. Dysbiosis was more pronounced in patients with gastrointestinal manifestations of SSc including pathological oesophageal function, $p = 0.036$ (**d**); at risk for malnutrition, $p = 0.005$ (**e**); low levels of P-transthyretin, $p = 0.045$ (**f**); increased levels of F-calprotectin, $p < 0.001$ (**g**); gastrointestinal symptoms present, $p = 0.019$ (**h**) or micronutrient deficiency $p = 0.009$ (**i**). Also, patients with pulmonary fibrosis, $p = 0.009$ (**j**); telangiectasias, $p = 0.020$ (**k**); or pitting scars, $p = 0.023$ (**l**) had more pronounced dysbiosis compared to other patients. *dcSSc* diffuse cutaneous SSc, *F-calprotectin* faecal calprotectin, *lcSSc* limited cutaneous SSc, *MUST* Malnutrition Universal Screening Tool

**Table 2** Correlation between the Dysbiosis Index Score and laboratory markers of inflammation, and disease characteristics, respectively

| | n | Spearman's correlation coefficient ($r_s$) | p value |
|---|---|---|---|
| *Laboratory markers of inflammation* | | | |
| C-reactive protein | 98 | 0.35 | <0.001 |
| Haptoglobin | 98 | 0.34 | <0.001 |
| Orosomucoid | 98 | 0.39 | <0.001 |
| $\alpha_1$-antitrypsin | 98 | 0.27 | 0.007 |
| Erythrocyte sedimentation rate | 98 | 0.16 | 0.156 |
| IgA | 98 | 0.13 | 0.266 |
| IgM | 98 | −0.05 | 0.654 |
| IgG | 98 | −0.05 | 0.632 |
| Faecal calprotectin | 83 | 0.38 | <0.001 |
| *Disease characteristics* | | | |
| Years since onset of RP | 94 | −0.07 | 0.501 |
| Years since the first non-RP symptom | 89 | 0.09 | 0.383 |
| Patient's age at dysbiosis analysis | 98 | 0.08 | 0.413 |
| modified Rodnan skin score | 98 | 0.05 | 0.659 |
| Dysmotility of oesophagus | 97 | 0.31 | 0.002 |

*Ig* immunoglobulin, *RP* Raynaud's phenomenon

RA, systemic lupus erythematosus, Sjögren's syndrome, and IBD [7, 8, 11, 28]. Among human IMIDs, dysbiosis has been most extensively studied in IBD. These patients display decreased diversity in their gut microbiota, increased numbers of bacteria driving inflammatory activity, and decreased numbers of bacteria with immunoregulatory effects [28]. An important question is whether IBD-associated dysbiosis is a primary or secondary phenomenon. In animal models of IBD both loss of immunoregulatory and addition of disease-promoting bacteria have been shown to contribute to disease activity, supporting a primary disease-driving role for dysbiosis [29]. In IBD patients, various strategies for manipulating the gut microbiota, including exclusive enteral nutrition, prebiotics, probiotics, postbiotics, and faecal microbiota transplantation have shown mixed but overall promising results [30].

Molecular analyses have revealed some similarities between the process of IBD-associated intestinal fibrosis and SSc-associated skin fibrosis, including transforming growth factor beta (TGF-β) and peroxisome proliferator-activated receptor-dependent pathways resulting in collagen I production by fibrocytes and fibroblasts [31, 32]. Furthermore, while inflammation can be treated by immunosuppressive therapy, these fibrotic processes are resilient also to modern therapy in both diseases. In IBD as well as SSc, elevated F-calprotectin levels are

common, indicating intestinal inflammation. Similar to data presented in this study, increased F-calprotectin levels have been associated with dysbiosis also in IBD [33].

Volkmann et al. recently reported altered microbial colonic mucosal composition in 17 SSc patients [16]. Our study comprising 98 SSc patients corroborates this finding, as we show a high incidence of dysbiosis in our patients. We also report low levels of the immunoregulatory bacteria *Faecalibacterium prausnitzii*, which is in agreement with studies in IBD [34]. In accordance with Volkmann et al., we report high levels of *Lactobacillus* in SSc patients, which contrasts this disease from several other IMIDs [4]. As previously suggested, this finding might raise novel questions regarding the usage of *Lactobacilli*-containing probiotics in SSc.

Our report is based on faecal analyses and not analyses on colonic lavage or intestinal biopsies. Consequently, a weakness of our approach is the inability to specifically focus on bacteria prevalent in the interface between the colonic mucosa and the intestinal lumen. It is noteworthy that even though different methodologies were used, our major finding is consistent with Volkmann's report.

Objective evaluation of GI disease in SSc is challenging. SSc can affect the GI tract in several different ways including dysmotility, malnutrition, inflammation, and fibrosis. In our study, we evaluated the GI tract by assessment of esophagus motility using barium cineradiography which has previously been suggested as the gold standard in objective evaluation of this disease [17]. We investigated malnutrition by laboratory markers including P-transthyretin, and anthropometric data using the MUST [19, 20]. While malnutrition in SSc has been suggested to be caused by malabsorption [35], additional mechanisms are likely to be involved including cachexia caused by the chronic inflammatory process [36].

A majority of our patients were prescribed PPI and usage of this medication was interestingly enough associated with dysbiosis. However, previous studies have failed to show that PPI usage per se causes significant aberrations in colonic microbiota composition [37]. In agreement with a previous study and interpretation by Krause et al. [36], we suggest that regular use of PPI primarily is an unspecific marker of symptomatic GI SSc. In this study, all patients were questioned about GI symptoms, and indeed, dysbiosis was more common in patients with GI symptoms indicating that a validated questionnaire, such as the UCLA SCTC GIT 2.0 should be included in future studies [38].

The primary aim of this study was to study the prevalence of dysbiosis in SSc. Unlike whole-genome sequencing studies, we have only limited data on specific bacterial genera. Furthermore, we do not have data on intestinal metabolic pathways used by the different microbiomes our patients harbor. Further studies encompassing such analyses are needed to further elucidate the intricate relationship between the host and the microbiome in SSc [39].

We can only speculate on the mechanisms behind the associations between dysbiosis and GI or extraintestinal manifestations of SSc. It can be hypothesised that several of these manifestations are indirect markers of severe disease. However, we were unable to identify an association between the mRSS, disease subtype, autoantibody profile, and immunosuppressive therapy. Taking this into consideration, we are therefore inclined to suggest that the relationship between the intestinal microbiome and SSc is multifactorial and related to factors independent of disease severity or autoantibody status. We note that dysbiosis is associated with increased serum levels of markers of inflammation and we suggest that further studies are warranted to elucidate the impact of GI dysbiosis on the immune system in SSc.

## Conclusions

Examining a large cross-sectional cohort of SSc patients we report that intestinal dysbiosis is prevalent in early as well as late disease, and associated with both GI and extraintestinal manifestations of SSc. Given our current knowledge from other IMIDs, we suggest that an aberration of the intestinal microbiota may contribute to the development of systemic inflammation and fibrosis, although causal relationships remain to be established.

## Abbreviations

ACA: anti-centromeric antibodies; ACR/EULAR: American Congress of Rheumatology/European League Against Rheumatism; ANA: anti-nuclear antibodies; ARA: anti-RNA-polymerase III antibodies; ATA: anti-topoisomerase antibodies; CRP: C-reactive protein; dcSSc: diffuse cutaneous SSc; ELISA: enzyme-linked immunosorbent assay; ESR: erythrocyte sedimentation rate; F-calprotectin: faecal calprotectin; GI: gastrointestinal; IBD: inflammatory bowel disease; Ig: immunoglobulin; IMID: immune-mediated inflammatory disease; lcSSc: limited cutaneous SSc; mRSS: modified Rodnan skin score; MUST: Malnutrition Universal Screening Tool; PAH: pulmonary arterial hypertension; PPI: proton pump inhibitor; RA: rheumatoid arthritis; RP: Raynaud's phenomenon; SSc: systemic sclerosis; TGF-β: transforming growth factor beta; TIBC: total iron-binding capacity

## Acknowledgements

The authors acknowledge the assistance from Ivana Kojic, Department of Laboratory Medicine, Malmö and Magnus Jöud and Maria Lundgren, Clinical Immunology and Transfusion Medicine, Region Skåne, Lund, Sweden for excellent assistance in the laboratory analyses.
We also acknowledge fruitful discussions with Professor Bodil Ohlsson and Associate Professor Thomas Mandl, Department of Clinical Sciences, Lund University.

## Funding

This study was supported by grants to researchers in public health care from the Swedish government (ALF for young researchers), Anna-Greta Crafoord Foundation, Lion Research Foundation, and Swedish Society of Medicine (to KA); Funding from Hedlund Foundation, Österlund Foundation, and grants to researchers in public health care from the Swedish government (ALF for young researchers) contributed to financing JM's research time.

## Authors' contributions

KA conceived and designed the study, analysed and interpreted the data and drafted the manuscript. ZA analysed and interpreted the data and reviewed the manuscript for intellectual content. AP acquired the data and organised the study and reviewed the manuscript for intellectual content. GJ analysed and interpreted the data and reviewed the manuscript for intellectual content. JM conceived the study, analysed and interpreted the data and helped drafting and revising the manuscript. All authors read and approved the final manuscript.

## Competing interests

The authors declare that they have no competing interests.

## Author details

[1]Section of Rheumatology, Department of Clinical Sciences, Lund University, Lund, Sweden. [2]Section of Infectious Diseases, Department of Clinical Sciences, Lund University, Lund, Sweden. [3]Department of Clinical Sciences, Lund University, Lund, Sweden. [4]Immunology Section, Lund University, Lund, Sweden. [5]Department of Gastroenterology, Skåne University Hospital, Lund, Sweden.

## References

1.  Gabrielli A, Avvedimento EV, Krieg T. Scleroderma. N Engl J Med. 2009;360(19):1989–2003.
2.  Qin J, Li R, Raes J, et al. A human gut microbial gene catalogue established by metagenomic sequencing. Nature. 2010;464(7285):59–65.
3.  Honda K, Littman DR. The microbiota in adaptive immune homeostasis and disease. Nature. 2016;535(7610):75–84.
4.  Forbes JD, Van Domselaar G, Bernstein CN. The gut microbiota in immune-mediated inflammatory diseases. Front Microbiol. 2016;7:1081.
5.  Andreasson K, Marsal J, Mansson B, Saxne T, Wollheim FA. Diet-induced arthritis in pigs: comment on the article by Scher et al. Arthritis Rheumatol. 2016;68(6):1568–9.
6.  Iebba V, Totino V, Gagliardi A, et al. Eubiosis and dysbiosis: the two sides of the microbiota. New Microbiol. 2016;39(1):1–12.
7.  Scher JU, Littman DR, Abramson SB. Microbiome in inflammatory arthritis and human rheumatic diseases. Arthritis Rheumatol. 2016;68(1):35–45.
8.  Hevia A, Milani C, Lopez P, et al. Intestinal dysbiosis associated with systemic lupus erythematosus. MBio. 2014;5(5):e01548–14.
9.  Rosser EC, Mauri C. A clinical update on the significance of the gut microbiota in systemic autoimmunity. J Autoimmun. 2016;74:85–93.
10. Costello ME, Ciccia F, Willner D, et al. Intestinal dysbiosis in ankylosing spondylitis. Arthritis Rheumatol. 2014. doi: 10.1002/art.38967. [Epub ahead of print].
11. de Paiva CS, Jones DB, Stern ME, et al. Altered mucosal microbiome diversity and disease severity in Sjogren syndrome. Sci Rep. 2016;6:23561.
12. Alipour B, Homayouni-Rad A, Vaghef-Mehrabany E, et al. Effects of Lactobacillus casei supplementation on disease activity and inflammatory cytokines in rheumatoid arthritis patients: a randomized double-blind clinical trial. Int J Rheum Dis. 2014;17(5):519–27.
13. Pineda Mde L, Thompson SF, Summers K, de Leon F, Pope J, Reid G. A randomized, double-blinded, placebo-controlled pilot study of probiotics in active rheumatoid arthritis. Med Sci Monit. 2011;17(6):CR347–54.
14. Marie I, Ducrotte P, Denis P, Menard JF, Levesque H. Small intestinal bacterial overgrowth in systemic sclerosis. Rheumatology (Oxford). 2009;48(10):1314–9.
15. Marie I, Leroi AM, Menard JF, Levesque H, Quillard M, Ducrotte P. Fecal calprotectin in systemic sclerosis and review of the literature. Autoimmun Rev. 2015;14(6):547–54.
16. Volkmann ER, Chang YL, Barroso N, et al. Association of systemic sclerosis with a unique colonic microbial consortium. Arthritis Rheumatol. 2016;68(6):1483–92.
17. Clements PJ, Becvar R, Drosos AA, Ghattas L, Gabrielli A. Assessment of gastrointestinal involvement. Clin Exp Rheumatol. 2003;21(3 Suppl 29):S15–8.
18. Andreasson K, Scheja A, Saxne T, Ohlsson B, Hesselstrand R. Faecal calprotectin: a biomarker of gastrointestinal disease in systemic sclerosis. J Intern Med. 2011;270(1):50–7.
19. Codullo V, Cereda E, Klersy C, et al. Serum prealbumin is an independent predictor of mortality in systemic sclerosis outpatients. Rheumatology (Oxford). 2016;55(2):315–9.

20. Baron M, Hudson M, Steele R. Canadian Scleroderma Research G. Malnutrition is common in systemic sclerosis: results from the Canadian scleroderma research group database. J. Rheumatol. 2009;36(12):2737–43.

21. Ingenbleek Y, Bernstein LH. Plasma transthyretin as a biomarker of lean body mass and catabolic states. Adv Nutr. 2015;6(5):572–80.

22. LeRoy EC, Black C, Fleischmajer R, et al. Scleroderma (systemic sclerosis): classification, subsets and pathogenesis. J Rheumatol. 1988;15(2):202–5.

23. Summerton SL. Radiographic evaluation of esophageal function. Gastrointest Endosc Clin N Am. 2005;15(2):231–42.

24. Clements P, Lachenbruch P, Siebold J, et al. Inter and intraobserver variability of total skin thickness score (modified Rodnan TSS) in systemic sclerosis. J Rheumatol. 1995;22(7):1281–5.

25. Moreno Chulilla JA, Romero Colas MS, Gutierrez MM. Classification of anemia for gastroenterologists. World J Gastroenterol. 2009;15(37):4627–37.

26. Manz M, Burri E, Rothen C, et al. Value of fecal calprotectin in the evaluation of patients with abdominal discomfort: an observational study. BMC Gastroenterol. 2012;12:5.

27. Casen C, Vebo HC, Sekelja M, et al. Deviations in human gut microbiota: a novel diagnostic test for determining dysbiosis in patients with IBS or IBD. Aliment Pharmacol Ther. 2015;42(1):71–83.

28. Miyoshi J, Chang EB. The gut microbiota and inflammatory bowel diseases. Transl Res. 2016;S1931–5244(16):30095.

29. Belkaid Y, Hand TW. Role of the microbiota in immunity and inflammation. Cell. 2014;157(1):121–41.

30. Dolan KT, Chang EB. Diet, gut microbes, and the pathogenesis of inflammatory bowel diseases. Mol Nutr Food Res. 2016. doi: 10.1002/mnfr. 201600129. [Epub ahead of print].

31. Manetti M, Neumann E, Milia AF, et al. Severe fibrosis and increased expression of fibrogenic cytokines in the gastric wall of systemic sclerosis patients. Arthritis Rheum. 2007;56(10):3442–7.

32. Manetti M, Neumann E, Muller A, et al. Endothelial/lymphocyte activation leads to prominent CD4+ T cell infiltration in the gastric mucosa of patients with systemic sclerosis. Arthritis Rheum. 2008;58(9):2866–73.

33. Shaw KA, Bertha M, Hofmekler T, et al. Dysbiosis, inflammation, and response to treatment: a longitudinal study of pediatric subjects with newly diagnosed inflammatory bowel disease. Genome Med. 2016;8(1):75.

34. Sokol H, Seksik P, Furet JP, et al. Low counts of Faecalibacterium prausnitzii in colitis microbiota. Inflamm Bowel Dis. 2009;15(8):1183–9.

35. Bishop V, Harrison E, Lal S, Herrick AL. Evidence for a clinical association between body mass index and malabsorption in patients with systemic sclerosis. Scand J Rheumatol. 2015;44(4):341–3.

36. Krause L, Becker MO, Brueckner CS, et al. Nutritional status as marker for disease activity and severity predicting mortality in patients with systemic sclerosis. Ann Rheum Dis. 2010;69(11):1951–7.

37. Tsuda A, Suda W, Morita H, et al. Influence of proton-pump inhibitors on the luminal microbiota in the gastrointestinal tract. Clin Transl Gastroenterol. 2015;6:e89.

38. Khanna D, Hays RD, Maranian P, et al. Reliability and validity of the University of California, Los Angeles Scleroderma Clinical Trial Consortium Gastrointestinal Tract Instrument. Arthritis Rheum. 2009;61(9):1257–63.

39. Abdollahi-Roodsaz S, Abramson SB, Scher JU. The metabolic role of the gut microbiota in health and rheumatic disease: mechanisms and interventions. Nat Rev Rheumatol. 2016;12(8):446–55.

# Multiplex serum protein analysis reveals potential mechanisms and markers of response to hyperimmune caprine serum in systemic sclerosis

Niamh Quillinan[1†], Kristina E. N. Clark[1†], Bryan Youl[2], Jeffrey Vernes[3], Deirdre McIntosh[3], Syed Haq[3] and Christopher P. Denton[1*]

## Abstract

**Background:** Hyperimmune caprine serum (HICS) is a novel biological therapy with potential benefit for skin in established diffuse cutaneous systemic sclerosis. Here we report multiplex protein analysis of blood samples from a placebo-controlled phase II clinical trial and explore mechanisms of action and markers of response.

**Methods:** Patients were treated with HICS ($n = 10$) or placebo ($n = 10$) over 26 weeks, with follow-up open-label treatment to 52 weeks in 14 patients. Serum or plasma samples at baseline, 26 and 52 weeks were analysed using multiplex or individual immunoassays for 41 proteins. Patterns of change were analysed by clustering using Netwalker 1.0, Pearson coefficient and significance analysis of microarrays (SAM) correction.

**Results:** Cluster analysis, SAM multiplex testing and paired comparison of individual analytes identified proteins that were upregulated or downregulated during treatment with HICS. There was upregulation of the hypothalamo-pituitary-adrenal axis after HICS treatment evidenced by increases in α-MSH and ACTH in cases treated with HICS. Interestingly, significant increase in PIIINP was associated with HICS treatment and improved MRSS suggesting that this may be a marker of extracellular matrix turnover. Other relevant factors reduced in HICS-treated patients compared with controls, although not reaching statistical significance included COMP, CCL2, IL6, TIMP2, Fractalkine and TGFβ1 levels.

**Conclusions:** Our results suggest mechanisms of action for HICS, including upregulation of α-MSH, that has been shown to be anti-fibrotic in preclinical models, and possible markers to be included in future trials targeting skin in diffuse cutaneous systemic sclerosis.

**Keywords:** Scleroderma, Clinical trial, Biomarker, Goat serum, Melanocortin

## Background

Hyperimmune caprine serum (HICS) has been reported to have beneficial effects in several disease settings with potential improvement in several neurological and inflammatory human diseases [1–5]. The mechanism of action in these conditions is poorly understood and

likely multifactorial. Proposed pharmacodynamic effects of HICS include an effect on ion channel function [6–9], immunosuppression and neuroendocrine modulation through the hypothalamo-pituitary axis [10].

Recently reported clinical data from a phase II study in established diffuse cutaneous systemic sclerosis (dcSSc) suggest possible treatment benefit of HICS for skin over 26 weeks for active treatment compared with placebo and meaningful improvement in 50% of cases, and improvement in modified Rodnan skin score (MRSS) in an extended dataset including subjects that

---

* Correspondence: c.denton@uc.ac.uk
†Equal contributors
[1]Centre for Rheumatology, UCL Division of Medicine, Royal Free Campus, Rowland Hill Street, London NW3 2PF, UK
Full list of author information is available at the end of the article

moved from placebo to active treatment after the first 26 weeks [11]. Here we report the effect of treatment on multiple serum proteins and examine the potential association between changes in analytes and modified Rodnan skin score in individual study subjects.

In addition to elucidating the effect of HICS, this systematic study of biologically relevant candidate molecular markers in a cohort of established dcSSc gives new insight to a phase of the disease that is associated with substantial morbidity and mortality, but that has often been excluded from clinical trials that generally focus on early diffuse systemic sclerosis (SSc). In this way we have highlighted the potential benefit of biological intervention/immunomodulation in established SSc and also demonstrated that information about skin treatment may be derived from this population.

## Methods

### Study cohort and clinical outcomes

This was a placebo-controlled study of 20 patients with established diffuse cutaneous SSc, defined by disease duration of at least 36 months from first non-Raynaud's symptom. Subjects were randomly allocated 1:1 to active treatment or placebo. The clinical and demographic features of the study cohort have been described in detail previously [11]. Of note, three patients withdrew from the study; one in the HICS group due to cerebral infarction unrelated to study medication and two in the placebo group due to progression of disease. After 26 weeks of blinded treatment, all patients were offered open-label treatment for a further 26 weeks. The blind of original treatment allocation was maintained to 52 weeks. The flow of subjects for the study is shown in Additional file 1: Figure S1. For the primary analysis, baseline and 26-week MRSS were compared and statistical difference between the active treatment and placebo-treated cases was compared. Secondary analysis differentiated responders from non-responders defined by improvement in skin score by at least 20% of baseline and four MRSS units. Post hoc analysis of MRSS change included seven placebo cases that moved to the active treatment and three cases that continued without medication.

### Serum and plasma protein analysis

Blood samples were obtained at baseline, week 0 (pre- and post-injection of medication), weeks 26 and 52. Serum and plasma samples were sent frozen to Quest Diagnostics (Valencia, CA, USA) for single-protein analysis or Quansys Biosciences (Logan, UT, USA) for multiplex analysis, as outlined below.

Single-analysis assays were used for analysis of procollagen III N-terminal propeptide (PIIINP), soluble interleukin-2 receptor (sIL-2R), cartilage oligomeric matrix protein (COMP), transforming growth factor beta 1 (TGF-β1) and

von Willebrand factor (vWF). vWF samples were plasma samples and an enzyme-linked immunosorbent assay (ELISA) (Cat. No. 84793; Aushon Biosystems, Inc., Billerica, MA, USA). Soluble IL-2R samples were serum samples and an ELISA (Cat. No. EH2IL2R; Thermo Fisher Scientific, Waltham, MA, USA). TGF-β1 samples were serum samples and an ELISA (Cat. No. DB100B; R&D Systems, Inc., Minneapolis, MN, USA). PIIINP samples were serum samples and a radioimmunoassay (Cat. No. 06098; Orion Diagnostica Ltd., Espoo, Finland).

Multiplex serum analysis was performed for αMSH, ACTH, ANG2, HGF, PDGF-bb, TIMP-1, TIMP-2, VEGF, FGF basic, Eotaxin, GRO-α, MCP-1, MCP-2, RANTES, I-309, TARC, IP-10, IL-1α, IL-1β, IL-2, IL-4, IL-6, IL-8, IL-10, IL-12p70, IL-13, IL-15, IL-17, IL-23, IFN-γ, TNF-α, TNF-β, IFN-α, IFN-β, Fractalkine and PARC by multiplex analysis. Samples were Quansys Biosciences by Q-Plex Array™ kits for Human Angiogenesis (No. 150251HU), Human Chemokine (No. 120251HU), and Human Cytokine (No. 110951HU). Both Fractalkine and PARC were custom developed from matched pair antibodies available from R&D Systems. The Q-Plex™ kits used in the sample testing have undergone extensive validation. Ranges for each assay were determined by dilutions determining upper ranges where high-end hook effect and apparent antibody saturation are avoided and lower ranges that are above detection limits. Antigen standard curves were performed in duplicate.

### Statistical analysis

For each analyte there was an individual comparison of baseline, 26 and 52 weeks and an integrated multiplex analysis to look for clusters of change in groups of cytokines that may reflect treatment with HICS or clinical differences in MRSS occurring during the study period. Unsupervised and supervised cluster analysis was undertaken to define baseline differences or changes over 26 and 52 weeks. Differences were compared between treatment groups and also for those with subgrouping strategies at baseline, longitudinally and linked to meaningful or numerical change in clinical variables. Permutation analysis was used to compare cytokine levels between the treatment arm and placebo arm. This was processed in EXCEL (Microsoft Corp., Redmond, WA, USA) and analysed using $t$ tests with significance analysis of microarray (SAM) correction. Normalisation of data points and hierarchical clustering were performed using Netwalker 1.0 (http://netwalkersuite.org), and heat map construction was performed using CIMminer (https://discover.nci.nih.gov/cimminer/). Scatter plots were used to explore the association between MRSS and individual analytes. Baseline and 26-week values were compared between HICS and control treatment arms in the extended dataset and changes were also examined in the subset of subjects that changed from placebo to HICS at 26 weeks and for those that received HICS over a total of 52 weeks.

In order to normalise data, the analyte titre was divided by the average titre for all patients at time point zero, and then log transformed. The normalized data were expressed as a value that is centred on the mean level of the analyte across all the samples examined. This is a well-established and validated method which permits comparison of multiple proteins in each subject and allows the levels to be compared for different proteins within the cohort – this both vertical and horizontal clustering can be achieved for the heat maps. We have expanded the "Methods" section of the revised manuscript to explain normalization methods included in our analysis in more detail. When using SAM analysis, the cutoff of significance is determined by tuning the parameter delta, and then selection based on the fold change and q value. This highlighted genes that were differentially expressed. A combination of fold change and q value together with level of statistical significance in univariable comparison for HICS treatment effect compared with placebo were used to select hallmark upregulated or downregulated analytes that are included in Table 1 and annotated on heat maps.

## Results
### Clinical outcome data for modified Rodnan skin score
This manuscript focuses on pre-specified analysis of multiple serum proteins over 52 weeks. For the first 26 weeks, the enrolled subjects ($n = 20$) were randomly assigned to self-administer twice weekly HICS by subcutaneous injection or matched placebo. Following this period, all subjects were offered the opportunity to receive 26 weeks of active HICS treatment. Three of the

study cohort did not elect to receive HICS during this second 26-week period. The primary efficacy end point for this trial was change in MRSS measured as a continuous variable and comparing baseline and 26-week values. The clinical data for the placebo-controlled trial have been previously reported [11]. Briefly, mean mRSS fell by $1.4 \pm 4.7$ units with active treatment but worsened by $2.1 \pm 6.4$ units on placebo ($p = 0.181$, unpaired $t$ test) when baseline values were compared with 26-week values. Responder analysis showed that 50% of HICS patients improved compared to 10% of placebo patients at 26 weeks ($p = 0.062$). We undertook further analysis of an extended dataset, comparing placebo patients who took medication on a compassionate basis after the double-blind phase of treatment for a further 26 weeks. Thus, skin score data were available for seven additional cases treated for 26 weeks with HICS, and from three cases that chose not to take the drug but that were observed for a further 26 weeks off treatment. Skin score data for this extended dataset comprising 13 subjects receiving placebo or no active therapy with the 17 subjects that received HICS for 26 weeks confirms statistically significant difference between active treatment and controls in a post hoc analysis, $p = 0.025$ (Fig. 1).

### Serum and plasma protein analysis
The data for the 26-week placebo-controlled phase of the study for PIIINP, vWF and sIL2R have been presented previously [11]. Here we show additional data to week 52 that confirm the earlier findings (Table 1). For the baseline measurements, there were 20 subjects, at 26 weeks there were $n = 10$ receiving placebo and $n = 9$ receiving HICS due to one patient discontinuing treatment early in the study. Fifty-two-week follow-up was on a compassionate basis

**Table 1** Representative serum analytes (mean [SD]) for subjects receiving HICS or placebo treatment over 26 weeks

| Direction of change | Change during study HICS | | | Change during study placebo | | | HICS versus placebo | | |
|---|---|---|---|---|---|---|---|---|---|
| | Basal | 26 wk | 26 wk versus basal p value | Basal | 26 wk | 26 wk versus basal p value | Fold change | q value | p value |
| Sample number | n = 10 | n = 9 | n = 9 | n = 10 | n = 10 | n = 10 | | | |
| UP | | | | | | | | | |
| α-MSH pg/ml | 3.7 [3.6] | 31.1 [35.8] | 0.0035 | 1.8 [0.9] | 2.2 [1.9] | 0.75 | 299.6 | 0 | 0.039 |
| ACTH pg/ml | 1.9 [2.4] | 27.6 [42.3] | 0.0099 | 1.1 [1.1] | 1.0 [0.7] | 0.97 | 176.6 | 0 | 0.05 |
| bFGF pg/ml | 3.4 [6.5] | 21.5 [21.9] | 0.0185 | 21.3 [43.3] | 23.6 [51.6] | 0.62 | 65 | 0 | 0.15 |
| PIIINP ug/ml | 6.9 [3.8] | 15.4 [10.1] | 0.0002 | 5.3 [2.7] | 5.9 [2.7] | 0.62 | 14.6 | 20 | 0.012 |
| DOWN | | | | | | | | | |
| COMP ng/ml | 1.8 [1.1] | 1.4 [0.3] | 0.055 | 1.3 [0.5] | 1.4 [0.6] | 0.7 | −3.38 | 36 | 0.265 |
| FRACT (CX3CL1) ng/ml | 3.7 [6.4 | 3.3 [6.1] | 0.108 | 1.1 [0.7] | 1.0 [0.6] | 0.79 | −6.1 | 43 | 0.318 |
| CCL2 (MCP1) pg/ml | 262.3 [101.1] | 202.4 [132.0] | 0.239 | 280.6 [133.6] | 325.8 [225.9] | 0.293 | −0.5 | 36 | 0.121 |
| TIMP2 ng/ml | 13.4 [1.9] | 13.0 [1.8] | 0.322 | 13.1 [1.8] | 13.9 [2.3] | 0.172 | −12.6 | 43 | 0.1044 |
| TGFβ1 ng/ml | 29.4 [7.9] | 27.8 [4.3] | 0.901 | 26.4 [4.4] | 25.4 [10.4] | 0.385 | −3.8 | 43 | 0.601 |
| Gro-α pg/ml | 35.0 [97.2] | 10.7 [17.1] | 0.076 | 3.6 [5.5] | 10.2 [15.1] | 0.939 | −2.3 | 36 | 0.206 |
| IL6 pg/ml | 4.6 [9.7] | 1.4 [1.4] | 0.309 | 25.4 [69.5] | 30.6 [66.8] | 0.128 | −0.04 | 36 | 0.053 |

*SD* standard deviation, *HICS* hyperimmune caprine serum

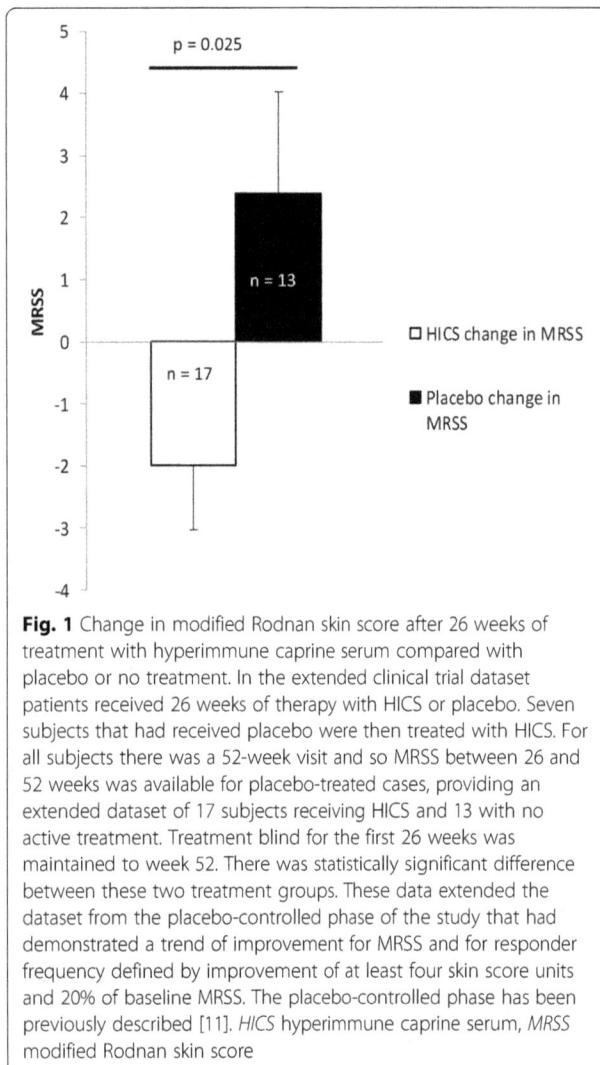

**Fig. 1** Change in modified Rodnan skin score after 26 weeks of treatment with hyperimmune caprine serum compared with placebo or no treatment. In the extended clinical trial dataset patients received 26 weeks of therapy with HICS or placebo. Seven subjects that had received placebo were then treated with HICS. For all subjects there was a 52-week visit and so MRSS between 26 and 52 weeks was available for placebo-treated cases, providing an extended dataset of 17 subjects receiving HICS and 13 with no active treatment. Treatment blind for the first 26 weeks was maintained to week 52. There was statistically significant difference between these two treatment groups. These data extended the dataset from the placebo-controlled phase of the study that had demonstrated a trend of improvement for MRSS and for responder frequency defined by improvement of at least four skin score units and 20% of baseline MRSS. The placebo-controlled phase has been previously described [11]. *HICS* hyperimmune caprine serum, *MRSS* modified Rodnan skin score

with safety review and so fewer samples were available. For clarification, the total study cohort was 20 subjects. There were samples available for assay from $n = 7$ subjects who had moved from placebo to HICS, $n = 6$ subjects continuing HICS treatment and $n = 2$ subjects who moved from HICS to no treatment and $n = 3$ subjects who were in the placebo arm and chose not to receive HICS from weeks 26 to 52. The flow of patients through the study is illustrated in the schematic in Additional file 1: Figure S1.

## Cluster analysis and heat maps

First, the dataset was examined using cluster analysis with generation of heat maps to identify differences in the protein levels for the study cohort at baseline or 26 weeks. Unsupervised analysis of absolute concentrations, scaled and normalized for the purposes of comparison, did not show any clear differences for baseline values (Fig. 2a) whilst the 26-week data are more clustered (Fig. 2b). Changes were examined to explore the

potential effect of HICS on serum protein levels of the large number of analytes and specifically focus on those cases that had shown a clinically meaningful improvement in MRSS (responders) compared to those that had stable or worsening skin score. Unsupervised clustering was first performed (Additional file 2: Figure S2) and later supervised analysis (Fig. 3). For these analyses the primary exploration was for data from the first placebo-controlled phase of the study, but the extended dataset including the additional seven patients treated for the first time with HICS over weeks 26 to 52 are also included as a secondary analysis to confirm and extend the data from the placebo-controlled phase. These are included in Additional file 3: Figure S3.

To provide a clearer signal of potential serum protein changes seen in the SSc subjects receiving active treatments in the placebo-controlled phase of the study, a summary heat map was generated for the placebo-controlled phase of the study. This demonstrates that some markers are shared and these may be markers of clinical change or response. In contrast the signature comparing HICS and placebo (Additional file 4: Figure S4) is more likely to be a direct effect of the HICS administration and may therefore be a better reflection of the impact of this novel therapy rather than the clinical changes occurring in MRSS, that might also provide insight into potential markers of change in skin severity that may be independent of treatment effect (Additional file 4: Figure S4). For the key analytes highlighted in Table 1 the heat maps are annotated showing that for almost all of these the change seen with HICS treatment compared with placebo was also observed in analysis based upon the responder status for MRSS.

## Statistical analysis of changes in serum proteins associated with HICS treatment

We next undertook statistical analysis of the whole dataset using SAM. The strength of this methodology is that it takes account of the multiple simultaneous analyses that are performed and corrects the data for false discovery risk. From this analysis a signature of proteins up- or downregulated by HICS emerged and these proteins were then subjected to a more detailed analysis of change over the 52 weeks of the study. These proteins are shown in Table 1 together with the basal and 26-week level, fold change and significance assessed by SAM and for individual statistical analysis of the analytes.

To further demonstrate the changes in proteins that are upregulated by HICS at 26 weeks, the change in cases that switched from placebo to active treatment between weeks 26 and 52 treatment effect individual patient data are plotted in Fig. 4 for key proteins included in Table 1. Congruity of mean and median values suggests near

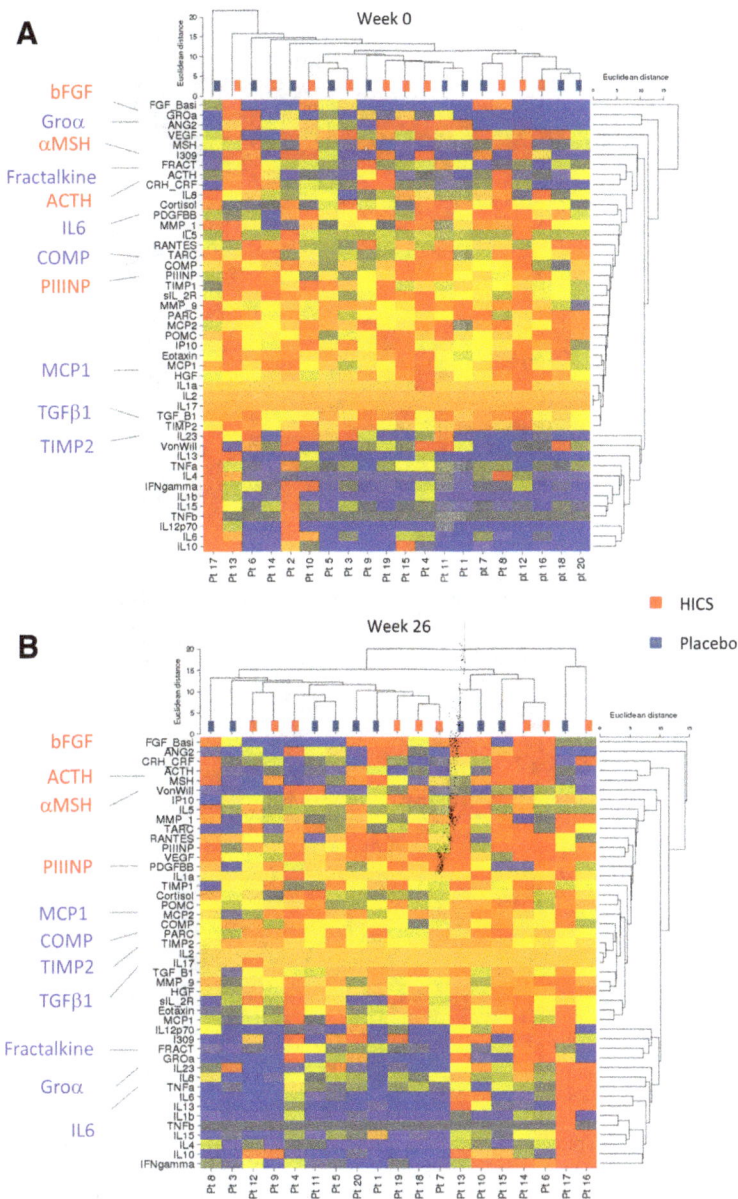

**Fig. 2** Unsupervised hierarchical cluster analysis for multiplex serum proteins at baseline and 26 weeks during the placebo-controlled trial of HICS. Unsupervised cluster analysis was undertaken to identify any subgroups within the study cohort at baseline based upon the serum levels of multiple protein analytes as described in text. The same analysis was repeated for serum samples after 26 weeks of treatment with HICS or placebo. The randomly assigned treatment allocation is shown for each subject. Data for baseline samples are shown in panel **a**. After 26 weeks of treatment there were clear changes in the patterns of protein analytes that were spread between the two treatment arms as shown in panel **b**. *HICS* hyperimmune caprine serum

normal distribution and non-parametric assessment and the results are not significantly different from the methods included in the current manuscript. As detailed below to avoid confusion and ensure consistency with the external statistical analysis included in our final study report, we prefer to keep the results of parametric testing in this manuscript. The most significant changes were observed for αMSH, ACTH, and PIIINP. This demonstrates patterns of change in the extended dataset and in subjects

moving from placebo to active treatment at 26 weeks and those receiving HICS over a 52-week period. For these analytes, individual subjects show clear evidence of increase similar to that seen over 24 weeks for actively treated subjects. Although the small numbers preclude formal statistical analysis, the data provide support to the effect seen in the first 26 weeks of the study and in the extended dataset. Mean and median values of relevant serum proteins, including COMP, CCL2, IL6, TIMP2,

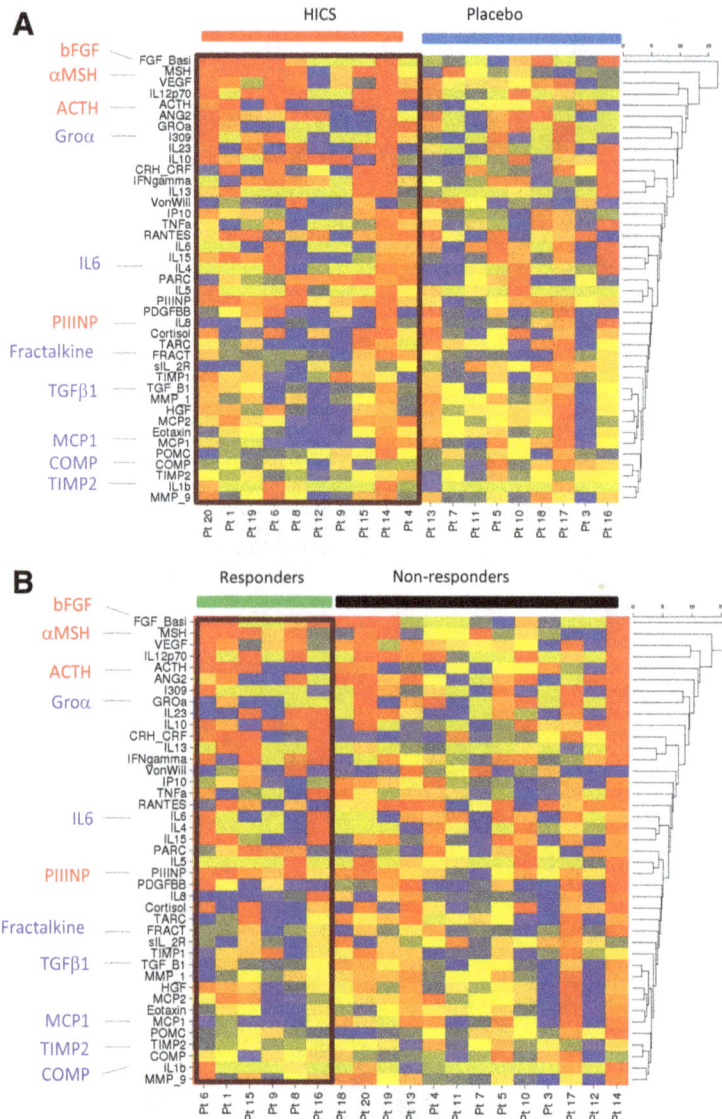

**Fig. 3** Supervised analysis for change in serum proteins according to treatment or responder status in the 26-week placebo-controlled trial of HICS. **a** Cluster analysis was undertaken for serum analytes after allocation to HICS or placebo during the 26-week parallel-group controlled phase of the clinical trial to identify any subgroups within the study cohort at baseline based upon the serum levels of multiple protein analytes as described in text. A pattern of upregulation or downregulation of specific proteins is seen more frequently in cases treated with HICS than controls. **b** The same analysis was repeated with subjects allocated to responder or non-responder categories based upon improvement in MRSS by at least four skin score units and 20% of baseline MRSS. Of the responders 5/6 were in the HICS-treated arm of the study. In this way groups of proteins that are clustered for similar patterns of change in response to HICS or associated with clinically meaningful improvement in MRSS

Fractalkine and TGFβ1were reduced in HICS-treated patients compared with controls, although not reaching statistical significance, and are shown in Table 1.

At an individual patient level levels of some analytes, including COMP, TGFβ1, αMSH and PIIINP that showed significant correlation for baseline MRSS confirming previous published data from other independent studies. However, there was no correlation between changes in these analytes and MRSS change during the study at an individual patient level (data not shown).

## Discussion

In this study we demonstrate the value of including biological analyses exploring potential markers and mechanisms of treatment effect in clinical trials of novel potential therapeutics, such as hyperimmune caprine serum [12]. By including later stage dcSSc we highlight the feasibility of recruiting this subgroup that may have some advantages (e.g. clinical homogeneity, acceptability of requiring no other immunosuppression and acceptability of a true placebo control) compared with early-stage

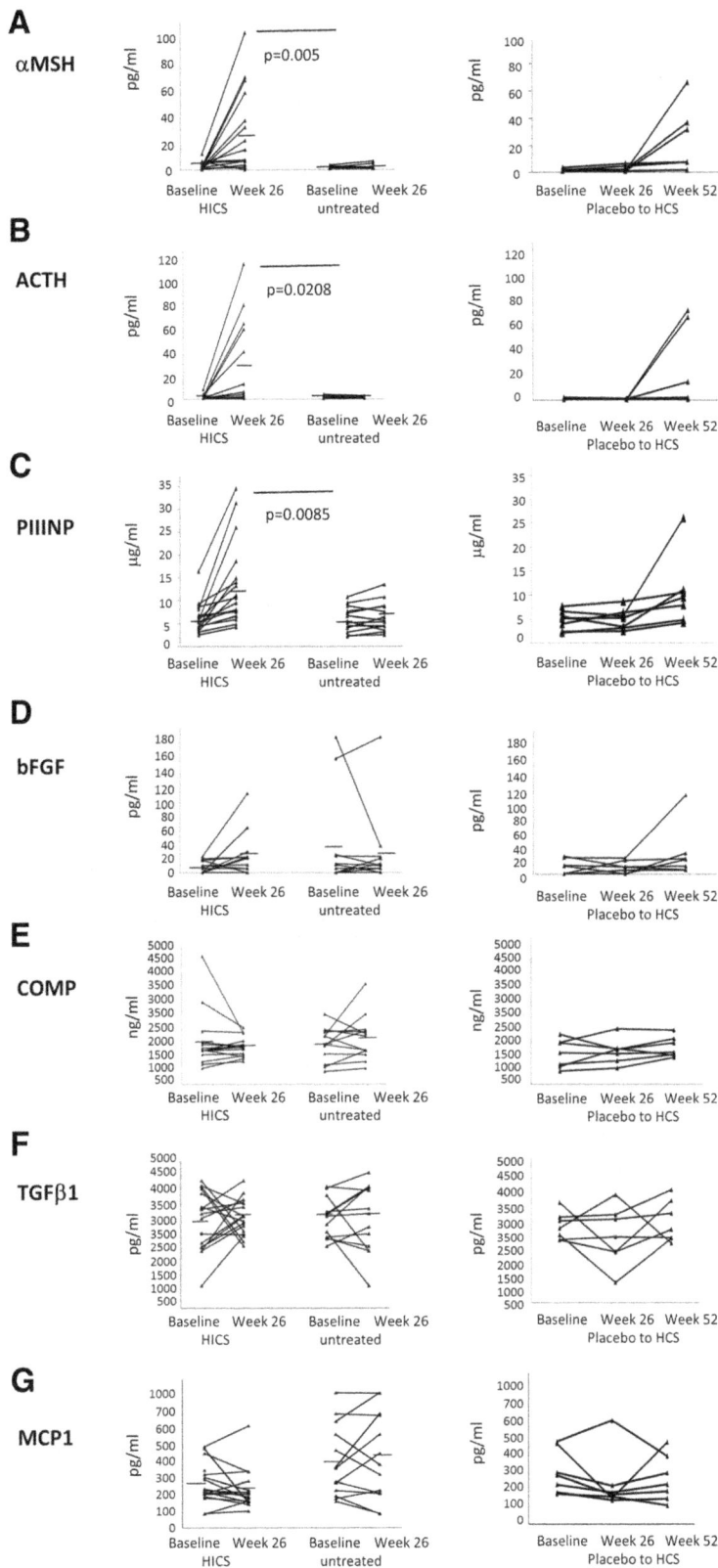

**Fig. 4** (See legend on next page.)

SSc [13]. It is notable that there was progression in the placebo group in this study that is contrary to recent suggestions that later stage dcSSc is likely to be in a regressive stage [14]. A potential explanation for this is that immunosuppressive treatments were withdrawn in the study subjects and this may have led to more active skin disease.

Simultaneous measurement of multiple analytes is a powerful approach that has been applied in cross-sectional analyses but few longitudinal studies [15, 16]. We identify a molecular signature of HICS response in SSc and correlate with potential treatment effect that includes proteins that increase with HICS treatment compared with untreated cases, especially PIIINP, αMSH and ACTH, and also proteins that showed trends of reduction in the HICS-treated subjects. Our findings suggest potential for development of composite serum biomarkers for HICS response in SSc and could inform development of a more generic composite serum biomarker for SSc [17–19]. This would complement other markers that include serum variables and tests of other available markers such as the enhanced liver fibrosis (ELF) test [20] and confirm the feasibility of this approach. Our study has the particular strength of having longitudinal sampling and simultaneous assessment of MRSS. The changes observed for HICS treatment are notable in the context of falling MRSS. For PIIINP, the changes are unexpected in that there is increase in the context of improved MRSS both in the overall treatment cohort for HICS and also in the responder analysis (Additional file 3: Figure S3). This suggests that PIIINP may be a marker of extracellular matrix (ECM) remodeling as well as fibrotic burden as discussed below. Other proteins showing significant change include markers of activation (αMSH and ACTH) with highly significant increase at 26 weeks suggesting sustained upregulation of the hypothalamic pituitary axis in response to HICS. COMP has previously been suggested as a marker of skin score in scleroderma and so a trend for reduction in HICS-treated cases but not controls in notable.

Several distinct possible effects of HICS that have previously been suggested are highly relevant to the study. First, HICS is likely to have an immunomodulatory effect. This may reflect the presence of proteins and cytokines that affect immune function [21],

including polyclonal immunoglobulin that has previously been suggested to be beneficial for some aspects of SSc. A recent retrospective single-centre observational study of 30 patients with refractory dcSSc receiving intravenous immunoglobulin (IVIG) showed significant reduction in MRSS at 24 months, indicating that it may be an effective adjunctive treatment [22]. To date, only one randomised double-blind trial has been completed. In this trial, a single 5-day course of IVIG did not show significant improvement but a retreatment with a second course showed an improvement in skin score [23]. Other recent reports suggest benefits in gastrointestinal symptoms and myositis in SSc patients receiving IVIG [24, 25].

One of the most compelling potential anti-fibrotic mechanisms for HICS is through stimulation of the hypothalmo-pituitary axis. It is notable that there is considerable evidence that stimulation of MSH pathways may benefit preclinical animal models of fibrosis and in vitro studies with human tissue [26–28]. For example, Bohm et al. described that human dermal fibroblasts express the MC1 receptor (MC1R) that binds α-MSH with high affinity and they found that α-MSH suppressed TGF-β-induced collagen synthesis in vitro [29, 30]. Furthermore, the authors used a bleomycin mouse model to investigate the effects of α-MSH on skin fibrosis and found that simultaneous administration of α-MSH with bleomycin suppressed the effects of bleomycin on HDF. ACTH was also found to have similar suppressive effects. α-MSH exerts its effects via a cAMP-driven pathway and not via Smad 2/3. α-MSH upregulates superoxide dismutase 2 and hemeoxygenase 1, which is protective against the effects of bleomycin on reactive oxygen species. They also confirmed the presence of POMC and the MC1R in affected skin from patients with SSc and dermal fibroblasts strongly expressed both POMC and MC1R [31]. In a recent study MC1-signalling-deficient mice were susceptible to bleomycin-induced fibrosis, whereas wild-type animals were not [32].

Strengths of this work include prospective definition of clinical phenotype, collection within the framework of a double-blind clinical trial and standardised assay methodology. Longitudinal sampling of candidate makers and placebo control data over a clinically meaningful duration allows more robust interpretation than in cross-sectional studies. There are also some limitations such as the relatively small number of study subjects in a heterogeneous disease so that subgroups may be distributed unevenly between the treatment groups. The need to use different platforms for some single-factor assays may be a limitation compared with using the same methods for all analyses. In addition, conclusions may only apply to late-stage diffuse cutaneous SSc. It would be useful in future work to extend this and include other stages and subsets of SSc such as limited cutaneous disease (lcSSc) or early diffuse SSc. The effect of previous immunosuppression cannot be reliably explored in this study but interplay between HICS and other more conventional immunomodulatory approaches that are in use as treatment for SSc or its complications could be addressed in future work.

## Conclusions

These findings provide important information about future potential for SSc molecular markers. They provide important insight into the potential biological effects of HICS in SSc and in other medical indications. The data are hypothesis generating and suggest potential future therapeutic avenues to explore such as the effect of HICS in a larger and more diverse clinical cohort, and possible development of new composite serum markers that reflect changes in MRSS in clinical trials across the disease spectrum.

## Additional files

**Additional file 1: Figure S1.** Subject progression in the clinical trials with serum sample time points. Schematic indicates how 20 subjects were randomly allocated to active treatment with hyperimmune caprine serum (HICS) or placebo. One patient withdrew from the HICS arm and was not available for follow-up. Other subjects were all followed to 52 weeks and at 26 weeks were offered open-label compassionate HICS. The study blind for 0–26 week treatment was maintained until after 52-week assessment. Serum and plasma samples were available for weeks 0, 26 and 52. Additional screening blood samples (pre-randomisation) were available for quality control purposes. (TIF 132 kb)

**Additional file 2: Figure S2.** Unsupervised hierarchical cluster analysis for multiplex serum proteins at baseline and 26 weeks for the extended dataset of 26 weeks treatment with HICS. Unsupervised cluster analysis was undertaken to identify any subgroups within the extended dataset of the study cohort at baseline, the end of placebo treatment period, or at 52 weeks based upon the serum levels of multiple protein analytes as described in text. This provided a larger sample size by including 17 subjects treated with HICS over 26 weeks and 13 subjects with 26 weeks of observation on placebo or no active treatment. The same analysis was repeated for serum samples after 26 weeks of treatment with HICS or placebo. The randomly assigned treatment allocation is shown for each subject. Data for baseline samples are shown in panel A together with treatment allocation. After 26 weeks of treatment there were clear changes in the patterns of protein analytes that were spread between the two treatment arms as shown in panel B. (TIF 1373 kb)

**Additional file 3: Figure S3.** Unsupervised cluster analysis for change in serum proteins from baseline to 26 weeks comparing treatment with hyperimmune caprine serum (HICS) with placebo over 26 weeks and in extended dataset at 52 weeks. (A) Unsupervised cluster analysis of change

in protein level during 26-week treatment phase of placebo-controlled trial reveals patterns of change that are reflected in the supervised analysis shown in Fig. 3. Thus, subjects receiving placebo show generally less treatment effect and those treated with HICS show the patterns consistent with the summary changes shown above. (B) Unsupervised cluster analysis is also performed for the extended 52-week dataset that includes subjects moving from placebo to active treatment (n = 7) in the second 26 weeks and three cases that have no active treatment and were previously on placebo. This complements the presentation of data for baseline and 26 weeks presented in Additional file 1: Figure S1 and shows close congruity for the two 26-week unsupervised heat maps in the extended dataset. (TIF 1444 kb)

**Additional file 4: Figure S4.** Average change in serum proteins comparing treatment with hyperimmune caprine serum (HICS) or placebo and for MRSS responders versus non-responder at 26 weeks. (A) Average change in serum protein was calculated for each treatment arm over 26 weeks and ranked according to fold change average after HICS treatment. (B) Similar analysis was undertaken for average protein changes in the subjects showing significant improvement of four skin score units and 20% of baseline MRSS score during the trial (responders) or these that did not demonstrate clinical response. These were ranked for the most increased proteins in responder cases. Key proteins that emerged as upregulated (red) or downregulated (blue) for HICS treatment, shown in Fig. 4, are annotated with asterisks. (TIF 761 kb)

## Abbreviations

COMP: cartilage oligomeric matrix protein; dcSSc: Diffuse cutaneous systemic sclerosis; ECM: Extracellular matrix; ELISA: Enzyme-linked immunosorbent assay; HICS: Hyperimmune caprine serum; IVIG: Intravenous immunoglobulin; MRSS: Modified Rodnan skin score; PIIINP: Procollagen III N-terminal propeptide; SAM: Significance analysis of microarray; SSc: Systemic sclerosis; TGF-β1: Transforming growth factor beta 1; vWF: von Willebrand factor

## Acknowledgements
The clinical trial was sponsored and funded by Daval International. Additional biomarker analysis and interpretation was supported by a research grant from EULAR as part of their Orphan Diseases Programme.

## Funding
Daval International sponsored this clinical trial and funded this work. Analysis and additional work was supported by European League Against Rheumatism (EULAR) through the Orphan Diseases Programme.

## Authors' contributions
NQ designed the study, collected, analysed and interpreted clinical and laboratory data, drafted the manuscript, critically revised the manuscript and approved the final version. KC analysed and interpreted multiplex cytokine data, drafted the manuscript, critically revised the manuscript and approved the final version. BY conceived and designed the study, analysed and interpreted data, critically revised the manuscript and approved the final version. JV analysed and interpreted statistical aspects of the data, critically revised the manuscript and approved the final version. DM designed the study, analysed and interpreted data, critically revised the manuscript and approved the final version. SH designed the study, analysed and interpreted data, critically revised the manuscript and approved the final version. CD conceived and designed the study, collected, analysed and interpreted data, drafted the manuscript, critically revised the manuscript and approved the final version.

## Competing interests
DM and JV are employees of Daval International. SH is a consultant for Daval International. No other competing interests.

**Author details**
[1]Centre for Rheumatology, UCL Division of Medicine, Royal Free Campus, Rowland Hill Street, London NW3 2PF, UK. [2]Department of Neurophysiology, Royal Free London NHS Foundation Trust, London, UK. [3]Daval International, London, UK.

## References

1. Mackenzie R, Kiernan M, McKenzie D, Youl BD. Hyperimmune goat serum for amyotrophic lateral sclerosis. J Clin Neurosci. 2006;13(10):1033–6.
2. Mackenzie RA. Follow-up study of hyper-immune goat serum (Aimspro) for amyotrophic lateral sclerosis (ALS). J Clin Neurosci. 2009;16(11):1508–9.
3. Youl BD, Ginsberg L. Goat serum product AIMSPRO® shows promise as an effective treatment in CIDP. London: BSCN meeting, National Hospital; 2004.
4. Youl BD, Crum J. Clinical improvement in Krabbe's disease case treated with hyperimmune goat serum product AIMSPRO®. J Neurol Sci. 2005;238:S110.
5. Youl BD, Angus-Leppan H, Hussein N, Brooman I, Fitzsimons RB. Rapid and sustained response to hyperimmune goat serum product in a patient with Myaesthenia Gravis. J Neurol Sci. 2005;238:S177.
6. Moore CEG, Hannan R, McIntosh D. In vivo, human peripheral nerve strength duration time constant changes with AIMSPRO® implicate altered sodium channel function as a putative mechanism of action. J Neurol Sci. 2005;238:S238.
7. Kiernan MC, Burke D, Bostock H. Nerve excitability measures: biophysical basis and use in investigation of peripheral nerve disease use in investigation of peripheral nerve disease. In: Dyck PJ, Thomas PK, editors. Peripheral Neuropathy. 4th ed. Philadelphia: Elsevier Saunders; 2005. p. 113–29.
8. Burke G, Cavey A, Matthews P, Palace J. The evaluation of a novel 'goat serum' (AIMSPRO®) in multiple sclerosis. J Neurol Neurosurg Psychiatr. 2005;76:1326.
9. Youl BD, White SDT, McIntosh D, Cadogan M, Dalgleish AG, Ginsberg L. Hyperimmune serum reverses conduction block in demyelinated human optic nerve and peripheral nerve fibres. J Neurol Neurosurg Psychiatr. 2004;76:615.
10. Youl BD, Orrell R. Goat serum product AIMSPRO® produces sustained improvement in muscle power in a patient with fascioscapulohumeral dystrophy. J Neurol Sci. 2005;238:S169.
11. Quillinan NP, McIntosh D, Vernes J, Haq S, Denton CP. Treatment of diffuse systemic sclerosis with hyperimmune caprine serum (AIMSPRO): a phase II double-blind placebo-controlled trial. Ann Rheum Dis. 2014;73(1):56–61.
12. Chung L, Denton CP, Distler O, Furst DE, Khanna D, Merkel PA. Clinical trial design in scleroderma: where are we and where do we go next? Clin Exp Rheumatol. 2012;30(2 Suppl 71):S97–102.
13. Khanna D, Furst DE, Allanore Y, Bae S, Bodukam V, Clements PJ, et al. Twenty-two points to consider for clinical trials in systemic sclerosis, based on EULAR standards. Rheumatology (Oxford). 2015;54(1):144–51.
14. Maurer B, Graf N, Michel BA, Müller-Ladner U, Czirják L, Denton CP, Tyndall A, Metzig C, Lanius V, Khanna D, Distler O. Prediction of worsening of skin fibrosis in patients with diffuse cutaneous systemic sclerosis using the EUSTAR database. Ann Rheum Dis. 2015;74:1124–31.
15. Beirne P, Pantelidis P, Charles P, Wells AU, Abraham DJ, Denton CP, et al. Multiplex immune serum biomarker profiling in sarcoidosis and systemic sclerosis. Eur Respir J. 2009;34(6):1376–82.
16. Vettori S, Cuomo G, Iudici M, D'Abrosca V, Giacco V, Barra G, et al. Early systemic sclerosis: serum profiling of factors involved in endothelial, T-cell, and fibroblast interplay is marked by elevated interleukin-33 levels. J Clin Immunol. 2014;34(6):663–8.
17. Pendergrass SA, Hayes E, Farina G, Lemaire R, Farber HW, Whitfield ML, et al. Limited systemic sclerosis patients with pulmonary arterial hypertension show biomarkers of inflammation and vascular injury. PLoS One. 2010;5(8):e12106.
18. Rice LM, Ziemek J, Stratton EA, McLaughlin SR, Padilla CM, Mathes AL, et al. A longitudinal biomarker for the extent of skin disease in patients with diffuse cutaneous systemic sclerosis. Arthritis Rheumatol. 2015;67(11):3004–15.
19. Chakravarty EF, Martyanov V, Fiorentino D, Wood TA, Haddon DJ, Jarrell JA, et al. Gene expression changes reflect clinical response in a placebo-controlled randomized trial of abatacept in patients with diffuse cutaneous systemic sclerosis. Arthritis Res Ther. 2015;17:159.
20. Abignano G, Cuomo G, Buch MH, Rosenberg WM, Valentini G, Emery P, et al. The enhanced liver fibrosis test: a clinical grade, validated serum test, biomarker of overall fibrosis in systemic sclerosis. Ann Rheum Dis. 2014;73(2):420–7.
21. Thacker JD, Brown MA, Rest RF, Purohit M, Sassi-Gaha S, Artlett CM. 1-Peptidyl-2-arachidonoyl-3-stearoyl-sn-glyceride: an immunologically active lipopeptide from goat serum (Capra hircus) is an endogenous damage-associated molecular pattern. J Nat Prod. 2009;72(11):1993–9.
22. Poelman CL, Hummers LK, Wigley FM, Anderson C, Boin F, Shah AA. Intravenous immunoglobulin may be an effective therapy for refractory, active diffuse cutaneous systemic sclerosis. J Rheumatol. 2015;42(2):236–42.
23. Takehara K, Ihn H, Sato S. A randomized, double-blind, placebo-controlled trial: intravenous immunoglobulin treatment in patients with diffuse cutaneous systemic sclerosis. Clin Exp Rheumatol. 2013;31(2 Suppl 76):151–6.
24. Raja J, Nihtyanova SI, Murray CD, Denton CP, Ong VH. Sustained benefit from intravenous immunoglobulin therapy for gastrointestinal involvement in systemic sclerosis. Rheumatology (Oxford). 2016;55(1):115–9.
25. Clark KE, Etomi O, Denton CP, Ong VH, Murray CD. Intravenous immunogobulin therapy for severe gastrointestinal involvement in systemic sclerosis. Clin Exp Rheumatol. 2015;33(4 Suppl 91):S168–70.
26. Lee TH, Jawan B, Chou WY, Lu CN, Wu CL, Kuo HM, et al. Alpha-melanocyte-stimulating hormone gene therapy reverses carbon tetrachloride induced liver fibrosis in mice. J Gene Med. 2006;8(6):764–72.
27. Zhang Z, Ma J, Yao K, Yin J. Alpha-melanocyte stimulating hormone suppresses the proliferation of human tenon's capsule fibroblast proliferation induced by transforming growth factor beta 1. Mol Biol (Mosk). 2012;46(4):628–33.
28. Luo LF, Shi Y, Zhou Q, Xu SZ, Lei TC. Insufficient expression of the melanocortin-1 receptor by human dermal fibroblasts contributes to excess collagen synthesis in keloid scars. Exp Dermatol. 2013;22(11):764–6.
29. Bohm M, Raghunath M, Sunderkotter C, Schiller M, Stander S, Brzoska T, et al. Collagen metabolism is a novel target of the neuropeptide alpha-melanocyte-stimulating hormone. J Biol Chem. 2004;279(8):6959–66.
30. Bohm M, Eickelmann M, Li Z, Schneider SW, Oji V, Diederichs S, et al. Detection of functionally active melanocortin receptors and evidence for an immunoregulatory activity of alpha-melanocyte-stimulating hormone in human dermal papilla cells. Endocrinology. 2005;146(11):4635–46.
31. Kokot A, Sindrilaru A, Schiller M, Sunderkotter C, Kerkhoff C, Eckes B, et al. alpha-melanocyte-stimulating hormone suppresses bleomycin-induced collagen synthesis and reduces tissue fibrosis in a mouse model of scleroderma: melanocortin peptides as a novel treatment strategy for scleroderma? Arthritis Rheum. 2009;60(2):592–603.
32. Bohm M, Stegemann A. Bleomycin-induced fibrosis in MC1 signalling-deficient C57BL/6 J-Mc1r(e/e) mice further supports a modulating role for melanocortins in collagen synthesis of the skin. Exp Dermatol. 2014;23(6):431–3.

# The 5-HT1A receptor agonist buspirone improves esophageal motor function and symptoms in systemic sclerosis: a 4-week, open-label trial

George P. Karamanolis[1*], Stylianos Panopoulos[2], Konstantinos Denaxas[1], Anastasios Karlaftis[1], Alexandra Zorbala[2], Dimitrios Kamberoglou[1], Spiros D. Ladas[1] and Petros P. Sfikakis[2]

## Abstract

**Background:** Acute administration of the oral 5-HT$_1$A receptor agonist buspirone, which is commonly used as an anxiolytic drug, may improve compromised lower esophageal sphincter function. In an open-label trial we assessed the effects of buspirone on esophageal motor function and symptoms in patients with esophageal involvement associated with systemic sclerosis (SSc).

**Methods:** Thirty consecutive patients with SSc and symptomatic esophageal involvement, despite treatment with proton pump inhibitors, underwent high resolution manometry and chest computed tomography for assessment of motor function and esophageal dilatation, respectively. Regurgitation, heartburn, dysphagia, and chest pain severity was subjectively scored by visual analog scales. Manometric parameters (primary endpoint) and symptom severity (secondary endpoint) were re-examined after 4-week daily administration of 20 mg buspirone. Other medications remained unchanged.

**Results:** Eight patients did not complete the trial because of buspirone-associated dizziness ($n = 2$), or nausea ($n = 2$), or reluctancy to undergo final manometry. In the remaining 22 patients lower esophageal sphincter (LES) resting pressure increased from $7.7 \pm 3.9$ to $12.2 \pm 4.6$ mmHg ($p = 0.00002$) after buspirone administration; other manometric parameters did not change. Statistical analysis revealed negative correlation between individual increases in resting LES pressure and supra-aortic esophageal diameter ($r = -0.589$, $p = 0.017$), suggesting a more beneficial effect in patients with less severely affected esophageal function. Heartburn and regurgitation scores decreased at 4 weeks compared to baseline ($p = 0.001$, and $p = 0.022$, respectively).

**Conclusion:** Our findings warrant more conclusive evaluation with a double-blind controlled study; however, buspirone could potentially be given under observation for objective improvement in all patients with SSc who report reflux symptoms despite undergoing standard treatment.

**Keywords:** Scleroderma, Buspirone, Esophageal motility, Reflux symptoms

**Abbreviations:** 5-HT, 5-hydroxytryptamine; CT, computed tomography; GERD, gastroesophageal reflux disease; HRM, high resolution manometry; IRP, integrated relaxation pressure; LES, lower esophageal sphincter; SSc, systemic sclerosis; VAS, visual analog scale

* Correspondence: georgekaramanolis@yahoo.co.uk
[1]Academic Department of Gastroenterology, "Laiko" Hospital, Athens Medical School National and Kapodistrian University, Athens, Greece
Full list of author information is available at the end of the article

## Background

Systemic sclerosis (SSc) is a chronic autoimmune fibrotic disease affecting the skin and other organs including the gastrointestinal tract. The esophagus is commonly affected in SSc and esophageal function is compromised in up to 90 % of patients [1, 2]. Symptoms of esophageal disease are due to gastroesophageal reflux disease (GERD) and esophageal motor dysfunction. Thus, heartburn, regurgitation and dysphagia have been reported by 80 % of patients with SSc [3, 4].

Although several medications are used in patients with symptomatic SSc and esophageal involvement, there is no universally effective treatment. The current therapeutic approach includes administration of proton pump inhibitors (PPIs) and prokinetics agents (including metoclopromide, erythromycin, cisapride and domperidone), although the evidence to support their use is limited [5]. It is well-known that there are many issues in the efficacy and long-term use of the currently available prokinetic drugs; use of metoclopromide or erythromycin or cisapride is restricted due to safety profile issues and administration route problems, while administration of domperidone has no effect on esophageal motor dysfunction in patients with symptomatic SSc [6].

Animal studies have identified serotonin (5-hydroxytryptamine, 5-HT) as one of the putative neurotransmitters involved in esophageal motor function making its receptors suitable therapeutic targets [7]. Studies in healthy volunteers show that acute administration of buspirone, a 5-HT$_1$A receptor agonist, has a strong stimulatory effect on esophageal peristalsis and lower esophageal sphincter (LES) function [8, 9]. Moreover, we have recently observed that acute administration of buspirone exerts a beneficial effect on esophageal motor dysfunction associated with SSc [6]. Thus, in order to investigate whether buspirone exerts a long-term effect in SSc-associated esophageal involvement we conducted a prospective 4-week open-label trial. The primary objective was to assess the efficacy of buspirone on LES dysfunction. The secondary efficacy endpoint was change in esophageal symptoms after buspirone administration.

## Methods

### Study population

Thirty consecutive consenting patients who fulfilled classification criteria for SSc [10] and were able to perform high resolution manometry (HRM) participated in this open-label, non-randomized study. The only inclusion criterion was the presence of symptoms associated with esophageal involvement, such as regurgitation, heartburn, dysphagia, and chest pain, despite standard treatment with PPIs. These symptoms were scored on a 100-point visual analog scale (VAS) ranging from 0 (absent) to 100 (very severe)..Other types of esophageal diseases that could explain patients'

symptoms were excluded because all patients had undergone gastroscopy in the past.

Eight patients did not complete the study; 4 patients reported adverse effects with buspirone administration (2 dizziness and 2 nausea) and 4 patients were reluctant to perform the second HRM examination. The remaining 22 patients (aged 52.5 ± 11.6 years, 19 women) were re-examined after 4 weeks. During the study period all patients continued their therapy unchanged, including administration of proton pump inhibitors. All patients were on single PPIs dose before and during the study period and none was on medications that could affect results, such as prokinetics or erythromycin.

Before proceeding to esophageal manometry studies all patients filled out a self-reported symptom questionnaire in order to assess the severity of esophageal symptoms. Severity of dysphagia, heartburn, regurgitation, and chest pain was measured on a VAS (0–100). The VAS score has been adopted in many other trials for evaluation of visceral symptoms and has been used as a tool for self-assessment of symptoms [11, 12], and any decrease in the score at week 4 versus baseline was considered an improvement. Demographic data and phenotypic characteristics of the disease were collected from the clinical charts. Moreover, in all patients the supra-aortic and infra-aortic coronal diameters of the esophagus were measured in chest computed tomography (CT) performed within the previous 3 months. Esophageal dilatation was deemed present when the diameter was >9 mm [13]. The study protocol was approved by the ethics committee of "Laikon" General Hospital and informed consent was obtained from all participating patients.

### High resolution manometry

All patients were fasted and were studied in the supine position. Esophageal manometry was performed with a water-perfused assembly with 22 pressure sensors (Solar GI HRM, MMS, Enschede, The Netherlands). The HRM catheter was passed trans-nasally and positioned to record from the hypopharynx to the stomach. The catheter was fixed in place by taping it to the nose. The manometric examination included a 30-sec period to assess basal LES pressure and 10 swallows of 5 mL water. Double swallows were discarded and these were repeated. The study was repeated 4 weeks after oral administration of 20 mg buspirone (10 mg twice a day). We recorded 1) amplitude, duration and velocity of contractions at the distal part of the esophagus (defined as the mean amplitude at 3 and 8 cm proximal to the LES upper border of the esophagus) and 2) resting and residual LES pressure and integrated relaxation pressure (IRP). The LES pressures were referenced to intragastric pressure and we reported the mean resting pressure values.

All HRM tracings were interpreted by the same investigator (GK), who was blinded to whether administration of buspirone was performed. Hypotensive LES was considered when LES resting pressure was ≤10 mmHg, whereas isobaric contour <20 mmHg was considered as the cutoff for esophageal hypomotility [14].

## Statistical methods

The paired-sample $t$ test was used to compare changes from baseline in manometric values and severity of symptoms after buspirone administration, as all data analyzed were normally distributed. The Spearman correlation coefficient was used to assess the relationship between increase in LES pressure and other clinical, manometric, and CT parameters, because of non-canonical data distribution. Values were expressed as mean ± SD. A $p$ value <0.05 was considered significant.

## Results

Table 1 summarizes demographic characteristics, expression and duration of disease, CT, baseline manometry, and severity of esophageal symptoms. The mean amplitude of distal esophageal contractions was 16.6 ± 9.6 mmHg, whereas esophageal hypomotility was identified in 19 patients (86 %). The mean resting pressure of the LES was 7.7 ± 3.9 mmHg, whereas a hypotensive LES was observed in 17 patients (77 %). Both esophageal body and LES abnormalities were found in 16 patients (73 %). According to the Chicago classification 16 patients had absent peristalsis, 5 patients had weak peristalsis and 1 patient had normal esophageal motility. On chest CT 12 patients (54.5 %) had supra-aortic esophageal dilatation, whereas almost all patients had infra-aortic esophageal dilatation (21/22, 95.5 %).

Heartburn and regurgitation were reported by almost all patients (91 % and 86 %, respectively), while dysphagia was reported by 54.5 % of patients. Only 36 % of patients reported chest pain as one of their symptoms. Moreover, regurgitation and heartburn were the most bothersome symptoms reported to a similar extent, followed by dysphagia and chest pain (Table 1).

## Effect of buspirone on manometric parameters

Following buspirone administration for 4 weeks the LES resting pressure significantly increased from 7.7 ± 3.9 to 12.2 ± 4.6 mmHg ($p < 0.00005$). Figure 1 increased LES resting pressure after buspirone administration was observed in 15 patients (68 %) with a range of 4–13 mmHg (41–220 %, accordingly). There were significantly fewer patients with hypotensive LES after compared to before buspirone administration (8/22 vs. 17/22, respectively, $p = 0.006$).

In contrast to LES resting pressure, buspirone administration had no effect on LES residual pressure or on IRP (Table 2). In addition, buspirone administration did

**Table 1** Demographic characteristics, disease characteristics, symptoms, and manometry in the study population ($n = 22$)

| Variable | Value |
|---|---|
| Age (years) | 52.5 ± 11.9 |
| Sex (female/male) | 19/3 |
| Duration of disease (years)[a] | 8.7 ± 6.7 |
| Diffuse SSc (n (%)) | 16 (72.7) |
| Pulmonary fibrosis[b] | 15 (68.1) |
| Digital ulcers[c] | 10 (45.5) |
| Anti-Scl 70 (%) | 9 (41 %) |
| ANA (%) | 19 (86.4 %) |
| ACA (%) | 2 (9.1 %) |
| CPK (> × 2 normal values) (%) | 2 (9.1 %)[d] |
| Supra-aortic coronal diameters (cm) | 12.4 ± 5.3 |
| Infra-aortic coronal diameters (cm) | 22.5 ± 11.1 |
| Frequency of symptoms (%) | |
| -dysphagia | 12 (54.5) |
| -heartburn | 20 (91.0) |
| -regurgitation | 19 (86.0) |
| -chest pain | 8 (36.4) |
| severity of symptoms (0–100) | |
| -dysphagia | 25.8 ± 30.7 |
| -heartburn | 27.1 ± 24.0 |
| -regurgitation | 39.3 ± 29.8 |
| -chest pain | 10.4 ± 2.1 |
| amplitude of distal contractions (mmHg) | 16.6 ± 9.6 |
| duration of distal contractions (cm) | 3.7 ± 2.4 |
| velocity of distal contractions (cm/sec) | 2.6 ± 1.9 |
| LES resting pressure (mmHg) | 7.7 ± 3.9 |
| LES residual pressure (mmHg) | 2.9 ± 1.9 |
| IRP (mmHg) | 3.1 ± 2.3 |

*SSc* systemic sclerosis, *ANA* antinuclear antibody, *ACA* anti-centromere antibody, *LES* lower esophageal sphincter, *IRP* integrated relaxation pressure, *HRCT*, High resolution computed tomography, *CPK*, creatinophosphokinase, *anti-Scl*, anti-topoisomerase I

[a]Disease duration was from first non-Raunaud's symptom
[b]Presence of interstitial lung disease was determined after evaluation of HRCT
[c]Five out of these ten patients had active digital ulcers at the time of the manometry
[d]None of the patients had clinical signs of myositis or skeletal myopathy

not increase the duration and velocity of esophageal body contractions or the amplitude of contractions, compared to baseline values (Table 2). Buspirone was well-tolerated by all patients who completed the study.

## Correlation between individual increase in LES pressure and other clinical, manometric and CT parameters

Table 3 summarizes the correlation between individual increase in LES pressure and other variables. There was moderate, but significant, inverse correlation between increased LES resting pressure and supra-aortic diameter

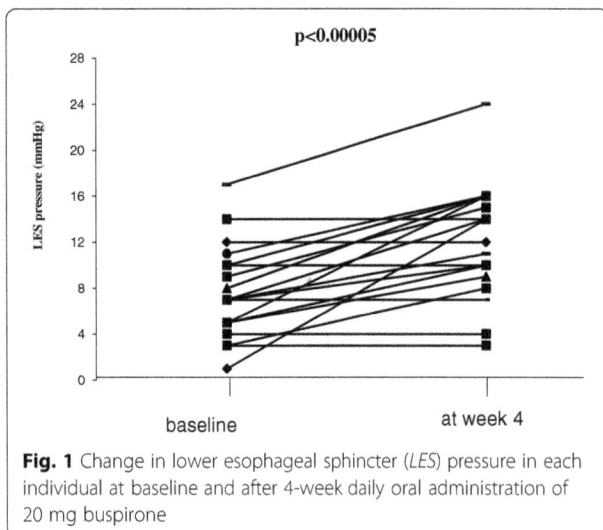

**Fig. 1** Change in lower esophageal sphincter (*LES*) pressure in each individual at baseline and after 4-week daily oral administration of 20 mg buspirone

**Table 3** Correlation between increase in LES pressure after 4-week daily administration of 20 mg buspirone and clinical, manometric and computed tomography parameters

|  | r | p |
|---|---|---|
| Baseline LES | -0.356 | 0.113 |
| Supra-aortic diameter | -0,589 | 0.017 |
| Infra- aortic diameter | -0.406 | 0.191 |
| Disease duration | -0.226 | 0.325 |
| Heartburn | 0.129 | 0.578 |
| Regurgitation | -0.188 | 0.415 |
| Chest pain | 0.103 | 0.657 |
| Dysphagia | 0.188 | 0.414 |

*r* Spearman correlation coefficient, *LES* lower esophageal sphincter

($p = 0.017$). The Pearson correlation coefficient was an r value of -0.589. In patients without supra-esophageal dilatation there was greater improvement in LES pressure ($83.9 \pm 38.1$ % vs. $19.2 \pm 26.8$ %, $p = 0.037$). There was no significant correlation between increased LES pressure and other measured parameters.

### Effect of buspirone on esophageal symptoms

The severity of regurgitation and heartburn significantly decreased from baseline following buspirone administration for 4 weeks ($39.3 \pm 29.8$ vs. $24.4 \pm 22.0$, $p = 0.02$ and $37.1 \pm 23.9$ vs. $21.9 \pm 21.2$, $p = 0.001$, respectively). There was no significant improvement in the scores for severity of chest pain and dysphagia ($10.4 \pm 23.1$ vs. $8.5 \pm 20.0$ and $25.8 \pm 30.7$ vs. $18.9 \pm 21.9$, $p = 0.203$, respectively).

Improvement in the severity of heartburn was reported by 70 % (14/20) of patients who had heartburn at baseline, while 58 % (11/19) of patients with regurgitation at baseline had improvement in the severity of regurgitation. Increased LES resting pressure was simultaneously observed in the majority of patients with improvement in heartburn and regurgitation (12/14 and 8/11, respectively). Half of the patients with baseline dysphagia reported improvement in their symptom severity, while a

**Table 2** Manometric parameters at baseline and after 4-week daily administration of 20 mg buspirone

|  | Baseline | After buspirone | p |
|---|---|---|---|
| Amplitude (mmHg) | $16.6 \pm 9.6$ | $17.5 \pm 9.6$ | 0.163 |
| Velocity (cm/sec) | $3.7 \pm 2.4$ | $3.4 \pm 1.9$ | 0.701 |
| Duration (sec) | $2.6 \pm 1.9$ | $3.1 \pm 2.3$ | 0.668 |
| LES resting pressure (mmHg) | $7.7 \pm 3.9$ | $12.2 \pm 4.6$ | 0.00002 |
| LES residual pressure (mmHg) | $2.9 \pm 1.9$ | $3.2 \pm 2.1$ | 0.157 |
| IRP (mmHg) | $3.1 \pm 2.3$ | $3.5 \pm 2.1$ | 0.143 |

*LES* lower esophageal sphincter, *IRP* integrated relaxation pressure

minority of patients (25 %) with baseline chest pain had an improvement in the severity of their symptoms.

### Discussion

Treatment of patients with symptomatic SSc and esophageal involvement is still an area of unmet need, as there is no available treatment with established efficacy. Administration of PPIs and prokinetic drugs do not appear to provide substantial symptomatic relief in patients with SSc and esophageal symptoms [5]. Pathophysiology of gastrointestinal dysmotility in SSc is multifactorial and different neurotransmitters could be involved in this process [15, 16]. Serotonin (5-HT) is considered a key neurotransmitter and acute studies, both in healthy subjects and patients with SSc, have shown that agonists of specific class of its receptors, such as 5-HT$_1$A, could be a putative therapeutic option [6, 8, 9]. Buspirone had been initially developed for clinical use in the treatment of depression and anxiety disorders. Its mechanisms of action are thought to include agonistic actions, mainly on 5-HT$_1$A receptors, but also on dopamine D2 receptors. Buspirone is absorbed rapidly and almost completely with a $t_{max} = 0.89 \pm 0.15$ h [17].

To the best of our knowledge no previous study has prospectively investigated whether a pharmaceutical agent may help patients with SSc and esophageal involvement. The results of our open-label, prospective 4-week trial suggest that the 5-HT$_1$A receptor agonist, buspirone, given orally for 4 weeks, significantly increases the LES resting pressure by 41 % to 220 % over the baseline values in almost 70 % of patients with SSc. Furthermore, patients with a less dilated esophagus as detected on chest CT had a better response to buspirone administration. This is an important aspect of our study, as patients with SSc undergo routine chest CT as a screening test for lung fibrosis. Many studies have suggested that measurement of esophageal coronal diameter on chest CT is a marker of the functional status of the esophagus in SSc and a dilated esophagus represents more severe visceral involvement [18, 19].

Herein, the 4-week administration of buspirone also alleviated heartburn and regurgitation in the majority of patients. Buspirone seems more effective for GERD-related symptoms, whereas symptoms related to esophageal hypomotility, such as dysphagia and chest pain are not affected. Thus, we could suggest that buspirone administration may be most helpful for the subgroup of SSc patients with reflux symptoms. An objective assessment of reflux response with pH-impedance measurement could certainly enhance our results.

As all patients were on PPIs before and during the study period, the strategy with add-on buspirone could be a worthwhile therapeutic option. Keeping in mind the anecdotal evidence that persistent reflux contributes significantly to the development of interstitial lung disease and/or progress, which is the leading cause of death in SSc, the potential beneficial effect of buspirone becomes more important. Buspirone-associated improvement in the severity of reflux symptoms can be explained by a strong stimulatory effect on LES resting pressure. However, other mechanisms cannot be excluded. Comorbid psychiatric diseases in patients with a chronic disorder, such as SSc, and especially anxiety, are common [20, 21]. Buspirone is used as anxiolytic drug in clinical practice. Therefore, a potential alteration in the sensitivity by decreasing the anxiety level may play a role in symptom improvement. As we did not include measurement of anxiety scores, this is a limitation of the present study. However, in the event that the main mechanism underlying symptom improvement with buspirone was the anxiolytic effect of the drug, other non-reflux symptoms should have been improved.

A limitation of the present study, due to restrictive regulatory rules that we were unable to overcome, is that it is not a randomized, placebo-controlled investigation and there is a lack of a control arm. Another limitation is the relatively small number of patients studied; however, we have to keep in mind that patients with SSc due to the chronic nature of their disease have several medical disabilities, making recruitment very challenging. The use of a validated questionnaire, such as the UCLA STCC SSc-GI [22] rather than a self-reported one could strengthen our results, however, this questionnaire, which covers a broad spectrum of gastrointestinal symptoms in patients with SSc, is not validated in Greek. Moreover, the majority of available questionnaires are focused on reflux symptoms rather than on dysmotility-associated symptoms characterizing SSc.

Buspirone was well-tolerated in the present study. Treatment interruption due to adverse effects (dizziness and nausea) was observed in only 4 out of 30 patients. Patients who completed the study reported sporadic and self-limited adverse effects that did not affect their daily activities.

## Conclusions

In conclusion, our study showed that 4-week daily administration of buspirone increases the LES resting pressure and improves esophageal symptoms in the majority of SSc patients with esophageal involvement. Furthermore, buspirone exerts a greater beneficial effect on patients with less severely affected esophageal function as detected on chest CT, suggesting a therapeutic role mainly in patients with earlier or less severe involvement. Although further evaluation in placebo-controlled studies is warranted, buspirone could potentially be given under observation for objective improvement in all patients with SSc who report reflux symptoms, despite undergoing standard treatment.

**Funding**
There is no funding for the manuscript.

**Authors' contributions**
GPK and PPS: conception and design, analysis and interpretation of the data, drafting of the article, and critical revision of the article for important intellectual content. SP: analysis and interpretation of the data, statistical analysis, and critical revision of the article for important intellectual content. KD, AK, AZ, and DK: analysis and interpretation of the data and critical revision of the article for important intellectual content. SLD: conception and design and critical revision of the article for important intellectual content. All authors approved the final manuscript.

**Competing interests**
The authors declare that they have no competing interests.

**Author details**
¹Academic Department of Gastroenterology, "Laiko" Hospital, Athens Medical School National and Kapodistrian University, Athens, Greece. ²Joint Academic Rheumatology Programme, Athens Medical School National and Kapodistrian University, Athens, Greece.

**References**
1. Varga J, Abraham D. Systemic sclerosis: a prototypic multisystem fibrotic disorder. J Clin Invest. 2007;117:557–67.
2. Clements PJ, Becvar R, Drosos AA, Ghattas L, Gabrielli A. Assessment of gastrointestinal involvement. Clin Exp Rheumatol. 2003;21 Suppl 29:S15–8.
3. Ebert EC. Esophageal disease in scleroderma. J Clin Gastroenterol. 2006;40:769–75.
4. Ntoumazios SK, Voulgari PV, Potsis K, Koutis E, Tsifetaki N, Assimakopoulos DA. Esophageal involvement in scleroderma: gastroesophageal reflux, the common problem. Semin Arthritis Rheum. 2006;36:173–81.
5. Sallam H, McNearney TA, Chen JD. Systematic review: pathophysiology and management of gastrointestinal dysmotility in systemic sclerosis (scleroderma). Aliment Pharmacol Ther. 2006;23:691–712.
6. Karamanolis G, Panopoulos S, Karlaftis A, Denaxas K, Kamberoglou D, Sfikakis PP, Ladas SD. Beneficial effect of the 5-HT$_{1A}$ receptor agonist buspirone on esophageal dysfunction associated with systemic sclerosis: a pilot study. United Eur Gastroenterol J. 2015;3:266–71.
7. Hempfling C, Neuhuber WL, Worl J. Serotonin-immunoreactive neurons and mast cells in the mouse esophagus suggest involvement of serotonin in both motility control and neuroimmune interactions. Neurogastroenterol Motil. 2012;24:e67–78.
8. Blonski W, Vela MF, Freeman J, Sharma N, Castell DO. The effect of oral buspirone, pyridostigmine, and bethanechol on esophageal function evaluated with combined multichannel esophageal impedance-manometry in healthy volunteers. J Clin Gastroenterol. 2009;43:253–60.

9.  Di Stefano M, Papathanasopoulos A, Blondeau K, Vos R, Boecxstaens V, Farré R, et al. Effect of buspirone, a 5-HT1A receptor agonist, on esophageal motility in healthy volunteers. Dis Esophagus. 2012;25:470–6.

10. van den Hoogen F, Khanna D, Fransen J, Johnson SR, Baron M, Tyndall A, et al. 2013 classification criteria for systemic sclerosis: an American college of rheumatology/European league against rheumatism collaborative initiative. Ann Rheum Dis. 2013;72(11):1747–55.

11. Geeraerts B, Vandenberghe J, Van Oudenhove L, Gregory LJ, Aziz Q, Dupont P, et al. Influence of experimentally induced anxiety on gastric sensorimotor function in humans. Gastroenterology. 2005;129:1437–44.

12. de Bortoli N, Martinucci I, Savarino E, Bellini M, Bredenoord AJ, Franchi R, et al. Proton pump inhibitor responders who are not confirmed as GERD patients with impedance and pH monitoring: who are they? Neurogastroenterol Motil. 2014;26:28–35.

13. Pitrez EH, Bredemeier M, Xavier RM, Capobianco KG, Restelli VG, Vieira MV, et al. Oesophageal dysmotility in systemic sclerosis: comparison of HRTC and scintigraphy. Br J Radiol. 2006;79:719–24.

14. Breedenoord AJ, Fox M, Kahrilas PJ, Pandolfino JE, Schwizer W, Smout AJ, International High Resolution Manometry Working Group. Chicago classification criteria of esophageal motility disorders defined in high resolution esophageal pressure topography. Neurogastroenterol Motil. 2012; 24 Suppl 1:57–65.

15. Gao F, Liao D, Drewes AM, Gregersen H. Modelling the elastin, collagen and smooth muscle contribution to the duodenal mechanical behaviour in patients with systemic sclerosis. Neurogastroenterol Motil. 2009;21:914–e68.

16. McNearney TA, Sallam HS, Hunnicutt SE, Doshi D, Wollaston DE, Mayes MD, Chen J. Gastric slow waves, gastrointestinal symptoms and peptides in systemic sclerosis patients. Neurogastroenterol Motil. 2009;21:1269–e120.

17. Loane C, Politis M. Buspirone: what is it all about? Brain Res. 2012;1461:111–8.

18. Vonk MC, Van Die CEV, Snoeren MM, Bhansing KJ, van Riel PL, Fransen J, van den Hoogen FH. Oesophageal dilatation on high-resolution computed tomography scan of the lungs as a sign of scleroderma. Ann Rheum Dis. 2008;67:1317–21.

19. Pandey AK, Wilcox P, Mayo JR, Moss R, Ellis J, Brown J, et al. Oesophageal dilatation on high-resolution CT chest in systemic sclerosis: What does it signify? J Med Imag Radiat Oncol. 2011;55:551–5.

20. Nguyen C, Ranque B, Baubet T, Bérezné A, Mestre-Stanislas C, Rannou F, et al. Clinical, functional and health-related quality of life correlates of clinically significant symptoms of anxiety and depression in patients with systemic sclerosis: a cross-sectional survey. PLoS One. 2014;9:e90484.

21. Malcarne VL, Fox RS, Mills SD, Gholizadeh S. Psychosocial aspects of systemic sclerosis. Curr Opin Rheumatol. 2013;25:707–13.

22. Khanna D, Hays RD, Maranian P, Seibold JR, Impens A, Mayes MD, et al. Reliability and validity of the University of California, Los Angeles Scleroderma Clinical Trial Consortium Gastrointestinal Tract Instrument. Arthritis Rheum. 2009;61(9):1257–63.

# miR-155 in the progression of lung fibrosis in systemic sclerosis

Romy B. Christmann[1*], Alicia Wooten[1], Percival Sampaio-Barros[2], Claudia L. Borges[3], Carlos R. R. Carvalho[2], Ronaldo A. Kairalla[2], Carol Feghali-Bostwick[4], Jessica Ziemek[1], Yu Mei[1], Salma Goummih[1], Jiangning Tan[5], Diana Alvarez[5], Daniel J. Kass[5], Mauricio Rojas[5], Thiago Lemos de Mattos[6], Edwin Parra[2], Giuseppina Stifano[1], Vera L. Capelozzi[2], Robert W. Simms[1] and Robert Lafyatis[1,5]

## Abstract

**Background:** MicroRNA (miRNA) control key elements of mRNA stability and likely contribute to the dysregulated lung gene expression observed in systemic sclerosis associated interstitial lung disease (SSc-ILD). We analyzed the miRNA gene expression of tissue and cells from patients with SSc-ILD. A chronic lung fibrotic murine model was used.

**Methods:** RNA was isolated from lung tissue of 12 patients with SSc-ILD and 5 controls. High-resolution computed tomography (HRCT) was performed at baseline and 2–3 years after treatment. Lung fibroblasts and peripheral blood mononuclear cells (PBMC) were isolated from healthy controls and patients with SSc-ILD. miRNA and mRNA were analyzed by microarray, quantitative polymerase chain reaction, and/or Nanostring; pathway analysis was performed by DNA Intelligent Analysis (DIANA)-miRPath v2.0 software. Wild-type and miR-155 deficient (miR-155ko) mice were exposed to bleomycin.

**Results:** Lung miRNA microarray data distinguished patients with SSc-ILD from healthy controls with 185 miRNA differentially expressed ($q < 0.25$). DIANA-miRPath revealed 57 Kyoto Encyclopedia of Genes and Genomes pathways related to the most dysregulated miRNA. miR-155 and miR-143 were strongly correlated with progression of the HRCT score. Lung fibroblasts only mildly expressed miR-155/miR-21 after several stimuli. miR-155 PBMC expression strongly correlated with lung function tests in SSc-ILD. miR-155ko mice developed milder lung fibrosis, survived longer, and weaker lung induction of several genes after bleomycin exposure compared to wild-type mice.

**Conclusions:** miRNA are dysregulated in the lungs and PBMC of patients with SSc-ILD. Based on mRNA-miRNA interaction analysis and pathway tools, miRNA may play a role in the progression of the disease. Our findings suggest that targeting miR-155 might provide a novel therapeutic strategy for SSc-ILD.

**Keywords:** Systemic Sclerosis, Lung fibrosis, Gene expression, microRNA, Biomarker, miR-155, Bleomycin

## Background

Systemic sclerosis (SSc) is a chronic autoimmune disease in which pulmonary involvement, particularly interstitial lung disease (SSc-ILD), is known to be the leading cause of mortality [1–3]. The prevalence of SSc-ILD is high and approximately 15–30 % of patients will progress to severe lung fibrosis. However, distinguishing those who will progress from those who will have slow or stable

disease remains challenging [4, 5]. Using mRNA expression analysis of lung tissue in a prospective cohort of patients with SSc-ILD, we recently described immune activation pathways and upregulated transforming growth factor-β (TGFβ)-induced signature genes associated with progressive lung fibrosis [6].

MicroRNA (miRNA) are small RNA that are of vital importance in regulating gene expression within cells, having critical roles in innate and adaptive immunity in general [7]. In addition, there is increasing evidence they play a role in fibrosis and are strongly associated with the pathogenesis of a wide range of human diseases [8, 9].

* Correspondence: romy.souza@gmail.com
[1]Boston University School of Medicine, E501, Arthritis Center, Medical Campus, 72 East Concord Street, Boston, MA 02118-2526, USA
Full list of author information is available at the end of the article

miRNA are remarkably stable and reliable for detection in the blood and urine and bring new hope to the development of clinical biomarkers. More importantly, disease-associated miRNA represent a new class of therapeutic targets.

Using high-throughput technology, we show that many miRNA are dysregulated in the lungs of patients with SSc-ILD. In addition, selected miRNA are associated with progressive lung fibrosis based on image lung score and lung function tests, with miR-155 as one of the best markers. miR-155-deficient mice survive longer and develop milder lung fibrosis. Therefore, miR-155 could be a potential novel therapeutic target for lung fibrosis in patients with SSc.

## Methods
### Study participants
Between January 2002 and July 2004, 28 consecutive patients with SSc-ILD, identified on HRCT as having associated respiratory symptoms and/or reduced performance on a pulmonary function test (PFT) underwent an open lung biopsy and were followed for at least 3 years. Twelve subjects involved in the previous study [6] were selected (sixteen samples were not included due to lack of lung material for miRNA isolation). The patients included in the current study were classified as having diffuse SSc (dSSc) (n = 7) and limited SSc (lcSSc) (n = 5), according to diagnostic [10] and subtype criteria [11]. Controls were five samples of normal histological healthy lung tissue obtained during lung cancer surgical resection. Lung explants from controls and patients with SSc-ILD were obtained from lung transplants at the University of Pittsburgh Medical Center (healthy controls, n = 6; SSc-ILD, n = 6) and used for fibroblast culture. Peripheral blood mononuclear cells (PBMC) were collected from healthy controls (n = 6) and patients with SSc-ILD (n = 13) from Boston University Medical Center. Informed consent was obtained from all patients and healthy subjects involved in the study. The Boston University Medical Center, the University of Sao Paulo, and the University of Pittsburgh Institutional Review Boards reviewed and approved the conduct of this study.

### Histological diagnosis
Two pathologists (VLC and ERP) classified the lung specimens as previously described [6].

### High-resolution computed tomography
Two pulmonologists (CRC and RC) performed blinded evaluation of the images. As described previously [6] each lung was divided into three zones: upper (lung apex to aortic arch); middle (aortic arch to inferior pulmonary veins); and lower (inferior

pulmonary veins to lung bases). For baseline and follow up HRCT, the extent of the pulmonary abnormality was scored as previously described [6]. The sum of all scores on the lung zones is referred to as FibMax. A delta FibMax, which is the difference between the follow-up FibMax and the baseline FibMax, was used to evaluate the progression of the lung fibrosis.

### Lung biopsy
Open lung biopsy was performed by formal thoracotomy, avoiding honeycombing areas [6].

### Follow up
Patients with evidence of non-specific interstitial pneumonia (NSIP) on lung biopsy were treated with monthly intravenous cyclophosphamide (0.5–1.0 g/m$^2$) for at least one year (see previous report for details [6]). HRCT and PFT were performed before biopsy and repeated 2–3 years after the one-year treatment (Fig. 1a).

### RNA and microRNA isolation and microarray analysis hybridization
Total RNA and miRNA from human lung biopsy tissue, lung fibroblasts, and PBMC were extracted using microRNeasy Mini Kits (Qiagen). RNA samples were stored at −80 °C.

### MicroRNA and messenger RNA quantitative PCR (qPCR)
Complementary DNA (cDNA) was transcribed using the TaqMan MicroRNA Reverse Transcription Kit (Life Technologies) and Reverse Transcriptase (Gibco BRL) and primers using 200 ng of total RNA and according to the manufacturer's protocol. Samples were diluted 1:15 and followed the TaqMan Universal PCR Master Mix (Life Technologies) protocol. Specific miRNA primers were used for miR-155, miR-21, miR-182, miR-15b, miR-193a, and RNU6B (Life Technologies). Specific mRNA primers were used for collagen type 3 alpha-1 (Col3a1), MS4A4A, periostin (POSTN), and 18S (Life Technologies). miRNA and mRNA qPCR was performed using the TaqMan assay and StepOne Plus Real Time PCR system (Applied Biosystems) in a 20-ul reaction for 40 cycles. Gene expression was analyzed using the difference in cycle threshold (ΔCt) method. The Ct values of the miRNAs were normalized to RNU6B and of the mRNA were normalized to 18S as an internal control using the equation:

ΔCt = Ct reference − Ct target and expressed as ΔCt.

### Microarray data clustering
All procedures were performed at Boston University Microarray Resource Facility as described in the Affymetrix GeneChip 3′IVT Express user manual (Affymetrix, Santa

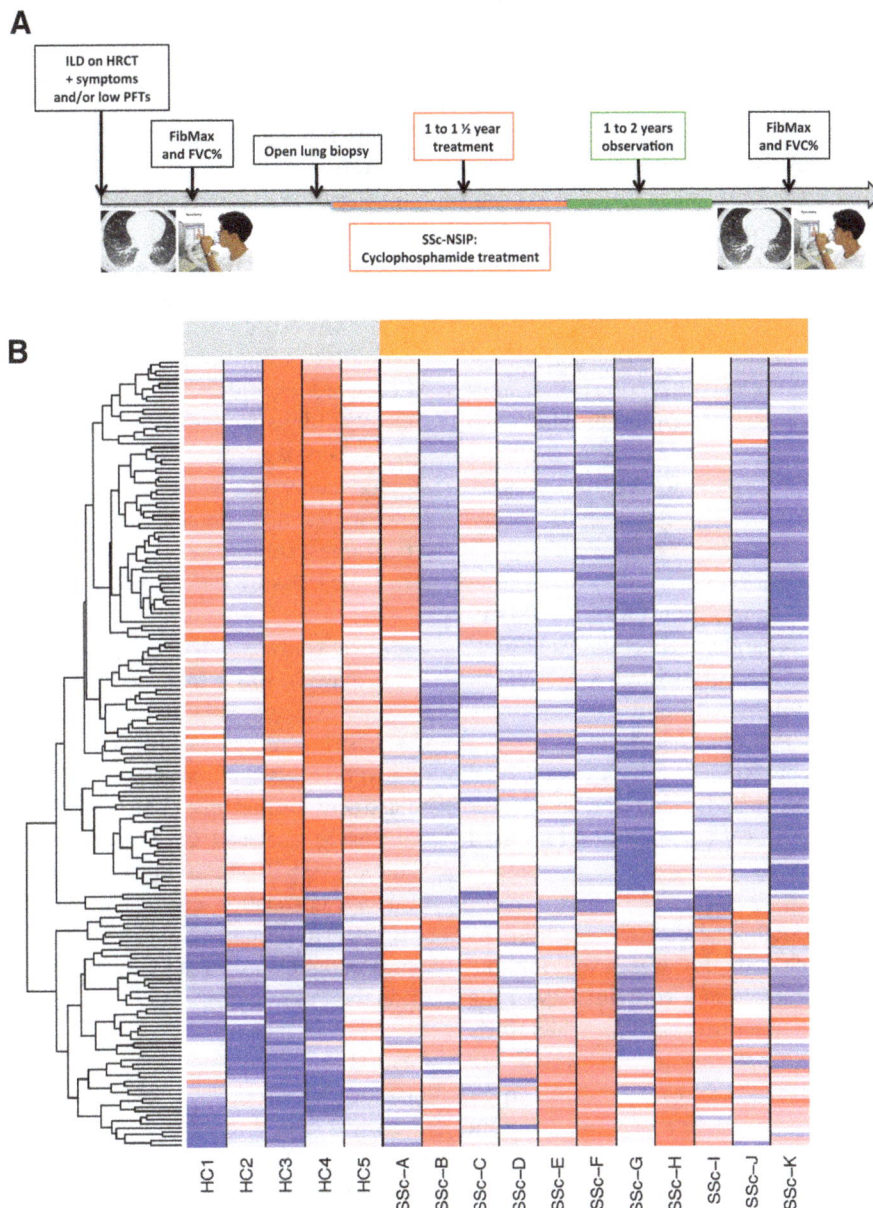

**Fig. 1** **a** Timeline of the study. See "Methods" for more details. **b** Heatmap of whole lung homogenate showing the expression of genes clustered using complete linkage hierarchical supervised clustering. *Gray* indicates healthy controls (*HC1* to *HC5*; n = 5); *orange* indicates patients with systemic sclerosis interstitial lung disease (SSc-ILD) (*SSc-A* to *SSc-K*; n = 12). Each miRNA was z-score-normalized across all samples and was scaled to *red* and *blue* (≥2 or ≤−2, respectively) and *white* indicating a z score of zero. *ILD* interstitial lung disease, HRCT high-resolution computer tomography, *PFT* pulmonary function test, *FibMax* HRCT lung score, *FVC%* percent forced vital capacity, *NSIP* non-specific interstitial pneumonia

Clara, CA, USA; www.affymetrix.com). For mRNA arrays biotin-labeled amplified total RNA was purified, fragmented, and hybridized to Affymetrix U133A 2.0 microarrays. The MAS5 algorithm with global scaling normalization was used to generate gene-level expression data. For miRNA arrays miRNA was purified, fragmented and hybridized to Affymetrix GenChip miRNA 3.0 microarrays. The signal of the samples was amplified and microarrays were immediately scanned using Affymetrix GeneArray Scanner 3000 7G Plus (Affymetrix, Santa Clara, CA, USA). The resulting CEL files were summarized using the Affymetrix Expression Console (current version 1.1). Clustering was performed using Cluster 3.0 software. Both mRNA and miRNA Affymetrix data [GEO:GSE81294] and SubSeries linked to GSE81294 [GEO:GSE81292; GEO:GSE81293] are available at the public repository Gene Expression Omnibus. Additional file 1: Table S1 and Additional file 2: Table S2 contain all the miRNA and mRNA, respectively, that were significantly different in patients with SSc-ILD and controls.

## Fibroblast culture

Lung tissue was minced and primary fibroblasts cultured using the outgrowth method as previously described [12]. Lung fibroblasts were cultured in DMEM supplemented with 10 % fetal bovine serum and penicillin/streptomycin and utilized at passages 2–4. Fibroblasts (100 % confluent) were incubated in serum-free DMEM overnight prior to stimulation with TGFß (R&D System; 2.5 ng/ml), recombinant human IL-13 (R&D Systems, 20 ng/ml), or interferon-alpha (IFN) (R&D Systems; 500 U/ml) for 18 hours. Total RNA from fibroblasts was transferred in Qiazol buffer and purified using the miR-Nease mini kit protocol (Qiagen). RNA samples were stored at −80 °C.

## Peripheral blood mononuclear cells

Blood was collected in cell preparation tubes (CPTs) designed for one-step cell separation (Becton Dickinson) from healthy controls and patients within 3 months of the date when the lung function tests were performed. The sample was immediately mixed and centrifuged at 1800 g at ambient temperature for 30 minutes. Total RNA from PBMC was extracted using the miRNease mini kit protocol (Qiagen). RNA samples were stored at −80 °C.

## MicroRNA Nanostring technology

RNA (100 ng from each sample) was used for the miRNA analysis. The miRNA library contains 800 of the most relevant miRNA described in the literature. Normalization was performed using the average of expression of the top 20 most-expressed miRNA in all samples. The minimal threshold for the detection of miRNA was considered as 50 counts.

## RNA Nanostring technology

RNA (100 ng of from each mouse) was used for RNA analysis. The lung gene panel was built based on a microarray analysis of the lungs of mice exposed to a bleomycin-pump compared to PBS in previous experiments (unpublished results). Normalization was performed using nine housekeeping genes that were not affected by the bleomycin-pump model.

DNA Intelligent Analysis (DIANA) DIANA-miRPath v2.0 utilizes miRNA targets based on DIANA-microT-CDS, which predicts miRNA-gene interaction including the binding region, position, and type, and/or miRNA-gene interaction experimentally validated from Tarbase v7.0 [13]. Combined analysis results for miRNA and pathway-related information was obtained from miRBase 18 [14] and the Kyoto Encyclopedia of Genes and Genomes

(KEGG) v58 [15]. The selected top 30 upregulated and downregulated miRNA were used (Additional file 1: Table S1).

## Bleomycin lung fibrosis model

C57BL/6 J (B6) and B6.Cg-Mir155$^{tm1.Rsky}$/J mice were purchased from The Jackson Laboratory (Bar Harbor, ME, USA). Age-matched and sex-matched mice were used in the experiments at 8 to 10 weeks. Mice were kept in pathogen-free conditions with food and water. The in vivo study was approved by the Animal Ethics Committee at the Boston University School of Medicine. Mice were chronically exposed to PBS or Bleomycin (90 U/Kg) by subcutaneous osmotic pump injections for 7 days. Mice were observed and sacrificed on day 28. The survival curve was calculated. Lungs were harvested for histology and gene expression. H&E and Masson's Trichrome staining were performed. The Ashcroft lung score was measured blinded by one investigator (RBC).

## Statistical analysis

Data analysis was performed using GraphPad Prism 6 software, version 6.0a (GraphPad Software, San Diego, CA, USA). Multiple group comparisons were analyzed by one-way analysis of variance (ANOVA) with Bonferroni adjustment for multiple comparisons. Two-group comparisons were analyzed by Student's $t$ test or the Mann-Whitney test. Correlation was tested and presented as Pearson's correlation coefficient ($r$). The survival fraction was calculated by the Kaplan-Meier test with 95 % confidence intervals computed by the asymmetrical method using the log-rank test.

# Results

## Baseline characteristics of patients with systemic sclerosis interstitial lung disease

A timeline of the study is summarized in Fig. 1a. We have previously described all the demographic and FibMax data of these patients with SSc-ILD before and after treatment [6]. Note that despite treatment, most patients with SSc-ILD developed progressive disease based on the FibMax, with a mean baseline score of $6.88 \pm 4.47$ compared to $12.76 \pm 6.59$ after treatment; $p = 0.006$. The delta FibMax was used to gauge the progression of lung fibrosis as previously described [6]. Healthy control lungs were obtained from cancer-free resected lungs.

## Patients with systemic sclerosis interstitial lung disease have distinct microRNA gene expression patterns

We analyzed lung tissue samples from healthy controls (n = 5) and patients with SSc-ILD (n = 12) using miRNA microarrays. Both middle and lower lobe samples were analyzed in five of the patients with SSc-ILD, while only the lower lobes were analyzed in seven patients. One patient was excluded from the miRNA analysis on the basis of poor quality metrics. To identify genes with differential expression associated with SSc-ILD, Student's two-sample $t$ test was performed to compare SSc-ILD (expression averaged for each gene from both lung biopsy sites) and control samples ($p < 0.05$). A false discovery rate (FDR)-corrected $p$ value ($q < 0.25$) was computed after removing miRNA present in $\leq 25$ % of the samples, to eliminate miRNA with low overall expression. A heatmap of the most informative miRNA ($n = 185$ genes) was created containing the miRNA with the most significant differential expression between SSc-ILD and control samples. Most of the miRNA were downregulated in patients compared to the healthy controls (Fig. 1b). The complete list of significantly different miRNA can be found in Additional file 1: Table S1.

We validated several miRNA that were upregulated in patients with SSc-ILD compared to the controls, by qPCR. miR-182 was highly expressed in the lung tissue from patients with SSc-ILD (mean fold-change $17.5 \pm 14.8$) compared to controls (mean fold-change $1.1 \pm 0.6$; $p = 0.001$. Fig. 2a). miR-155 was upregulated in patients with SSc-ILD (mean fold-change $7.6 \pm 9.2$) compared to controls (mean fold-change $1.0 \pm 0.5$; $p = 0.003$. Fig. 2b), and miR-21 was upregulated in patients with SSc-ILD (mean fold-change $3.4 \pm 2.6$) compared to controls (mean fold-change $1.1 \pm 0.7$; $p = 0.06$), although not statistically significant (Fig. 2c).

## Validation of relevant gene signatures in systemic sclerosis interstitial lung disease

In order to better understand the potential mRNA targeted by altered lung miRNA expression, we analyzed all samples for mRNA expression by microarray. We identified genes with differential expression associated with SSc-ILD, using Student's two-sample $t$ test ($p < 0.05$) corrected by FDR ($q < 0.25$). These microarray data confirmed the altered expression of hundreds of genes in SSc-ILD that we reported previously [6], such as chemokine C-C motif ligand 18 (CCL18), several collagens (types I and III), macrophage activation markers (for example, CD163 and MS4A4A), secreted phosphoprotein 1/osteopontin (SPP1), and others (Additional file 2: Table S2). Using qPCR, we validated several of the top upregulated genes in lung tissue from patients with SSc-ILD, such as COL3a1 ($p = 0.004$), MS4A4A ($p = 0.02$), and POSTN ($p = 0.006$) Fig. 2d-f.

## Messenger RNA and microRNA: a complex network

Taking advantage of our simultaneous analysis of mRNA and miRNA in the same cohort of patients with SSc-ILD

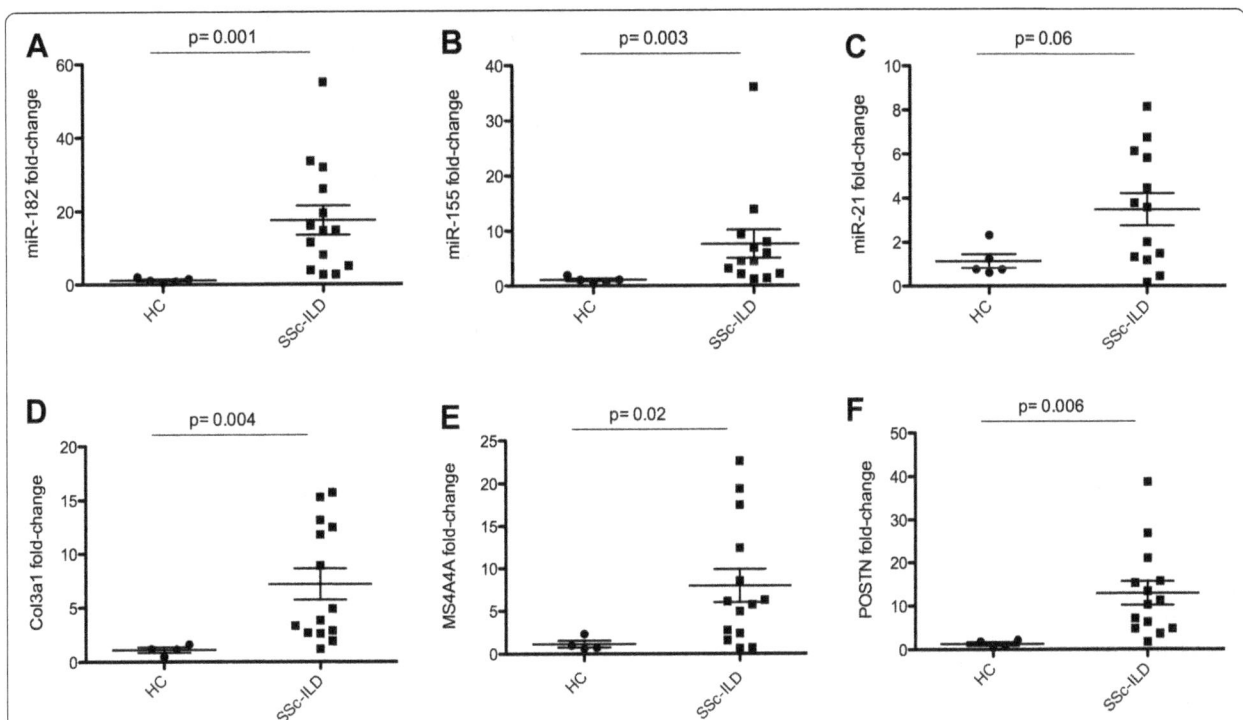

**Fig. 2** Whole lung homogenate with miRNA and mRNA expression by qPCR of miR-182 (**a**), miR-155 (**b**), miR-21 (**c**), collagen type 3 alpha-1 (*Col3a1*) (**d**), MS4A4A (**e**), and periostin (*POSTN*) (**f**) in healthy controls (*HC*) (n = 5) and patients with systemic sclerosis interstitial lung disease (*SSc-ILD*) (n = 14). Data are expressed as fold-change normalized to miRNA (RNU6B) or mRNA (18S) average expression in HC samples. Student's *t* test; *p* < 0.05 was considered significant

and healthy controls we further investigated interactions between mRNA and miRNA lung expression. Pearson's correlation was tested between selected upregulated and downregulated miRNA (see Additional file 1: Table S1) and the most highly upregulated and downregulated mRNA in SSc-ILD (see Additional file 2: Table S2) by microarray analysis, based on average fold-change gene expression compared to controls. miR-155, miR-21, and miR-4459 were the miRNA that were most strongly correlated and their interactions are shown in Table 1.

### RNA and microRNA: pathway analysis

We selected the top upregulated and downregulated miRNA in patients with SSc-ILD compared to the controls (see Additional file 1: Table S1) for pathway analysis. First, we applied the DIANA-Tarbase v7.0 database in order to identify miRNA target genes experimentally validated in the literature (see "Methods"). Only a few miRNA from the selected group had validated target genes: miR-155, miR-21, miR-125a, miR-31, miR-205, miR-20a, let-7f, miR-182, let-7e, miR-199b, miR-199a, miR-663, and miR-193a. miR-155 (n = 812) and miR-21 (n = 581) had the largest list of target genes already validated.

To gain further insight into the function of the top dysregulated miRNA and their targets, DIANA-microT-CDS miRPath was applied to identify the significant KEGG pathways (see "Methods"): 57 KEGG biological processes were significantly enriched ($p < 0.05$, FDR-corrected) in SSc-ILD (Additional file 3: Figure S1). The 10 most highly implicated processes identified using this approach, with their related miRNA, can be found in Table 2.

### miR-155 lung expression correlates with progressive systemic sclerosis interstitial lung disease

There is an urgent need for a biomarker that predicts the progression of lung fibrosis in patients with SSc. miRNA are known to regulate a complex network; therefore, we tested the correlation between miRNA microarray lung gene expression and changes in the lung fibrosis score FibMax, the sum of all fibrotic scores in the six lung zones (see "Methods"). The delta FibMax of each patient, when available, was correlated with corresponding patient lung miRNA microarray fold-change gene expression (see Additional file 1: Table S1). Surprisingly, only four miRNA correlated positively with the delta FibMax ($r > 0.4$) with miR-155 having the strongest correlation ($r = 0.65$, $p < 0.001$, Fig. 3a), followed by miR-182 ($r = 0.49$, $p = 0.06$), miR-27a ($r = 0.49$, p = 0.06), and miR-21 ($r = 0.47$, $p = 0.07$). Five miRNA correlated negatively with the delta FibMax, with miR-143 having the strongest negative correlation ($r = -0.64$, $p < 0.01$), followed by miR-4270 ($r = -0.59$, $p = 0.01$), miR-4530 ($r = -0.54$,

$p = 0.03$), miR-19b ($r = -0.51$, $p = 0.05$), and miR-4459 ($r = -0.50$, $p = 0.05$).

### miR-155 expression by peripheral blood mononuclear cells is correlated with progressive systemic sclerosis interstitial lung disease

PBMC gene expression has been used as a surrogate for rarely available lung tissue to further investigate lung complications in SSc, such as SSc-ILD and SSc pulmonary arterial hypertension (SSc-PAH) [16]. Therefore, we analyzed miRNA expression in SSc-ILD (n = 13) and control PBMC (n = 5) by Nanostring; demographic features are shown in Additional file 4: Table S3. Among the miRNA that were upregulated in the lungs of patients with SSc-ILD (Additional file 1: Table S1) let-7d ($p = 0.01$), miR-15b ($p = 0.05$), and miR-21 ($p = 0.1$) were the most expressed in PBMC from SSc-ILD compared to controls (Additional file 5: Table S4) based on fold-change expression.

More importantly, we observed that miR-155 expression on SSc-ILD PBMC was strongly negatively correlated with both %FVC ($r = -0.60$; $p = 0.01$) and %DLCO ($r = -0.58$; p = 0.02). let-7d was also strongly negatively correlated with %FVC ($r = -0.65$; $p = 0.007$) and with %DLCO ($r = -0.56$; $p = 0.02$). miR-21 PBMC expression did not correlate with lung function tests (%FVC $r = 0.14$; %DLCO $r = 0.18$; both $p > 0.05$).

### Activated lung fibroblasts have minor influence on the microRNA signature in systemic sclerosis interstitial lung disease

In order to elucidate whether fibroblasts might be responsible for the miRNA expression in SSc-ILD we stimulated healthy lung fibroblasts (n = 6) and fibroblasts from the lungs of patients with SSc-ILD (n = 6) with cytokines known to be involved in the progression of lung disease: TGFβ, IL-13, and IFN [6]. Fibroblasts were stimulated for 18 hours and miRNA expression was analyzed by Nanostring technology (Additional file 6: Table S5) and confirmed in a larger number of samples by qPCR (see "Methods").

Expression of miR-21 was in general slightly increased after IFN and TGFβ stimulation of fibroblasts in SSc-ILD, although not statistically significant (Fig. 3d, $p > 0.05$). On the other hand, miR-155 expression was reduced overall after all three stimuli of fibroblasts in SSc-ILD, although not statistically significant (Fig. 3e, $p > 0.05$). There was mild expression of miR-193a and miR-15b in lung fibroblasts in both groups after all three stimuli (Additional file 7: Figure S2A and B, respectively).

### The absence of miR-155 protects mice from bleomycin-induced lung fibrosis

We observed that miR-155 expression in the lungs and in the blood of patients with SSc-ILD are strongly

**Table 1** Strongest positive and negative correlation between the most expressed messenger RNA (top upregulated and downregulated genes) and miR-155/miR-21/miR-4459 lung expression

| Abbreviation | Gene name | Fold-change | r (miR-155) | r (miR-21) | r (miR-4459) |
|---|---|---|---|---|---|
| MMP1 | Matrix metallopeptidase 1 (interstitial collagenase) | 14.1 | 0.13 | 0.24 | **-0.52** |
| MMP7 | Matrix metallopeptidase 7 (matrilysin, uterine) | 12.0 | **0.57** | **0.54** | **-0.85** |
| KRT15 | Keratin 15 | 7.1 | 0.27 | 0.40 | **-0.51** |
| S100A2 | S100 calcium binding protein A2 | 6.6 | 0.29 | 0.45 | **-0.57** |
| PDIA3 | Protein disulfide isomerase family A, member 3 | 6.2 | **0.67** | **0.52** | **-0.76** |
| CDH3 | Cadherin 3, type 1, P-cadherin (placental) | 5.6 | **0.60** | **0.60** | **-0.82** |
| IL13RA2 | Interleukin 13 receptor, alpha 2 | 5.6 | **0.75** | **0.81** | **-0.78** |
| IGHM | Immunoglobulin heavy constant mu | 5.5 | **0.67** | **0.52** | **-0.63** |
| SPP1 | Secreted phosphoprotein 1 | 5.1 | **0.69** | **0.55** | **-0.74** |
| GPR87 | G protein-coupled receptor 87 | 4.7 | 0.29 | 0.32 | -0.45 |
| RRM2 | Ribonucleotide reductase M2 | 4.7 | **0.72** | **0.59** | **-0.57** |
| CTSE | Cathepsin E | 4.4 | **0.66** | **0.66** | **-0.91** |
| AADAC | Arylacetamide deacetylase | 4.4 | **0.60** | 0.48 | **-0.76** |
| CXCL6 | Chemokine (C-X-C motif) ligand 6 (granulocyte chemotactic protein 2) | 4.3 | 0.34 | 0.34 | -0.30 |
| CR2 | Complement component (3d/Epstein Barr virus) receptor 2 | 4.2 | **0.61** | 0.37 | -0.42 |
| TYMS | Thymidylate synthetase | 4.2 | **0.72** | **0.58** | **-0.75** |
| CXCL13 | Chemokine (C-X-C motif) ligand 13 | 4.1 | **0.77** | **0.59** | -0.48 |
| SCG5 | Secretogranin V (7B2 protein) | 4.1 | **0.76** | **0.70** | **-0.70** |
| MEOX1 | Mesenchyme homeobox 1 | 3.9 | **0.59** | **0.52** | **-0.51** |
| TOP2A | Topoisomerase (DNA) II alpha 170 kDa | 3.7 | **0.68** | **0.62** | **-0.64** |
| POSTN | Periostin, osteoblast specific factor | 3.7 | **0.74** | **0.70** | **-0.74** |
|  | Pearson's correlation >0.5 or < -0.5 | total | n = 16 | n = 14 | n = 17 |
| IL6 | Interleukin 6 (interferon, beta 2) | -45.2 | **-0.50** | -0.44 | **0.54** |
| SERPINE1 | Plasminogen activator inhibitor type 1, member 1 | -21.9 | -0.45 | -0.36 | **0.60** |
| FOSB | FBJ murine osteosarcoma viral oncogene homolog B | -18.4 | **-0.69** | **-0.66** | **0.73** |
| MT1M | Metallothionein 1 M | -15.8 | **-0.50** | -0.41 | **0.54** |
| DDX3Y | DEAD (Asp-Glu-Ala-Asp) box polypeptide 3, Y-linked | -14.3 | -0.17 | **-0.51** | 0.33 |
| RND1 | Rho family GTPase 1 | -13.6 | -0.46 | -0.37 | 0.40 |
| IL8 | Interleukin 8 | -12.8 | -0.40 | -0.26 | 0.37 |
| NXF3 | Nuclear RNA export factor 3 | -12.0 | **-0.80** | **-0.75** | **0.89** |
| CSF3 | Colony stimulating factor 3 (granulocyte) | -11.8 | **-0.50** | -0.34 | 0.48 |
| CCL2 | Chemokine (C-C motif) ligand 2 | -11.6 | -0.47 | -0.36 | **0.54** |
| PTX3 | Pentraxin 3, long | -11.4 | -0.15 | -0.02 | 0.27 |
| IL12A | Interleukin 12A | -11.1 | **-0.70** | **-0.64** | **0.85** |
| CCL20 | Chemokine (C-C motif) ligand 20 | -9.5 | -0.25 | -0.17 | 0.15 |
| GADD45B | Growth arrest and DNA-damage-inducible, beta | -9.5 | **-0.50** | -0.42 | **0.54** |
| ESM1 | Endothelial cell-specific molecule 1 | -8.6 | **-0.52** | -0.36 | 0.48 |
| CXCL2 | Chemokine (C-X-C motif) ligand 2 | -8.5 | -0.40 | -0.44 | 0.46 |
| SLC6A4 | Solute carrier family 6 (neurotransmitter transporter, serotonin), member 4 | -8.4 | **-0.82** | **-0.87** | **0.72** |
| SLCO4A1 | Solute carrier organic anion transporter family, member 4A1 | -8.3 | **-0.62** | **-0.50** | **0.64** |
| KDM5D | Lysine (K)-specific demethylase 5D | -8.2 | -0.15 | -0.48 | 0.37 |
| S100A12 | S100 calcium binding protein A12 | -8.2 | -0.45 | -0.33 | **0.53** |
| HAS2 | Hyaluronan synthase 2 | -8.2 | -0.29 | -0.27 | 0.30 |
|  | Pearson's correlation >0.5 or < -0.5 | total | n = 9 | n = 6 | n = 10 |

In sequence: gene symbol, gene name, average fold-change expression in SSc-ILD compared to healthy controls, r values for correlation between each gene and specific miRNA

**Table 2** Top 10 Kyoto Encyclopedia of Genes and Genomes (KEGG) pathways related to the most expressed microRNA in the lungs of patients with systemic sclerosis interstitial lung disease compared to controls

| KEGG pathway | p value | #genes | miRNA | | | | |
|---|---|---|---|---|---|---|---|
| ECM-receptor interaction (hsa04512) | <1e-16 | 16 | 3 | let-7e, | miR-4459, | let-7f | |
| Ubiquitin mediated proteolysis (hsa04120) | <1e-16 | 76 | 9 | miR-182, | miR-141, | miR-125a, | miR-379, | miR-4484, |
| | | | | miR-574, | miR-3613, | miR-4739, | miR-20a | |
| Wnt signaling pathway (hsa04310) | <1e-16 | 79 | 10 | miR-155, | miR-205, | miR-1224, | let-7e, | miR-4459, |
| | | | | miR-762, | miR-4668, | let-7f, | miR-3613, | miR-20a |
| MAPK signaling pathway (hsa04010) | <1e-16 | 132 | 13 | miR-21, | miR-155, | miR-125a, | let-73, | miR-4530, |
| | | | | miR-1207, | miR-149, | miR-762, | let-7f, | miR-199a, |
| | | | | miR-199b, | miR-3613, | miR-20a | | |
| Pathways in cancer (hsa05200) | <1e-16 | 166 | 15 | miR-21, | miR-155, | miR-182, | miR-205, | miR-1224, |
| | | | | let-7e, | miR-4459, | miR-4484, | let-7f, | miR-199a, |
| | | | | miR-574, | miR-199b, | miR-3613, | miR-4739, | miR-20a |
| Axon guidance (hsa04360) | 7.77E-16 | 72 | 11 | miR-155, | miR-205, | miR-1224, | miR-379, | miR-4741, |
| | | | | miR-762, | miR-4689, | miR-4484, | miR-3613, | miR-4739, |
| | | | | miR-20a | | | | |
| PI3K-Akt signaling pathway (hsa04151) | 2.74E-14 | 137 | 12 | miR-155, | miR-182, | let-7e, | miR-379, | miR-4459, |
| | | | | miR-149, | miR-4668, | let-7f, | miR-199a, | miR-199b, |
| | | | | miR-3613, | miR-20a | | | |
| TGF-beta signaling pathway (hsa04350) | 5.88E-14 | 41 | 10 | miR-21, | miR-205, | let-7e, | miR-4668, | miR-451a, |
| | | | | miR-4484, | let-7f, | miR-3613, | miR-20a, | miR-455 |
| ErB signaling pathway (hsa04012) | 1.17E-13 | 40 | 12 | miR-155, | miR-205, | miR-193a, | miR-200b, | miR-4530, |
| | | | | miR-451a, | miR-4484, | miR-199a, | miR-199b, | miR-200c, |
| | | | | miR-3613, | miR-20a | | | |
| Transcriptional misregulation in cancer (hsa05202) | 1.23E-13 | 83 | 11 | miR-182, | miR-205, | miR-1224, | let-7e, | miR-1207, |
| | | | | miR-149, | miR-4668, | let-7f, | miR-3613, | miR-20a, |
| | | | | miR-455 | | | | |

In sequence: pathway names, significance levels based on p value, number of targeted genes, number of miRNA targeting each pathway, and list of miRNA related to each pathway

correlated with progressive lung disease identified by image and by lung function tests, respectively. Therefore, we tested the bleomycin model of chronic lung fibrosis in mice deficient in miR-155 (miR-155 knockout (KO)) compared to wild-type mice (WT). miR-155 KO mice had a 100 % survival rate over the course of 28 days after starting bleomycin compared to a 45 % survival rate in WT mice; $p < 0.001$, log-rank test (Fig. 4a). WT (n = 7) and miR-155 KO (n = 6) mice exposed to PBS were used as controls. WT (n = 11) and miR-155 KO (n = 11) mice were exposed to bleomycin and three WT mice were found dead on days 8, 13, and 17, respectively. One WT mouse exposed to bleomycin was killed on day 20 due to poor conditions and was included in the lung Nanostring analysis. miR-155 KO mice (n = 11) developed milder fibrosis in the lungs as measured by the Ashcroft lung score (Fig. 4b, $p < 0.001$) compared to the WT (n = 7) exposed to bleomycin on day 28.

We tested the effect of miR-155 deletion on bleomycin-induced gene expression using a custom-designed Nanostring that we developed to detect pro-inflammatory and profibrotic genes upregulated in the lungs of bleomycin-treated lung tissue and lung tissue from patients with SSc-ILD. Overall, bleomycin-induced lung gene expression was lower in miR-155 KO mice (Additional file 8: Figure S3). Arginase-1 lung gene expression was strongly induced in the WT mice and correlated positively with the Ashcroft score ($r = 0.70$, $p < 0.001$). Arginase-1, a marker of M2 macrophages (Fig. 4c), and tissue inhibitor of metalloproteinase-1 (TIMP1) lung expression (Fig. 4d) were induced significantly less after bleomycin in miR155 KO mice compared to WT mice. Expression of other bleomycin-induced genes was blunted in miR-155 KO lungs compared to WT mice and clustered with Arginase-1 and TIMP1 (Fig. 4e). On the other hand, expression of CD68, a general marker

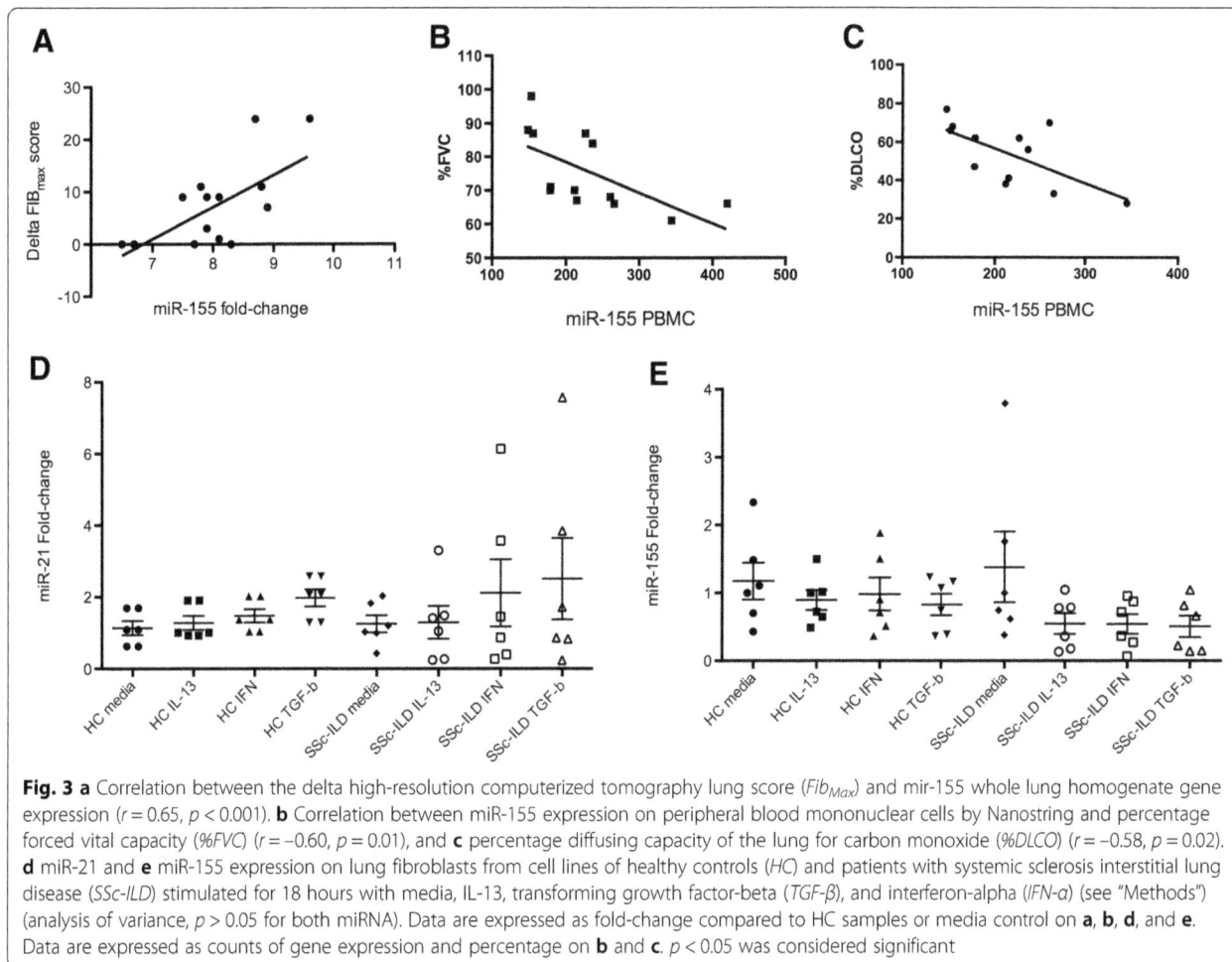

**Fig. 3 a** Correlation between the delta high-resolution computerized tomography lung score (Fib$_{Max}$) and mir-155 whole lung homogenate gene expression ($r = 0.65$, $p < 0.001$). **b** Correlation between miR-155 expression on peripheral blood mononuclear cells by Nanostring and percentage forced vital capacity (%FVC) ($r = -0.60$, $p = 0.01$), and **c** percentage diffusing capacity of the lung for carbon monoxide (%DLCO) ($r = -0.58$, $p = 0.02$). **d** miR-21 and **e** miR-155 expression on lung fibroblasts from cell lines of healthy controls (HC) and patients with systemic sclerosis interstitial lung disease (SSc-ILD) stimulated for 18 hours with media, IL-13, transforming growth factor-beta (TGF-β), and interferon-alpha (IFN-α) (see "Methods") (analysis of variance, $p > 0.05$ for both miRNA). Data are expressed as fold-change compared to HC samples or media control on **a**, **b**, **d**, and **e**. Data are expressed as counts of gene expression and percentage on **b** and **c**. $p < 0.05$ was considered significant

of macrophages, was induced similarly in both groups exposed to bleomycin ($p > 0.05$).

## Discussion

Dysregulation of the immune system is critical for the development of skin and lung involvement in SSc. In this regard, we have recently shown that this inappropriate inflammatory response in the lungs is strongly correlated with progressive lung fibrosis [6], along with a profibrotic TGFβ signature. miRNA are a new class of regulators that tightly control the overall inflammatory response. We show here that miRNA are intensely dysregulated in the lungs and in PBMC in patients with SSc-ILD. Moreover, we found that dysregulated gene expression of only a few miRNA, including miR-155, are strongly associated with progressive lung disease and that the absence of miR-155 is protective for the bleomycin-lung fibrotic model.

miR-155 controls differentiation of CD4+ T cells into its several subtypes to regulate B-cell differentiation and antibody production, and is highly expressed in activated monocytes/macrophages [17]. miR-155 is upregulated in

several autoimmune disorders, such as rheumatoid arthritis [18], multiple sclerosis [19], systemic lupus erythematosus [20, 21], and ulcerative colitis [22]. In our cohort, we showed that miR-155 expression correlates highly with profibrotic gene expression, such as SPP1 and POSTN. We also observed strong correlation between miR-155 PBMC expression in patients with SSc-ILD and lung function tests. On the other hand, lung fibroblasts seem not to be the most relevant cell type driving the strong expression of miR-155 in the lungs in patients with SSc-ILD.

We showed the functional relevance of miR-155 in lung fibrotic disease where miR-155 KO mice survived longer and developed substantially less aggressive lung fibrosis based on lung phenotype and on a comprehensive lung gene expression analysis. This protective effect might be underestimated as three mice in the WT bleomycin group did not survive until day 28 and neither the lung score nor the lung gene expression were considered in the analysis. In addition, the absence of miR-155 in the model blocked the alternative activation of lung macrophages, which correlates strongly with

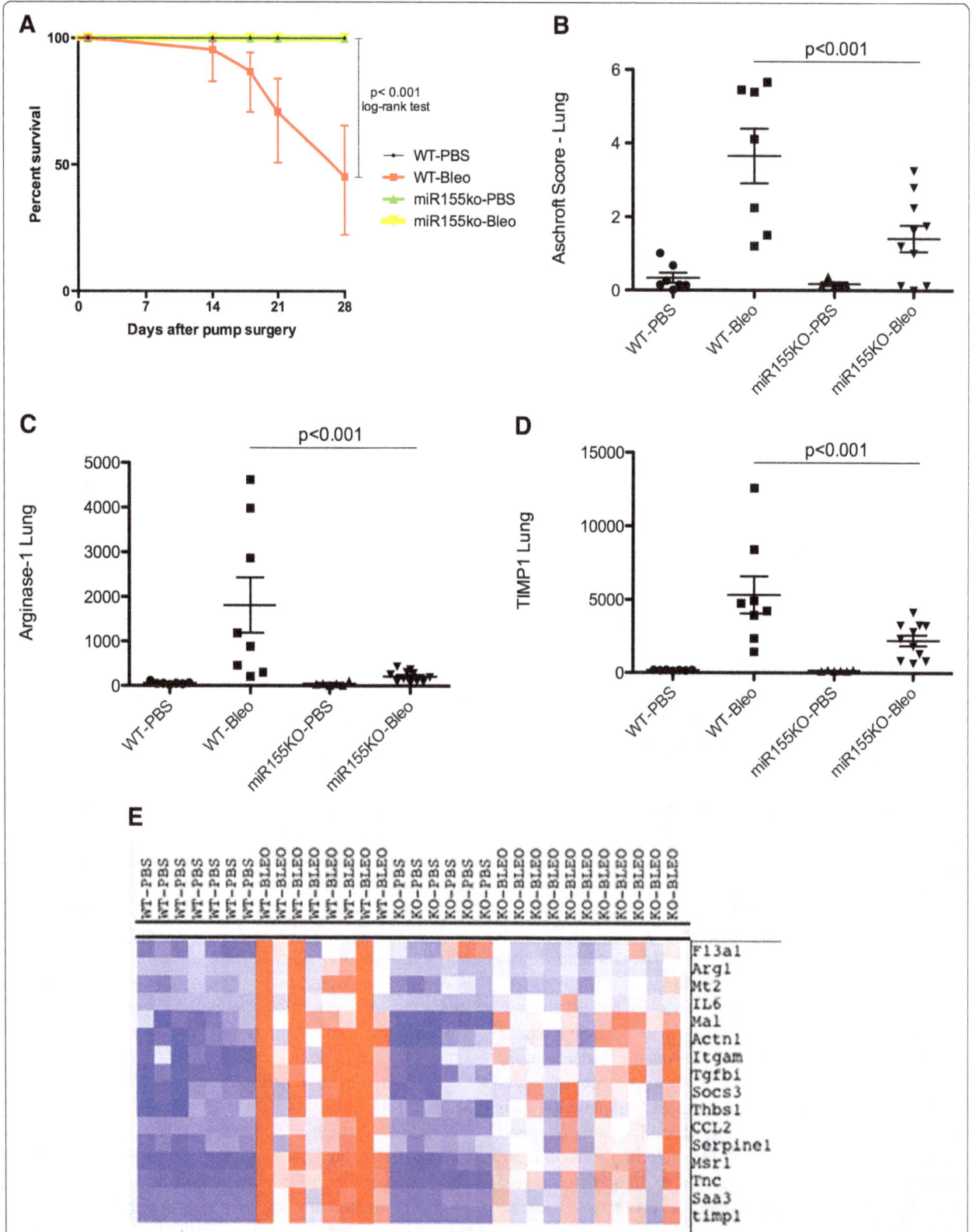

**Fig. 4** (See legend on next page.)

(See figure on previous page.)
**Fig. 4** Milder lung fibrosis in miR-155 knockout (*KO*) mice. **a** Percent survival rate by Kaplan-Meier, log-rank test. **b** Ashcroft lung score assessed by Masson's trichrome staining. Lung gene expression by Nanostring of Arginase-1 (**c**) and tissue inhibitor of metalloproteinase-1 (*TIMP1*) (**d**). **e** Cluster of the most affected genes by the absence of miR-155 (*blue*). Data are expressed by counting gene expression on **c** and **d**. Each microRNA was z-score-normalized across all samples and scaled to *red* and *blue* ($\geq 2$ or $\leq -2$, respectively) and *white* indicating a z score of zero. Analysis of variance; $p < 0.05$ was considered significant. *WT* wild-type, *Bleo* bleomycin

progressive lung fibrosis in patients with SSc-ILD [6] and with the Ashcroft lung fibrotic score in our murine model. Yan et al. [23] recently showed protection of bleomycin cutaneous fibrosis in miR-155-deficient mice and reduced skin thickness after topical antagomiR-155 treatment in mice primed with subcutaneous bleomycin [23]. In the intratracheal bleomycin murine lung model miR-155 was upregulated and correlated with the degree of lung fibrosis [24]. Altogether, our observations reinforce the hypothesis of a strong immune activation in SSc-ILD with miR-155 as a key regulator.

Our observations that miR-21 is upregulated in the lungs of patients with SSc-ILD suggest that modulating miR-21 might be a future therapeutic strategy for SSc-ILD. miR-21 has been extensively studied in fibrosis, with increased expression observed in the lungs of bleomycin-treated mice and in the lungs of patients with idiopathic pulmonary fibrosis (IPF) in whom it is mainly localized in myofibroblasts [25]. More importantly, restoring miR-21 to normal levels inhibits bleomycin-induced pulmonary fibrosis [25]. miR-21 is also upregulated in the skin and fibroblasts from patients with both diffuse and limited subtypes of SSc [26]. miR-21 is induced by TGFβ in stellate hepatic cells and in a feed-forward loop it amplifies its signal, eventually promoting fibrosis [27]. Lung fibroblasts might not be the main cell type responsible for the miRNA signature in SSc-ILD, as we observed only a slight increase in miR-21 expression after TGFβ stimulation. Although our data on lung tissues in SSc-ILD do not permit a direct assessment of intracellular pathways, we showed that several upregulated profibrotic genes, such as Col3a1 and POSTN, correlate positively with miR-21 lung expression. In addition to being well-established as a profibrotic-miR, miR-21 is also central to many inflammatory pathways, and most importantly, in controlling the Toll-like receptor signaling with strong connection with miR-155 [28].

We also showed for the first time that miR-182 is upregulated in the lungs of patients with SSc-ILD. miR-182 has been implicated in several types of cancer and it is known to regulate proliferation, invasion, and migration of cancer cells [29]. Interestingly enough, some of the recently identified miR-182 targets are strong inhibitors of extracellular matrix degradation [30]. miR-4484 and miR-4459 were significantly downregulated in our cohort of patients with

SSc-ILD and neither of them have validated target genes based on Tarbase v7.0 [13].

Our study has limitations. Our cohort was small and our results should ideally be validated in a larger group. The suggested mRNA-miRNA interactions and pathways are mainly predicted, although our agnostic and unbiased analysis using algorithmic tools guided us in similar directions, which support the validity of our results.

## Conclusions

Our unique approach of analyzing the relevance of miRNA in SSc-ILD using gene expression, pathway analysis, and functional studies, revealed a selected group of miRNA that might mediate the development and/or the progression of SSc-ILD. miR-155 and miR-21 were the most relevant miRNA having in common a close involvement in altered pathways observed in fibrotic diseases. mir-155 regulates the development of lung fibrosis in mice, thus, opening a new drug development opportunity.

## Additional files

**Additional file 1: Table S1.** The 185 differential miRNA expression (present in $\geq 25$ % of samples, $q < 0.25$) in average fold-change observed in SSc-ILD compared to healthy controls. In sequence: transcript ID, fraction of samples. Top 30 upregulated and downregulated miRNA (present in >80 % of samples, $p < 0.05$) are highlighted in bold. (XLSX 55 kb)

**Additional file 2: Table S2.** List of mRNA gene expression in SSc-ILD compared to healthy controls. In sequence: gene symbol, gene name, and average fold-change expression in SSc-ILD compared to healthy controls. (XLSX 15 kb)

**Additional file 3: Figure S1.** List of the 57 KEGG pathways related to the most expressed miRNA in the lungs of patients with SSc-ILD compared to controls. In sequence: pathway names, significance levels based on $p$ value, number of targeted genes, number of miRNA targeting each pathway. (PDF 1456 kb)

**Additional file 4: Table S3.** Demographic data of patients with SSc-ILD and healthy controls for the miRNA analysis in PBMC. *%FVC* percentage forced vital capacity. *%DLCO* percentage diffusing capacity of the lung for carbon monoxide, *LSSc* limited systemic sclerosis, *DSSc* diffuse systemic sclerosis. (XLSX 35 kb)

**Additional file 5: Table S4.** miRNA expression in PBMC by Nanostring analysis. Data are expressed as counts ofgenes and fold-change of the average on PBMC in SSc-ILD compared to the average of the controls (column U). (XLSX 167 kb)

**Additional file 6: Table S5.** miRNA expression in lung fibroblasts by Nanostring analysis. Healthy control lung fibroblasts (HC) and SSc-ILD lung fibroblasts were stimulated with media, interleukin-13 (IL-13), interferon alpha (IFN), and TGF-beta for 18 hours. Data are expressed as counts of gene expression. (XLSX 56 kb)

**Additional file 7: Figure S2.** miRNA expression of miR-193a (A) and miR-15b (B) on lung fibroblasts from cell lines of healthy controls (HC) and patients with SSc-ILD stimulated for 18 hours with media, IL-13, TGF-beta, and IFN-alpha. Data are expressed as fold-change compared to HC samples or media control. ANOVA, $p > 0.05$ for both miRNAs. (TIF 1112 kb)

**Additional file 8: Figure S3.** Cluster of genes analyzed on lungs from wild-type and miR-155 KO mice exposed to PBS or bleomycin (see "Methods"). Two main clusters of genes upregulated (A) and downregulated (B) on lungs from wild-type mice exposed to bleomycin on day 28 of the model. Each miRNA was z-score-normalized across all samples and scaled to *red* and *blue* ($\geq 2$ or $\leq -2$; respectively) and *white* indicating a z-score of zero. (TIF 3423 kb)

## Abbreviations
%DLCO, percentage of diffusing capacity of the lungs for carbon monoxide; %FVC, percentage of forced vital capacity; ANOVA, analysis of variance; CCL18, chemokine C-C motif ligand 18; cDNA, complementary DNA; Col3a1, collagen type 3 alpha-1; Ct, cycle threshold; DIANA, DNA Intelligent Analysis; DMEM, Dulbecco's modified Eagle's medium; dSSc, diffuse systemic sclerosis; H&E, hematoxylin and eosin; FDR, false discovery rate; FiBMax, high-resolution computed tomography lung score; HRCT, high-resolution computed tomography; IFN, interferon alpha; IL-13, interleukin 13; KEGG, Kyoto Encyclopedia of Genes and Genomes; KO, knockout; lSSc, limited systemic sclerosis; mRNA, messenger RNA; miRNA, micro RNA; MS4A4A, membrane-spanning 4-domains, subfamily A, member 4A; NSIP, non-specific interstitial pneumonia; PBMC, peripheral blood mononuclear cells; PBS, phosphate-buffered saline; PFT, pulmonary function tests; POSTN, periostin; SPP1, osteopontin-1; SSc, systemic sclerosis; SSc-ILD, systemic sclerosis interstitial lung disease; TGF-beta, transforming growth factor beta; TIMP-1, tissue inhibitor of metalloproteinases type-1; WT, wild-type; IPF, idiopathic pulmonary fibrosis

## Acknowledgements
We thank Yuriy Alekseyev, Ph.D. (Department of Pathology and Laboratory Medicine) and Adam Gower, Ph.D. (Clinical and Translational Science Institute) of Boston University Microarray Resource Core Facility for supervising all microarray-based experiments and help with data analysis. CTSI award U54-TR001012. This work was supported by 1P50AR060780-01 (RL) and 2R01AR051089-06A1 NIH/NIAMS grants (RL and RS), by the Fundação de Amparo à Pesquisa do Estado de São Paulo (FAPESP) 2013/14277-4 (VLC), by Universal National Council for Scientific and Technological Development (CNPq) 483005/2012-6 (VLC), and by Coordenação de Aperfeiçoamento de Pessoal de Nível Superior (CAPES), Foundation Ministry of Education of Brazil (TLM). This work was also supported in part by 5T32AI007309-25 NIAID training grant entitled "Research Training in Immunology" (AW), by K-08 Mentored Clinical Scientist Research Career Development Award, 2014 #1K08AR065507 (RBC), by Department of Medicine Career Investment Award, Boston University School of Medicine (RBC), by P30 AR061271 (CFB, SG, and RL), and by R01HL126990 (DJK).

## Authors' contributions
All authors participated in the preparation of the manuscript in a significant way. RBC participated in the design and the coordination of the study, carried out material collection, executed the experiments, performed data analysis, and drafted the manuscript. AW and TLM participated in the design of the study and sample collection. JT and DA executed the lung fibroblast culture experiments. YM carried out the murine model experiments and sample collection. SG executed the lung staining. PSB, CLB, CRRC, and RAK participated in the design of the study and in the collection of the clinical data from baseline and follow up of the patients with SSc-ILD. VLC and EP participated in the design of the study and in the lung histologic diagnosis. JZ and GS carried out material collection and coordinated the study. CFB, DK, and MR provided the lung fibroblasts and participated in the design of the study. RS and RL participated in the design and coordination of the study. All authors read and approved the manuscript after revising it critically for relevant scientific content.

## Competing interests
The authors declare that they have no competing interests.

## Author details
[1]Boston University School of Medicine, E501, Arthritis Center, Medical Campus, 72 East Concord Street, Boston, MA 02118-2526, USA. [2]Hospital das Clinicas da Faculdade de Medicina da Universidade de São Paulo, São Paulo, SP, Brazil. [3]Universidade CEUMA, São Luís do Maranhão, MA, Brazil. [4]Medical University of South Carolina, Charleston, SC, USA. [5]University of Pittsburgh, Division of Pulmonary, Allergy, and Critical Care Medicine, and the Dorothy P. and Richard P. Simmons Center for Interstitial Lung Disease, Pittsburgh, PA, USA. [6]Universidade do Estado do Amazonas, Manaus, AM, Brazil.

## References
1. Ioannidis JP, Vlachoyiannopoulos PG, Haidich AB, Medsger Jr TA, Lucas M, Michet CJ, et al. Mortality in systemic sclerosis: an international meta-analysis of individual patient data. Am J Med. 2005;118(1):2–10.
2. Tyndall AJ, Bannert B, Vonk M, Airo P, Cozzi F, Carreira PE, et al. Causes and risk factors for death in systemic sclerosis: a study from the EULAR Scleroderma Trials and Research (EUSTAR) database. Ann Rheum Dis. 2010;69(10):1809–15.
3. Sampaio-Barros PD, Bortoluzzo AB, Marangoni RG, Rocha LF, Del Rio AP, Samara AM, et al. Survival, causes of death, and prognostic factors in systemic sclerosis: analysis of 947 Brazilian patients. J Rheumatol. 2012;39(10):1971–78.
4. Roth MD, Tseng CH, Clements PJ, Furst DE, Tashkin DP, Goldin JG, et al. Predicting treatment outcomes and responder subsets in scleroderma-related interstitial lung disease. Arthritis Rheum. 2011;63(9):2797–08.
5. Steen VD, Medsger TA. Changes in causes of death in systemic sclerosis, 1972-2002. Ann Rheum Dis. 2007;66(7):940–4.
6. Christmann RB, Sampaio-Barros P, Stifano G, Borges CL, de Carvalho CR, Kairalla R, et al. Association of Interferon- and transforming growth factor beta-regulated genes and macrophage activation with systemic sclerosis-related progressive lung fibrosis. Arthritis Rheumatol. 2014; 66(3):714–25.
7. Baumjohann D, Ansel KM. MicroRNA-mediated regulation of T helper cell differentiation and plasticity. Nat Rev Immunol. 2013;13(9):666–78.
8. Pandit KV, Milosevic J, Kaminski N. MicroRNAs in idiopathic pulmonary fibrosis. Transl Res. 2011;157(4):191–99.
9. Booton R, Lindsay MA. Emerging role of MicroRNAs and long noncoding RNAs in respiratory disease. Chest. 2014;146(1):193–04.
10. Preliminary criteria for the classification of systemic sclerosis (scleroderma). Subcommittee for scleroderma criteria of the American Rheumatism Association Diagnostic and Therapeutic Criteria Committee. Arthritis Rheum. 1980;23(5):581-90.
11. Furst DE, Clements PJ, Steen VD, Medsger Jr TA, Masi AT, D'Angelo WA, et al. The modified Rodnan skin score is an accurate reflection of skin biopsy thickness in systemic sclerosis. J Rheumatol. 1998;25(1):84–8.
12. Hsu E, Shi H, Jordan RM, Lyons-Weiler J, Pilewski JM, Feghali-Bostwick CA. Lung tissues in patients with systemic sclerosis have gene expression patterns unique to pulmonary fibrosis and pulmonary hypertension. Arthritis Rheum. 2011;63(3):783–94.
13. Vlachos IS, Paraskevopoulou MD, Karagkouni D, Georgakilas G, Vergoulis T, Kanellos I, et al. DIANA-TarBase v7.0: indexing more than half a million experimentally supported miRNA:mRNA interactions. Nucleic Acids Res. 2015;43(Database issue):D153–159.
14. Kozomara A, Griffiths-Jones S. miRBase: integrating microRNA annotation and deep-sequencing data. Nucleic Acids Res. 2011;39(Database issue):D152–7.
15. Kanehisa M, Goto S, Sato Y, Furumichi M, Tanabe M. KEGG for integration and interpretation of large-scale molecular data sets. Nucleic Acids Res. 2012;40(Database issue):D109–14.
16. Christmann RB, Hayes E, Pendergrass S, Padilla C, Farina G, Affandi AJ, et al. Interferon and alternative activation of monocyte/macrophages in systemic sclerosis-associated pulmonary arterial hypertension. Arthritis Rheum. 2011;63(6):1718–28.
17. Elton TS, Selemon H, Elton SM, Parinandi NL. Regulation of the MIR155 host gene in physiological and pathological processes. Gene. 2013;532(1):1–12.
18. Leah E. Rheumatoid arthritis: miR-155 mediates inflammation. Nat Rev Rheumatol. 2011;7(8):437.
19. Moore CS, Rao VT, Durafourt BA, Bedell BJ, Ludwin SK, Bar-Or A, et al. miR-155 as a multiple sclerosis-relevant regulator of myeloid cell polarization. Ann Neurol. 2013;74(5):709–20.
20. Wang G, Tam LS, Li EK, Kwan BC, Chow KM, Luk CC, et al. Serum and urinary cell-free MiR-146a and MiR-155 in patients with systemic lupus erythematosus. J Rheumatol. 2010;37(12):2516–22.

21. Zhou S, Wang Y, Meng Y, Xiao C, Liu Z, Brohawn P, et al. In Vivo Therapeutic Success of MicroRNA-155 (miR-155) Antagomir in a Mouse Model of Lupus Alveolar Hemorrhage. Arthritis Rheumatol. 2015. doi:10.1002/art.39485 [Epub ahead of print].

22. Takagi T, Naito Y, Mizushima K, Hirata I, Yagi N, Tomatsuri N, et al. Increased expression of microRNA in the inflamed colonic mucosa of patients with active ulcerative colitis. J Gastroenterol Hepatol. 2010;25 Suppl 1:S129–133.

23. Yan Q, Chen J, Li W, Bao C, Fu Q. Targeting miR-155 to treat experimental scleroderma. Sci Rep. 2016;6:20314.

24. Pottier N, Maurin T, Chevalier B, Puissegur MP, Lebrigand K, Robbe-Sermesant K, et al. Identification of keratinocyte growth factor as a target of microRNA-155 in lung fibroblasts: implication in epithelial-mesenchymal interactions. PLoS One. 2009;4(8), e6718.

25. Liu G, Friggeri A, Yang Y, Milosevic J, Ding Q, Thannickal VJ, et al. miR-21 mediates fibrogenic activation of pulmonary fibroblasts and lung fibrosis. J Exp Med. 2010;207(8):1589–97.

26. Zhu H, Li Y, Qu S, Luo H, Zhou Y, Wang Y, et al. MicroRNA expression abnormalities in limited cutaneous scleroderma and diffuse cutaneous scleroderma. J Clin Immunol. 2012;32(3):514–22.

27. Zhang Z, Zha Y, Hu W, Huang Z, Gao Z, Zang Y, et al. The autoregulatory feedback loop of microRNA-21/programmed cell death protein 4/activation protein-1 (MiR-21/PDCD4/AP-1) as a driving force for hepatic fibrosis development. J Biol Chem. 2013;288(52):37082–93.

28. Quinn SR, O'Neill LA. A trio of microRNAs that control Toll-like receptor signalling. Int Immunol. 2011;23(7):421–25.

29. Kouri FM, Hurley LA, Daniel WL, Day ES, Hua Y, Hao L, et al. miR-182 integrates apoptosis, growth, and differentiation programs in glioblastoma. Genes Dev. 2015;29(7):732–45.

30. Sachdeva M, Mito JK, Lee CL, Zhang M, Li Z, Dodd RD, et al. MicroRNA-182 drives metastasis of primary sarcomas by targeting multiple genes. J Clin Invest. 2014;124(10):4305–19.

# Exercise echocardiography for the assessment of pulmonary hypertension in systemic sclerosis

Rui Baptista[1,2]* (ID), Sara Serra[3], Rui Martins[1], Rogério Teixeira[1,2], Graça Castro[1], Maria João Salvador[3], José António Pereira da Silva[2,3], Lèlita Santos[2,4], Pedro Monteiro[1,2] and Mariano Pêgo[1]

## Abstract

**Background:** Pulmonary arterial hypertension (PAH) complicates the course of systemic sclerosis (SSc) and is associated with poor prognosis. The elevation of systolic pulmonary arterial pressure (sPAP) during exercise in patients with SSc with normal resting haemodynamics may anticipate the development of PAH. Exercise echocardiography (ExEcho) has been proposed as a useful technique to identify exercise-induced increases in sPAP, but it is unclear how to clinically interpret these findings. In this systematic review, we summarize the available evidence on the role of exercise echocardiography to estimate exercise-induced elevations in pulmonary and left heart filling pressures in patients with systemic sclerosis.

**Methods:** We conducted a systematic review of the literature using MEDLINE, Cochrane Library and Web of Knowledge, using the vocabulary terms: ('systemic sclerosis' OR 'scleroderma') AND ('exercise echocardiography') AND ('pulmonary hypertension'). Studies including patients with SSc without a prior diagnosis of PAH, and subjected to exercise echocardiography were included. All searches were limited to English and were augmented by review of bibliographic references from the included studies. The quality of evidence was assessed by the Effective Public Health Practice Project system.

**Results:** We identified 15 studies enrolling 1242 patients, who were mostly middle-aged and female. Several exercise methods were used (cycloergometer, treadmill and Master's two step), with different protocols and positions (supine, semi-supine, upright); definition of a positive test also varied widely. Resting estimated sPAP levels varied from 18 to 35 mm Hg, all in the normal range. The weighted means for estimated sPAP were $22.2 \pm 2.9$ mmHg at rest and $43.0 \pm 4.3$ mmHg on exercise; more than half of the studies reported mean exercise sPAP $\geq 40$ mmHg. The assessment of left ventricular diastolic function on peak exercise was reported in a minority of studies; however, when assessed, surrogate variables of left ventricular (LV) diastolic dysfunction were associated with higher sPAP on exercise.

**Conclusions:** We found very high heterogeneity in the methods, the protocols and the estimated sPAP response to exercise. LV diastolic dysfunction was common and was associated with greater elevation of sPAP on exercise.

**Keywords:** Exercise, Echocardiography, Systemic sclerosis, Pulmonary hypertension, Scleroderma

* Correspondence: rui.baptista@fmed.uc.pt
[1]Department of Cardiology, Centro Hospitalar e Universitário de Coimbra, Praceta Mota Pinto, 3000-001 Coimbra, Portugal
[2]Faculty of Medicine, University of Coimbra, Coimbra, Portugal
Full list of author information is available at the end of the article

## Background

Systemic sclerosis (SSc) is an autoimmune disorder characterised by autoantibody production, microvascular lesions and collagen deposition [1] and can be complicated by pulmonary arterial hypertension (PAH) in 8 to 20 % of patients [2]. PAH remodelling affects the small pulmonary arteries, leading to progressive increase in pulmonary vascular resistance (PVR) and right heart failure [3]. Importantly, histopathological evidence of pulmonary arteriopathy has been reported in up to 72 % of patients with SSc, raising the possibility that subclinical features are present well before the PAH diagnosis [4]. Therefore, early diagnosis is of importance, not only because of the rapid progression of the disease but also because it is critical to initiate early treatment [5].

Echocardiography is a useful tool for pulmonary hypertension (PH) screening, as it estimates systolic PAP (sPAP), assesses right ventricular remodelling, identifies morphological abnormalities that can indicate the aetiology and may be used to evaluate treatment effectiveness [6]. However, a resting echocardiogram has limited accuracy to diagnose elevations in pulmonary pressures in SSc [7–9]. Stress tests performed during exercise have been used increasingly in cardiology to better characterise haemodynamic changes and therefore, a strong rationale exists to suggest that reduced pulmonary vascular reserve may signal a subclinical phase of pulmonary vascular disease (PVD) [10]. The definition of exercise-induced PH (EIPH) has been present in former PH guidelines, being defined by a mean PAP (mPAP) >30 mmHg. However, it has been abandoned due to lack of standardisation, prognostic impact assessment and overlap with normal subjects [11]. Nonetheless, performing an exercise echocardiogram may be an advantageous approach, as it allows not only estimation of exercise-induced changes in sPAP but also quantification of changes in cardiac output (CO) and left ventricular (LV) diastolic filling pressures, two determinants of variation in pulmonary pressure. Some authors suggest that this early exercise PAH phase is more amenable to treatment; others suggest it may be stable with no pathological implications [12, 13].

In this systematic review, we summarize the available evidence on the role of exercise echocardiography to estimate exercise-induced elevations in pulmonary pressures and in left heart filling pressures in patients with SSc without resting PH.

## Methods

The methods used conformed to the Meta-analysis of Observational Studies in Epidemiology [14] and the Cochrane Collaboration [15] recommendations.

## Selection criteria and search strategy

The literature search was conducted between January 2013 and December 2015 and comprised peer-reviewed original research that investigated estimated EIPH as a primary endpoint in patients with SSc using exercise echocardiography. The search resources included MEDLINE, Cochrane Library and Web of Knowledge, using the search terms: ('systemic sclerosis' OR 'scleroderma') AND ('exercise echocardiography') AND ('pulmonary hypertension'). Studies that were already known to the authors of this review (based on previous work or familiarity with the research area) were also included in the review. The search was limited to English language articles published from 1995 onwards. Publications reporting no original data or without a clear description of the research methods were excluded. Studies that did not present estimated sPAP results for patients with SSc were excluded. Conference abstracts or results posted in trial registries were excluded. The grey literature was not searched.

## Data extraction and assessment

Study selection was performed by the investigators RB (cardiologist) and SS (rheumatologist). References were managed using Mendeley Desktop software (V.1.12.3). We contacted the authors who reported sPAP by groups of patients defined by a cutoff for exercise-induced sPAP, but not for overall patients. Retrieved papers were hand-searched for additional references. Details of the literature search process are outlined in the flow chart (Fig. 1). Eligible studies included adult (18 years old or more) patients with SSc (either diffuse or limited), subjected to a stress protocol with exercise echocardiography. Patients were enrolled consecutively in all but one study, where only patients at high risk of developing PAH were included. As the main goal of exercise echocardiography in SSc is to identify patients with pre-capillary (PAH) elevations in pulmonary pressures, most authors aimed to exclude patients at high risk of group-2 PH, as those with uncontrolled systemic hypertension or a history or evidence of significant cardiovascular or lung disease (including coronary artery disease, LV hypertrophy, myocardial ischaemia and severe valvular conditions). A prior PAH diagnosis was also a criterion for study exclusion.

All studies had a similar design. Patients were submitted to echocardiography at rest (before exercise) and during or immediately (within the first minute) after exercise. The following variables were extracted when available: year of publication, sample size, gender ratio, age, lung function test parameters (forced vital capacity (FVC), forced expiratory volume in the first second ($FEV_1$) and total lung capacity (TLC)), carbon monoxide diffusion capacity ($DL_{CO}$), type and date of SSc diagnosis, exercise

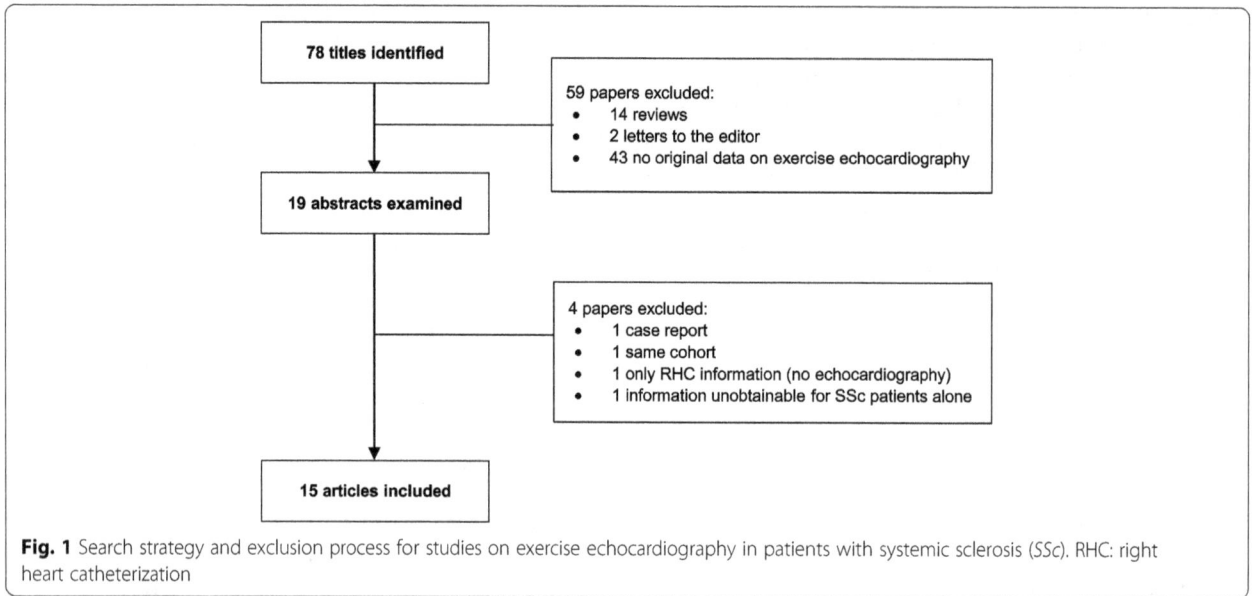

**Fig. 1** Search strategy and exclusion process for studies on exercise echocardiography in patients with systemic sclerosis (*SSc*). RHC: right heart catheterization

method, time of exercise-induced estimated sPAP measurement, maximum achieved workload in metabolic equivalent of task (MET), patient position (supine or upright), feasibility and intra and inter-observer variability (the latter two parameters are presented in Additional file 1). Cardiovascular variables collected included estimated resting right atrial pressure (RAP), tricuspid regurgitation-derived estimated sPAP (at rest and peak exercise), heart rate (HR) (at rest and peak exercise), estimated CO and cardiac index (CI) (at rest and peak exercise) and estimated pulmonary vascular resistance (PVR). In addition, diastolic dysfunction markers were retrieved when available, namely the ratio of early diastolic (E) and late diastolic (A) transvalvular velocities (E/A) for each ventricle and the ratio of early diastolic (E) and tissue Doppler-derived early (e') and atrial (a') diastolic mitral annular velocity to early diastolic (E) wave (E/e'). All data retrieved from the studies were relevant to the population characteristics, study design, type of exercise endured and outcomes of interest. In the scope of this review, the weighted mean and standard deviation for estimated sPAP (both at rest and peak exercise) was also calculated.

### Grading the quality of evidence of included studies

The Effective Public Health Practice Project (EPHPP) was used by two of the authors (RB and SS) to rate the quality of the evidence in the reviewed studies (Additional file 2) [16]. Each study was assigned a score category of strong, moderate or weak. Studies were graded by independent reviews; when the original ratings disagreed, they underwent a resolution review consensus. Double entry of data was performed for three studies (20 % of studies) and demonstrated a high level of accuracy (98.7 %).

## Results

A total of 78 publications were identified in the literature search. Of these, 19 were retrieved and analysed for eligibility. A total of 15 studies were eligible for inclusion in the review, and these were published between 1996 and 2015 (Fig. 1) [8, 17–30]. The characteristics of each eligible study are presented in Table 1.

### Demographic variables

The demographic characteristics are presented in Table 1. A total of 1242 patients was assessed, with a large female majority (range 76–100 %). The mean age in each study ranged from 50–58 years and the mean time since SSc diagnosis varied from 16 months to 12 years.

### Stress protocols and measurements

Exercise echocardiography protocols and maximum workload levels are described in Additional file 3. Of the selected studies, 10 used a cycloergometer in the supine or semi-supine position. Half of the studies estimated exercise-induced sPAP immediately after or within one to two minutes after exercise. HR was measured in 10 of the selected studies. At rest, mean HR ranged between 71 and 82 bpm. Mean peak exercise HR varied between 115 and 150 bpm, signalling for moderate intensity exercise, given the mean age of the population (54 years) and the expected maximum HR for this age group (approximately 166 bpm).

Mean estimated sPAP is shown by study in Fig. 2. Resting sPAP varied from 18–35 mmHg, all in the normal range. At peak exercise, mean sPAP ranged from 30–51 mmHg, with half of the studies reporting a mean exercise sPAP $\geq$40 mmHg (Fig. 3). The weighted means for estimated sPAP were $22.2 \pm 2.9$ mmHg at rest and $43.0 \pm 4.3$ mmHg at peak exercise. Most of the studies

**Table 1** Main characteristics of studies and patients

| First author | Publication year | Condition | Sample size | Female gender (%) | Age (years) | Mean time since diagnosis | Enrolment criteria |
|---|---|---|---|---|---|---|---|
| Mininni [25] | 1996 | SSc | 9 | 78 % | 56 | 27 m | Consecutive |
| Alkotob [17] | 2006 | SSc | 65 | 86 % | 51 | — | Consecutive |
| Collins[a][21] | 2006 | DSSc | 9 | 100 % | 59 | — | Consecutive |
| Collins[b][21] | 2006 | LSSc | 10 | 100 % | 52 | — | |
| Pignone [26] | 2007 | LSSc | 27 | 89 % | 50 | 7 y | Consecutive |
| Huez [24] | 2007 | SSc | 8 | 92 % | 54 | 16 m | Consecutive |
| Callejas-Rubio [29] | 2008 | SSc | 41 | – | 53 | 9 y | Consecutive |
| Steen [27] | 2008 | SSc | 54 | 94 % | 53 | — | At high risk of PH[d] |
| Reichenberger [8] | 2009 | SSc | 33 | 94 % | 54 | 9 y | Consecutive |
| D'Alto [22] | 2010 | SSc | 172 | 90 % | 52 | — | Consecutive |
| Ciurzynski [20] | 2011 | SSc | 67 | 96 % | 57 | — | Consecutive |
| Baptista [18] | 2013 | SSc | 23 | 96 % | 58 | — | Consecutive |
| Gargani [23] | 2013 | SSc | 164 | 91 % | 58 | 11 y | Consecutive |
| Voilliot [29] | 2014 | SSc | 45 | 76 % | 54 | — | Consecutive |
| Suzuki [28] | 2014 | SSc | 494 | 89 % | 56 | — | Consecutive |
| Nagel[c][30] | 2015 | SSc | 21 | 84 % | 58 | 12 y | Consecutive |

Quantitative variables (age) reported as means. Female and male patients represented by counts. [a]Results for patients with diffuse systemic sclerosis (DSSc). [b]Rresults for patients with limited systemic sclerosis (LSSc). [c]Results are for the full population studied (including patients unaware of having pulmonary hypertension). [d]Dyspnea on exertion, carbon monoxide diffusion capacity ($DL_{CO}$) <60 % of predicted, forced vital capacity (FVC) <60 % of predicted, FVC %/DLCO % >1.6, or resting right ventricular systolic pressure on echocardiogram >30 mmHg but <50 mmHg. *m* months, *SSc* systemic sclerosis, *y* years

defined a minimum cutoff for EIPH that would define a clinically relevant hypertensive response (a "positive test") for the exercise echocardiographic study. These thresholds are shown in Additional file 4; the proportion of positive tests ranged from 12–67 %.

Patients who exercised in an upright position on a treadmill had numerically smaller elevation in sPAP than patients assessed on a cycloergometer in a semi-supine position ($40 \pm 7$ vs. $47 \pm 4$ mmHg) (Additional file 5). However, this might be due to the fact that upright echocardiographic assessments of patients on the treadmill were always performed immediately after exercise. In the studies where measurements were taken at peak exercise, mean sPAP was $45 \pm 5$ mmHg, whereas in studies were it was collected immediately after exercise was $40 \pm 3$ mmHg.

### Left ventricular diastolic dysfunction markers

As SSc commonly affects the LV, the elevation of sPAP during exercise might also be due to backward transmission of elevated LV end-diastolic pressure (LVEDP). Therefore, the assessment of a surrogate of LVEDP is critical during the exercise test. Table 2 shows the results from eight studies that reported these markers among patients with and without positive tests in the exercise echocardiogram in resting conditions (described in Additional file 5 for each study). Most studies report signs of resting LV diastolic dysfunction in the group of patients who exhibited EIPH. Only three studies reported

LV E/e' during peak exercise; all demonstrated a higher exercise E/e' in the patients with a positive exercise test.

### Cardiac output, cardiac index and pulmonary vascular resistance

Table 3 shows the studies that evaluated CO, CI and PVR at rest and during/after exercise, with some performing comparisons between patients with and without a positive test. Baptista et al. [18] observed higher mean resting CO in patients with positive tests. Suzuki et al. and Voilliot et al. [28, 29] also observed higher mean PVR in patients with positive tests, both for resting and peak exercise PVR. Gargani et al. [23] also observed a difference, but for peak exercise PVR only and they also measured the ratio between changes in mean PAP (mPAP) and changes in CO (mPAP/CO) induced by exercise. Patients with positive tests had higher ratios compared with the remaining patients ($p < 0.05$). D'Alto et al. [22] also identified higher $\Delta$sPAP/$\Delta$CI ratios in patients with SSc, compared with controls; Voilliot et al. [29] demonstrated positive correlation between PVR and exercise sPAP.

### Lung function tests

$DL_{CO}$ and spirometry measures are presented in Additional file 5. On evaluating the association between these parameters and sPAP, Steen et al. [27] reported that patients with $DL_{CO}$ <50 % or with FVC %/$DL_{CO}$ ratio >1.6 were more likely to have an increase in sPAP ≥20 mmHg at peak

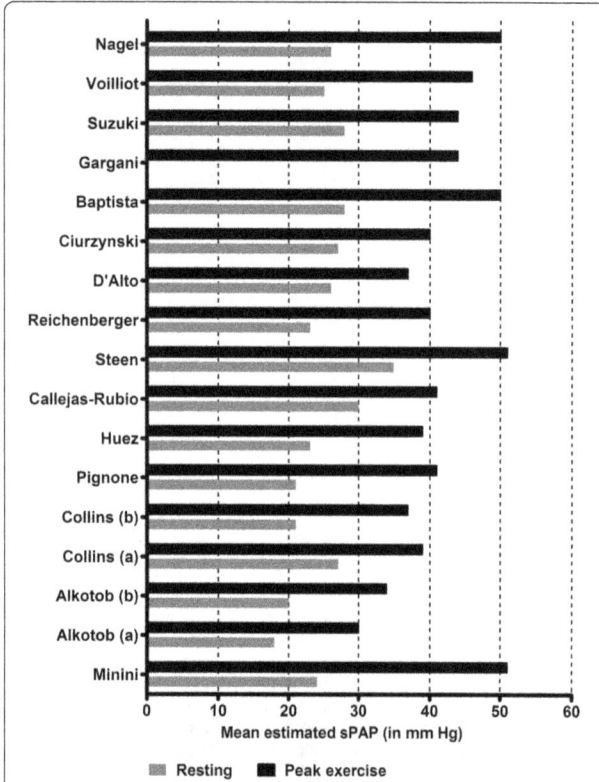

**Fig. 2** Mean pulmonary arterial systolic pressure by study. Results from Alkotob et al. are divided into (a) patients with pulmonary fibrosis and (b) patients without pulmonary fibrosis. Results from Collins et al are divided into (a) patients with diffuse systemic sclerosis and (b) patients with limited systemic sclerosis. The weighted mean for estimated systolic pulmonary arterial pressure (sPAP) was $22.2 \pm 2.9$ mmHg at rest and $43.0 \pm 4.3$ mmHg at peak exercise

exercise ($p < 0.001$). Callejas-Rubio et al. [19] also observed negative correlation between exercise sPAP and $DL_{CO}$.

## Discussion

We conducted a systematic review of the scientific literature assessing estimated sPAP by echocardiography during

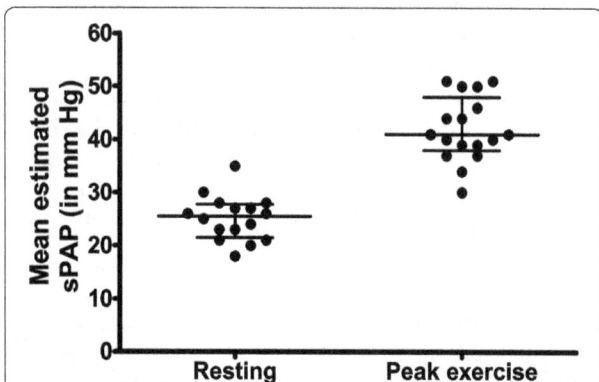

**Fig. 3** Median systolic pulmonary arterial pressure (sPAP) (with interquartile range) estimated by exercise echocardiography in resting and peak exercise conditions for each study

exercise in patients with SSc. The results demonstrate very high heterogeneity in (1) the methodology used to exercise the patients and to estimate pressures, (2) the definition of what is a positive response and (3) the assessment of the LV diastolic performance at rest and during exercise. Further, robust outcome data from patients with EIPH are also lacking, making it difficult to establish prognostic correlation.

### Methodology of the test

Several exercise methods, positions and protocols were used among the studies. It is well-known that the cardiopulmonary circulatory responses are different if patients exercise in the supine or upright position and may relate differently to symptoms; also, Doppler-derived parameters can change with position and are challenging to assess in the upright position [31–33]. However, we observed several methods (cycloergometer, Master's two step and treadmill) and several positions (upright, supine and semi-supine) used for exercise. Moreover, the different stress protocols did not specify a predefined level of exertion to be achieved to define a test as being positive, as in other clinical scenarios such as coronary ischaemic disease, in a classical treadmill test. In combination, these factors may have accounted for the significant variability found in the workload and peak exercise heart rate among the different studies, and consequently, in the increased cardiac work necessary to elicit a significant haemodynamic response. Besides different workloads, Doppler-derived parameters can change with position. For instance, when a patient moves from the supine to the upright position, the E/e' ratio can change, as both parameters are preload-dependent [34]. Additionally, correct Doppler assessment of the tricuspid regurgitant velocity needs correct alignment of the Doppler beam, something that can be difficult to achieve in a patient exercising upright on a treadmill. Therefore, the most reproducible approach is probably semi-supine exercise on a cycloergometer with a ramped stress protocol, as recently proposed [35].

Another important aspect is the timing of imaging acquisition. In most, but not all studies, estimated pressures were collected during and at peak exercise, while the patient was still exercising. However, some authors assessed the patient one or two minutes after the end of exercise. CO and heart rate pressure rapidly return to normal after cessation of exertion (due to reversal of splanchnic vasoconstriction and decreased venous return), and these findings may underestimate sPAP elevation (or the severity of diastolic dysfunction) [36]. In comparison with the other studies, the low proportion of patients with a positive test reported by Ciurzynski et al. may be due to the fact that sPAP was not measured during but after exercise [31–33]. Using a ramp protocol with a cycloergometer, the load can be

**Table 2** Echocardiographic diastolic dysfunction markers

| Condition | | Alkotob (n = 65) | Pignone (n = 27) | | | Huez (n = 25) | D'Alto (n = 172) | Baptista (n = 23) | | | Gargani (n = 164) | | Voilliot (n = 45) | | | Suzuki (n = 494) | | |
|---|---|---|---|---|---|---|---|---|---|---|---|---|---|---|---|---|---|---|
| | | Total | Total | ≤40 mmHg | >40 mmHg | Total | Total | Total | <50 mHg | ≥50 mmHg | <50 mmHg | ≥50 mmHg | Total | ≤50 mmHg | >50 mmHg | Total | <50 mmHg | ≥50 mmHg |
| Rest | RV E/A | | | | | | 0.9 | | | | 1.0* | 0.7* | | | | | | |
| | LV E/A | 1.2 | 1.1 | 1.2 | 1.0 | 1.3 | 1.2 | 1.1 | 1.1 | 1.1 | | | 1.1 | 1.1 | 1.1 | 1.2 | 1.2* | 1.1* |
| | E/e' | | | | | | | 10.2 | 9.9 | 10.5 | 6.6* | 7.5* | 6.0 | 5.5* | 6.8* | 9.6 | 9.2* | 10.7* |
| Exercise | RV E/A | | | | | | 0.7 | | | | | | | | | | | |
| | LV E/A | | | | | | | 1.2 | 1.3 | 1.1 | | | 1.1 | 1.1 | 1.0 | | | |
| | E/e' | | | | | | | 10.0 | 9.4 | 10.5 | | | 6.8 | 5.7* | 9.2* | 10.7 | 10.3* | 11.8* |

Results presented as means. *Comparison between patients with maximum exercise-induced systolic pulmonary arterial pressure (sPAP) <50 mmHg and ≥50 mmHg statistically significantly different ($p < 0.05$). E/A ratio of early diastolic (E) and late diastolic (A) transvalvular velocities, E/e' ratio of early diastolic (E) and early diastolic mitral annular velocity (e'), LV left ventricle, RV right ventricle

**Table 3** Echocardiographic-derived cardiac output, cardiac index and pulmonary vascular resistance

| First author | Resting CO (L.min⁻¹) | Exercise CO (L.min⁻¹) | Resting CI (L.min⁻¹.m²) | Exercise CI (L.min⁻¹.m²) | Resting PVR (WU) | Exercise PVR (WU) |
|---|---|---|---|---|---|---|
| Huez | | | | | | |
|   Total | 3.0 | 8.7 | | | | 2.9 |
| D'Alto | | | | | | |
|   Total | | | 3.0 | 5.8 | | |
| Baptista | | | | | | |
|   Total | 3.6 | 9.2 | | | | |
|   sPAP <50 mmHg | 3.8* | 8.5 | | | | |
|   sPAP ≥50 mmHg | 5.1* | 9.9 | | | | |
| Suzuki | | | | | | |
|   Total | 5.5 | 7.6 | | | 1.7 | 1.9 |
|   sPAP <50 mmHg | 5.5 | 7.6 | | | 1.6* | 1.8* |
|   sPAP ≥50 mmHg | 5.5 | 7.6 | | | 1.9* | 2.3* |
| Voilliot | | | | | | |
|   Total | 3.7 | 7.2 | | | 1.9 | 2.5 |
|   sPAP ≥50 mmHg | 3.9 | 7.7 | | | 1.4* | 2.1* |
|   sPAP >50 mmHg | 3.5 | 6.5 | | | 2.6* | 3.6* |
| Gargani | | | | | | |
|   sPAP <50 mmHg | | | 2.5 | 4.6 | 1.7 | 2.0* |
|   sPAP ≥50 mmHg | | | 2.7 | 4.9 | 1.7 | 2.3* |

Results are presented as means. *Comparison between patients with maximum exercise-induced systolic pulmonary arterial pressure (sPAP) <50 mmHg and ≥50 mmHg statistically significantly different (p < 0.05). *CI* cardiac index, *CO* cardiac output, *PVR* pulmonary vascular resistance, *WU* Wood units

maintained constant over approximately three minutes (at a pedalling rate of 55–65 bpm), enabling imaging acquisition during peak exercise (or when symptoms develop) instead of post-exercise measurements [35].

### Interpretation of an exercise echocardiography test

Importantly, exercise sPAP cannot be interpreted without information on two other determinants of pressure: flow and LVEDP [37]. Pulmonary flow was reported in six studies. In comparison to baseline CO, peak exercise CO ranged between twofold and threefold the baseline value, a small increase taking into consideration the expected increase in CO in healthy subjects (fourfold to tenfold) [38]. This may signify either (1) a limited capacity in patients with SSc to increase the CO during exercise or (2) an inability of patients with SSc to exercise to a higher workload due to other mechanisms such as lung fibrosis, osteoarticular issues, anaemia or deconditioning.

In general, the mean increase in sPAP across all studies was 15 mmHg, to a weighted mean level of 43 mmHg; most studies reported a value >40 mmHg. This elevation in pressure is probably higher than would be expected from the concomitant elevation in CO in this group of patients with SSc, taking into consideration that in normal individuals, exercise leads to smaller increases in sPAP (mean $34.3 \pm 7.5$ mmHg) under large elevations of CO (approximately 20 L.min⁻¹) [38]. The importance of taking

CO into consideration when reporting exercise haemodynamics is of paramount importance. In a study by Argiento et al., 19 of 25 normal individuals had an elevation of estimated sPAP >40 mmHg. However, the mean CO at peak exercise was $18.0 \pm 4.2$ L.min⁻¹ [39], much higher than the values achieved by the patients with SSc. Therefore, for a CO <8–10 L.min⁻¹ (similar to the ones reported in the SSc studies we reviewed), mPAP should be <30 mmHg (corresponding to an sPAP of approximately 47 mmHg), a threshold surpassed in the majority of the studies performed in patients with SSc.

LV diastolic dysfunction is a critical determinant of EIPH. As the LVEDP can contribute with more than 75 % to sPAP during exercise in patients with resting PH due to LV diastolic dysfunction [40], any analysis of exercise sPAP without concomitant assessment of a surrogate of LVEDP is difficult to interpret [41]. The studies that analysed resting and exercise LV diastolic parameters mostly used E/e' as a marker of diastolic function [42]. Although arguably useful in the resting estimation of LV filling pressures, the use of E/e' in exercise protocols is debatable and used in isolation, E/e' is probably not sufficient to form conclusions about exercise-induced diastolic dysfunction [35, 43]. However, taking into consideration those limitations, most studies found that higher elevations of sPAP were associated with higher levels of either resting or peak E/e', and many conclude that there is an association between impaired relaxation of the LV and an increase in sPAP, both at rest and on peak exercise. Therefore, one cannot diagnose the presence of pulmonary vascular disease based only on sPAP elevation upon exercise, as diastolic dysfunction is very prevalent in patients with SSc (at least when assessed using E/e'). In the future, multiparametric algorithms may enable a more accurate diagnosis of diastolic dysfunction [35], namely, not only based on a single parameter, but also including clinical factors (such as the presence of hypertension, atrial fibrillation, diabetes or obesity), electrocardiographic data and echocardiographic markers of long-standing elevated LV filling pressures (such as LA area or the presence of LV hypertrophy) [44].

Due to the concurrent need for assessing CO along with pulmonary pressures and the limitations of establishing a diagnosis with only one sPAP value collected at some time point, a better method for evaluating the pressure-flow relationship in the pulmonary circulation might be by the analysis of $\Delta$PAP/$\Delta$CO slopes (i.e., total pulmonary resistance, TPR), calculated by the measurement of several pressure-flow points throughout the exercise period [10, 45]. An abnormal response to exercise is signalled by an mPAP >30 mmHg with an mPAP/CO slope >3 mmHg.L.$^{-1}$.min$^{-1}$ [3]. Steeper slopes were found in patients with SSc compared with controls [46]. Importantly, this calculation does not take in consideration LVEDP; therefore, it is unable to differentiate pre-capillary from post-capillary EIPH.

## Definition of a positive result on exercise echocardiography

The invasive right heart catheterization-based definition of EIPH (mPAP >30 mmHg) was abandoned in 2008 due to limited supporting data [11]. Similarly, for echo-derived sPAP, there is no consensus on an sPAP cutoff to identify a "hypertensive response". This led to different definitions of what was a positive test in almost all studies. Some assessed the proportion of patients who achieved a predetermined exercise sPAP over a cutoff (mostly in the 40–50 mmHg range), whereas others analysed the variation/increase in sPAP during exercise. RAP estimation also varied among studies, adding more variability. These variable definitions are important limitations of exercise echocardiography.

Additionally, for a result be considered positive, it should be correlated with a clinical outcome, such as faster progression to resting PAH. However, there are few data on the natural history of EIPH. Two RHC-based studies, with a total of 66 patients with pre-capillary EIPH, observed a PAH incidence of 8–19 % after 2 years [47, 48]. Two recent echocardiographic-based studies are available. A 3.5-year follow up of 170 patients from the cohort of D'Alto et al. identified 6 patients (3.5 %) with incident resting PH [49]. Of these, three developed group-2 PH, one developed

group-3 PH and three developed PAH. Among the three patients with PAH, only one had an increase in sPAP >18 mmHg during the index exercise echocardiogram. Recently, another study followed up 40 patients with SSc who had previously undergone exercise echocardiography [50]. After 2 years, 28 % developed resting PH, all belonging to the group of patients with EIPH at the index evaluation. In this cohort, the development of resting PH was associated with factors suggestive of latent LV diastolic dysfunction. The large variation in PH incidence might be related to the absence of confirmation of resting PH by RHC in this latter study. In summary, any variable used to define a positive exercise echocardiographic test has to (1) accurately reflect the pulmonary vascular reserve, which may be achieved using multipoint $\Delta$PAP/$\Delta$CO slopes instead of an isolated sPAP cutoff [51]; (2) integrate information on diastolic function markers, which may be accomplished using a multi-parametric approach for the estimation of LV filling pressures, using E/e' but also other imaging targets, such as mitral propagation velocity (Vp), diastolic times, pulmonary vein flow measurements or twist analysis [35]; and (3) to be related to outcomes [52]. The $\Delta$PAP/$\Delta$CO slope method that is associated with a comprehensive diastolic function assessment is probably the best suited to comply with all those requirements.

## Other factors to consider

There are also other factors that may influence the results, such as differences in age, gender, athletic capability or levels of adrenergic response among patients [8, 17, 53, 54]. Interstitial lung disease and persistent hypoxia and/or systemic hypertension may also interfere with exercise-induced sPAP [4, 17, 22, 23]. Usually, $DL_{CO}$ is lower in patients with SSc-associated PAH that than in those with idiopathic PAH [55]. This marker, therefore, is considered a valuable predictor of future PAH in SSc, decreasing for 10–15 years before a diagnosis of PAH is made and reaching a mean of 35 % of the predicted value at the time of diagnosis [56–58]. Two authors reported association between lower $DL_{CO}$ and greater risk of developing exercise-induced elevation in estimated sPAP [19, 27]. Although this finding may suggest a common pathophysiological mechanism for both $DL_{CO}$ impairment and exercise PH, further longitudinal studies need to be performed to clarify this relationship.

Lung fibrosis is also associated with a pulmonary hypertensive response to exertion. In the study by D'Alto et al. patients with moderate interstitial lung disease had higher estimated sPAP on exertion than patients without lung disease (39.7 $\pm$ 9.3 vs. 36.0 $\pm$ 8.4 mm Hg, $p = 0.016$). Once more, several mechanisms can contribute to the elevation of pulmonary pressures during exercise and it is difficult to clearly quantify the contribution of each one of them alone.

## Limitations

As with most systematic reviews, our study is limited by publication bias that may have supported the utility of exercise echocardiography for this indication. We tried to minimize the risk of bias by conducting an extensive search for potentially relevant studies and reviewing all bibliographic references.

## Future perspectives

There is increasing recognition that EIPH may represent a preclinical sign of resting PAH. The standardization of exercise echocardiography for this indication is underway, with several multi-centric initiatives promoting development of a simple and reliable protocol. Concurrently, prospective studies are progressively validating the concept that abnormal responses to exercise, measured with the integration of pressure and flow variables, are associated with a higher incidence of PAH. These studies will provide data to define diagnostic cutoffs that will stratify risk in individual patients and indicate which mechanisms of EIPH (reduced pulmonary reserve or diastolic dysfunction) are the most important in each subject, therefore guiding targeted treatments. Ideally, exercise should be performed in a semi-supine cycloergometer using a ramp protocol, aiming to measure pressure-flow relationships during exertion. Further research will then focus on prophylactic therapeutic interventions aiming to reduce the incidence of PAH in patients at risk.

## Conclusions

In summary, although exercise echocardiography has a strong rationale in the setting of patients with SSc, we found relevant heterogeneity in the methods, the protocols, the expected response to yield a positive result, and critically, no robust data on the prognostic validation of the EIPH concept. Also, the mechanisms whereby pulmonary pressures increase during exercise (either due to PVD, LV diastolic dysfunction, lung disease or a high CO) must be clearly defined and quantified for each patient before the results are to be translated into clinical practice. Current research is addressing those issues to provide a safe, non-invasive tool for preclinical screening of pulmonary vascular disease in patients with systemic sclerosis in the near future.

## Abbreviations

CI, cardiac index; CO, cardiac output; $DL_{CO}$, diffusion capacity of carbon monoxide; E/A, ratio of early diastolic (E) and late diastolic (A) transvalvular velocities; E/e', ratio of early (e') diastolic mitral annular velocity to early diastolic (E) wave; EIPH, exercise-induced pulmonary hypertension; FEV1, forced expiratory volume in the first second; FVC, forced vital capacity; HR, heart rate; LV, left ventricle; LVEDP, left ventricular end-diastolic pressure; MET, metabolic equivalent of task; mPAP, mean pulmonary arterial pressure; PAH, pulmonary arterial hypertension; PH, pulmonary hypertension; PVD, pulmonary vascular disease; PVR, pulmonary vascular resistance; RAP, right atrial pressure; sPAP, systolic pulmonary arterial pressure; SSc, systemic sclerosis; TLC, total lung capacity; TPR, total pulmonary resistance

## Acknowledgements

This work was supported by grants from the Portuguese Foundation for Science and Technology no. SFRH/SINTD/60112/2009 (R.B.) and from an unrestricted grant from Bayer Portugal (RB; SS).

## Authors' contributions

RB conceived of the study, participated in its design and coordination, performed the statistical analysis, collected the data and helped to draft the manuscript; SS participated in its design and coordination, collected the data and helped to draft the manuscript; RM participated in its design and revised the manuscript; RT participated in its design and helped to draft the manuscript; GC participated in its design and revised the manuscript; MJS participated in its design and revised the manuscript; LS participated in its design and revised the manuscript; JAPS participated in its design and helped to draft and to revise the manuscript; PM participated in its design and revised the manuscript; MP: participated in its design and coordination and helped to draft the manuscript. All authors read and approved the manuscript.

## Competing interests

The authors declare that they have no competing interests.

## Author details

[1]Department of Cardiology, Centro Hospitalar e Universitário de Coimbra, Praceta Mota Pinto, 3000-001 Coimbra, Portugal. [2]Faculty of Medicine, University of Coimbra, Coimbra, Portugal. [3]Department of Rheumatology, Centro Hospitalar e Universitário de Coimbra, Coimbra, Portugal. [4]Department of Internal Medicine, Centro Hospitalar e Universitário de Coimbra, Coimbra, Portugal.

## References

1. Barnes J, Mayes MD. Epidemiology of systemic sclerosis: incidence, prevalence, survival, risk factors, malignancy, and environmental triggers. Curr Opin Rheumatol. 2012;24(2):165–70.
2. Steen VD, Medsger TA. Changes in causes of death in systemic sclerosis, 1972-2002. Ann Rheum Dis. 2007;66:940–4.
3. Lewis GD, Bossone E, Naeije R, Grunig E, Saggar R, Lancellotti P, et al. Pulmonary vascular hemodynamic response to exercise in cardiopulmonary diseases. Circulation. 2013;128(13):1470–9.
4. Saggar R, Khanna D, Furst DE, Shapiro S, Maranian P, Belperio JA, et al. Exercise-induced pulmonary hypertension associated with systemic sclerosis: four distinct entities. Arthritis Rheum. 2010;62(12):3741–50.
5. Hachulla E, Gressin V, Guillevin L, Carpentier P, Diot E, Sibilia J, et al. Early detection of pulmonary arterial hypertension in systemic sclerosis: a French nationwide prospective multicenter study. Arthritis Rheum. 2005;52:3792–800.
6. Howard LS, Grapsa J, Dawson D, Bellamy M, Chambers JB, Masani ND, et al. Echocardiographic assessment of pulmonary hypertension: standard operating procedure. Eur Respir Rev. 2012;21:239–48.
7. Grunig E, Weissmann S, Ehlken N, Fijalkowska A, Fischer C, Fourme T, et al. Stress Doppler echocardiography in relatives of patients with idiopathic and familial pulmonary arterial hypertension: results of a multicenter European analysis of pulmonary artery pressure response to exercise and hypoxia. Circulation. 2009;119(13):1747–57.
8. Reichenberger F, Voswinckel R, Schulz R, Mensch O, Ghofrani HA, Olschewski H, et al. Noninvasive detection of early pulmonary vascular dysfunction in scleroderma. Respir Med. 2009;103(11):1713–8.
9. Coghlan JG, Denton CP, Grunig E, Bonderman D, Distler O, Khanna D, et al. Evidence-based detection of pulmonary arterial hypertension in systemic sclerosis: the DETECT study. Ann Rheum Dis. 2014;73:1340–9.
10. Herve P, Lau EM, Sitbon O, Savale L, Montani D, Godinas L, et al. Criteria for diagnosis of exercise pulmonary hypertension. Eur Respir J. 2015;46(3):728–37.
11. Galiè N, Humbert M, Vachiery JL, Gibbs S, Lang I, Torbicki A, et al. 2015 ESC/ERS Guidelines for the diagnosis and treatment of pulmonary hypertension:

The Joint Task Force for the Diagnosis and Treatment of Pulmonary Hypertension of the European Society of Cardiology (ESC) and the European Respiratory Society (ERS): Endorsed by: Association for European Paediatric and Congenital Cardiology (AEPC), International Society for Heart and Lung Transplantation (ISHLT). Eur Heart J. 2016;37(1):67–119.

12. Saggar R, Khanna D, Shapiro S, Furst DE, Maranian P, Clements P, et al. Brief report: effect of ambrisentan treatment on exercise-induced pulmonary hypertension in systemic sclerosis: a prospective single-center, open-label pilot study. Arthritis Rheum. 2012;64(12):4072–7.

13. Tolle JJ, Waxman AB, Van Horn TL, Pappagianopoulos PP, Systrom DM. Exercise-induced pulmonary arterial hypertension. Circulation. 2008;118(21):2183–9.

14. Stroup DF, Berlin JA, Morton SC, Olkin I, Williamson GD, Rennie D, et al. Meta-analysis of observational studies in epidemiology: a proposal for reporting. Meta-analysis Of Observational Studies in Epidemiology (MOOSE) group. JAMA. 2000;283(15):2008–12.

15. Maxwell L, Santesso N, Tugwell PS, Wells GA, Judd M, Buchbinder R. Method guidelines for Cochrane Musculoskeletal Group systematic reviews. J Rheumatol. 2006;33(11):2304–11.

16. Thomas BH, Ciliska D, Dobbins M, Micucci S. A process for systematically reviewing the literature: providing the research evidence for public health nursing interventions. Worldviews Evid Based Nurs. 2004;1(3):176–84.

17. Alkotob ML, Soltani P, Sheatt MA, Katsetos MC, Rothfield N, Hager WD, et al. Reduced exercise capacity and stress-induced pulmonary hypertension in patients with scleroderma. Chest. 2006;130(1):176–81.

18. Baptista R, Serra S, Martins R, Salvador MJ, Castro G, Gomes M, et al. Exercise-induced pulmonary hypertension in scleroderma patients: a common finding but with elusive pathophysiology. Echocardiography. 2013;30(4):378–84.

19. Callejas-Rubio JL, Moreno-Escobar E, de la Fuente PM, Perez LL, Fernandez RR, Sanchez-Cano D, et al. Prevalence of exercise pulmonary arterial hypertension in scleroderma. J Rheumatol. 2008;35(9):1812–6.

20. Ciurzynski M, Bienias P, Irzyk K, Rymarczyk Z, Kostrubiec M, Szewczyk A, et al. Usefulness of echocardiography in the identification of an excessive increase in pulmonary arterial pressure in patients with systemic sclerosis. Kardiol Pol. 2011;69(1):9–15.

21. Collins N, Bastian B, Quiqueree L, Jones C, Morgan R, Reeves G. Abnormal pulmonary vascular responses in patients registered with a systemic autoimmunity database: pulmonary hypertension assessment and screening evaluation using stress echocardiography (PHASE-I). Eur J Echocardiogr. 2006;7(6):439–46.

22. D'Alto M, Ghio S, D'Andrea A, Pazzano AS, Argiento P, Camporotondo R, et al. Inappropriate exercise-induced increase in pulmonary artery pressure in patients with systemic sclerosis. Heart. 2011;97(2):112–7.

23. Gargani L, Pignone A, Agoston G, Moreo A, Capati E, Badano LP, et al. Clinical and echocardiographic correlations of exercise-induced pulmonary hypertension in systemic sclerosis: a multicenter study. Am Heart J. 2013;165(2):200–7.

24. Huez S, Roufosse F, Vachiery JL, Pavelescu A, Derumeaux G, Wautrecht JC, et al. Isolated right ventricular dysfunction in systemic sclerosis: latent pulmonary hypertension? Eur Respir J. 2007;30(5):928–36.

25. Mininni S, Diricatti G, Vono MC, Giglioli C, Margheri M, Olivo G, et al. Noninvasive evaluation of right ventricle systolic pressure during dynamic exercise by saline-enhanced Doppler echocardiography in progressive systemic sclerosis. Angiology. 1996;47(5):467–74.

26. Pignone A, Mori F, Pieri F, Oddo A, Galeota G, Fiori G, et al. Exercise Doppler echocardiography identifies preclinic asymptomatic pulmonary hypertension in systemic sclerosis. Ann NY Acad Sci. 2007;1108:291–304.

27. Steen V, Chou M, Shanmugam V, Mathias M, Kuru T, Morrissey R. Exercise-induced pulmonary arterial hypertension in patients with systemic sclerosis. Chest. 2008;134(1):146–51.

28. Suzuki K, Izumo M, Kamijima R, Mizukoshi K, Takai M, Kida K, et al. Influence of pulmonary vascular reserve on exercise-induced pulmonary hypertension in patients with systemic sclerosis. Echocardiography. 2015;32(3):428–35.

29. Voilliot D, Magne J, Dulgheru R, Kou S, Henri C, Laaraibi S, et al. Determinants of exercise-induced pulmonary arterial hypertension in systemic sclerosis. Int J Cardiol. 2014;173(3):373–9.

30. Nagel C, Henn P, Ehlken N, D'Andrea A, Blank N, Bossone E, et al. Stress Doppler echocardiography for early detection of systemic sclerosis-associated pulmonary arterial hypertension. Arthritis Res Ther. 2015;17:165.

31. Badruddin SM, Ahmad A, Mickelson J, Abukhalil J, Winters WL, Nagueh SF, et al. Supine bicycle versus post-treadmill exercise echocardiography in the detection of myocardial ischemia: a randomized single-blind crossover trial. J Am Coll Cardiol. 1999;33(6):1485–90.

32. Cotrim C, Joao I, Fazendas P, Almeida AR, Lopes L, Stuart B, et al. Clinical applications of exercise stress echocardiography in the treadmill with upright evaluation during and after exercise. Cardiovasc Ultrasound. 2013;11:26.

33. Saggar R, Lewis GD, Systrom DM, Champion HC, Naeije R, Saggar R. Pulmonary vascular responses to exercise: a haemodynamic observation. Eur Respir J. 2012;39(2):231–4.

34. Rustad LA, Amundsen BH, Slordahl SA, Stoylen A. Upright bicycle exercise echocardiography in patients with myocardial infarction shows lack of diastolic, but not systolic, reserve: a tissue Doppler study. Eur J Echocardiogr. 2009;10(4):503–8.

35. Erdei T, Smiseth OA, Marino P, Fraser AG. A systematic review of diastolic stress tests in heart failure with preserved ejection fraction, with proposals from the EU-FP7 MEDIA study group. Eur J Heart Fail. 2014;16(12):1345–61.

36. Nagueh SF, Appleton CP, Gillebert TC, Marino PN, Oh JK, Smiseth OA, et al. Recommendations for the evaluation of left ventricular diastolic function by echocardiography. J Am Soc Echocardiogr. 2009;22(2):107–33.

37. Naeije R, Vanderpool R, Dhakal BP, Saggar R, Saggar R, Vachiery JL, et al. Exercise-induced pulmonary hypertension: physiological basis and methodological concerns. Am J Respir Crit Care Med. 2013;187(6):576–83.

38. Kovacs G, Berghold A, Scheidl S, Olschewski H. Pulmonary arterial pressure during rest and exercise in healthy subjects: a systematic review. Eur Respir J. 2009;34:888–94.

39. Argiento P, Chesler N, Mule M, D'Alto M, Bossone E, Unger P, et al. Exercise stress echocardiography for the study of the pulmonary circulation. Eur Respir J. 2010;35(6):1273–8.

40. Borlaug BA, Nishimura RA, Sorajja P, Lam CS, Redfield MM. Exercise hemodynamics enhance diagnosis of early heart failure with preserved ejection fraction. Circ Heart Fail. 2010;3(5):588–95.

41. Baptista R, Teixeira R. Exercise-induced pulmonary hypertension in systemic sclerosis: a multifactorial entity. Am Heart J. 2013;166:e13.

42. Mullens W, Borowski AG, Curtin RJ, Thomas JD, Tang WH. Tissue Doppler imaging in the estimation of intracardiac filling pressure in decompensated patients with advanced systolic heart failure. Circulation. 2009;119(1):62–70.

43. Santos M, Rivero J, McCullough SD, West E, Opotowsky AR, Waxman AB, et al. E/e' ratio in patients with unexplained dyspnea: lack of accuracy in estimating left ventricular filling pressure. Circ Heart Fail. 2015;8(4):749–56.

44. Rosenkranz S, Gibbs JS, Wachter R, De Marco T, Vonk-Noordegraaf A, Vachiéry JL. Left ventricular heart failure and pulmonary hypertension. Eur Heart J. 2016;37(12):942–54.

45. Gabriels C, Lancellotti P, Van De Bruaene A, Voilliot D, De Meester P, Buys R, et al. Clinical significance of dynamic pulmonary vascular resistance in two populations at risk of pulmonary arterial hypertension. Eur Heart J Cardiovasc Imaging. 2015;16(5):564–70.

46. Lau EMT, Manes A, Celermajer DS, Galiè N. Early detection of pulmonary vascular disease in pulmonary arterial hypertension: time to move forward. Eur Heart J. 2011;32:2489–98.

47. Bae S, Saggar R, Bolster MB, Chung L, Csuka ME, Derk C, et al. Baseline characteristics and follow-up in patients with normal haemodynamics versus borderline mean pulmonary arterial pressure in systemic sclerosis: results from the PHAROS registry. Ann Rheum Dis. 2012;71(8):1335–42.

48. Condliffe R, Kiely DG, Peacock AJ, Corris PA, Gibbs JS, Vrapi F, et al. Connective tissue disease-associated pulmonary arterial hypertension in the modern treatment era. Am J Respir Crit Care Med. 2009;179(2):151–7.

49. Codullo V, Caporali R, Cuomo G, Ghio S, D'Alto M, Fusetti C, et al. Stress doppler echocardiography in systemic sclerosis: evidence for a role in the prediction of pulmonary hypertension. Arthritis Rheum. 2013;65(9):2403–11.

50. Voilliot D, Magne J, Dulgheru R, Kou S, Henri C, Caballero L, et al. Prediction of new onset of resting pulmonary arterial hypertension in systemic sclerosis. Arch Cardiovasc Dis. 2016;109(4):268–77.

51. Chin K, Mathai SC. Exercise echocardiography in connective tissue disease. J Am Coll Cardiol. 2015;66(4):385–7.

52. Kusunose K, Yamada H. Rest and exercise echocardiography for early detection of pulmonary hypertension. J Echocardiogr. 2016;14(1):2–12.

53. Mahjoub H, Levy F, Cassol M, Meimoun P, Peltier M, Rusinaru D, et al. Effects of age on pulmonary artery systolic pressure at rest and during exercise in normal adults. Eur J Echocardiogr. 2009;10(5):635–40.

54. Vachiery JL, Pavelescu A. Exercise echocardiography in pulmonary hypertension. Eur Heart J Suppl. 2007;9(Supplement H):H48–53.

55. Steen VD, Champion H. Is exercise-induced pulmonary hypertension ready for prime time in systemic sclerosis? Int J Clin Pract Suppl. 2011;169:1–3.
56. Chatterjee S. Pulmonary hypertension in systemic sclerosis. Semin Arthritis Rheum. 2011;41(1):19–37.
57. Nathan SD, Shlobin OA, Ahmad S, Urbanek S, Barnett SD. Pulmonary hypertension and pulmonary function testing in idiopathic pulmonary fibrosis. Chest. 2007;131(3):657–63.
58. Steen V, Medsger TA. Predictors of isolated pulmonary hypertension in patients with systemic sclerosis and limited cutaneous involvement. Arthritis Rheum. 2003;48(2):516–22.

# B cell depletion therapy upregulates Dkk-1 skin expression in patients with systemic sclerosis: association with enhanced resolution of skin fibrosis

Dimitrios Daoussis[1][*], Athanassios Tsamandas[2], Ioannis Antonopoulos[1], Alexandra Filippopoulou[1], Dionysios J. Papachristou[3], Nicholaos I. Papachristou[3], Andrew P. Andonopoulos[1] and Stamatis-Nick Liossis[1]

## Abstract

**Background:** Rituximab (RTX) may favorably affect skin and lung fibrosis in patients with systemic sclerosis (SSc); however, the underlying molecular mechanisms remain unknown. We aimed to explore the hypothesis that RTX may mediate its antifibrotic effects by regulating the expression of Dickkopf-1 (Dkk-1), an inhibitor of the Wnt pathway.

**Methods:** Fourteen patients with SSc and five healthy subjects were recruited. Dkk-1 expression was immunohistochemically assessed in skin biopsies obtained from 11 patients with SSc (8 treated with RTX and 3 with standard treatment), whereas DKK1 gene expression was assessed in 3 patients prior to and following RTX administration.

**Results:** In baseline biopsies obtained from all patients with SSc but not in healthy subjects, Dkk-1 was undetectable in skin fibroblasts. Following RTX treatment, four out of eight patients had obvious upregulation of Dkk-1 skin expression. Similarly, RTX treatment correlated with a significant 4.8-fold upregulation of DKK1 gene expression ($p = 0.030$). In contrast, TGFβ expression in the upper dermis was significantly attenuated following treatment. Moreover, this decreased expression of TGFβ in the skin was significantly more pronounced in the subgroup of patients with Dkk-1 upregulation. In this subgroup TGFβ was downregulated by 50.88 % in contrast to only 15.98 % in patients who did not have Dkk-1 upregulation ($p = 0.022$).

**Conclusions:** This is the first study demonstrating a link between B cell depletion and skin Dkk-1 upregulation in patients with SSc. RTX-mediated B cell depletion may mechanistically function via the recently established TGFβ-Dkk-1 axis in improving skin fibrosis.

**Keywords:** Systemic sclerosis, Scleroderma, Rituximab, B cell depletion, Dickkopf-1, Dkk-1, TGFβ, Fibrosis, Skin

## Background

Systemic sclerosis (SSc) is a complex systemic rheumatic disease characterized by autoimmunity, vasculopathy, and aberrant fibroblast activation, eventually leading to fibrosis, tissue damage, and organ failure [1]. The therapeutic armamentarium for SSc is very restricted; numerous therapies have been tested and either failed or had a modest effect. However, an increasing amount of clinical evidence accumulated over the last few years suggests that B cell depletion therapy may favorably affect skin and lung fibrosis in patients with SSc [2]. We have previously reported that RTX treatment improves skin thickening and lung function in patients with SSc [3]; this effect seems to be further enhanced following long-term treatment [4, 5]. Similar data have been also reported by other research groups [6–8]. Most importantly, recent large-scale multi-center studies, including one from the European League against Rheumatism Scleroderma Trial and Research group, reported encouraging results, thus, supporting the

* Correspondence: jimdaoussis@hotmail.com
[1]Division of Rheumatology, Department of Internal Medicine, Patras University Hospital, University of Patras Medical School, Rion, Patras 26504, Greece
Full list of author information is available at the end of the article

concept of B cell depletion therapy in SSc [9, 10]. It is currently not known how RTX may mediate its potential beneficial effects in SSc. However, experimental evidence indicates that B cells are critically involved in the fibrotic process [11–14].

SSc is a disease characterized by enhanced fibroblast activation leading to increased collagen production and eventually tissue fibrosis. There have been many theories related to the drivers of aberrant fibroblast activation in SSc; recent studies have provided strong experimental data pointing to the direction of the canonical Wnt pathway as a central mediator of the fibrotic process in SSc [15–18]. The Wnt pathway is a developmental pathway with β-catenin serving as the main signaling molecule. The activation of the Wnt pathway is strictly controlled by several soluble inhibitors such as Dickkopf-1 (Dkk-1) [19]. Experimental data indicate that the Wnt pathway is highly activated in the skin in scleroderma. Dkk-1 is virtually undetectable in the skin of patients with SSc in sharp contrast to healthy skin where it is clearly expressed. Moreover, it was found that transforming growth factor β (TGFβ), the most potent profibrotic molecule that is crucially involved in the pathophysiology of SSc, downregulates Dkk-1 expression [20]. These data have unraveled a previously unknown link between TGFβ and the Wnt pathway (TGFβ → downregulation of Dkk-1 → upregulation of the Wnt pathway → fibrosis) and have highlighted the role of Dkk-1 in the fibrotic process.

In our study we aimed to explore the hypothesis that B cell depletion therapy may mediate its antifibrotic effects via the Wnt pathway. More specifically, we aimed to assess (1) expression of Dkk-1 and TGFβ in the skin and circulating levels in patients with SSc prior to and following B cell depletion therapy and (2) DKK1 gene expression in cultured fibroblasts obtained from patients with SSc prior to and following B cell depletion therapy.

We report herein that Dkk-1 is upregulated following B cell depletion therapy in a subset of patients with SSc; these patients exhibit the most profound reduction in skin fibrosis following treatment.

## Methods

### Patients

Fourteen patients with SSc, fulfilling the preliminary American College of Rheumatology criteria for the classification of the disease [21], were recruited. Eleven patients were originally enrolled in a proof of concept study performed in our institution, assessing the clinical efficacy of RTX in SSc [3]. In this study, eight patients were randomized to the treatment arm and received two courses of RTX (at baseline and at 6 months), and six patients were randomized to the control arm and received standard therapy. Skin biopsies from clinically involved

skin were obtained from all patients in the treatment group ($n = 8$) and in three patients in the control group (at baseline and at 6 months). Skin biopsies from these 11 patients were immunohistochemically assessed. Three additional patients with SSc treated with RTX, were similarly subjected to skin biopsies at baseline and at 6 months; these biopsies were used for fibroblast extraction and gene expression analysis.

Demographic and clinical characteristics of the study subjects and clinical outcomes following treatment have already been reported in detail elsewhere [3]. Briefly, all patients had diffuse disease, were anti-Scl70 positive, and had no change in medication and/or dosage of treatment administered during the last 12 months before enrollment. Patients in the RTX group had a significant improvement in pulmonary function tests (PFTs) and skin thickening at 1 year (following two courses of RTX treatment) compared to baseline. There was a significant increase in forced vital capacity (FVC) (mean ± SD $68.13 ± 19.69$ vs $75.63 ± 19.73$, at baseline vs 1 year, respectively, $p = 0.0018$) and diffusing lung capacity for carbon monoxide (DLco) (mean ± SD $52.25 ± 20.71$ vs. $62 ± 23.21$, at baseline vs 1 year, respectively, $p = 0.017$) in the RTX group. The modified Rodnan skin score (MRSS) also improved significantly in the RTX group compared to the baseline score (mean ± SD, $13.5 ± 6.84$ vs $8.37 ± 6.45$, at baseline vs 1 year, respectively, $p < 0.001$).

As a disease control group for the current study we used three patients from the control arm of the original study, for whom skin biopsies were available. Two of these patients were receiving cyclophosphamide, whereas the third patient received no treatment. Skin biopsies from five age-matched and sex-matched healthy subjects were evaluated as healthy controls.

The study has been approved by a local Ethics Committee (Patras University Hospital, Patras, Greece) and written informed consent was obtained from all participating individuals.

### Assessment of circulating levels of Dkk-1, TGFβ and IL-6

Circulating Dkk-1, TGFβ and IL-6 levels were measured using a solid phase immunoassay, according to the manufacturer's instructions (R&D Systems, MN, USA). All measurements were performed in triplicates for each sample and the mean value was calculated.

### Skin histology and immunohistochemistry

Skin biopsies of 5 mm were taken from skin affected by lesions on the forearm. All biopsies were fixed in 10 % neutral buffered formalin and embedded in paraffin. Dkk-1 and TGFβ expression were immunohistochemically assessed using mouse anti-human monoclonal antibodies (R&D Systems, MN, USA); analysis was performed separately for the upper and lower dermis. Masson's trichrome was used for skin collagen visualization and fibrosis evaluation. Computerized image analysis using the Image J software was used to quantify the results as previously described [3, 22].

### Extraction and culture of skin fibroblasts

Biopsies were mechanically minced using a scalpel and then fibroblasts were extracted using a standard protocol. Fibroblasts were cultured in EMEM supplemented with 10 % FBS and antibiotics (penicillin (100 U/ml), streptomycin (100 mg/ml)); fibroblasts from the third to the fifth passages were used for experiments. In some experiments fibroblasts (obtained from healthy subjects and patients with SSc) were treated with serum obtained from patients with SSc ($n = 3$) prior to and 6 months after treatment with RTX or serum obtained from healthy controls. These experiments were performed to explore whether soluble factors affect DKK1 expression in skin fibroblasts. In these experiments fibroblasts were subjected to 24 hours starvation prior to treatment with 10 % human serum for another 24 hours.

### Fibroblast lysis, RNA extraction and DKK1 gene expression

Cells were detached using trypsin, lysed, and subjected to mRNA extraction according to a standard protocol (RNeasy Mini Kit, Qiagen) following manufacturer's instructions. RNA purity was confirmed using a NanoDrop Spectrophotometer (Thermo Scientific). cDNA synthesis was carried out using the iScript cDNA synthesis kit (Bio-Rad Laboratories, Hercules, CA, USA) from 1 μg of total RNA. DKK1, Thrombospondin 1 (THBS1) and glyceraldehyde 3-phosphate dehydrogenase (GAPDH) mRNA relative expression levels were assessed, using the iTaq Universal SYBR Green supermix (Bio-Rad Laboratories) with CFX96 Touch Real-time System (Bio-Rad Laboratories). For human DKK1, THBS1 and GAPDH gene-specific KiCqStart™ primers were purchased from Sigma-Aldrich Co. The relative expression level of the gene of interest was calculated with the comparative $2^{\Delta\Delta CT}$ method and all samples were normalized to GAPDH. All experiments were independently performed in duplicate three times, each time using 1 μg of template RNA.

### Statistical analysis

Statistical analysis was performed using the GraphPad Prism software version 5. Data are presented as mean ± SEM, median (lower and upper quartile values), or percentages, as appropriate. Student's $t$ test was used for comparisons between groups. Significance was defined as $p < 0.05$ (two-tailed).

## Results

### Dkk-1 deficiency in the skin of patients with scleroderma is restored following B cell depletion therapy

Dkk-1 was expressed in the epidermis, appendices, and fibroblasts in the dermis in all the biopsies obtained from healthy subjects. In sharp contrast, in all baseline biopsies obtained from patients with SSc ($n = 11$), Dkk-1 was virtually undetectable in skin fibroblasts. In fact, weak Dkk-1 staining was detected at the epidermis in only two patients (one from the RTX and one from the disease control group). Representative histological analysis of normal skin and the human colon (used as a positive control for Dkk-1 expression) is shown in Fig. 1. These data confirm previously reported results [20].

Following B cell depletion therapy, four out of eight patients had obvious expression of Dkk-1 in skin fibroblasts, in sharp contrast to the disease control group in whom there was no Dkk-1 expression seen in fibroblasts in the follow-up biopsies. Representative histological analysis from a patient showing Dkk-1 upregulation after RTX treatment is shown in Fig. 2. Histological analysis of biopsies from all remaining patients is shown in the Additional files (see Additional file 1: Figures S1-S3 for depiction of patients with Dkk-1 upregulation after RTX treatment, Additional file 2: Figures S4-S6 and Additional file 3: Figure S7 for depiction of patients with no Dkk-1 upregulation after RTX treatment, and Additional file 4: Figures S8-S10 for depiction of patients in the disease control group).

### B cell depletion therapy significantly induces DKK1 gene expression in skin

We first evaluated the expression of the DKK1 gene in scleroderma compared to normal fibroblasts. There was significant 4.1-fold downregulation of DKK1 expression in fibroblasts from patients with scleroderma compared to normal fibroblasts ($p < 0.001$) as shown in Fig. 3a. We next assessed whether B cell depletion therapy affects the expression of the DKK1 gene in the skin. To address this question we analyzed DKK1 gene expression in fibroblasts extracted from skin biopsies from three patients with SSc treated with RTX (at baseline and 6 months after treatment). All three patients responded clinically with a significant decline of >30 % in the MRSS. There was significant 4.2-fold upregulation of DKK1 expression following RTX treatment ($p = 0.030$) as shown in Fig. 3b.

### Levels of Dkk-1 and TGFβ expression in skin from patients with SSc are inversely correlated

Taking into account recently reported data indicating that TGFβ regulates Dkk-1 expression, we next asked whether TGFβ skin expression is modified following B cell depletion therapy. In skin, TGFβ expression (assessed immunohistochemically) in fibroblasts from the upper dermis was significantly attenuated following RTX treatment (mean ± SEM 32.72 ± 4.67 vs 20.21 ± 3.08, at baseline and at 6 months, respectively, $p = 0.01$). However, the downregulation of TGFβ expression in skin was significantly more pronounced in the subgroup of patients ($n = 4$)

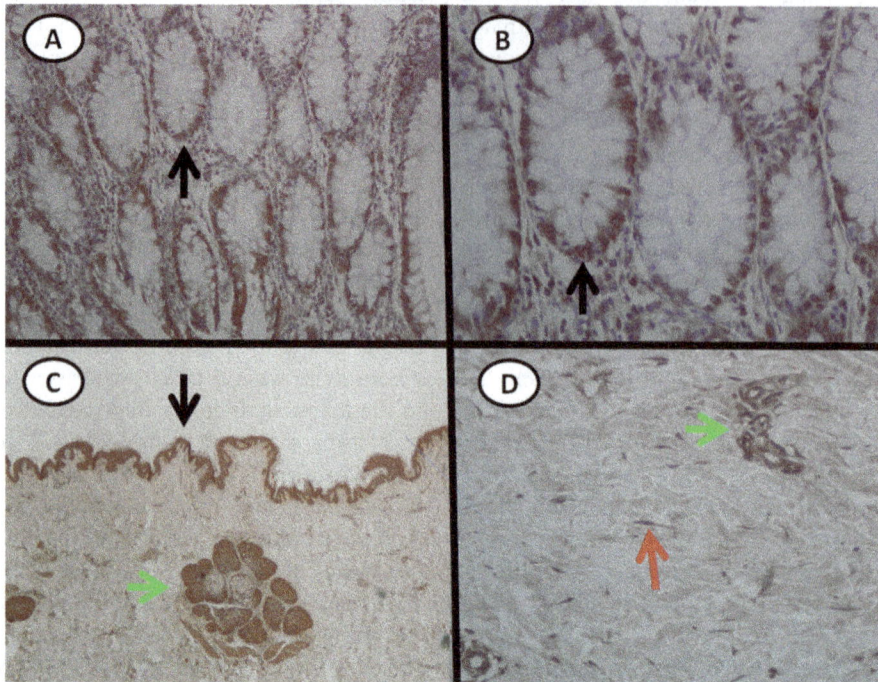

**Fig. 1** Dickkopf-1 (Dkk-1) is expressed in the normal colon and skin. Dkk-1 expression in a section from a positive control (normal colon) (**a, b**). Note the cytoplasmic expression in the basis of crypt epithelium (*black arrows*). Streptavidin biotin peroxidase: magnification × 20 (**a**), × 400 (**b**). Dkk1-expression in a section from normal skin (**c, d**). Dkk-1 is clearly expressed at the epidermis (*black arrows*), appendices (*green arrows*) and spindle-like cells (*red arrow*). Streptavidin biotin peroxidase: magnification × 20 (**c**), × 400 (**d**)

with upregulation of Dkk-1. More specifically, in this subgroup TGFβ was downregulated by a mean percentage (± SEM) of 50.88 % (±10.81) in sharp contrast to only 15.98 % (±3.73) in patients with no upregulation of Dkk-1 ($p = 0.02$) (Fig. 4e). Representative histological analysis from a patient with significant downregulation of TGFβ expression in skin is also shown in Fig. 4a-d. In the disease control group there was no change in TGFβ expression in the upper dermis (mean ± SEM 27.37 ± 6.76 vs 29.0 ± 2.15, at baseline and at 6 months, respectively, $p$ value not significant). There were no changes in TGFβ expression in the lower dermis in either patient group. We

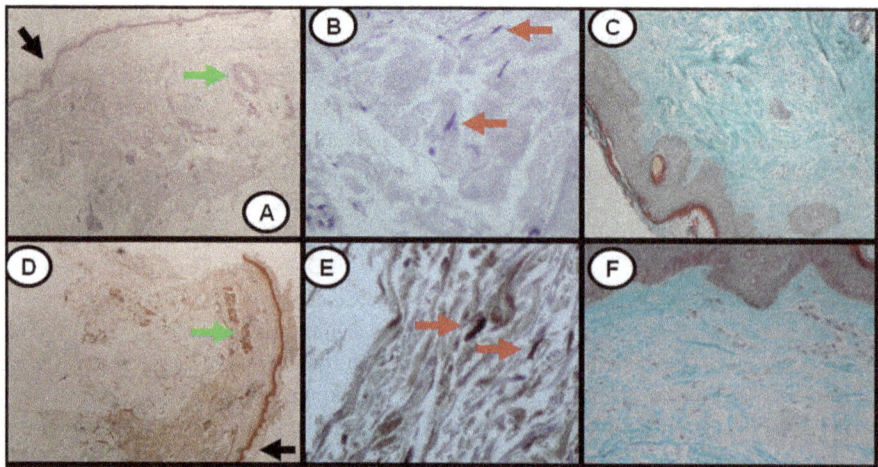

**Fig. 2** Dickkopf-1 (Dkk-1) is upregulated responders to rituximab (RTX) therapy. In the baseline biopsy (**a, b**) Dkk-1 is not expressed in the epidermis (*black arrow*), appendices (*green arrow*), and spindle-like cells (*red arrows*). Following RTX treatment (**d, e**) there is clear expression of Dkk-1 in the epidermis (*black arrow*), appendices (*green arrow*) and spindle-like cells (*red arrows*). Streptavidin biotin peroxidase: magnification × 20 (**a, d**), × 400 (**b, e**). Upregulation of Dkk-1 expression is associated with a decrease in collagen accumulation (prior to (**c**) and after (**f**) RTX treatment). Masson's trichrome × 100

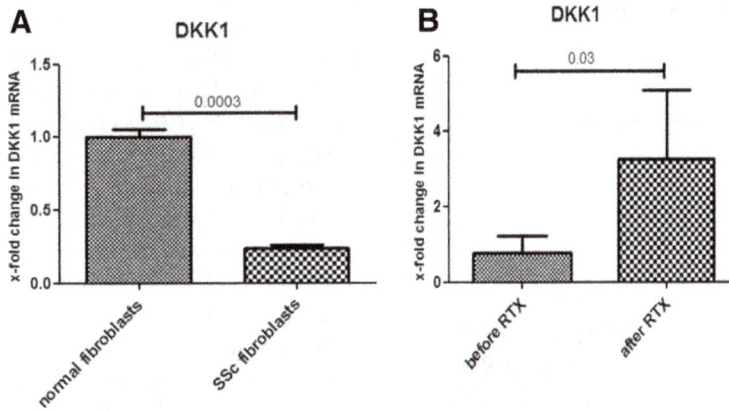

**Fig. 3** Dickkopf-1 (*DKK1*) gene is downregulated in scleoderma fibroblasts. Rituximab (*RTX*) treatment upregulates DKK1 gene expression in the skin. Fibroblasts from patients with systemic sclerosis had 4.1-fold downregulation of DKK1 gene expression compared to normal fibroblasts ($p < 0.001$) (**a**). RTX treatment mediates significant 4.2-fold upregulation of skin DKK1 gene expression ($p = 0.030$) (**b**)

further analyzed the expression of THBS1, a well-known target of TGFβ, in skin fibroblasts obtained from two patients with SSc prior to and 6 months after treatment with RTX. THBS1 expression was downregulated (by 37.93 % and 50.90 %, respectively) in both patients. Collectively these data indicate that B cell depletion therapy is associated with downregulation of TGFβ expression in skin; this downregulation is more pronounced in the subset of SSc patients with upregulation of Dkk-1.

## Upregulation of Dkk-1 in skin is associated with enhanced resolution of skin fibrosis

We further explored potential differences in histologic response between patients who had and those who did not have upregulation of Dkk-1. Patients with upregulation of Dkk-1 skin expression ($n = 4$) had an enhanced histologic response in the resolution of skin fibrosis. More specifically, on histologic analysis of skin from these patients, Dkk-1 upregulation was associated with a significant decrease in collagen accumulation in the upper dermis by a mean ± SEM 49.47 ± 10.63 %, compared to 18.18 ± 6.67 % in patients who did not have upregulation of Dkk-1 ($p = 0.04$) (Fig. 5). Histologic data matched the clinical data; the MRSS at 1 year (following two cycles of RTX treatment at baseline and at 6 months) decreased by a median of 63.33 % (24.34–72.92) in the subgroup with Dkk-1 upregulation compared to only 28.08 % (27.35–44.64) in the subgroup with undetectable Dkk-1;

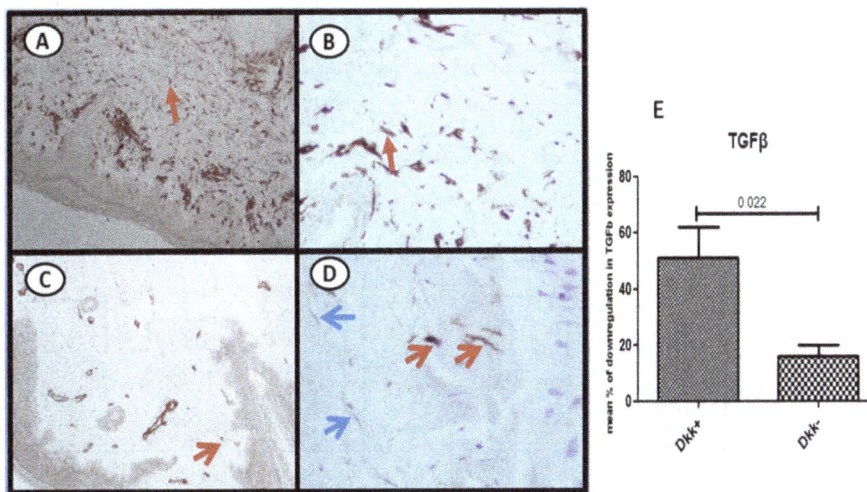

**Fig. 4** Rituximab (RTX) treatment correlates with significant attenuation of transforming growth factor β (*TGFβ*) expression in the skin. TGFβ is strongly expressed in the vast majority of spindle-like cells at baseline (*red arrows*) (**a**, **b**). Following RTX treatment significant attenuation of TGFβ expression is seen; many spindle-like cells do not express TGFβ (*blue arrows*) (**c**, **d**). Streptavidin biotin peroxidase: magnification × 20 (**a**, **c**), × 400 (**b**, **d**). Downregulation of TGFβ expression is more pronounced in the subgroup of patients with upregulation of Dkk-1 following RTX treatment (*Dkk+*) compared to the subgroup of patients who did not have upregulation of Dkk-1 following RTX treatment (*Dkk-*) (**e**)

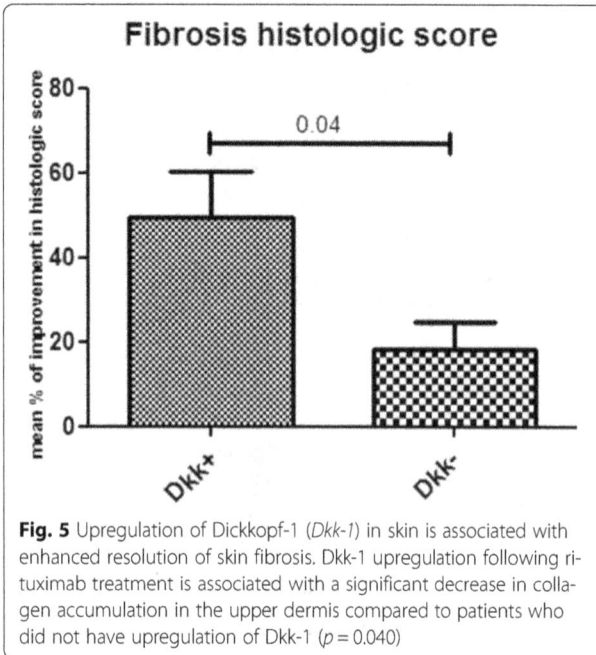

## Fibrosis histologic score

**Fig. 5** Upregulation of Dickkopf-1 (*Dkk-1*) in skin is associated with enhanced resolution of skin fibrosis. Dkk-1 upregulation following rituximab treatment is associated with a significant decrease in collagen accumulation in the upper dermis compared to patients who did not have upregulation of Dkk-1 ($p = 0.040$)

however this was not statistically significant. PFTs improved following RTX treatment, irrespective of Dkk-1 expression in skin.

### B cell depletion in skin is associated with Dkk-1 upregulation following RTX treatment

We next explored potential mechanisms of DKK1 upregulation in the skin following RTX treatment. We first aimed to explore whether circulating factors participate; to do so we assessed circulating levels of Dkk-1, TGFβ and IL-6 prior to and following B cell depletion therapy. Circulating levels of Dkk-1 did not change following treatment (mean ± SEM optical density (OD) $0.17 \pm 0.04$ vs $0.19 \pm 0.03$, prior to and following treatment, respectively,

$p$ value not significant). Serum TGFβ levels remained unchanged (mean ± SEM OD: $2.01 \pm 0.38$ vs $2.41 \pm 0.36$, prior to and following treatment respectively, $p$ value not significant). This was also true for IL-6 levels (mean ± SEM OD $0.35 \pm 0.07$ vs $0.37 \pm 0.11$, prior to and following treatment, respectively, $p$ value not significant). To assess whether other circulating factors may mediate DKK1 upregulation we treated normal fibroblasts and fibroblasts from patients with scleroderma with serum obtained from patients with SSc ($n = 3$) prior to and 6 months after RTX treatment. DKK1 gene expression in fibroblasts treated with serum obtained from patients with SSc prior to RTX treatment was similar to DKK1 gene expression in fibroblasts treated with serum obtained from SSc patients after RTX treatment, as shown in Fig. 6a (normal fibroblasts) and 6b (fibroblasts from patients with SSc).

We further assessed whether skin B cell depletion may correlate with DKK1 upregulation. Skin-infiltrating B cells were present in all patients with SSc in relatively small numbers; details have been previously reported [3, 5]. Briefly, RTX treatment effectively depleted skin-infiltrating B cells in four out of eight patients assessed. In the subgroup of patients who had Dkk-1 upregulation following RTX treatment ($n = 4$); three patients also had effective B cell depletion in the skin. In sharp contrast, in the subgroup of patients who did not have upregulation of Dkk-1 ($n = 4$), effective B cell depletion in the skin was evident in one patient only. These data suggest a potential link between skin B cell depletion and Dkk-1 upregulation.

### Discussion

Even though clinical data pointing to the direction of a beneficial role of RTX in SSc continue to emerge, the critical question of how B cell depletion therapy may mediate its antifibrotic effects remains largely unanswered. In animal models of SSc, B cells exhibit a disturbed

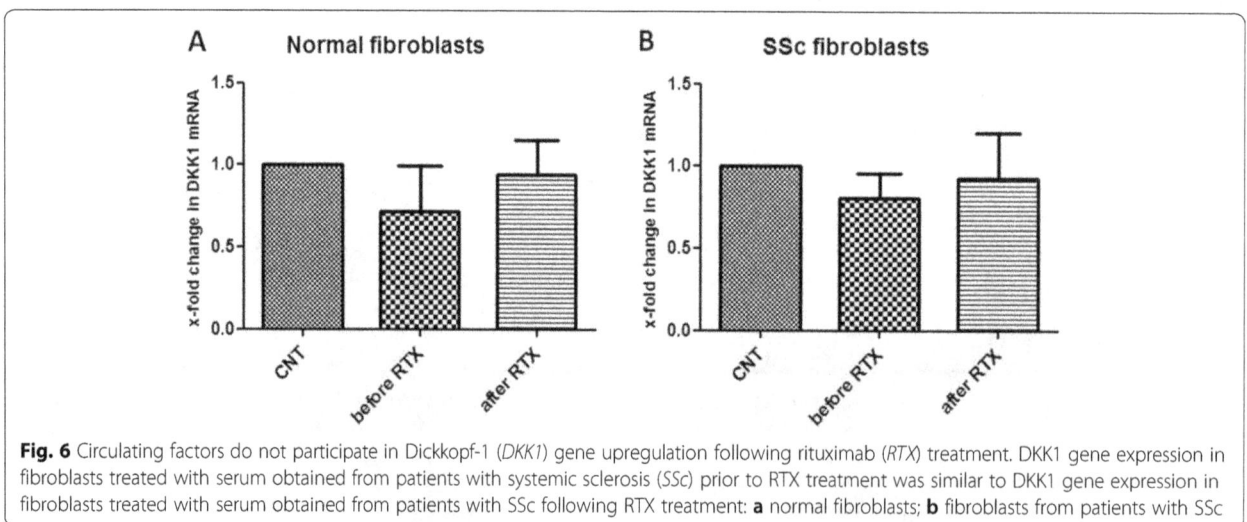

**Fig. 6** Circulating factors do not participate in Dickkopf-1 (*DKK1*) gene upregulation following rituximab (*RTX*) treatment. DKK1 gene expression in fibroblasts treated with serum obtained from patients with systemic sclerosis (*SSc*) prior to RTX treatment was similar to DKK1 gene expression in fibroblasts treated with serum obtained from patients with SSc following RTX treatment: **a** normal fibroblasts; **b** fibroblasts from patients with SSc

phenotype by displaying increased CD19 signaling and hyper-responsiveness [23]. There is strong evidence that RTX effectively ameliorates collagen accumulation in these models [13], indicating a link between B cells and the fibrotic process.

Evidence from patients with SSc indicate that B cells are present locally in fibrotic tissue in both skin [24] and lung [25]; most importantly, gene expression analysis has revealed a B cell signature in the skin in scleroderma [26]. Even though these data suggests that B cells are active players in fibrosis, the exact mechanisms involved are not entirely known. In order to reveal these mechanisms one must explore how B cells may directly or indirectly interact with fibroblasts, the cell type responsible for collagen overproduction.

There are three potential ways whereby B cells may interact with fibroblasts [27]. First, B cells may produce agonistic fibroblast-stimulating auto-antibodies (Abs), such as anti-platelet-derived growth factor receptor (PDGFR) Abs [28]. A second way is by producing soluble mediators; B cells can produce TGFβ and IL-6, which are cytokines strongly involved in the pathophysiology of fibrosis. Finally, recent evidence suggests that B cells can stimulate fibroblasts in vitro via a contact-dependent mechanism. Francois et al. have shown that when scleroderma fibroblasts are co-cultured with B cells, there is significant upregulation of collagen production [29]. Interestingly, the effect of B cells on collagen production in this experimental model was comparable to that of TGFβ, one of the most important profibrotic molecules known. Moreover, it was shown that the effect of B cells on fibroblasts in this experimental model is contact-dependent and at least partially mediated by TGFβ.

In this study we provide experimental evidence, at both protein and gene expression level, that RTX treatment may affect Dkk-1 skin expression in patients with SSc. This is the first study to suggest a link between B cell depletion and Dkk-1 expression in skin. Dkk-1 is strikingly absent from the skin in scleroderma; however, in a subset of patients with SSc, this molecule is upregulated following RTX treatment. More importantly, the patients with Dkk-1 upregulation have the more profound histologic response to B cell depletion therapy. Our data indicate that the upregulation of Dkk-1 may represent a specific effect of RTX treatment, as it was not observed in patients with SSc who were receiving standard treatment including cyclophosphamide; however, our results should be interpreted with caution, taking into account the limited number of patients assessed. These data reinforce existing evidence that Dkk-1 is a crucial mediator of the fibrotic process.

A critical question is how RTX may affect the expression of Dkk-1 in skin. It is currently unknown whether RTX mediates its potential antifibrotic effects by depleting B cells or by other mechanisms; it is known that RTX has a broad effect on the immune system [30]. In this study we found a strong association between skin B cell depletion and Dkk-1 upregulation/histologic response. This strong association suggests that B cells in skin, or other, so far unknown factor(s), may potentially suppress Dkk-1 expression in fibroblasts and therefore, effective B cell depletion in skin alleviates this suppression, leading to Dkk-1 upregulation. If indeed this is true and B cells are responsible for the striking lack of Dkk-1 expression in fibroblasts from patients with scleroderma, the next question is how B cells mediate this effect. Our data suggest that this may be a TGFβ-dependent effect. It is also of interest that circulating levels of Dkk-1 and TGFβ did not change following treatment, indicating that the whole process is taking place in the affected tissues such as the skin; this is in accordance with previously reported data [31].

Our study has several potential limitations. The first one is the relatively small number of patients assessed, therefore, definite conclusions cannot be drawn. The second limitation is that the expression of TGFβ in skin was assessed mainly by immunohistochemical analysis, which cannot distinguish between active and latent forms of TGFβ. Therefore, the evidence provided in our study implicating TGFβ in the regulation of Dkk-1 expression should not be considered powerful. Further studies are needed to clarify the potential role of TGFβ in this process. Moreover, an additional limitation is that Wnt pathway activation in the skin was not assessed.

## Conclusions

This is the first study that demonstrates a link between B cell depletion and upregulation of Dkk-1 in the skin of patients with SSc. Moreover, patients with upregulation of Dkk-1 following RTX treatment have the best histologic response to treatment. Large-scale randomized controlled studies assessing the efficacy of RTX in SSc are highly needed.

## Additional files

**Additional file 1: Figures S1-S3.** In the baseline biopsy (**A** and **B**) Dkk-1 is not expressed in epidermis (*black arrow*), appendices (*green arrow*) and spindle-like cells (*red arrows*). In the follow up biopsy (**C** and **D**) there is clear expression of Dkk-1 in epidermis (*black arrow*), appendices (*green arrow*) and spindle-like cells (*red arrows*). All three patients responded to RTX treatment. Streptavidin biotin peroxidase (**A** and **D** × 20, **B** and **E** × 400) (ZIP 5323 kb)

**Additional file 2: Figures S4-S6.** Dkk-1 is not expressed in epidermis (*black arrow*), appendices (*green arrow*) and spindle-like cells (*red arrows*) prior to (**A** and **B**) and following RTX treatment (**D** and **E**). These patients did not respond to RTX treatment. Streptavidin biotin peroxidase (**A** and **D** × 20, **B** and **E** × 400) (ZIP 5591 kb)

**Additional file 3: Figure S7.** Dkk-1 is not expressed in epidermis (*black arrow*), appendices (*green arrow*) and spindle-like cells (*red arrows*) in both baseline (**A** and **B**) and follow up biopsy (**D** and **E**) in a non responder. Streptavidin biotin peroxidase (**A** and **D** × 20, **B** and **E** x400). RTX treatment had no effect on collagen accumulation (**C** and **F**, prior to and following RTX treatment, respectively). Masson's trichrome × 100 (TIF 876 kb)

**Additional file 4: Figures S8-S10.** Dkk-1 is not expressed in epidermis (*black arrow*), appendices (*green arrow*) and spindle-like cells (*red arrows*) in the control patient group at baseline (**A** and **B**) and follow up biopsies (**D** and **E**). Streptavidin biotin peroxidase (**A** and **D** × 20, **B** and **E** × 400) (ZIP 5018 kb)

## Abbreviations

Dkk-1: Dickkopf-1; DLCO: diffusing lung capacity for carbon monoxide; FBS: fetal bovine serum; FVC: forced vital capacity; GAPDH: glyceraldehyde 3-phosphate dehydrogenase; IL-6: intrleukin-6; MRSS: modified Rodnan skin score; OD: optical density; PDGFR: platelet-derived growth factor receptor; PFT: pulmonary function test; RTX: rituximab; SEM: standard error of the mean; SSc: systemic sclerosis; TFGβ: transforming growth factor β.

## Competing interests

The authors declare that they have no competing interests.

## Authors' contributions

DD conceived the idea for the study, designed the study, performed the skin biopsies, analyzed the data, and drafted the manuscript. AT carried out the immunohistochemical analysis and assisted in manuscript drafting. IA extracted fibroblasts from skin biopsies and participated in data analysis and manuscript drafting. AF performed the RT-PCR assays and assisted in manuscript drafting. DJP assisted in the processing of skin biopsies and assisted in manuscript drafting. NIP assisted in fibroblast culture, provided crucial technical assistance, and assisted in manuscript drafting. APA participated in data analysis, patient recruitment, and manuscript drafting. SNL participated in data analysis, patient recruitment, study design, and manuscript drafting. All authors read and approved the manuscript.

## Acknowledgements

This study was partially funded by the Hellenic Society for Rheumatology-Professional Organization for Rheumatologists (a non profitable organization, which did not interfere in any part of the study).

## Author details

[1]Division of Rheumatology, Department of Internal Medicine, Patras University Hospital, University of Patras Medical School, Rion, Patras 26504, Greece. [2]Department of Pathology, Patras University Hospital, University of Patras Medical School, Patras, Greece. [3]Department of Anatomy-Histology-Embryology, Laboratory of Bone and Soft Tissue Studies, University of Patras Medical School, Patras, Greece.

## References

1. Varga J, Abraham D. Systemic sclerosis: a prototypic multisystem fibrotic disorder. J Clin Invest. 2007;117(3):557–67.
2. McQueen FM, Solanki K. Rituximab in diffuse cutaneous systemic sclerosis: should we be using it today? Rheumatology (Oxford). 2015;54(5):757–67.
3. Daoussis D, Liossis SN, Tsamandas AC, Kalogeropoulou C, Kazantzi A, Sirinian C, et al. Experience with rituximab in scleroderma: results from a 1-year, proof-of-principle study. Rheumatology (Oxford). 2010;49(2):271–80.
4. Daoussis D, Liossis SN, Tsamandas AC, Kalogeropoulou C, Kazantzi A, Korfiatis P, et al. Is there a role for B-cell depletion as therapy for scleroderma? A case report and review of the literature. Semin Arthritis Rheum. 2010;40(2):127–36.
5. Daoussis D, Liossis SN, Tsamandas AC, Kalogeropoulou C, Paliogianni F, Sirinian C, et al. Effect of long-term treatment with rituximab on pulmonary function and skin fibrosis in patients with diffuse systemic sclerosis. Clin Exp Rheumatol. 2012;30(2 Suppl 71):S17–22.
6. Bosello S, De Santis M, Lama G, Spano C, Angelucci C, Tolusso B, et al. B cell depletion in diffuse progressive systemic sclerosis: safety, skin score modification and IL-6 modulation in an up to thirty-six months follow-up open-label trial. Arthritis Res Ther. 2010;12(2):R54.
7. Smith V, Van Praet JT, Vandooren B, Van der CB, Naeyaert JM, Decuman S, et al. Rituximab in diffuse cutaneous systemic sclerosis: an open-label clinical and histopathological study. Ann Rheum Dis. 2010;69(1):193–7.
8. Smith V, Piette Y, van Praet JT, Decuman S, Deschepper E, Elewaut D, et al. Two-year results of an open pilot study of a 2-treatment course with rituximab in patients with early systemic sclerosis with diffuse skin involvement. J Rheumatol. 2013;40(1):52–7.
9. Jordan S, Distler JH, Maurer B, Huscher D, van Laar JM, Allanore Y, et al. Effects and safety of rituximab in systemic sclerosis: an analysis from the European Scleroderma Trial and Research (EUSTAR) group. Ann Rheum Dis. 2015;74(6):1188–94.
10. Keir GJ, Maher TM, Ming D, Abdullah R, de Lauretis A, Wickremasinghe M, et al. Rituximab in severe, treatment-refractory interstitial lung disease. Respirology. 2014;19(3):353–9.
11. Daoussis D, Liossis SN, Yiannopoulos G, Andonopoulos AP. B-cell depletion therapy in systemic sclerosis: experimental rationale and update on clinical evidence. Int J Rheumatol. 2011;2011:214013.
12. Hasegawa M, Fujimoto M, Takehara K, Sato S. Pathogenesis of systemic sclerosis: altered B cell function is the key linking systemic autoimmunity and tissue fibrosis. J Dermatol Sci. 2005;39(1):1–7.
13. Hasegawa M, Hamaguchi Y, Yanaba K, Bouaziz JD, Uchida J, Fujimoto M, et al. B-lymphocyte depletion reduces skin fibrosis and autoimmunity in the tight-skin mouse model for systemic sclerosis. Am J Pathol. 2006;169(3):954–66.
14. Sato S, Fujimoto M, Hasegawa M, Takehara K, Tedder TF. Altered B lymphocyte function induces systemic autoimmunity in systemic sclerosis. Mol Immunol. 2004;41(12):1123–33.
15. Beyer C, Schramm A, Akhmetshina A, Dees C, Kireva T, Gelse K, et al. beta-catenin is a central mediator of pro-fibrotic Wnt signaling in systemic sclerosis. Ann Rheum Dis. 2012;71(5):761–7.
16. Beyer C, Reichert H, Akan H, Mallano T, Schramm A, Dees C, et al. Blockade of canonical Wnt signalling ameliorates experimental dermal fibrosis. Ann Rheum Dis. 2013;72(7):1255–8.
17. Dees C, Schlottmann I, Funke R, Distler A, Palumbo-Zerr K, Zerr P, et al. The Wnt antagonists DKK1 and SFRP1 are downregulated by promoter hypermethylation in systemic sclerosis. Ann Rheum Dis. 2014;73(6):1232–9.
18. Bergmann C, Akhmetshina A, Dees C, Palumbo K, Zerr P, Beyer C, et al. Inhibition of glycogen synthase kinase 3beta induces dermal fibrosis by activation of the canonical Wnt pathway. Ann Rheum Dis. 2011;70(12):2191–8.
19. Daoussis D, Andonopoulos AP. The emerging role of Dickkopf-1 in bone biology: is it the main switch controlling bone and joint remodeling? Semin Arthritis Rheum. 2011;41(2):170–7.
20. Akhmetshina A, Palumbo K, Dees C, Bergmann C, Venalis P, Zerr P, et al. Activation of canonical Wnt signalling is required for TGF-beta-mediated fibrosis. Nat Commun. 2012;3:735.
21. Preliminary criteria for the classification of systemic sclerosis (scleroderma). Subcommittee for scleroderma criteria of the American Rheumatism Association Diagnostic and Therapeutic Criteria Committee. Arthritis Rheum. 1980;23(5):581–90.
22. Daoussis D, Tsamandas AC, Liossis SN, Antonopoulos I, Karatza E, Yiannopoulos G, et al. B-cell depletion therapy in patients with diffuse systemic sclerosis associates with a significant decrease in PDGFR expression and activation in spindle-like cells in the skin. Arthritis Res Ther. 2012;14(3):R145.
23. Saito E, Fujimoto M, Hasegawa M, Komura K, Hamaguchi Y, Kaburagi Y, et al. CD19-dependent B lymphocyte signaling thresholds influence skin fibrosis and autoimmunity in the tight-skin mouse. J Clin Invest. 2002;109(11):1453–62.
24. Lafyatis R, Kissin E, York M, Farina G, Viger K, Fritzler MJ, et al. B cell depletion with rituximab in patients with diffuse cutaneous systemic sclerosis. Arthritis Rheum. 2009;60(2):578–83.
25. Lafyatis R, O'Hara C, Feghali-Bostwick CA, Matteson E. B cell infiltration in systemic sclerosis-associated interstitial lung disease. Arthritis Rheum. 2007;56(9):3167–8.
26. Whitfield ML, Finlay DR, Murray JI, Troyanskaya OG, Chi JT, Pergamenschikov A, et al. Systemic and cell type-specific gene expression patterns in scleroderma skin. Proc Natl Acad Sci USA. 2003;100(21):12319–24.
27. Daoussis D, Liossis SN. B cells tell scleroderma fibroblasts to produce collagen. Arthritis Res Ther. 2013;15(6):125.
28. Baroni SS, Santillo M, Bevilacqua F, Luchetti M, Spadoni T, Mancini M, et al. Stimulatory autoantibodies to the PDGF receptor in systemic sclerosis. N Engl J Med. 2006;354(25):2667–76.

# Permissions

All chapters in this book were first published in AR&T, by BioMed Central; hereby published with permission under the Creative Commons Attribution License or equivalent. Every chapter published in this book has been scrutinized by our experts. Their significance has been extensively debated. The topics covered herein carry significant findings which will fuel the growth of the discipline. They may even be implemented as practical applications or may be referred to as a beginning point for another development.

The contributors of this book come from diverse backgrounds, making this book a truly international effort. This book will bring forth new frontiers with its revolutionizing research information and detailed analysis of the nascent developments around the world.

We would like to thank all the contributing authors for lending their expertise to make the book truly unique. They have played a crucial role in the development of this book. Without their invaluable contributions this book wouldn't have been possible. They have made vital efforts to compile up to date information on the varied aspects of this subject to make this book a valuable addition to the collection of many professionals and students.

This book was conceptualized with the vision of imparting up-to-date information and advanced data in this field. To ensure the same, a matchless editorial board was set up. Every individual on the board went through rigorous rounds of assessment to prove their worth. After which they invested a large part of their time researching and compiling the most relevant data for our readers.

The editorial board has been involved in producing this book since its inception. They have spent rigorous hours researching and exploring the diverse topics which have resulted in the successful publishing of this book. They have passed on their knowledge of decades through this book. To expedite this challenging task, the publisher supported the team at every step. A small team of assistant editors was also appointed to further simplify the editing procedure and attain best results for the readers.

Apart from the editorial board, the designing team has also invested a significant amount of their time in understanding the subject and creating the most relevant covers. They scrutinized every image to scout for the most suitable representation of the subject and create an appropriate cover for the book.

The publishing team has been an ardent support to the editorial, designing and production team. Their endless efforts to recruit the best for this project, has resulted in the accomplishment of this book. They are a veteran in the field of academics and their pool of knowledge is as vast as their experience in printing. Their expertise and guidance has proved useful at every step. Their uncompromising quality standards have made this book an exceptional effort. Their encouragement from time to time has been an inspiration for everyone.

The publisher and the editorial board hope that this book will prove to be a valuable piece of knowledge for researchers, students, practitioners and scholars across the globe.

# List of Contributors

**Christopher R. Pasarikovski, Adrienne M. Roos, Saghar Sadeghi, Amie T. Kron and Cathy Chau**
Toronto Scleroderma Program, Mount Sinai Hospital, Toronto Western Hospital, Division of Rheumatology, Department of Medicine, Faculty of Medicine, University of Toronto, Ground Floor, East Wing, Toronto Western Hospital, 399 Bathurst Street, Toronto, ON M5T 2S8, Canada

**Sindhu R. Johnson**
Toronto Scleroderma Program, Mount Sinai Hospital, Toronto Western Hospital, Division of Rheumatology, Department of Medicine, Faculty of Medicine, University of Toronto, Ground Floor, East Wing, Toronto Western Hospital, 399 Bathurst Street, Toronto, ON M5T 2S8, Canada
University Health Network Pulmonary Hypertension Programme, Toronto General Hospital, Division of Respirology, Department of Medicine, Faculty of Medicine, University of Toronto, Toronto, ON, Canada
Institute of Health Policy, Management and Evaluation, University of Toronto, Toronto, ON, Canada

**John T. Granton**
University Health Network Pulmonary Hypertension Programme, Toronto General Hospital, Divisions of Respirology and Critical Care Medicine, Department of Medicine, Faculty of Medicine, University of Toronto, Toronto, ON, Canada

**John Thenganatt**
University Health Network Pulmonary Hypertension Programme, Toronto General Hospital, Division of Respirology, Department of Medicine, Faculty of Medicine, University of Toronto, Toronto, ON, Canada

**Jakov Moric**
University Health Network Pulmonary Hypertension Programme, Toronto General Hospital, Division of Respirology, Women's College Hospital, Department of Medicine, Faculty of Medicine, University of Toronto, Toronto, ON, Canada

**A. Sulli, B. Ruaro, S. Paolino, C. Pizzorni and M. Cutolo**
Research Laboratory and Academic Division of Clinical Rheumatology, Department of Internal Medicine, University of Genova, Viale Benedetto XV, n° 6, AOU IRCCS San Martino, 16132 Genova, Italy

**V. Smith**
Department of Rheumatology, Ghent University Hospital, Department of Internal Medicine, Ghent University, Ghent, Belgium

**G. Pesce**
Laboratory of Autoimmunity, Department of Internal Medicine, University of Genova, IRCCS A.O.U, San Martino, Genoa, Italy

**Janine Schniering, Renate E. Gay, Steffen Gay, Oliver Distler and Britta Maurer**
Department of Rheumatology, University Hospital Zurich, Gloriastrasse 25, 8091 Zurich, Switzerland

**Falk Moritz**
Department of Rheumatology, University Hospital Zurich, Gloriastrasse 25, 8091 Zurich, Switzerland
Department of Oncology, St. Georg Hospital, Leipzig, Germany

**Jörg H. W. Distler**
Department of Internal Medicine 3,University Hospital, Erlangen, Germany

**Carol M. Artlett and Sihem Sassi-Gaha**
Department of Microbiology and Immunology, Drexel University College of Medicine, 2900 Queen Lane, Philadelphia, PA 19129, USA

**Jennifer L. Hope and Peter D. Katsikis**
Department of Microbiology and Immunology, Drexel University College of Medicine, 2900 Queen Lane, Philadelphia, PA 19129, USA
Department of Immunology, Erasmus University Medical Center, Rotterdam, The Netherlands

**Carol A. Feghali-Bostwick**
Division of Rheumatology & Immunology, Medical University of South Carolina, Charleston, SC, USA

**David Prior**
Department of Medicine, The University of Melbourne at St Vincent's Hospital, 41 Victoria Parade, Fitzroy, 3065 Melbourne, Victoria, Australia

**Kathleen Morrisroe, Molla Huq and Mandana Nikpour**
Department of Medicine, The University of Melbourne at St Vincent's Hospital, 41 Victoria Parade, Fitzroy, 3065 Melbourne, Victoria, Australia
Department of Rheumatology St Vincent's Hospital, 41 Victoria Parade, Fitzroy, 3065 Melbourne, Victoria, Australia

**Wendy Stevens**
Department of Rheumatology St Vincent's Hospital, 41 Victoria Parade, Fitzroy, 3065 Melbourne, Victoria, Australia

**Jo Sahhar and Gene-Siew Ngian**
Monash University and Monash Health, 246 Clayton Road, Clayton 3168, Victoria, Australia

**David Celermajer**
The University of Sydney at Royal Prince Alfred Hospital, Missenden Road, Camperdown 2050, NSW, Australia

**Jane Zochling**
Department of Rheumatology, Menzies Institute for Medical Research, Hobart, Australia

**Susanna Proudman**
Rheumatology Unit, Royal Adelaide Hospital, North Terrace, Adelaide, SA 5000, Australia
Discipline of Medicine, University of Adelaide, Adelaide, SA 5000, Australia

**Corrado Campochiaro, Korsa Khan, David J. Abraham, Voon H. Ong and Christopher P. Denton**
Centre for Rheumatology and Connective Tissue Diseases, University College London, London, UK

**Emma C. Derrett-Smith**
Centre for Rheumatology and Connective Tissue Diseases, University College London, London, UK
University Hospitals Birmingham NHS Foundation Trust, Birmingham, UK

**Viktor Martyanov, Tammara A. Wood and Michael L. Whitfield**
Department of Molecular and Systems Biology, Geisel School of Medicine at Dartmouth, Hanover, NH, USA

**Cecilia B. Chighizola and Pier Luigi Meroni**
Experimental Laboratory of Immunological and Rheumatologic Researches, IRCCS Istituto Auxologico Italiano, University of Milan, Milan, Italy

**Pia Moinzadeh**
Department of Dermatology and Venerology, University of Cologne, Cologne, Germany

**Robert Lafyatis**
Division of Rheumatology and Clinical Immunology, University of Pittsburgh Medical Center, Pittsburgh, PA, USA

**Huayong Zhang, Jun Liang, Xiaojun Tang, Dandan Wang, Xuebing Feng, Fan Wang, Bingzhu Hua, Hong Wang and Lingyun Sun**
Department of Rheumatology and Immunology, The Affiliated Drum Tower Hospital of Nanjing University Medical School, 321 Zhongshan Road, Nanjing 210008, China

**Sabine Adler and Peter M. Villiger**
Department of Rheumatology, Immunology and Allergology, University Hospital and University of Bern, Freiburgstrasse 4, 3010 Bern, Switzerland

**Dörte Huscher**
German Rheumatism Research Center, A Leibniz Institute, Berlin, Germany
Department of Rheumatology and Clinical Immunology, Charité University Hospital, Berlin, Germany

**Elise Siegert**
Department of Rheumatology and Clinical Immunology, Charité University Hospital, Berlin, Germany

**Yannick Allanore**
Department of Rheumatology A, Descartes University, APHP, Cochin Hospital, Paris, France

**László Czirják**
Department of Rheumatology and Immunology, University of Pecs, Pecs, Hungary

**Francesco DelGaldo**
University of Leeds, Leeds, UK

**Christopher P. Denton**
UCL Division of Medicine, Centre for Rheumatology, Royal Free Hospital, London, UK

**Oliver Distler**
Department of Rheumatology, University Hospital Zurich, Zurich, Switzerland

**Marc Frerix, Ulf Mueller-Ladner and Ingo-Helmut Tarner**
Department of Rheumatology and Clinical Immunology, Osteology and Physical Therapy, Justus-Liebig-University Giessen, Kerckhoff Klinik, Bad Nauheim, Germany

**Marco Matucci-Cerinic**
Department Experimental and Clinical Medicine, Division of Rheumatology AOUC, University of Florence, Florence, Italy

**Gabriele Valentini**
Department of Rheumatology, Second University of Naples, Naples, Italy

**Ulrich A. Walker**
Department of Rheumatology, University of Basel, Basel, Switzerland

**Gabriela Riemekasten**
Department of Rheumatology, University Medical Center Schleswig-Holstein, Kiel, Germany

**Silvia Bosello, Stefano Alivernini, Barbara Tolusso, Elisa Gremese and Gianfranco Ferraccioli**
Unità Operativa Complessa di Reumatologia, Istituto di Reumatologia e Scienze Affini, Università Cattolica del Sacro Cuore, Rome, Italy
Fondazione Policlinico Universitario Agostino Gemelli, Via G. Moscati, 31-00168 Rome, Italy

**Cristiana Angelucci, Gina Lama and Gabriella Proietti**
Istituto di Istologia ed Embriologia, Università Cattolica del Sacro Cuore, Rome, Italy

**Gigliola Sica, A. Mitropoulos, H. Crank and M. Klonizakis**
Centre for Sport and Exercise Science, Collegiate Campus, Sheffield Hallam University, Collegiate Crescent, Sheffield S10 2BP, UK

**A. Gumber**
Centre for Health and Social Care Research, Sheffield Hallam University, Sheffield, UK

**M. Akil**
Rheumatology Department, Royal Hallamshire Hospital, Sheffield, UK

**Ulrich A. Walker and Veronika K. Jaeger**
Department of Rheumatology, University Hospital Basel, Petersgraben 4, 4032 Basel, Switzerland

**Katharina M. Bruppacher**
Bellikon, Switzerland

**Rucsandra Dobrota and Oliver Distler**
Department of Rheumatology, University Hospital Zurich, Zurich, Switzerland

**Lionel Arlettaz**
Institut Central—Hôpital du Valais, Sion, Switzerland

**Martin Banyai**
Kantonsspital Luzern, Luzern, Switzerland

**Jörg Beron**
Actelion Pharma Schweiz AG, Baden, Switzerland

**Carlo Chizzolini**
Immunology & Allergy, University Hospital and School of Medicine, Geneva, Switzerland

**Ernst Groechenig**
Kantonsspital Aarau, Aarau, Switzerland

**Rüdiger B. Mueller**
Kantonsspital St. Gallen, St. Gallen, Switzerland

**François Spertini**
Division of Immunology and Allergy, Centre Hospitalier Universitaire Vaudois, Lausanne, Switzerland

**Peter M. Villiger**
Department of Rheumatology, Immunology and Allergology, University Hospital and University of Bern, Bern, Switzerland

**Alfredo Guillén-Del-Castillo, Carmen Pilar Simeón-Aznar, Serafín Alonso-Vila, Vicente Fonollosa-Pla and Albert Selva-O'Callaghan**
Department of Systemic Autoimmune Diseases, Hospital Universitari Vall d'Hebron, Universitat Autònoma de Barcelona, Passeig Vall d'Hebron 119– 129, 08035 Barcelona, Spain

**Eduardo L. Callejas-Moraga and Carles Tolosa-Vilella**
Department of Internal Medicine, Corporació Sanitària Universitària Parc Taulí, Universitat Autònoma de Barcelona, Sabadell, Barcelona, Spain

**Christine T. Luu and Coline A. Gentil**
Division of Clinical Research, Fred Hutchinson Cancer Research Center, 1100 Fairview Ave N, Seattle, WA 98109, USA

**Hilary S. Gammill**
Division of Clinical Research, Fred Hutchinson Cancer Research Center, 1100 Fairview Ave N, Seattle, WA 98109, USA
Department of Obstetrics and Gynecology, University of Washington, Seattle, WA, USA

**J. Lee Nelson**
Division of Clinical Research, Fred Hutchinson Cancer Research Center, 1100 Fairview Ave N, Seattle, WA 98109, USA
Division of Rheumatology, University of Washington, Seattle, WA, USA

**Maureen D. Mayes**
Division of Rheumatology and Clinical Immunogenetics, University of Texas Health Science Center at Houston, Houston, TX, USA

**Dan E. Furst**
Division of Rheumatology, University of California, Los Angeles, CA, USA

**James Esposito and Mandana Nikpour**
1Department of Medicine, The University of Melbourne at St Vincent's Hospital (Melbourne), 41 Victoria Parade, Fitzroy, VIC 3065, Australia
Department of Rheumatology, St Vincent's Hospital (Melbourne), 41 Victoria Parade, Fitzroy, VIC 3065, Australia

**Zoe Brown, Wendy Stevens and Candice Rabusa**
Department of Rheumatology, St Vincent's Hospital (Melbourne), 41 Victoria Parade, Fitzroy, VIC 3065, Australia

**Joanne Sahhar**
Department of Rheumatology, Monash Health and Monash University, 246 Clayton Road, Clayton, VIC 3168, Australia
Department of Medicine, Monash Health and Monash University, 246 Clayton Road, Clayton, VIC 3168, Australia

**Jane Zochling**
Department of Rheumatology, Menzies Institute for Medical Research, Private Bag 23, Hobart, TAS 7001, Australia

**Janet Roddy**
Department of Rheumatology, Royal Perth Hospital, 197 Wellington Street, Perth, WA 6001, Australia

**Jennifer Walker**
Department of Rheumatology, Flinders Medical Centre, Flinders Drive, Bedford Park, SA 5042, Australia

**Susanna M. Proudman**
Rheumatology Unit, Royal Adelaide Hospital, North Terrace, Adelaide, SA 5000, Australia
Discipline of Medicine, University of Adelaide, Adelaide, SA 5000, Australia

**Valentina Lacconi, Stefania Lenna, Michael York, Maria Trojanowska and G. Alessandra Farina**
Rheumatology, Boston University School of Medicine, Arthritis Center, 72 E. Concord Street, E-5, Boston, MA 02118, USA

**Antonella Farina**
Rheumatology, Boston University School of Medicine, Arthritis Center, 72 E. Concord Street, E-5, Boston, MA 02118, USA
Department of Experimental Medicine, Sapienza University, Rome, Italy

**Alberto Faggioni and Stefania Morrone**
Department of Experimental Medicine, Sapienza University, Rome, Italy

**Giovanna Peruzzi**
Istituto Italiano di Tecnologia, CLNS@Sapienza, Rome, Italy

**Silvia Quarta and Edoardo Rosato**
Department of Clinical Medicine, Sapienza University, Rome, Italy

**Anna Rita Vestri**
Department of Public Health, Sapienza University, Rome, Italy

**David H. Dreyfus**
Department of Pediatrics, Yale, New Haven, CT, USA

**Kristofer Andréasson, Zaid Alrawi and Anita Persson**
Section of Rheumatology, Department of Clinical Sciences, Lund University, Lund, Sweden

**Göran Jönsson**
Section of Infectious Diseases, Department of Clinical Sciences, Lund University, Lund, Sweden

**Jan Marsal**
Department of Clinical Sciences, Lund University, Lund, Sweden
Immunology Section, Lund University, Lund, Sweden
Department of Gastroenterology, Skåne University Hospital, Lund, Sweden

**Niamh Quillinan, Kristina E. N. Clark and Christopher P. Denton**
Centre for Rheumatology, UCL Division of Medicine, Royal Free Campus, Rowland Hill Street, London NW3 2PF, UK

**Bryan Youl**
Department of Neurophysiology, Royal Free London NHS Foundation Trust, London, UK

**Jeffrey Vernes, Deirdre McIntosh and Syed Haq**
Daval International, London, UK

**George P. Karamanolis, Konstantinos Denaxas, Anastasios Karlaftis, Dimitrios Kamberoglou and Spiros D. Ladas**
Academic Department of Gastroenterology, "Laiko" Hospital, Athens Medical School National and Kapodistrian University, Athens, Greece

**Stylianos Panopoulos, Alexandra Zorbala and Petros P. Sfikakis**
Joint Academic Rheumatology Programme, Athens Medical School National and Kapodistrian University, Athens, Greece

**Romy B. Christmann, Alicia Wooten, Jessica Ziemek, Yu Mei, Salma Goummih, Giuseppina Stifano and Robert W. Simms**
Boston University School of Medicine, E501, Arthritis Center, Medical Campus, 72 East Concord Street, Boston, MA 02118-2526, USA

**Robert Lafyatis**
Boston University School of Medicine, E501, Arthritis Center, Medical Campus, 72 East Concord Street, Boston, MA 02118-2526, USA
University of Pittsburgh, Division of Pulmonary, Allergy, and Critical Care Medicine, and the Dorothy P. and Richard P. Simmons Center for Interstitial Lung Disease, Pittsburgh, PA, USA

**Percival Sampaio-Barros, Carlos R. R. Carvalho, Ronaldo A. Kairalla, Edwin Parra and Vera L. Capelozzi**
Hospital das Clinicas da Faculdade de Medicina da Universidade de São Paulo, São Paulo, SP, Brazil

**Claudia L. Borges**
Universidade CEUMA, São Luís do Maranhão, MA, Brazil

**Carol Feghali-Bostwick**
Medical University of South Carolina, Charleston, SC, USA

**Jiangning Tan, Diana Alvarez, Daniel J. Kass and Mauricio Rojas**
University of Pittsburgh, Division of Pulmonary, Allergy, and Critical Care Medicine, and the Dorothy P. and Richard P. Simmons Center for Interstitial Lung Disease, Pittsburgh, PA, USA

**Thiago Lemos de Mattos**
Universidade do Estado do Amazonas, Manaus, AM, Brazil

**Graça Castro, Rui Martins and Mariano Pêgo**
Department of Cardiology, Centro Hospitalar e Universitário de Coimbra, Praceta Mota Pinto, 3000-001 Coimbra, Portugal

**Rui Baptista, Rogério Teixeira and Pedro Monteiro**
Department of Cardiology, Centro Hospitalar e Universitário de Coimbra, Praceta Mota Pinto, 3000-001 Coimbra, Portugal
Faculty of Medicine, University of Coimbra, Coimbra, Portugal

**José António Pereira da Silva**
Faculty of Medicine, University of Coimbra, Coimbra, Portugal
Department of Rheumatology, Centro Hospitalar e Universitário de Coimbra, Coimbra, Portugal

**Lèlita Santos**
Faculty of Medicine, University of Coimbra, Coimbra, Portugal
Department of Internal Medicine, Centro Hospitalar e Universitário de Coimbra, Coimbra, Portugal

**Maria João Salvador and Sara Serra**
Department of Rheumatology, Centro Hospitalar e Universitário de Coimbra, Coimbra, Portugal

**Dimitrios Daoussis, Ioannis Antonopoulos, Alexandra Filippopoulou, Andrew P. Andonopoulos and Stamatis-Nick Liossis**
Division of Rheumatology, Department of Internal Medicine, Patras University Hospital, University of Patras Medical School, Rion, Patras 26504, Greece

**Athanassios Tsamandas**
Department of Patholology, Patras University Hospital, University of Patras Medical School, Patras, Greece

**Dionysios J. Papachristou and Nicholaos I. Papachristou**
Department of Anatomy-Histology-Embryology, Laboratory of Bone and Soft Tissue Studies, University of Patras Medical School, Patras, Greece

# Index

## A

Acetylcholine, 84, 87

Ankylosing Spondylitis, 144, 149

Anorexigen, 2, 7

Antiphospholipid Antibodies, 36-37, 42

Atrial Fibrillation, 2-3, 187

Azathioprine, 47, 51-52, 56, 61-62, 66, 68-69, 71-72, 119, 123, 145

## B

Bleomycin, 15, 17-18, 21-22, 24, 27-31, 158, 160, 167, 170, 172, 174-175, 177-178

Buspirone, 161-166

## C

C-reactive Protein, 65, 68, 71, 122-123, 125, 127-128, 145, 148-149

Calcium Channel Blocker, 2

Capillaroscopic Skin Ulcer, 95-101, 110

Cardiovascular Diseases, 16

Chemokines, 129, 140

Computer Tomography, 35, 39, 42, 169

Coronary Artery Disease, 2-3, 142, 181

Cutaneous Systemic Sclerosis, 8-9, 11, 13-14, 36, 42, 44, 49, 52-53, 59, 71, 83, 92, 105, 130, 133-134, 137-139, 141-142, 151, 159-160, 198

Cyclophosphamide, 54-55, 59, 61-62, 66, 68-69, 71-72, 74, 78, 119, 123, 168, 192, 197

## D

Diabetic Retinopathy, 16

Digital Ulceration, 2, 45-46

Dorsum, 8, 10

Dysbiosis, 143-150

## E

Echocardiography, 75, 102-107, 109-110, 119, 123, 144, 180-182, 184, 186-190

Endothelial Cells, 15-16, 18, 20, 24-25, 59, 81, 90, 140

Endothelin Receptor Antagonist, 2

Epoprostenol, 35, 43

Erythrocyte Sedimentation Rate, 65, 71, 76, 82, 117-118, 123, 125, 145, 148-149

Extractable Nuclear Antigens, 36, 42, 119

## F

Faecal Calprotectin, 144, 147-149

## G

Gastric Antral Vascular Ectasia, 38, 42, 103, 119, 123, 125

Gastrointestinal Tract, 12, 150, 162, 166

Green Fluorescent Protein, 27

## H

Hemodynamic Measurements, 2

Hierarchical Clustering, 44, 49, 152

Human Leukocyte Antigen, 55, 59, 111, 116

Hyalinised Collagen, 12

Hydroxychloroquine, 36-37, 39, 42, 47, 51, 123

Hydroxyproline Assays, 27

Hyperimmune Caprine Serum, 60, 151, 153-156, 158-160

Hyperlipidemia, 2-3

Hypocomplementaemia, 117-118, 120-127

Hypoxia, 15-17, 21, 24-25, 102, 187, 189

## I

Iloprost, 35, 47, 51, 60, 74, 87, 89, 91, 94

Imunosuppressive Treatment, 61

Inflammasome Orchestrates, 26

Interleukin, 26-27, 31-33, 54, 59-60, 62, 72, 82, 118, 127-128, 133-134, 141, 160, 173, 177-178

Interquartile Range, 13, 97-98, 101, 104, 106, 109, 121, 145, 184

Interstitial Lung Disease, 1-4, 6, 34, 39, 42-43, 46-47, 51, 54, 56-57, 59-62, 71-72, 85, 102-103, 105-106, 109, 117, 123, 125, 163, 165, 167, 169-172, 174-175, 178, 187, 198

## M

Macitentan, 35, 37, 60

Macrophages, 73-74, 79, 81-83, 129-130, 132-133, 137-142, 174-175, 178

Matrix Metalloproteinases, 15

Mesenchymal Stem Cells, 54-55, 59-60, 94

Methotrexate, 47, 51, 54, 56, 59-62, 66, 68-69, 71-72, 119, 123, 145

Microangiopathy Evolution, 9-10, 13

Micrornas, 26, 178-179

Microvascular Perturbations, 102

Modified Rodnan Skin Score, 8-9, 13-14, 47, 51-52, 54-57, 59, 62-63, 65, 71, 75, 83, 96, 98, 100, 123, 125, 128, 130, 144-145, 148-149, 151-154, 159, 178, 192, 198

Mycophenolate Mofetil, 36-37, 42-43, 54, 56, 59, 61-62, 66, 68-69, 71-72, 145

**N**

Nailfold Videocapillaroscopy, 8-10, 13, 25, 102-107, 109-110

**O**

Oedematous Phase, 12

**P**

Pericytes, 15-16

Perivascular Cells, 15

Phosphodiesterase Inhibitors, 2

Phosphodiesterase-5-inhibitors, 36

Placebo, 31, 52, 60, 71-72, 144, 149, 151-156, 158-160, 165

Plasmapheresis, 54-56, 58-60

Polybrene, 27

Polymerase Chain Reaction, 26-27, 130-131, 133, 141, 167

Prostaglandin Analogue, 2

Pulmonary Arterial Hypertension, 1, 3-7, 27, 34, 37, 39-40, 42-43, 45-47, 49, 51, 102, 105-110, 117, 123, 125, 127, 141, 144, 149, 160, 172, 178, 180-181, 188-190

Pulmonary Vascular Resistance, 2-3, 6, 35, 42, 65, 71, 103, 109, 181-183, 186, 188-189

**R**

Retrovirus, 27, 30

Rituximab, 14, 55, 62, 66, 71-72, 74, 78, 81, 83, 191, 194-196, 198

**S**

Scleroderma, 1, 4, 6-7, 14, 24-25, 32-36, 40, 42-46, 49, 52, 59-60, 62, 64-65, 69-75, 79-83, 85, 92-94, 101-103, 105, 109-110, 116-130, 141, 149-151, 158, 160-161, 165-166, 178-181, 189, 191-193, 196-198

Scleroderma Renal Crisis, 1, 4, 46, 70, 72, 103, 105, 109, 128

Sodium Nitroprusside, 84, 89

Systemic Lupus Erythematosus, 7, 41, 55, 60, 117, 124, 128, 141-142, 144, 148-149, 175, 179

Systemic Sclerosis, 1, 3-11, 13-15, 19-20, 24-26, 28-29, 32-34, 36-45, 47, 49, 51-54, 57-62, 70-74, 77-84, 90, 92-97, 101-103, 105, 109-111, 113-114, 116-117, 126-130, 133-134, 137-139, 141-146, 149-152, 159-163, 165-167, 169-172, 174-175, 177-178, 180-184, 188-191, 195-196, 198

**T**

T Cells, 73, 80-81, 83, 111, 115, 175

Teleangiectasias, 16, 19

Toll-like Receptor, 129-130, 133, 135-136, 141-142, 177, 179

Topoisomerase I, 2-3, 6, 65, 68, 71, 98, 103-105, 113, 163

Transforming Growth Factor, 27, 31-33, 44, 49, 52-54, 58-60, 82, 148-149, 152, 159-160, 167, 175, 178, 192, 195, 198

Transthoracic Echocardiogram, 35, 42

Tumor Necrosis Factor, 54, 59, 69, 82, 131, 134, 136, 141

**V**

Vascular Endothelial Growth Factor, 15-16, 20, 24-25, 54-55, 58-59, 103, 109

Vascular Smooth Muscle Cells, 15

**W**

Warfarin, 2, 7, 36-38, 40-41, 43

**Z**

Zygoma, 8, 10-11

www.ingramcontent.com/pod-product-compliance
Lightning Source LLC
Chambersburg PA
CBHW082027190326
41458CB00010B/3298